HISTOLOGY

Fourth Edition

THOMAS S. LEESON, M.D., Ph.D.

Professor and Chairman, Department of
Anatomy, University of Alberta, Edmonton,
Alberta, Canada

C. ROLAND LEESON, M.D., Ph.D.

Professor of Anatomy, School of Basic
Medical Sciences and School of Life
Sciences, University of Illinois, Urbana, Illinois

1981   W. B. SAUNDERS COMPANY/PHILADELPHIA/LONDON/TORONTO

W. B. Saunders Company: West Washington Square
Philadelphia, PA   19105

1 St. Anne's Road
Eastbourne, East Sussex BN21 3UN, England

Cedro 512
Mexico 4, D.F. Mexico

9 Waltham Street
Artarmon, N.S.W. 2064, Australia

Ichibancho, Central Bldg., 22-1
Chiyoda-ku, Tokyo 102, Japan

1 Goldthorne Avenue
Toronto, Ontario M8Z 5T9, Canada

Cover photography courtesy of the authors

Front and back cover: Light photomicrograph of the retina at
the fovea centralis. (Iron hematoxylin; low power.)

Listed below is the latest translated edition of this book together
with the language of the translation and the publisher:

Italian (2nd Edition) — Societa Editrice Universo, Rome, Italy

Spanish (3rd Edition) — Nueva Editorial Interamericana S.A. de C.V.
Mexico 4 D.F., Mexico

French (3rd Edition) — Masson & Cie, Paris, France

Portuguese (3rd Edition) — Editora Interamericana Ltda, Rio de Janeiro,
Brazil

Histology   ISBN   7216-5704-4

Last digit is the print number: 9   8   7   6   5   4   3   2   1

PREFACE

The first edition of this textbook was published in 1966 in an attempt to offer a viable alternative to the well-established but lengthy textbooks then in use. It was written for students in the fields of biomedicine and biology, and we were encouraged by its ready acceptance by both students and teachers. The second (1970) and third (1976) editions involved major revisions and changes in the illustrative material. The wide acceptance of these editions has justified our decision to prepare a textbook that was concise, yet comprehensive.

Since publication of the third edition, knowledge of the subject has expanded and, in undertaking this revision, we have found it necessary to review and revise all chapters carefully. We were aided greatly in this task by the suggestions for changes and additions we received from students and faculty at many institutions. One change relates to the publication of our *Brief Atlas of Histology* (1979). The sequence and number of chapters in the textbook now are identical to those in the atlas. As in previous editions, there is a division of the subject matter into two parts. Part I covers the cell, its structure and its various components and functions, and the primary tissues; the student is urged to acquire a firm knowledge of this material before proceeding to a study of the various organ systems that constitutes Part II. In some chapters there are relatively few changes in the text, but in others, for example, Chapter 1 (The Cell), Chapter 6 (Muscle), and Chapter 17 (Organs of Special Sense), the material has been virtually rewritten.

The number of light photomicrographs in this edition has been increased, particularly those from sections of plastic-embedded material. In the past decade many institutions have introduced such material into their slide collections, realizing, as we do, that they provide better detail than that found in paraffin-embedded material and that they facilitate correlation between light and electron microscopy. Several of the new photomicrographs are of sections from our own material, but many others were kindly loaned to us by Dr. A. Kokko-Cunningham of the School of Basic Medical Sciences, University of Illinois, Urbana, to whom we extend our thanks. No additional color photomicrographs have been included because color photomicrographs are fully represented in the *Brief Atlas of Histology*. Conversely, because the atlas contains few electron micrographs (it is basically a color atlas of light microscopy), the number of electron micrographs, scanning micrographs, and micrographs of freeze-etch material in this text has been increased when deemed appropriate. Several colleagues have been kind enough to provide this material. We are grateful to all of them and particularly to Dr. P. M. Andrews of the University of Texas Southwestern Medical School (Dallas); Dr. T. Fujita of the University of Nigata, Japan; Dr. S. Bullivant of the University of Auckland, New Zealand; Dr. L. Orci of the University of Geneva, Switzerland; and Dr. D. H. Dickson of Dalhousie University, Halifax, Canada. We are also grateful to Leona M. Allison for preparation of many of the new diagrams in this edition.

As we noted in the preface to our *Brief Atlas of Histology*, details of histological structure cannot be portrayed by photomicrographs alone, nor indeed by a study of prepared material. The interpretation of histological structure requires an inquiring mind, an understanding of the three-dimensional character of the material, and an appreciation of its physiological activity. Since the publication of the first edition of this textbook, the discipline of histology has experienced a tremendous and exciting increase in breadth. As a result, the relationship of histology to other disciplines, principally physiology, biochemistry, and pathology, necessarily must be emphasized. We hope that the evolution of this textbook over four editions reflects the evolution of the discipline over the past two decades.

We wish to express our thanks for secretarial assistance to Ms. Joan Junkus, Mrs. Lorrie Pearson, and Mrs. Brenda Jensen, and our sincere gratitude to the representatives of our publishers for their patience, encouragement, and suggestions. Those representatives include John Dusseau (during preparation of the first edition), Robert Rowan, Jack Hanley, and Brian Decker (during preparation of the second and third editions), and Roberta Kangilaski (during the present edition).

To all students, both those we know and those we probably never will meet, we hope this textbook will facilitate your comprehension of histology and we wish you well in your studies.

C. ROLAND LEESON
THOMAS S. LEESON

CONTENTS

V

PART II HISTOLOGY OF THE ORGAN SYSTEMS

INTRODUCTION

Histology is a term derived from the Greek *histos*, meaning tissue, and *logia*, meaning "the study of" or knowledge. Literally, then, it refers to the knowledge, or science, of tissues, both plant and animal. This textbook is restricted, in the main, to a consideration of human histology.

What does the term "histology" encompass today? Anatomy can be subdivided into that which is visible to the naked eye, gross anatomy, and that which can be seen only with the aid of a microscope, microscopic anatomy. The latter can be further subdivided into organology (the study of organs), histology (tissues), and cytology (cells). Today the term "histology" is used loosely to include all subdivisions of microscopic anatomy, and it is in this sense that the term is used here.

Histology involves, therefore, the study not only of tissues but of individual cells and organ systems. And since histology refers to the study of cells, tissues, and organs, it embraces a study of function as well as of structure. Thus, a study of histology not only complements the study of gross anatomy but provides a structural basis for the study of physiology. The correlation between structure and function perhaps provides the reason why histology is such an intriguing and readily understandable subject. The student will find that if he examines a structure he can deduce much about its function; conversely, if he knows the function of an organ or tissue, he can forecast much of its microscopic structure.

A knowledge of the normal is a necessary prelude to the study of the abnormal (pathology), which deals with the alterations in structure and function of the body and of its organs, tissues, and cells caused by disease. Hence the study of histology is fundamental within the medical and dental curriculum. For biology students not proceeding to professional degrees, it provides a reservoir of valuable knowledge. Too often in many special fields of biological science the student becomes involved in problems of a functional nature without sufficient consideration of the underlying microscopic structure.

In our study of histology, there are two important considerations with regard to methodology: the kind of microscope used and the preparation of the tissue or organ in a manner suitable for viewing with the microscope. In general, the development of histological techniques has lagged behind the technical achievements made in connection with various types of microscopes. Perhaps the best example of this applies to the electron microscope. Although the electron microscope was developed in the early 1930s, it was not utilized to any extent in biological work until the late 1940s and early 1950s when methods of thin sectioning were developed.

Microscopy dates from the seventeenth century when Robert Hooke and Marcello Malpighi employed simple lenses in the study of various structural features. Between 1673 and 1716, Leeuwenhoek developed compound lenses and published a series of observations upon protozoa, bacteria, muscle, nerve, and many other structures. Microscopic anatomy developed slowly during the eighteenth century, and by the early nineteenth century the compound microscope had become highly developed. Robert Brown (1831) dis-

1

covered the nucleus, and Schleiden (1838) and Schwann (1839) enunciated the "cell theory." In 1841 Henle published the first comprehensive (for that time) account of human histology. Although the term "tissues," for different groups of cells, was introduced initially by Bichat (1802) on the basis of observation of gross postmortem specimens, it was Virchow (1863) who described the human body as a "cell state" and listed specialized categories of cells. In the latter part of the nineteenth century, microtomes were developed commercially, and hand in hand with their appearance came the development of fixing, embedding, and staining techniques. The latter are still in the process of development, particularly with regard to their application to the newer forms of microscopy.

In the study of histology, the student will be introduced to the results obtained from various forms of microscopy and of histological technique. How these results were obtained should always be borne in mind since it will influence their interpretation. Thus, it is important for the student to understand the applications and limitations of the various types of microscopes in use today and the basic principles underlying the different methods of preparation of tissues.

MICROSCOPY

Several types of microscopes are available for the study of biological material. Basically they may be classified by the type of light source used. In most general use, of course, is the optical microscope using visible light. There are certain modifications of this, namely the polarization, phase contrast, interference, and dark-field microscopes. Microscopes which utilize invisible radiation, the ultraviolet, x-ray, and electron microscopes, are more recent developments.

The usefulness of any type of microscope depends not only upon its ability to magnify but, more important, upon its ability to resolve detail. Beyond certain limits, magnification adds no new details. The useful magnification of an ordinary light micro-

scope is about 1500×. The resolving power is a measure of the capacity of the microscope to separate clearly two points close together. Beyond the resolving power of any microscope, two points will appear as one. The resolution with lens systems is limited by the wavelength of light and by the numerical aperture, or light-gathering capacity, of the objective lens. The resolving power of a well-constructed light microscope is about 0.2 μm. (See footnote, p. 4.)

The Light (or Optical) Microscope

Basically the light microscope acts as a two-stage magnifying device. An objective lens provides the initial magnification, and an ocular lens is placed so as to magnify the primary image a second time. Total magnification is obtained by multiplying the magnifying power of the objective and ocular lenses. An additional condensing lens is normally employed beneath the stage of the microscope to concentrate the light from its source into a very bright beam illuminating the object, thus providing sufficient light for the inspection of the magnified image.

The Polarizing Microscope

This instrument was developed by mineralogists who employ it in their studies of crystalline materials. Many natural objects, including crystals and fibers, exhibit an optical property known as double refraction, or birefringence. In histological material, birefringence is caused by the orientation of particles too small to be resolved even by the best lenses. Thus an examination of birefringence permits deductions to be made concerning the organization of structure not demonstrable by regular methods of microscopy.

In its simplest form, the polarizing microscope is a conventional microscope in which a Nicol prism (or Polaroid sheet) is interposed in the light path below the condenser. This "polarizer" converts all light passing through the instrument into plane polarized light, or light which vibrates in one optical plane only. A similar, second prism, termed the "analyzer," is placed within the barrel of the microscope above the objective lens. When the analyzer is orientated so that its polarizing direction is parallel to that of the polarizer below, one sees the regular image. However, if the analyzer is rotated until its axis is perpendicular to that of the polarizer, no light can pass through the ocular lens and the field is black. The field will remain black if an *isotropic*, or singly refractive, object is placed on the stage. A birefringent object, however, will appear light upon a dark background when examined in this manner. Birefringence, or *anisotrophy*, is exhibited by many biological structures, for example, muscle fibers, certain connective tissue fibers, lipid droplets within the adrenal cortex, and the rods and cones of the retina.

The Phase Contrast Microscope

Lack of contrast has always been a problem in biological work because the refractive indices of cytoplasm and of its inclusions are similar. In normal microscopy, one overcomes this problem by staining differentially, but this is subject to numerous limitations. Phase microscopy provides a method whereby contrast is created by purely optical means.

The refractive index is a measure of the optical density of an object, or the speed with which it is traversed by a light wave. Air, for instance, has a refractive index of approximately 1.0, water about 1.3, and glass about 1.5. In other words, light travels fastest in air, more slowly in water, and slower still in glass. Light waves traversing equal distances through air, water, and glass will not emerge at the same time; they will emerge out of phase with each other. The phase contrast apparatus consists of optical plates placed within the condenser and objective lenses which convert the phase differences into amplitude differences. Briefly, therefore, differences in refractive index are rendered

directly visible. Objects ordinarily transparent become visible through contrast differences. The phase contrast microscope is of no particular assistance in the study of fixed and stained preparations in which transparency differences are not important. The instrument finds its application chiefly in the study of living cells and of unstained tissues.

The Interference Microscope

The interference microscope, like the phase contrast microscope, depends upon the ability of an object to retard light. Unlike the phase microscope, which depends upon the specimen diffracting light, the interference microscope sends through the specimen two separate beams of light which then are combined in the image plane. After recombination, difference in retardation of the light results in interference that can be used to measure the thickness or refractive index of the object under investigation.

The Dark-Field Microscope

This microscope utilizes a strong, oblique light that does not enter the objective lens. A special dark-field condenser, in which no light passes through the center of the lens, is employed. Light thus reaches the object to be viewed at an angle so oblique that none of it can enter the objective lens. The field is therefore dark. Small particles present in the field will reflect some light into the objective lens and appear as glistening spots. Thus it is possible to visualize particles far below the limits of bright light resolution. The effect is similar to the phenomenon of dust particles "seen" in a beam of sunlight entering a darkened room. Dark-field examination is also of use in the examination of small transparent objects such as chylomicrons, which are invisible in the glare of bright field illumination, and of microincineration specimens.

The microscopes just discussed all utilize visible light. However, images can be formed by rays other than visible light and in this instance, since the images cannot be viewed directly, they are made visible by means of a suitably sensitized photographic film. In general the rays used in these special microscopes all have a shorter wavelength than that of visible light and thus permit higher resolution.

The Ultraviolet Microscope

Since ordinary optical lenses are nearly opaque to ultraviolet light, quartz lenses are used throughout the lens system. In principle, this system allows an improvement in resolution about twice that of the ordinary microscope (0.1 μ or μm).

Ultraviolet light is also employed in *fluorescence microscopy*. Many substances have the property of emitting visible light when irradiated by invisible rays. When ultraviolet light is focused upon such a specimen, it glows and can be observed by its emitted fluorescence. Fluorescence may be naturally occurring within the specimen or may result from the introduction of fluorescent dyes bound to certain specific components of the specimen.

The X-Ray Microscope

X-rays have a shorter wavelength than visible or ultraviolet light and therefore a greater penetration and theoretically a higher resolving power. Preparation techniques similar to those used in light microscopy allow the specimen to be placed upon a photographic emulsion and exposed to soft x-irradiation. The small x-ray picture obtained is subsequently magnified optically. This process is known as contact microradiography. In *projection x-ray microscopy*, a point source of x-rays casts an enlarged image of a nearby object upon a distant fluorescent screen or photographic plate. It is the contrast obtained as a result of differences in x-ray absorption that is utilized in these procedures. Resolution in either case is not particularly high and with the instruments currently available is still far from the theoretical limits.

The Electron Microscope

The transmission electron microscope (TEM) utilizes a system which in principle is analogous to that of the light microscope. In the electron microscope, the illuminating source is a beam of high velocity electrons accelerated in a vacuum. The beam is passed through the specimen and is focused upon a fluorescent screen or photographic plate by a series of electromagnetic or electrostatic fields. The wavelength of the electrons depends upon the acceleration voltage used. At the voltages used routinely, the wavelengths of the electrons are of the order of 0.05. Å.* The electric or magnetic fields used as lenses are imperfect and do not have the numerical aperture of optical lenses. Thus the practical limit of resolution of the electron microscope is about 2 Å (0.2 nm), and the usual limit for biological preparations about 3.5 Å (0.35 nm).

The electron microscope permits the observation of cell and tissue structure beyond that seen with the light microscope. Structures smaller than individual macromolecules can now be visualized. To describe this particular level of structure requires the use of some special term. The one most commonly used is *fine structure*, which refers to those elements of structure which can be visualized only with the electron microscope. The term *ultrastructure*, which is used by many workers in this field, is better avoided since literally it means *beyond structure*.

Scanning electron microscopy (SEM) is a more recent development, and un-

---

Units of measurement: In the past, the terms micron (μ, one-thousandth of a millimeter), millimicron (mμ, one-thousandth of a micron), and angstrom unit (Å, one-tenth of a millimicron) received general acceptance as units of measurement in microscopy. Recently they have been replaced by units that relate more directly to the metric system.

Old terminology	New terminology
Micron (μ)	Micrometer (μm)
Millimicron (mμ)	Nanometer (nm)
Angstrom unit (Å)	0.1 nm

Thus, 0.05 Å (referred to above) becomes 0.005 nm in the new terminology. Since students will encounter both terminologies in their reading of the literature, they should be familiar with both.

LIGHT MICROSCOPE

ELECTRON MICROSCOPE

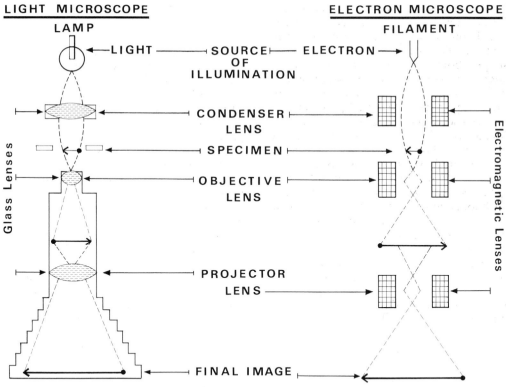

Figure 1. Diagrammatic comparison of the optical systems of light and electron microscopes. For ease of comparison the system of the light microscope has been inverted and a camera attachment added.

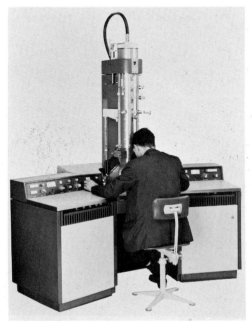

Figure 2. A modern electron microscope. (Courtesy of Philips Electronic Instruments.)

like transmission electron microscopy, it does not depend upon electrons passing through the specimen under examination. The scanning electron microscope bombards the surface of a specimen with a finely focused beam of electrons. As the beam strikes a point on the specimen, deflected primary and emitted secondary electrons which originate from the surface are collected by a detector. The resulting signals are accumulated from many points to build up an image that is displayed on a cathode ray tube. Since the scanning electron microscope is characterized by a great depth of focus, it permits the direct observation of the surface of a bulky specimen.

Just as with light microscopy, transmission and scanning electron microscopy require special techniques for preparing specimens for examination. These will be discussed in the following section.

THE PREPARATION OF TISSUES

It will be obvious to the student that cells, tissues, and organs cannot be studied to advantage unless they are suitably prepared for microscopic examination. The methods of preparation fall logically into two groups: methods involving the direct observation of living cells and methods employed with dead cells (fixed or preserved). In his or her personal study of histology, the student will employ, in the main, fixed and stained preparations of tissues and organs which are permanent. Living tissues are usually more difficult to handle and are valuable for a short period only. Nevertheless, it is important that the student be aware of the methods by which living cells may be observed and understand the ways in which they differ from fixed cells. In the living cell, structure and function may be studied simultaneously. Living cells may be seen to move, to ingest foreign material, occasionally to divide, and to carry on other functions.

Observation of Living Tissue

Unicellular organisms and, occasionally, free cells from a complex organism may be studied directly under the microscope while they still are alive. Free cells are colorless and structures within them lack contrast. This difficulty may be overcome by using a phase contrast microscope. Human blood cells are easy to obtain and can be studied in thin films while surrounded by their natural environment, plasma. In this way ameboid and phagocytic activity may be recognized within white blood cells.

Membranes may be thin enough to be viewed directly under the microscope: for instance, the web of the frog foot, the wing of the bat, and the buccal pouch of the hamster. Thin sections of relatively thick organs such as liver and kidney may be viewed by *transillumination* with quartz rods, which produce a cold light and avoid coagulation of protoplasm. *Glass windows* may be inserted

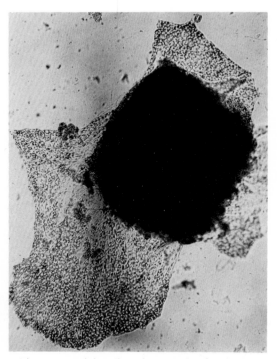

Figure 3. Light microphotograph of a tissue culture preparation. A guinea pig kidney explant (dark mass) is surrounded by sheets of epithelial cells which have grown out from the explant into the surrounding nutrient medium. × 50. (Courtesy of F. Jacoby.)

into ears or backs of animals and so permit extended study of processes such as tissue regeneration or vascular activities. Small pieces of tissue for microscopic examination may be excised, placed in some relatively harmless liquid such as serum or an 0.85 per cent aqueous solution of sodium chloride, and teased apart gently with needles of fine steel or glass.

Prolonged preservation of living cells outside the body can be achieved by a technique known as *tissue culture*. Fragments of tissue are removed aseptically, transferred to a physiological medium, and kept at a temperature normal for the animal from which the tissue was taken. The cultures are placed in thin glass vessels or in hanging drops on a coverglass mounted over a hollow slide. In this way they are available for observation under the microscope. In such cultures, growth, multiplication, and, in some cases, differentiation of cells into other cell types can be observed directly. Tissue culture is a valuable method for the study of cancer and of many viruses.

Microdissection involves the use of an instrument that moves very fine glass needles with precision under the microscope. In this way small portions of a cell such as a nucleus can be removed and the effect observed.

Two staining methods have been applied successfully to living animals or surviving cells. In *vital staining*, dyes are injected into the living animal. The activity of certain cells will result in the selective absorption of the coloring material by these cells. An example of this procedure is the staining by trypan blue of macrophages on the basis of their ability to phagocytose foreign particles. *Supravital staining* involves the addition of a dyestuff to a medium of cells already removed from the organism. Examples of this technique are the staining of mitochondria in living cells by Janus green, of lysosomes by neutral red, and of nerve fibers and cells by methylene blue.

Finally, motion picture records aid in the understanding of cellular activities. Lapsed time films made of individual living cells or of tissue cultures help to analyze processes such as mitosis, phagocytosis, and ameboid movement. Slow-motion films of such rapid processes as the beating of cilia permit analysis of the action.

Preparation of Dead Tissue

Light Microscopy. The most convenient way to study histology is to use *sections,* each of which is a more or less permanent preparation. A section is prepared by cutting a thin slice from a small piece of fixed tissue, which is then stained, mounted in a medium of suitable refractive index upon a slide, and finally covered with a coverslip. The various ways in which sections can be prepared constitute *histological technique*, about which many books have been written. Detailed information of this kind is not required by the student of histology, but he should be aware of the general principles involved so that he may use the material intelligently. The production of a histological section involves the following steps:

Removal of the Specimen. For cytological purposes, and for the best histological preparations, the material should be removed from an anesthetized animal or immediately after death of the animal. In the case of human material this is scarcely ever possible. Surgical material represents the best source of human material since frequently some normal tissue is removed together with the abnormal or diseased tissue.

Fixation. The primary objective of fixation is to preserve protoplasm with the least alteration from the living state. Fixing fluids act as preservatives, inhibiting autolytic changes and bacterial growth. They coagulate protoplasm, thus rendering it insoluble, and harden the tissue so that sectioning is facilitated. They may or may not preserve carbohydrates and lipids. Many fixatives also increase the affinity of protoplasm for certain stains.

The reagents that are employed most commonly as fixing agents are formalin, alcohol, mercuric bichloride, potassium bichromate, and certain acids (picric, acetic, osmic). No single fixative possesses all the desirable qualities, and many reagents are used in mixtures such as Bouin's fluid, Zenker's fluid, and Susa's fluid. The choice of a fixative is usually determined by the particular tissue or component that is to be studied and by the staining method to be used.

Embedding. The purpose of embedding is to provide rigid support to the tissue blocks so that they may be cut into thin sections. Prior to embedding, the fixed tissue is washed to remove excess fixative and then dehydrated by passing it through increasing strengths of alcohol or some other dehydrating agent. The tissue is then *"cleared."* This process involves the removal of the dehydrating agent and its replacement by some fluid which is miscible both with the dehydrating agent and with the embedding medium. *Clearing agents* include xylol, chloroform, benzene, and cedarwood oil. After clearing, the tissue is infiltrated with the embedding agent, usually paraffin or celloidin. After infiltration, the embedding agent is made to solidify so that a firm homogeneous mass containing the embedded tissue is obtained.

For special studies, tissue can be embedded in paraffin without subjecting it to preliminary treatment with fixatives, dehydrating solutions, or clearing agents. This is known as the *freeze-drying* method in which the fresh tissue is frozen rapidly and dehydrated, while still frozen, in vacuum at a low temperature. The dried tissue is then embedded. In the *freeze-substitution* modification of this method, the ice within the frozen tissue is replaced by alcohol at a very low temperature prior to embedding.

Sectioning. Tissue embedded in paraffin may be sliced very thin. For the majority of microscopic work, the sections are between 3 and 10 microns (or micrometers) thick. To cut such sections, a *microtome* is used. Each section is transferred to a clean glass microscope slide on which a little egg albumen has been smeared. Water is run under the section and the slide placed on a warming stage. The water evaporates and the section settles down onto the glass surface, to which it becomes attached. The mounted section is now ready for staining.

Staining. The purpose of staining is to enhance natural contrast and to make more evident various cell and tissue components and extrinsic material. Most stains are employed in aqueous solution, and thus to stain a paraffin section it is necessary to remove the paraffin by placing the section in a paraffin solvent or *decerating agent*, usually xylol or toluol. This step is omitted in the case of a section which has been embedded in celloidin. The section is then passed through descending strengths of alcohol prior to staining.

Mounting. After staining, excess dye is removed by washing with water or alcohol, depending upon the solvent of the dye, and the section is dehydrated through ascending grades of alcohol. Following absolute alcohol, the section is transferred to a solution of a clearing agent. After removal from the clearing agent, a drop of mounting medium, for instance Canada balsam, which has a refractive index similar to that of glass, is placed on the section. The preparation is covered with a coverslip and allowed to dry.

Electron Microscopy. In general, the method of preparation of sections for electron microscopy is similar to that employed for light microscopy. There are some important points of difference. Much smaller pieces of tissue are used since preservation and fixation of cell fine structure is more critical and requires rapid interaction with the fixative. Blocks are commonly about 1 cu mm or less in size. Tissue must be obtained fresh since postmortem changes are more obvious at the higher resolution of the electron microscope. The procedures of fixation, dehydration, and embedding, though similar to those employed in light microscopy, are effected rapidly because of the small pieces of tissue involved. Since paraffin is not suitable for very thin sectioning, it is replaced as an embedding medium by some agent, usually a plastic material such as Epon or Araldite, which produces a firm block. The sections, cut upon a special, precision-built microtome with glass or diamond knives, are minute, about 0.25 mm square and about 300 to 500 Å (30 to 50 nm) thick. They are mounted on perforated copper grids for viewing in the electron microscope.

Thick sections, about 0.2 to 1.0 micron (0.2 to 1.0 micrometer) thick, of

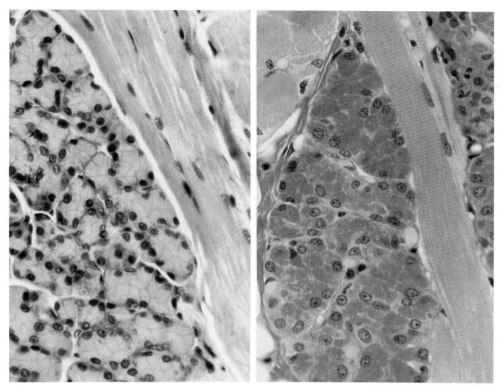

Figure 4. Comparison of the results obtained after routine preparation for light microscopy (paraffin embedding, *left*) and after preparation as for electron microscopy (plastic embedding, *right*). The clarity of detail generally is better in the latter and is the result of better fixation, less tissue shrinkage during preparation, and thinness of the section. In both sections (tongue, × 300), skeletal muscle fibers and glands, groups of secretory end-pieces (acini), are present. Secretory granules are well preserved in the plastic section.

such plastic embedded material can be mounted on glass slides, stained, and examined by light microscopy. Although such sections initially were used to overcome sampling problems encountered in electron microscopic studies, they now are finding increasing usage in light microscopy studies and in general histological laboratories. Several photomicrographs of this type of preparation are to be found in this textbook.

Freeze-etching is another method of preparation of material for electron microscopy. This method involves a purely physical preparation which may allow examination of specimens virtually free of artifacts. The specimen is frozen, cut into small pieces, briefly warmed to etch the cut surface by vacuum-sublimation, and a replica of the surface made by heavy metal shadowing. The frozen specimen is thawed and the replica can then be placed on a specimen grid and viewed in either a transmission or scanning electron microscope. The latter method helps to distinguish natural from artificial structures and allows examination of the surface of single cells or of such structures as cytoplasmic membrane systems.

For *scanning electron microscopy*, the specimen is fixed and dehydrated by special procedures that depend upon the nature of the specimen. Following drying, the specimen is coated evenly with a layer of metal, for example, gold or platinum, prior to viewing in the microscope. This technique allows the biologist to record accurately in three dimensions the surface features of cells and tissues.

Autoradiography. Autoradiography is a special technique which employs the microscope, either light or electron, only as a visual aid. The technique is coming into increasing prominence in histology as a method of chemical localization. Tracer isotopes introduced in the organism either by feeding or by injection follow the same metabolic pathways as do the naturally occurring elements. Their presence in an organ or tissue can be detected by autoradiography. After administration of a tracer isotope, the organ or tissue under investigation is removed and processed for light or electron microscopy in the normal manner. The section is placed in close contact with a photographic emulsion and allowed to remain in the dark for a certain period of time. After subsequent photographic development of the sensitive emulsion, the radioactive tracer elements will appear as dark areas lying over the cells or components of cells in which the radioactivity is located. Some excellent results have been achieved by this method: for instance, the localization of radioiodine in the thyroid gland and of phosphorus (using radiostrontium as a substitute) in bone, and the use of radioactive thymidine, which is specifically taken up by cells about to divide, in the study of the turnover of cell populations.

THE EXAMINATION AND INTERPRETATION OF SECTIONS

The ability to interpret histological sections is a skill which the student has to develop. In gross anatomy, structure is studied in three dimensions. Histology must be learned principally from a study of sections which, for all practical purposes, have no depth. *It is important to reconstruct a three-dimensional mental picture of cells, tissues, and organs from the two-dimensional sections.* In this respect, the plane of sectioning must be borne in mind. A single section of an organ may give a false impression of its architecture. Thus it is important to use several sections taken in different planes in order to make an interpretation of the structure of complex organs.

Nor are the mere identification and notation of structures sufficient. One must strive to interpret the functional significance of what one observes. Dead structures are examined for the purpose of throwing light upon their condition in life. Conditions which are dynamic in life have been converted to a static form in the permanent histological section.

It must be appreciated also that not all sections are perfect. Owing to the techniques used in preparation, sections may not be accurate representations. These alterations are termed *artifacts,* and they should be recognized as such by the student. They may be due to different chemicals used in the histological technique, resulting in shrinkage, or due to sectioning, leading to folding or wrinkling of the section, or to defects caused by an imperfect knife.

During the study of a collection of microscopic slides, the student often is confused by the varying appearance of different constituents of cells and tissues due to the use of a number of different staining techniques. With any microscopic preparation, interpretation involves also an appreciation of the staining techniques used. Although it is not necessary for the student to be conversant with details of the various staining techniques used, he should understand the general principles, uses, and results of the common staining procedures.

STAINS

In general the dyes used are complex organic chemicals which often show some variability in performance. They may be classified in numerous ways, but the simplest approach is to base the classification upon use, with regard to tissue and cell components. Dyes may be of general use, staining either the nucleus or the cytoplasm, or they may be more specific with regard to particular components. It must be emphasized that many dyes require special methods of fixation and preparation of the tissue, and the reader is referred to a textbook of histological and histochemical techniques for the details.

Stains in general use are considered to be either acids or bases, but in fact they are neutral salts having both acidic and basic radicals. When the coloring property of the dye is in the basic radical of the neutral salt, the stain is referred to as a basic dye and structures that stain with it are termed *basophil.* In most instances, the basophil substances which attract the basic dyes are them-

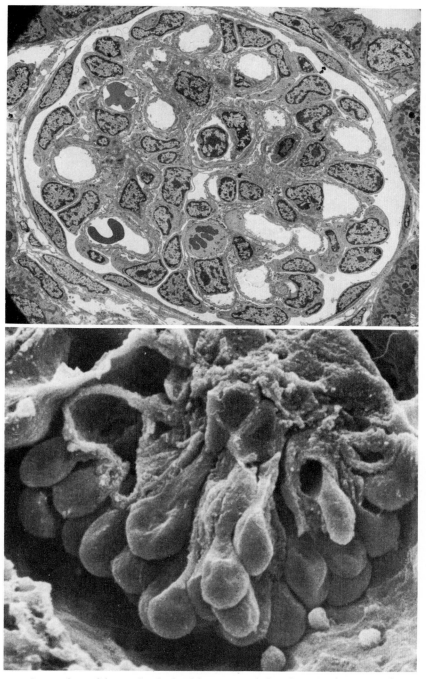

Figure 5. Comparison of the results obtained from transmission electron microscopy (above) and from scanning electron microscopy (below). Both micrographs are of a renal glomerulus. In the upper illustration, sectioned capillary loops of the glomerulus appear empty; in the lower illustration, the glomerulus is seen in three dimensions and a few capillary loops have been cut open. (Courtesy of Professor M. Miyoshi.)

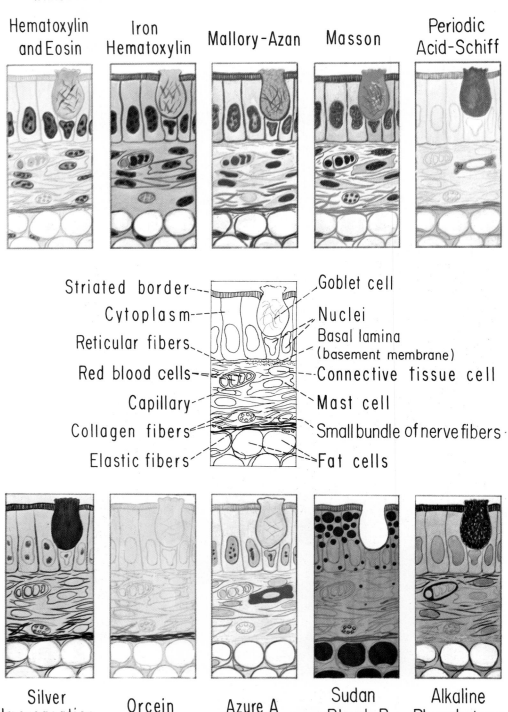

Hematoxylin and Eosin Iron Hematoxylin Mallory–Azan Masson Periodic Acid–Schiff

Striated border ---
Cytoplasm ---
Reticular fibers ---
Red blood cells ---
Capillary ---
Collagen fibers ---
Elastic fibers ---

--- Goblet cell
--- Nuclei
Basal lamina (basement membrane)
--- Connective tissue cell
--- Mast cell
--- Small bundle of nerve fibers
--- Fat cells

Silver Impregnation Orcein Azure A Sudan Black B Alkaline Phosphatase

Figure 6. Diagrammatic representation of a section (partly hypothetical) of a portion of intestine wall as it would appear after different staining procedures. Hematoxylin and eosin stains nuclei dark blue and both cytoplasm and connective tissue fibers pink-red. Iron hematoxylin stains nuclei a dark purple-black. It also stains red blood cells. With less differentiation after staining (see text) it would make visible also such cellular components as mitochondria. Mallory-Azan and Masson are examples of trichrome methods of staining which are useful in differentiating between cytoplasm and connective tissue fibers. In the former method, collagen fibers are stained bright blue; in the latter, green. Periodic acid–Schiff stains the brush

Legend continued on the opposite page.

selves acids, for instance, the nucleic acids of the nucleus and the acidic components of the cytoplasm such as ribonucleic acid (RNA). Similarly, when the staining property is in the acidic radical of the neutral salt, the stain is spoken of as an acid dye and the structures stained (for instance, the general cytoplasm) as *acidophil*.

The nuclear stain in most common use is hematoxylin, the staining property of which depends upon the presence in solution of its oxidation product, hematein. (Thus, a freshly prepared solution of hematoxylin must be allowed to "ripen" or "age" for oxidation to occur prior to use.) When stained with such a dye, nuclei appear blue. Iron hematoxylin, which stains nuclei dark blue or black, has a wide application. In most methods employing iron hematoxylin, one overstains with the dye and regressively differentiates in a weak acid or in a ferric salt solution. By careful *differentiation*, which may be viewed directly under the microscope, such organelles as chromosomes, mitochondria, Golgi apparatus, and the contractile elements of muscle may be visualized. The basic aniline dyes are a group of stains used extensively. This group includes azure A, toluidine blue, and methylene blue, stains that are employed also in the identification of mucopolysaccharides which stain *metachromatically* (*meta*, beyond; *chroma*, color). This means that mucopolysaccharides, when stained with one of these dyes, will take on a color different from that of the dye employed. It is thought that substances which demonstrate metachromasia do so because they are capable of concentrating the dye or of altering its molecular state. Mucin, matrix of cartilage, and

the granules of mast cells are demonstrated readily by their metachromatic staining. Other basic aniline dyes in common use are brilliant cresyl blue, neutral red, and Janus green, all of which are nontoxic and may be used also as vital or supravital stains.

Acidic dyes, commonly employed to stain the general cytoplasm, include eosin, picric acid, acid azo dyes such as chromotrope, and the acid diazo dyes, trypan blue and trypan red. The latter two are used also as vital stains.

Most histological sections are stained with both a basic stain and an acidic stain. The commonest combination is *hematoxylin and eosin* (H and E), in which nuclear structures are stained dark purple or blue, and practically all cytoplasmic structures and intercellular substances are stained pink. Trichrome methods, such as Mallory's connective tissue stain and the Mallory-Azan method, possess the advantage that they differentiate between cytoplasmic structures and intercellular materials. They stain certain connective tissue fibers bright blue, nuclei red or orange, and various cell constituents blue, red, orange, or purple. Masson's staining procedure is another trichrome method of general use in which connective tissue fibers are stained green, nuclei blue or purple, and cytoplasmic structures red. Although there is no truly specific stain for collagen, it is best shown by the acid aniline dyes in a trichrome method. Elastic fibers are brilliantly acidophil and can be stained selectively with orcein or with resorcin fuchsin. Reticulin can be demonstrated specifically by precipitation of silver from an alkaline solution. Hence these fibers are termed *argyrophil*. It must be realized that special methods of stain-

---

Figure 6 *Continued.*
border, mucus within the goblet cell, the basal lamina, and cytoplasmic granules of the mast cell positively. All other structures on the section are negative with this stain. Silver impregnation and orcein are examples of stains used to differentiate between the various types of connective tissue fibers. Impregnation with silver outlines reticular fibers; hence, commonly, they are termed *argyrophil*. Elastic fibers are stained selectively with orcein (and with resorcin fuchsin). Azure A is one of the group of basic aniline dyes which stains nuclei blue and also is employed in the identification of mucopolysaccharides which stain metachromatically as do the granules of the mast cell here (see text). Sudan black B is a dye which is absorbed by fat and thus stains it selectively. It requires a method of preparation of tissue which avoids the use of fat solvents. Alkaline phosphatase is an enzyme which can be localized by a histochemical method (see text). Hence there is a positive reaction in the brush border and, as often happens, in the cytoplasm of endothelium lining blood vessels. (After Garvin.)

ing are necessary to demonstrate certain constituents of cells and formed extracellular fibers, and that a single staining method does not suffice to demonstrate everything present within a section.

HISTOCHEMISTRY

The fact that deposition of specific stains in certain regions is a result of chemical or physical properties inherent in the tissue forms the basis of histochemistry. This is a field of research which has expanded rapidly and has as its goal the localization within specific areas or cell components of the chemical compounds known already by biochemical analysis to be present. Histochemical methods are now available for many inorganic and organic substances. An example of the former is the adaptation of the Prussian blue reaction for the detection of ferric iron. In sections treated with potassium ferrocyanide, deposits are colored blue.

The *Feulgen reaction* for the identification of deoxyribonucleic acid (DNA) is an example of a histochemical test which requires preliminary treatment of the section so that the substance under investigation either is liberated or produces a substance for which a specific test exists. Basic fuchsin is a magenta colored dye which can be bleached by treatment with hydrochloric acid and sodium bisulfite. Reaction with the aldehydes produces, in the bleached dye, a new, colored compound, also magenta. Mild hydrolysis of a section with hydrochloric acid will produce aldehydes from DNA. If the section is then immersed in the colorless form of basic fuchsin, the aldehydes formed from DNA will react with the dye and exhibit the magenta color. Since both deoxyribonucleic acid (DNA) and ribonucleic acid (RNA) are basophil, the Feulgen reaction allows a distinction to be made as to which basophil material is DNA. A method which employs a similar histochemical technique is the *periodic acid–Schiff reaction* (PAS reaction). Periodic acid is an oxidizing agent which will produce from certain polysaccharides aldehydes that are insoluble. These then react with the

Schiff reagent, which is the colorless form of basic fuchsin.

Not all reactions in histochemistry rely upon chemical affinities. Fat can be detected in sections which have not been exposed to fat solvents by stains such as Sudan III, Sudan IV, and Sudan black B. These stains have a physical affinity for lipid and are adsorbed by the fat. Use of such dyes forms the basis for the term *sudanophilia*, the ability to stain substances with this group of dyes.

Enzymes may be detected by histochemical methods which in principle attempt to localize the site of a specific enzyme by a chemical process similar to that performed by the enzyme *in vivo*. The section under examination is incubated at body temperature in the pres-

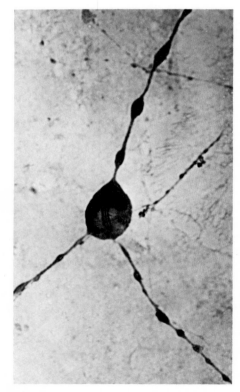

Figure 7.   An example of immunocytochemical localization using peroxidase-antiperoxidase (PAP). Angiotensin II (AII) neurons cultured from fetal rat brain were localized with a specific primary antiserum to AII followed by second antibody (against the primary antibody), PAP and a diaminobenzidine reaction with peroxidase. Positive AII immunoreactivity is observed in the perikaryon of the neuron (neuronal soma) and in processes containing prominent varicosities. × 3000. (Courtesy of Dr. J. Weyhenmeyer.)

ence of a suitable substrate, and the product of the resultant chemical reaction with the enzyme is converted into a chemical substance of a definite color. For example, to demonstrate the enzyme alkaline phosphatase, glycerophosphate is used as the substrate in an alkaline medium and the phosphate liberated by the action of the enzyme is deposited in the presence of calcium ions as calcium phosphate. The deposit of calcium phosphate is converted to an easily visualized black precipitate of cobalt sulfide (or metallic silver) by immersing the section in cobalt acetate (or silver acetate) and then rinsing in ammonium sulfide. Methods are available now for a wide variety of enzymes including phosphatases, lipases, oxidases, and esterases.

Glycogen is stained by Best's carmine stain or by the periodic acid–Schiff reagent. In either case, glycogen can be differentiated from other polysaccharides by the fact that the staining property of the latter substances is resistant to digestion by salivary amylase.

Immunocytochemistry is one branch of histochemistry that has received considerable attention recently. At the light microscopic level, the fluorescent antibody technique is a sensitive method for the localization of specific polysaccharides or proteins. The basis of this technique is the fact that the body reacts to foreign protein substances, the *antigens*, by elaborating specific substances, the *antibodies*, which combine with and inactivate the antigens. Fluorescent dye molecules are chemically linked to antibody molecules and the sites of their reaction with antigens can be visualized in the ultraviolet microscope. The method has been used to identify the cells of origin of protein hormones, the intracellular localization of various enzymes, and the sites of proteins such as myosin. The method has been adapted for use with the electron microscope by conjugating an antibody with a metalloprotein such as *ferritin*, which naturally possesses a distinct appearance in the electron microscope. This method enables the investigator to localize precisely the site of the antibody-antigen reaction.

REFERENCES

Baker, J. R.: Principles of Biological Microtechnique. London, Methuen, 1970.

Bancroft, J. D., and Stevens, A. (editors): Theory and Practice of Histological Techniques. Edinburgh, Churchill Livingstone, 1977.

Bullivant, S.: Freeze-etching and freeze fracturing. *In* Advanced Techniques in Biological Electron Microscopy, edited by J. Koehler. New York, Springer-Verlag, 1973, p. 66.

Coons, A. H.: Fluorescent antibody methods. *In* General Cytochemical Methods, edited by J. F. Danielli. New York, Academic Press, 1958, p. 400.

Elias, H.: Three-dimensional structure identified from single sections. Science, *174*:993, 1971.

Hall, C. A.: How to Use the Microscope, ed. 4. New York, Macmillan Co., 1955.

Hayat, M. A.: Principles and Techniques of Electron Microscopy: Biological Applications. Vol. 1. New York, Van Nostrand Reinhold Co., 1970.

Hollenburg, M. J., and Erickson, A. M.: The scanning electron microscope: potential usefulness to biologists. A review. J. Histochem. Cytochem., *21*:109, 1973.

Journal of the Royal Microscopical Society. Issue in celebration of the Tercentenary of "The Microscope in Living Biology," *83*:1–229, 1964.

Leeson, T. S., and Rennie, I. M.: A simplified method for routine use of glycol methacrylate, including hematoxylin and eosin staining. Can. J. Med. Technol., *37*:190, 1975.

Lewis, W. H., and Lewis, M. R.: Behavior of cells in tissue cultures. *In* General Cytology, edited by E. V. Cowdry. Chicago, University of Chicago Press, 1924, p. 385.

McManus, J. F. A., and Mowry, R. W.: Staining Methods: Histologic and Histochemical. New York, Paul B. Hoeber, Inc., 1960.

Oster, G., and Pollister, A. W. (editors): Physical Techniques in Biological Research. New York, Academic Press, 1955–1957, Vols. 1–3.

Parker, R. C.: Methods of Tissue Culture, ed. 3. New York, Paul B. Hoeber, Inc., 1961.

Pearse, A. G. E.: Histochemistry: Theoretical and Applied. Edinburgh, Churchill Livingstone, 1972.

Pease, D. C.: Histological Techniques for Electron Microscopy, ed. 3. New York, Academic Press, 1968.

Rogers, A. W.: Techniques of Autoradiography. New York, American Elsevier Publishing Co., 1967.

Rogers, A. W.: Recent developments in the use of autoradiographic techniques with electron microscopy. Phil. Trans. R. Soc. Lond. B., *261*:159, 1971.

Sjöstrand, F. S.: Electron Microscopy of Cells and Tissues. Vol. 1, Instrumentation and Techniques. New York, Academic Press, 1967.

Sternberger, L. A.: Electron microscopic immunocytochemistry: a review. J. Histochem. Cytochem., *15*:139, 1967.

Wyckoff, R. W. G.: Optical methods in cytology. *In* The Cell: Biochemistry, Physiology, Morphology, edited by J. Brachet and A. E. Mirsky. New York, Academic Press, 1959, Vol. 1, p. 1.

GENERAL PRINCIPLES AND PRIMARY TISSUES

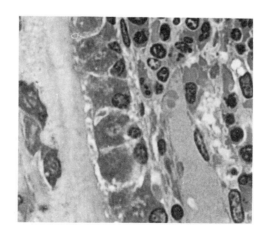

THE CELL

COMPONENTS OF THE BODY

The body is composed of three different elements: cells, intercellular substance, and the body fluids.

The body fluids include blood, confined within the vascular system; tissue (intercellular) fluid, which is located between and around cells and in which there is a free exchange of materials with blood on the one side and with intracellular fluid on the other; and lymph, draining tissue fluid into a closed system of fine tubes that eventually drain back into the venous system. These fluid components, with the exception of the formed elements (cells) of the blood, usually are not seen in histological sections because they are lost during preparation.

The obvious feature of most tissue sections is the presence of cells, although their entire outlines may not be discernible. Each cell exists as a discrete entity and is enclosed by a membrane which "isolates" it from its environment. The cell consists of *protoplasm,* that is, living material, existing as a heterogeneous aqueous phase in which are found both the chemical machinery for metabolic processes and the material of heredity. In very primitive cells such as bacteria, the metabolic and hereditary components are mixed. These are termed prokaryotic cells. In all cells of higher plants and animals, called eukaryotes, the bulk of the hereditary material is isolated in a membrane-bound nucleus lying in the remainder of the cell, or cytoplasm. It should be emphasized that in sections the nucleus may not be seen, and in some cells the cytoplasm may be nondiscernible. The nucleus, which occasionally is multiple, usually is regularly ovoid or spherical and darkly staining, while the surrounding cytoplasm is more lightly staining. There is great variation in the appearance, size, and shape of cells, which reflects the different functions of different cell types.

Intercellular substance, as the name suggests, is that material which lies between and supports the cells. It is primarily responsible for the firmness of tissues, and in histology we recognize two main types of intercellular material, formed and amorphous. The formed type includes the material called collagen (for example, the white, fibrous tissue that is found in meat and is tough to chew) and elastin, which is largely responsible for the elasticity of tissues. Amorphous intercellular material, or ground substance, is composed of a group of substances termed proteinpolysaccharides, long-chain polymers of protein-sugar complexes. These intercellular substances are described in detail in the following chapter.

PROTOPLASM

Cells are composed of protoplasm, which has been described as the physical basis for life, each cell being a living, dynamic entity. Approximately 75 per cent of protoplasm is water, partly free and thus available for metabolic processes, and partly bound to protein as a structural component of protoplasm. Salts account for about 1 per cent of body materials, and particularly impor-

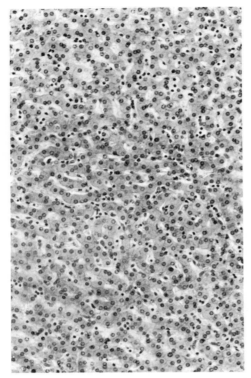

Figure 1–1. Photomicrograph of a section of the rat liver showing irregular cords of cells, each with a spherical nucleus. Cell boundaries are not distinct at this magnification. × 125.

tant are the cations potassium and magnesium and the anions phosphate and bicarbonate. Other components are the three basic food materials: proteins (10 to 20 per cent), lipids (2 to 3 per cent), and carbohydrates (1 per cent). Proteins are molecules of high molecular weight composed of amino acids, of which there are some 20 kinds. Lipids occur as structural components and as food reserves, all of which are soluble in fat solvents and thus are removed in routine histological preparations. Special techniques are used to preserve them. Carbohydrates are present in protoplasm as mono-, di-, and polysaccharides and as protein-polysaccharide complexes. Another important component of protoplasm is vitamins, required in small amounts for the growth and normal metabolism of cells.

Both the vital, living protoplasm of cells and the nonliving materials between cells (intercellular substance) exist in the colloidal state. It is difficult to define a colloid exactly, but the basic feature of a colloidal solution is that its particles are of such a size that they cannot be filtered through natural membranes, the membrane acting as a

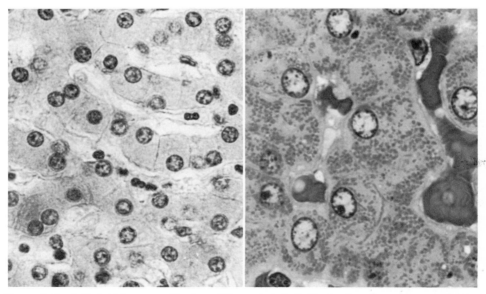

Figure 1–2. *Left:* A higher magnification of Figure 1–1. Individual cell outlines are recognizable and chromatin masses and nucleoli are visible in the nuclei. Several cells contain two nuclei. × 750. *Right:* A plastic section of liver. Cytoplasmic and nuclear details are more obvious. The small ovoid cytoplasmic bodies are mitochondria. × 1100.

sieve and holding back the particles. Crystalloids, e.g., glucose, can pass through such membranes. Proteins show all the characteristics of the colloidal state, and some can exist either as sols or as gels. Fluid solutions of colloids are sols, but they are viscous to some degree, e.g., egg albumen (egg "white"). If, however, the egg albumen is heated or subjected to a change in hydrogen ion concentration, it becomes solid; i.e., it has been transformed into the gel state. In the protoplasm of cells, such sol-gel transformations can occur and often are reversible, as is the case in the "setting" and "melting" of a solution of gelatin.

Substances that mainly are responsible for the form and organization of the protoplasm are the *macromolecules*. These are constructed from smaller organic building blocks, the *monomers*, linked together repetitively by covalent bonds. Proteins, for instance, are composed of amino acids linked by bonds. Polysaccharides are composed of sugar monomers. The degree of polymerization refers to the number of monomer units linked in a single macromolecule. Within animal cells, macromolecules fall into three principal classes: polysaccharides, proteins, and nucleic acids.

Polysaccharides. Polysaccharides of biological importance include glycogen and protein-polysaccharides. Glycogen, a highly branched polymer of *d*-glucose, constitutes a storage depot from which glucose, needed for many chemical activities within the cell, may be released readily upon demand. Protein-polysaccharides commonly encountered in histological material include hyaluronic acid, often found in association with the connective tissue protein collagen, and chondroitin sulfates, present in large quantities within the ground substance of cartilage.

Proteins. Proteins are large molecules composed of a variety of amino acid monomers linked by peptide bonds in a definite sequence. They occur either as structural proteins or as enzymes. Structural proteins include collagen, the keratins of hair and nails, and the muscle proteins. Enzymes constitute an important group of proteins which function as catalysts in many chemical processes, whether synthetic or degradative. Many hormones such as insulin and gonadotrophin also are proteins.

Nucleic Acids. Nucleic acids are the most restricted geographically of the macromolecules and are concerned with protein synthesis. There are two main classes, known as DNA (deoxyribonucleic acid) and RNA (ribonucleic acid). Each is composed of an alternating sequence of two units, a phosphate group and a sugar group. Attached to each sugar group is a base, either a purine or a pyrimidine. In DNA, the sugar is deoxyribose and the bases are of only four kinds, adenine, thymine, guanine, and cytosine, which follow each other in an irregular order. In RNA, the sugar is ribose, and the bases also are four in number and identical to those of DNA, with the exception that uracil replaces thymine. In metazoan cells, DNA is found principally in the nucleus, in which it constitutes the genetic material. RNA is found both within the nucleus and in the cytoplasm.

In addition to the macromolecules, protplasm contains lipids, which are smaller molecules and are important, since they often interact with proteins to constitute a structural basis of biological membrane formation. Lipids are composed of long aliphatic chains capable of orienting themselves at water interfaces into monomolecular layers. The complex of lipid-protein-water is found in membrane systems of nerve myelin sheaths, mitochondria, Golgi apparatus, and endoplasmic reticulum. The combination of two such complexes back to back constitutes a *unit membrane* (see later).

Metabolism

Metabolism can be defined as the chemical processes of the cell by which nutrition is effected. Metabolism may involve the breakdown of cell protoplasm itself or of the materials brought to the cell as food supply. In this case it is termed *catabolic*, energy being released. Alternatively, energy may be utilized by the cell to produce materials that may remain in the cell or be released. This type of metabolism is termed *anabolic*.

Cell Function

Protoplasm has a variety of physiological properties which indicate the functions of cells. The functions of any particular type of cell are a direct expression of one or more of these properties of its protoplasm, and they include the following:

Irritability. Irritability is the capacity of protoplasm to respond to a stimulus, the response of the cell being detected by one of the other properties of protoplasm. Irritability is an expression of life itself, and disappears with cell death.

Conductivity. Conductivity indicates that protoplasm can transmit a wave of excitation (an electrical impulse) throughout the cell from the point of stimulus. This property is highly developed in the cell membrane of nerve and, to a lesser extent, of muscle cells.

Contractility. Contractility is the property of changing shape, usually in the sense of shortening, and is highly developed in muscle cells.

Respiration. Respiration is the process whereby food substances and oxygen within the cell interact chemically to produce energy, carbon dioxide, and water. This process, of course, is essential for life.

Absorption. Absorption involves the imbibition of certain dissolved substances which later may be assimilated by the cell, the cell utilizing such material for metabolism. Fluids may diffuse directly into the cell through the plasma membrane or may be engulfed in bulk, a droplet of fluid passing into the cytoplasm being limited by a pinched-off portion of the plasma membrane to form a vacuole. This latter process is called *pinocytosis.* Cells also have the ability to take up particulate matter, this process being called *phagocytosis.*

Secretion and Excretion. Secretion and excretion are the processes by which a cell can extrude material. If the material passed out from the cell is a useful product, e.g., a digestive enzyme or a hormone, then the process is called secretion, but if waste materials are extruded, then the term excretion is applied to the process.

Growth and Reproduction. While cells vary in size, most human cells are in the range of 5 to 50 microns (micrometers). Diffusion between cells is rapid and this is correlated with cell size. As size increases, the surface area available for diffusion increases by the square of the diameter, but the volume of protoplasm increases by the cube. Thus, while some cells can grow in size, the maximum size is limited by the surface area and if further growth of a tissue occurs, it necessitates an increase in the number of cells. This involves division of cells, a process which will be discussed later.

COMPONENTS OF THE CELL

It is important to appreciate that there are many different kinds of cells in the body — different in size, shape, and function — but that each cell is composed of nucleus and cytoplasm. In the ordinary histological slide, these two components of a cell will be differentially stained; i.e., the cytoplasm will appear to be a different color from that of the nucleus (see page 10). As mentioned previously, the cytoplasm may be small in amount, or very lightly stained, and therefore difficult to see.

CYTOPLASM

With the light microscope, cytoplasm generally has an even, homogeneous, amorphous appearance but may show granular, fibrillar, or vacuolated areas. It does, in fact, contain many small bodies of varying types and functions. Variations in function of cell types, e.g., an enzyme-secreting cell or a nerve cell, are reflected by different appearances of the cytoplasm, which in turn is consequent upon variations in the number and type of these small cytoplasmic bodies. Variations in appearance of a cell type also are dependent on the metabolic activity of the cell. These cytoplasmic bodies are of two main types: *organelles,* which are living, structural components of the cell, and *inclusions,* which are best considered as nonliving accumulations of metabolites or cell products.

Cytoplasm in most cells is regionally specialized. Near the nucleus usually are

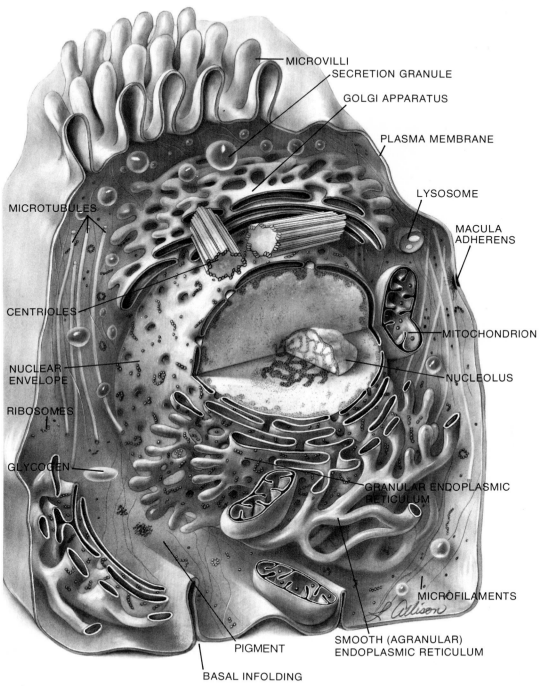

Figure 1–3. Schematic diagram of the cell to show many of the organelles and inclusions as they would be seen on electron microscopy.

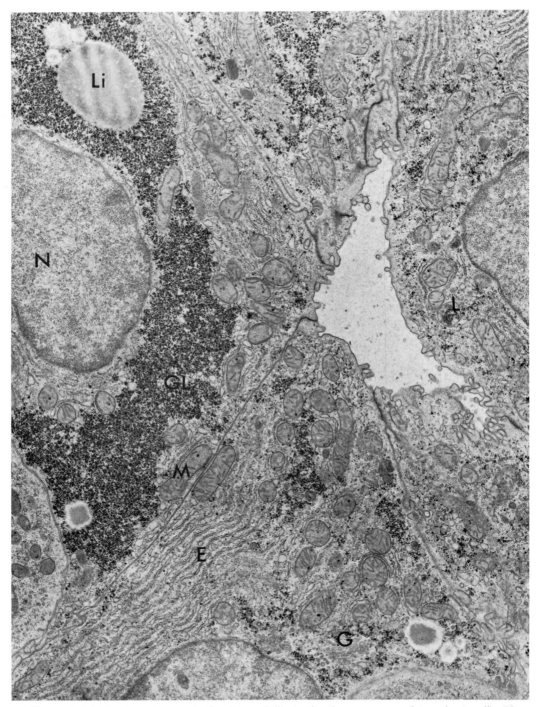

Figure 1–4. Electron micrograph of rat liver cells illustrating the appearance of several organelles: N = nucleus, M = mitochondrion, G = Golgi apparatus, E = granular endoplasmic reticulum, L = lysosome, GL = glycogen, Li = lipid. The clear space in the center is a bile canaliculus. × 13,000. (Courtesy of J. Steiner.)

situated the centrosome, or cell center, and the Golgi apparatus. Lysosomes often are closely adjacent to the Golgi apparatus and, in a cell which secretes protein, for example, granular endoplasmic reticulum and mitochondria are concentrated in basal (subnuclear) cytoplasm with the centrosome on the apical side of the nucleus and secretory droplets or granules in apical cytoplasm. Other organelles such as microtubules, microfilaments, and the contractile proteins of muscle cells are arranged in particular arrays. Each cell, of course, is bounded by a plasma membrane, or plasmalemma, which is one of the organelles.

Cell (Plasma) Membrane

All cells are enveloped by a plasma membrane or plasmalemma that is only 7.5 nm thick, and thus often it is invisible by light microscopy. However, it may be seen if it is sectioned obliquely, thus increasing its thickness, or if its staining is enhanced by the presence of associated material on its external surface. For general purposes, the cell or plasma membrane is defined as the thinnest layer resolved at the cell surface by light microscopy. It provides a selective barrier that regulates the transport of materials into and out of the cell.

All membranes, including intracytoplasmic membranes as well as the plasmalemma, are composed mainly of lipid and protein with a small amount of carbohydrate. The thickness varies a little from cell type to cell type and internal membranes usually are somewhat thinner than the plasmalemma. On electron microscopy, all show the so-called *"unit membrane"* structure of two dense lines, each about 2.5 nm thick, separated by a lucent intermediate layer of about 3 nm.

Several models have been proposed for the plasma membrane. The Davson-Danielli model postulates a lipid center with a coat of protein on each surface. Membrane lipids, mostly phospholipids, have a hydrophilic phosphate (polar) end, and a hydrophobic, nonpolar end (fatty acid "tail"), and in the membrane the phospholipids are arranged in two monomolecular layers with the hydro-

philic phosphate ends on the surface contacting the protein layers and the hydrophobic tails apposed to each other in the center of the membrane. The two dense lines of the unit membrane would represent the two protein surface sheets with the central lipid layer as the central lucent region. However, the "fluid mosaic model" of Singer and Nicholson is now generally accepted and proposes that membrane proteins are globular and float like icebergs in a sea of lipid. Recent studies have shown that integral membrane proteins have hydrophobic and hydrophilic regions, and that probably the hydrophobic parts are embedded within the central lipid of the membrane, with the hydrophilic regions exposed at the surface. This would explain the appearance seen on using the freeze-etch technique which demonstrates the presence of intramembranous particles of 6 to 12 nm diameter. Thus, these particles represent integral or intrinsic membrane proteins that, dependent on size, may be exposed on one surface of the membrane or extend completely through it. Additionally, some peripheral proteins probably are associated with the surfaces of the bilayer, lying between the protruding integral proteins.

While study of electron micrographs and freeze-etch replicas may give the impression that the plasma membrane is a rigid structure, many components, particularly membrane proteins, probably are in motion constantly in the plane of the membrane.

The plasma membrane presents a lipid barrier to the passage of some substances, partly determined by their lipid solubility. The maintenance of the intracellular environment requires selective membrane transport that is both active and passive, with nutrients passing into the cell and other materials passing out. Physiologically, it is believed that there are pores in the membrane, although these have not been demonstrated morphologically. They may be represented by channels in those proteins that traverse the full thickness of the membrane. The plasma membrane also receives signals from hormones and neurotransmitters. Hormones, at a "target" cell, either must penetrate the plasma membrane (which occurs with steroid hormones, probably

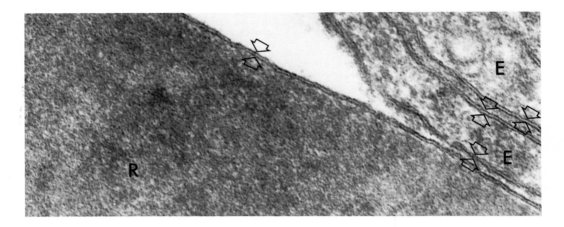

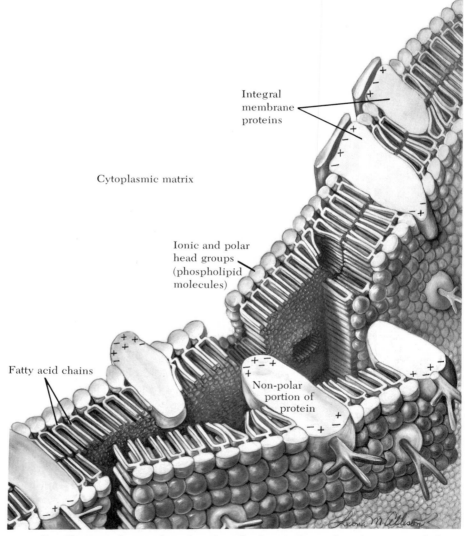

Figure 1–5. *Top:* Electron micrograph to show the trilaminar (unit membrane) structure of plasma membranes (between arrowheads). Seen are part of an erythrocyte (R) and cytoplasmic processes of endothelium (E) lining a blood vessel. × 110,000. *Bottom:* Diagram of the fluid mosaic model of the plasma membrane, after S. J. Singer and G. L. Nicolson.

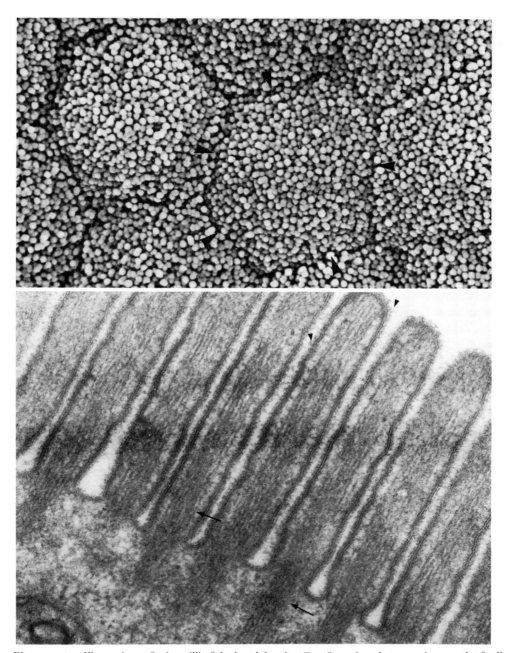

Figure 1–6. Illustrations of microvilli of the brush border. *Top:* Scanning electron micrograph of cells of the monkey gallbladder. Note cell outlines (arrowheads). × 4,000. (Courtesy of Dr. Peter Andrews.) *Bottom:* Microvilli of lining epithelial cells of the duodenum. Note the trilaminar plasma membrane with associated glycocalyx (arrowheads) and bundles of filaments (arrows) in the cores of the microvilli. × 125,000.

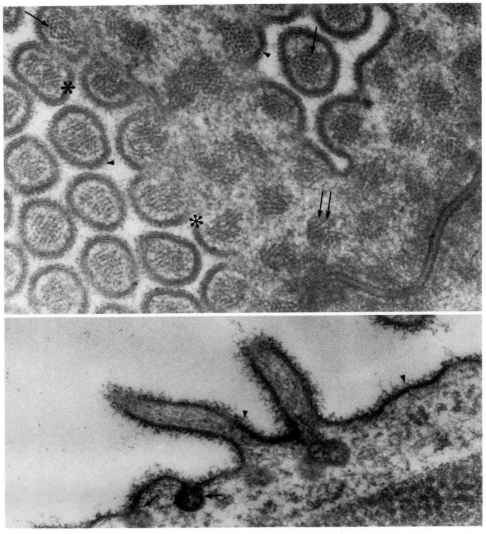

Figure 1–7. Electron micrographs of microvilli. *Top*: Brush border microvilli of duodenal lining epithelial cells, in transverse section. Note trilaminar plasma membrane (asterisks) and associated glycocalyx (arrowheads), core of filaments in the microvilli (arrows) extending into apical cytoplasm (double arrow). × 125,000. *Bottom*: Mesothelial cell of pleura showing occasional microvilli, glycocalyx associated with the plasma membrane (arrowheads), and micropinocytotic vesicles, two as invaginations (arrows) of the surface plasma membrane. × 115,000.

because they are lipid-soluble) or must transmit their message across it without penetrating (which occurs with glycoprotein hormones that bind to specific receptors on the outer cell surface).

The plasma membrane differs from other membranes in that its external surface is covered with glycoprotein, the *cell coat* or *glycocalyx*. It varies greatly in thickness but can be demonstrated in some cells by the PAS technique, for example, on the luminal surface of intestinal epithelium where it is associated

with small, finger-like protrusions of the cell surface called microvilli. On electron microscopy, it appears as a fine, filamentous material. The surfaces of probably all cells show a glycocalyx, although it may be thin, and it is absent only in areas of specialized cell contact (see page 88). It is formed by carbohydrate chains of glycoproteins of the plasma membrane that protrude from the external surface, probably associated with other polysaccharides synthesized by the cells. This cell coat confers a negative charge on the cell surface that probably is important in cellular contacts and adhesion, most cells being separated by a regular interval of about 20 nm.

Although the membrane is a bilayer structure, it is not symmetrical. Morphologically, as shown above, glycoproteins, glycopeptides, and glycolipids are situated in the outer layer, and there also are differences in composition of lipids between the two layers.

Larger molecules can enter the cell by a process of *pinocytosis,* a local invagination of the plasma membrane enclosing fluid or other material and then pinching off to form a membrane-bound vesicle in the cell. A similar process involving particulate material is called *phagocytosis.* Both are examples of *endocytosis;* the reverse of the process, i.e., extrusion of material, is called *exocytosis.*

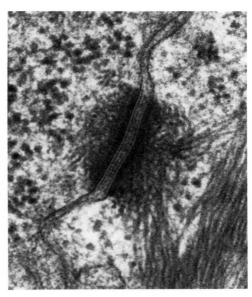

Figure 1–9. Electron micrograph of a spot desmosome (macula adherens) on a cellular interface of epithelial cells (epidermis). Note associated cytoplasmic filaments and density of the two plasma membranes. × 64,000.

Here, the membrane bounding an excretory granule or droplet, for example, fuses with the plasmalemma and releases its contents to the exterior. These processes are associated with the presence in the cytoplasm of vesicular structures, although other vesicular bodies also are present.

Micropinocytotic vesicles or *caveolae intracellulares* are only about 50 nm in diameter and are involved in transport of proteins and other molecules. They are particularly prominent in endothelial and mesothelial cells (lining vascular spaces and the body cavities) and in smooth muscle cells.

In many cell types, there are modifications in the form of the plasma membrane, the majority of these being visible only on electron microscopy. For example, in cells specialized for absorption there are at the apical (luminal) surface a series of small, finger-like processes or *microvilli.* These are simple, tubular evaginations of the plasma membrane with a cytoplasmic core in which there are collections of microfibrils. If the microvilli are regular and closely packed they collectively form a "brush" or "striated" border, visible on light microscopy, and obviously greatly increase

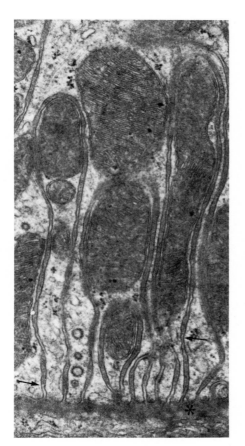

Figure 1–8. Electron micrograph of basal infoldings (arrows) of the plasma membrane in an epithelial cell of a kidney tubule. Amorphous basal lamina material is marked with asterisk. × 25,000.

surface area. In addition, the surface area of cells is often increased by numerous infoldings of the basal plasmalemma. Between cells, i.e., at lateral borders, adjacent plasma membranes are separated by a narrow gap of about 20 nm and, while the interface may be straight and regular with adjacent plasmalemmae parallel, often it is highly irregular with a system of interlocking tongues and grooves. This is termed a "jigsaw" or "zipper" interlocking and is a factor in cell adhesion. Other specializations of the cell surface are discussed later in relation to epithelial cells (see page 88). They include *maculae adherentes* or *spot desmosomes* that appear as small densities scattered along cell interfaces. Occasionally, the intercellular space is widened to form "intercellular canals," usually with microvillus or pseudopodial projections of adjacent cells into the intercellular space.

Rough-Surfaced (Granular) Endoplasmic Reticulum

By light microscopy, in some cell types, there are areas of cytoplasm that stain blue with basic stains, such regions being termed the *basophilic component* of the cytoplasm, *chromidial substance,* or *ergastoplasm* (ergastoplasm indicates work, i.e., that component of the cytoplasm involved in synthesis). On electron microscopy, these areas of cytoplasm contain large numbers of small electron-dense particles called *ribosomes,* usually attached to membranes arranged as a three-dimensional network or reticulum of channels in the form of cisternae or flattened sacs, tubules, and vesicles. The membrane of the reticulum shows a unit membrane or trilaminar structure, usually is 6 to 7 mm thick, and encloses a lumen or intracisternal space that may contain some flocculent material of moderate electron density that represents newly synthesized protein. The membranes of the reticulum thus enclose an intracellular compartment that segregates newly synthesized products. Attached to the outer surfaces of the membrane are the ribosomes; hence the term granular endoplasmic reticulum. The amount of granular reticulum in cells varies from one or two flattened cisternae to widely distributed, interconnected, parallel stacks of cisternae, and only in mature erythrocytes is granular reticu-

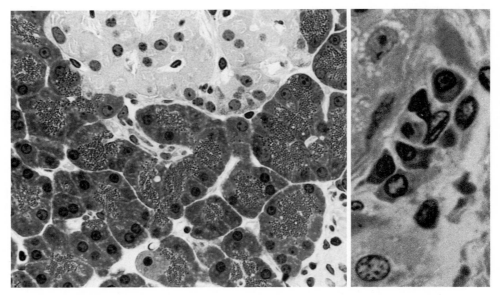

Figure 1–10.   Photomicrographs to illustrate cytoplasmic basophilia. The zymogen-secreting cells of the pancreas *(left)* are arranged in groups or acini. The basal cytoplasm of each cell stains intensely basophil owing to the presence of numerous ribosomes associated with the endoplasmic reticulum: the apical cytoplasm contains secretory (zymogen) droplets or granules. Compare the intense basophilia of these cells with the lack of it in endocrine cells of an islet of Langerhans (above). In the intertubular connective tissue of the testis *(right)* are several isolated cells also with intensely basophil cytoplasm. These are plasma cells. Both are plastic sections. Left, × 450; right, × 750.

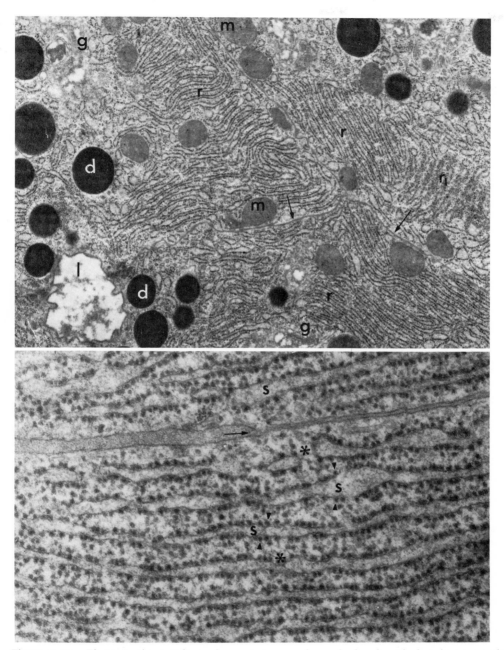

Figure 1–11.   Electron micrographs to demonstrate granular endoplasmic reticulum in pancreatic acinar cells. *Top:* Large collections of parallel cisternae of granular reticulum are seen (r), also sectioned *en face* at center right (r₁). Also seen are mitochondria (m), Golgi apparatus (g), secretory droplets (d), plasma membranes at cell interfaces (arrows), and the lumen (l) of an acinus. × 8,000. *Bottom:* Parts of two cells with a cell interface (arrow), parallel cisternae of granular reticulum with lumina or intracisternal spaces (s) containing some flocculent material and bounded by membranes studded with ribosomes (arrowheads) on their cytoplasmic surfaces. Note pores or fenestrae (asterisks), i.e., discontinuities in the cisternae. × 80,000.

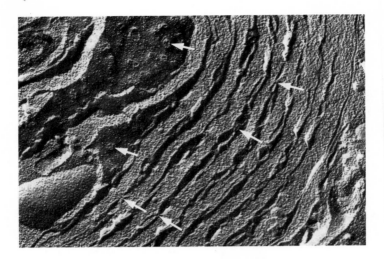

Figure 1–12. Freeze etch preparation of granular endoplasmic reticulum in transverse and longitudinal fracture planes in pancreatic acinar cell of the spiny mouse. Arrows point to fenestrae or pores. × 33,000. (Courtesy of Dr. L. Orci.)

lum totally absent. The amount is related to protein synthesis; for example, it is very extensive in pancreatic acinar cells that produce enzymes. This system of intracytoplasmic membranes may connect with the plasmalemma in a few cell types and with the nuclear envelope (discussed later), and in some cells it shows continuity also with the smooth or agranular endoplasmic reticulum. It communicates also with the Golgi apparatus by small vesicles.

When cells are disrupted or fragmented during homogenization and subjected to differential centrifugation, the endoplasmic reticulum is broken up and forms *microsomes,* small membrane-bound vesicles with their external surfaces studded with ribosomes and their lumina representing the intracisternal space and containing the secretory product of the reticulum.

As indicated already, the main function of the granular endoplasmic reticulum is synthesis of a secretory protein and its segregation from the remainder of the cytoplasm within the intracisternal space. In some cells, e.g., pancreatic acinar cells, concentration of the product also occurs within the reticulum, although concentration usually occurs mainly in the Golgi apparatus.

Ribosomes

As indicated above, ribosomes are responsible for cytoplasmic basophilia and contain RNA and protein. Ribosomes are sites where amino acids are incorporated into peptides and proteins, i.e., sites of protein synthesis. They are found in all cells except mature erythrocytes and may be attached to, and part of, the granular endoplasmic reticulum or lie free within the general cytoplasm. Ribosomes in both locations have a similar structure and appear on electron microscopy as small, dense particles of about 15 nm diameter, roughly spherical but irregular, and each is formed by two subunits, one large and one small. In man and all other mammals, the ribosome has a characteristic sedimentation coeffecient of 80S, with the larger, heavier subunit of 60S and the smaller subunit of 40S. Single ribosomes are seen lying free in the cytoplasm, but usually they occur in groups or rosettes, several ribosomes being strung on a fine thread of messenger RNA. Similarly, on the membranes of granular reticulum, they form spiral collections. Such groups of ribosomes connected by a strand of messenger RNA are called *polysomes* or *polyribosomes.* Polysomes vary in number of associated ribosomes and, in general, the larger the strand of messenger RNA, the greater the number of attached ribosomes and the longer the polypeptide chain that is produced.

Also, polysomes attached to endoplasmic reticulum are concerned with the production of proteins for secretion, the protein being passed into the intracis-

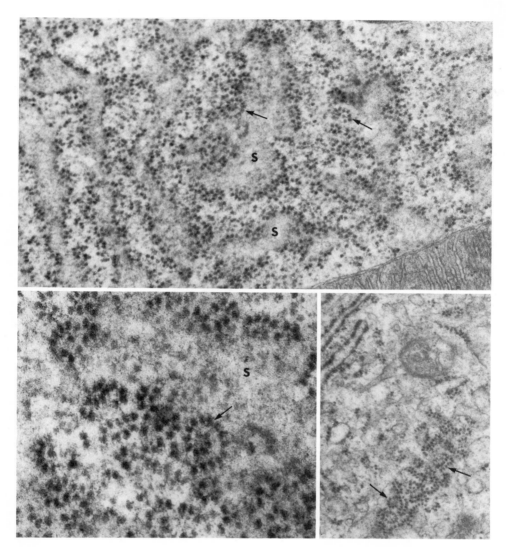

Figure 1–13. Electron micrographs to illustrate polysomes. *Top:* Cisternae of granular reticulum cut *en face* showing intracisternal spaces (s) with polysomes (arrows) associated with cisternal membranes. Pancreatic acinar cell, × 28,000. *Bottom left:* A higher magnification of the above, × 84,000. *Bottom right:* Intestinal epithelial cell, numerous polysomes (arrows), and two cisternae of granular reticulum (top left). × 22,000.

ternal space of the reticulum. Free cytoplasmic polysomes are involved in the main in the synthesis of proteins for intracellular use. They are numerous, for example, in rapidly growing and dividing cells, and may be in sufficient numbers in these cells to result in cytoplasmic basophilia.

The role of ribosomes and granular endoplasmic reticulum in protein synthesis is discussed in more detail at the end of this chapter (page 74).

Smooth-Surfaced (Agranular) Endoplasmic Reticulum

Smooth or agranular endoplasmic reticulum is composed of smooth-surfaced membranes unassociated with ribosomes and usually is tubular or vesicular in form rather than cisternal. The membranes are similar to those of granular reticulum, being 6 to 7 nm thick, with a tubular lumen of about 50 nm.

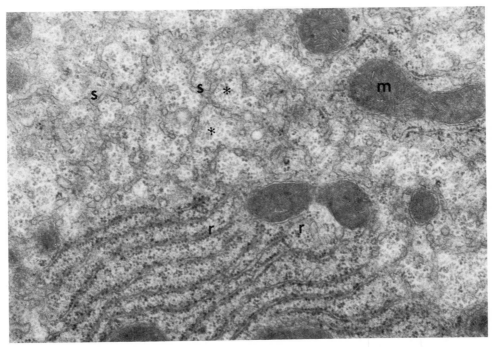

Figure 1–14. Electron micrograph of part of a parenchymal cell of the liver to show smooth or agranular endoplasmic reticulum (above, s) and granular reticulum (below, r). Also seen are mitochondria (m) and, associated with the smooth reticulum, glycogen particles (asterisks). × 22,000.

Tubular elements frequently show branching and may connect directly with the granular reticulum and indirectly with the Golgi apparatus via small vesicles. The amount of agranular reticulum varies with the cell type: it may be the most prominent organelle, e.g., in steroid-secreting cells, or may be represented by a few elements only. In different cell types it performs different functions. The smooth reticulum functions in the biosynthesis of steroid hormones and is found in abundance in, for example, Leydig cells of the testis that secrete testosterone, cells of the adrenal cortex that secrete corticosteroids, and progesterone-secreting cells of the corpus luteum of the ovary. In hepatic parenchymal cells, it is associated with glycogen breakdown to glucose and with lipid synthesis and is also concerned with the metabolism of several lipid-soluble drugs such as the barbiturates. In the columnar absorptive cells lining the intestine, it is associated with lipid absorption, resynthesizing triglycerides from monoglycerides and fatty acids that are absorbed into the cells,

and passing the triglycerides into intestinal lymphatic vessels. In striated and cardiac muscle, where it is termed *sarcoplasmic reticulum,* it actively regulates

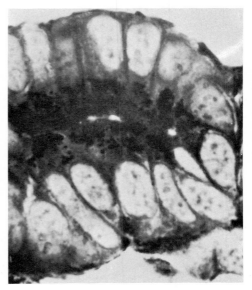

Figure 1–15. Pancreatic acinar cells stained to show the Golgi apparatus (black). Nuclei appear pale. Golgi silver stain. × 600.

the calcium level around the myofibrils (contractile elements).

The agranular reticulum must be distinguished from other smooth, membranous elements in the cytoplasm such as the Golgi apparatus and vesicles. The fact that it often is connected to cisternae of the rough endoplasmic reticulum suggests that it is derived from the rough reticulum.

Golgi Apparatus

Also termed the Golgi complex or region, this organelle may be visible by light microscopy as either a "positive" or "negative" image. After silver impregnation or prolonged exposure to osmium tetroxide, it is seen as a darkly staining network of canals or vacuoles or as an irregular granular mass located

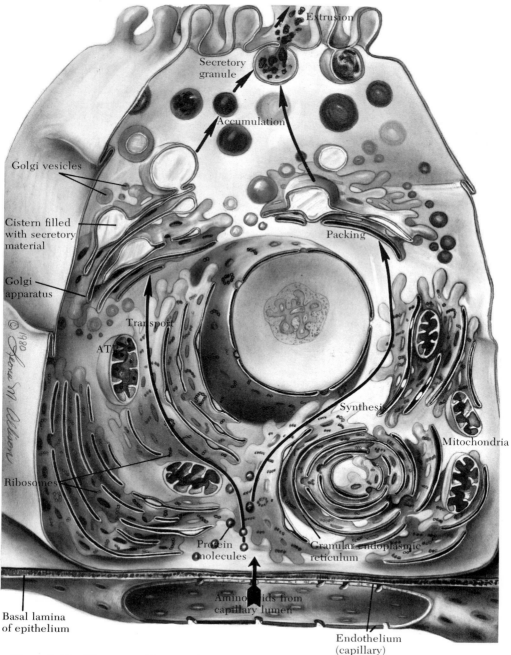

Figure 1–16. Diagram to illustrate the Golgi apparatus of a secretory cell and its participation in protein and glycoprotein secretion.

near the nucleus and sometimes multiple. Its appearance and location, however, do vary with cell type. In secretory cells, for example, it is supranuclear, but in nerve cells it usually forms a net around the entire nucleus. After routine H and E staining, in cells with intensely basophil cytoplasm such as osteoblasts and plasma cells the Golgi apparatus is indicated as a pale, clear area. This is a "negative" image; the "positive" image is seen after special techniques as indicated above.

With the electron microscope, three membranous components are seen in the Golgi complex: cisternae (flattened plates) or saccules, small vesicles, and larger vacuoles, all lacking ribosomes; the whole is situated in an area of cytoplasm devoid of other cytoplasmic components. The cisternae are flattened, curved, smooth-surfaced membranes arranged in parallel in stacks of 3 to 12 with a regular spacing of 20 to 30 nm between adjacent cisternae. Peripherally, a cisterna often shows pores or fenestrae and tubular expansions. Each stack has the form of a shallow bowl with a convex forming (immature) face and a concave or mature (secreting) face. The cisternal membrane at the forming face is thinner (about 6 to 7 nm) and similar to that of endoplasmic reticulum, whereas that at the mature face is thicker (7.5 to 10 nm) and similar to the plasmalemma. The cisternal lumen is about 15 nm wide but dilatation occurs, particularly at the periphery or rim of the saccules. Electron-dense material may be present within cisternae. The term *dictyosome* describes such a stack of cisternae and this may be the entire Golgi apparatus in a cell, although more usually several dictyosomes are present.

Associated with the cisternae are vesicles and vacuoles. Vesicles are small spheres of about 40 nm diameter, most smooth-surfaced but some with a bristle-like coat of fine filaments radiating from the surface ("coated vesicles"). Vacuoles vary in diameter up to 0.5 micrometer and may contain secretory products of varying density. The larger ones have a dense, homogeneous content and are termed "condensing" or secretory vacuoles. The location of vesicles and vacuoles in relation to the cisternal stack often is asymmetrical.

The Golgi apparatus is not static but

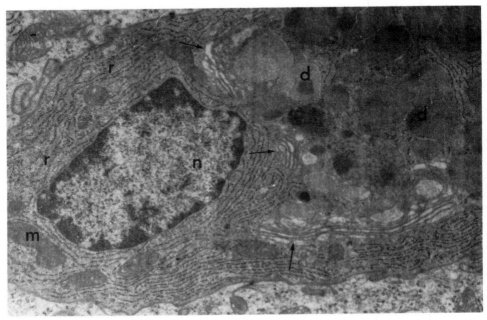

Figure 1–17.   Electron micrograph of a goblet (mucus-secreting) cell of the duodenum to show several dictyosomes (arrows) of an extensive Golgi apparatus. The base of the cell is to the left, with nucleus (n) and extensive granular endoplasmic reticulum (r) and mitochondria (m) in basal cytoplasm and apical cytoplasm (right) largely occupied by mucous secretory droplets (d). × 6,500. (See also Figure 1–11.)

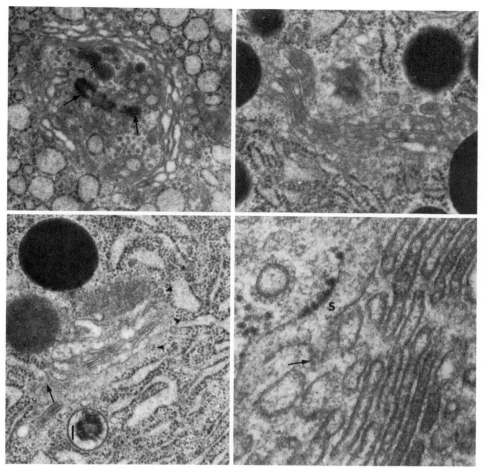

Figure 1–18. Electron micrographs of the Golgi apparatus. *Top left:* Intestinal epithelial cell with Golgi cisternae in a cup or bowl shape, forming face externally, mature face internally, with secretory droplets (asterisk) and centrioles (arrows) within the cup. × 16,000. *Top right:* Pancreatic acinar cell, forming face below, and cisternae containing secretory material with dense secretory droplets. × 24,000. *Lower left:* Pancreatic acinar cell, the dictyosome surrounded by granular endoplasmic reticulum with transfer vesicles (arrowheads) and one element of granular reticulum lacking ribosomes (arrow) where it was adjacent to the Golgi apparatus. A lysosome (l) also is seen. × 24,000. *Lower right:* Jejunal epithelial cell showing lack of ribosomes on an element of granular reticulum adjacent to the Golgi apparatus (s is the intracisternal space) and a transfer vesicle (arrow) budding from it to pass to the Golgi apparatus (right). × 66,000.

changes continually. Elements of granular reticulum adjacent to the Golgi apparatus lack ribosomes and from these elements small "transfer" vesicles "bud" off, enclosing some of the content of the reticulum, and pass toward and then fuse with a Golgi element, often a cisterna at the forming face, thus releasing the contents into the saccule. Also, secretory vacuoles are formed at the mature face and pass to the cell periphery. The Golgi apparatus, then, appears to accept vesicles from the endoplasmic reticulum, modify their contents and their enclosing membrane, and pass the

products in the form of secretory vesicles and lysosomes to other parts of the cell. This involves a movement or "flow" of membrane through the Golgi stack from forming to mature face, the membranes "maturing" from a type similar to endoplasmic reticulum to one similar to the plasmalemma. This process, as secretory vacuoles fuse with the plasmalemma and release their contents by exocytosis, would result in an increase in area of the plasmalemma; it is believed that to balance it some plasmalemma is internalized by endocytosis and then digested by lysosomal action. In contrast to this concept of "*membrane flow*" and to recognize the fact that there are differences between the membranes of the endoplasmic reticulum, Golgi apparatus, and plasmalemma, there is an alternative theory of "*membrane shuttle.*" This hypothesis postulates that the membrane types do not mix but that on the immature face, transfer vesicles release their content into the Golgi saccule and then shuttle back to the reticulum to repeat the process. On the mature face a similar shuttle mechanism transports secretory material to the surface via secretory vacuoles.

In some types of secretory cell, concentration of the secretory protein occurs by removal of water, and although this process starts in the Golgi apparatus, it usually continues after formation of the secretory granule or droplet, which becomes increasingly dense as it matures. In cells in which the secretory product is glycoprotein, some sugars are added to the polypeptide in the endoplasmic reticulum, but synthesis is completed in the Golgi apparatus by the addition of other sugar residues. The Golgi apparatus is involved too in the synthesis of sulfated mucopolysaccharides, e.g., in goblet cells of the intestinal mucosa. In β cells of the pancreas, proinsulin synthesized in the endoplasmic reticulum is cleaved into insulin (the active product) and C-peptide within the Golgi apparatus. The Golgi apparatus is responsible for the packaging of hydrolytic enzymes into lysosomes, at least in some cells, in a process similar to the formation of secretory vacuoles. In some cells, it may be that a type of smooth reticulum situated near the forming face of the Golgi apparatus is involved in the formation of lysosomes (and possibly also secretory vacuoles), without the involvement of the Golgi apparatus. This reticulum, because of its location, nature, and assumed function is called GERL (Golgi, Endoplasmic Reticulum, and Lysosome).

Thus, the Golgi apparatus is involved in membrane flow, in transport and concentration of secretory materials and their release from the cell, in synthesis of certain secretory products, particularly glycoproteins and mucopolysaccharides, and probably in lysosome formation.

Lysosomes

Lysosomes are small membrane-bound bodies that contain a variety of acid hydrolases. They constitute an intracellular digestive system capable of breaking down material originating both outside and within the cell. Owing to their involvement in digestion, their appearance depends upon their functional state, and this results in a great variety of appearances, or pleomorphism. Although variable in size, they usually range from 0.2 to 0.4 μm in diameter. Lysosomes are found in all cells except erythrocytes but are numerous particularly in macrophages, neutrophil leukocytes, hepatic cells, and cells of the proximal tubule of the kidney. They can be identified by electron cytochemistry using a modified Gomori technique for acid phosphatase but, in addition to phosphatases, they contain also proteases, nucleases, lipases, glycosidases, phospholipases, and sulfatases.

Lysosomes can be divided into two main groups, called *primary* and *secondary.* A primary lysosome is one that is "resting" and has yet to function in enzymatic activity, and as indicated above, probably arises in the Golgi complex. A secondary lysosome is engaged actively in digestion and occurs after fusion of a primary lysosome with some other membrane-bound body arising from within or outside the cell. Substances of extracellular origin that enter the cell by endocytosis do so as membrane-bound bodies. The cytoplasmic vacuole so formed by engulfing extracellular material may contain fluid with material in solution or suspension; this process is termed *pinoctyosis.* If a relatively large, solid material such as a microorganism is included in the vacuole, the process is called *phagocytosis.* The vacuole so formed by internalization of material from the exterior is referred to as a *phagosome* or *heterophagosome.* A similar process that involves segregation of a cell's own components, such as mitochondria, granules, or even small areas of cytoplasm, by enclosing them in a membrane (probably derived from endoplasmic reticulum or the Golgi apparatus) to form a vacuole is termed *autophagy,* and the resulting vacuole is an *autosome* or *autophagosome.* Fu-

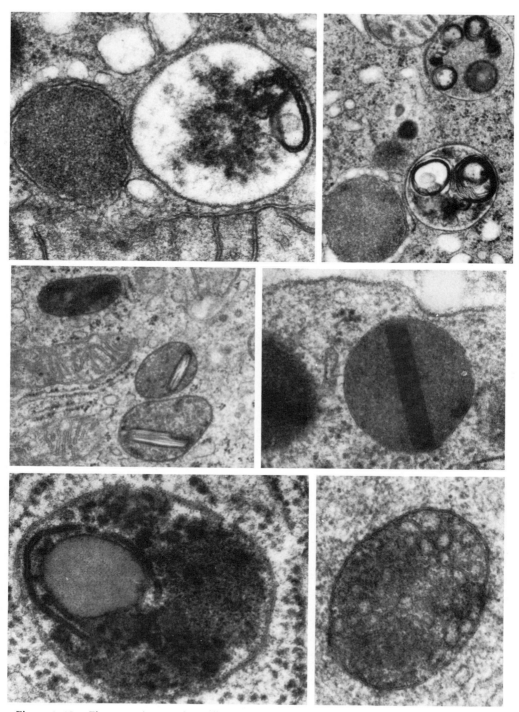

Figure 1–19. Electron micrographs to illustrate primary lysosomes (*top left and right*), secondary lysosomes (*center left and bottom left*), a lysosome ("specific granule") of an eosinophil leukocyte (*center right*), and a multivesicular body (*bottom right*). Top left, kidney tubule cell, × 65,000. Top right, kidney tubule cell, × 31,000. Center left, duodenal epithelial cell, × 21,000. Center right, eosinophil leukocyte, × 28,000. Lower left, pancreatic acinar cell, × 68,000. Lower right, duodenal epithelial cell, × 68,000.

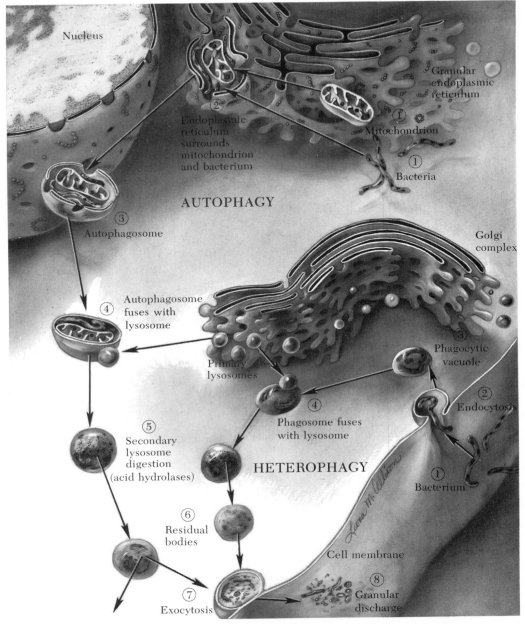

Figure 1–20. Diagram illustrating probable lysosomal pathways in the cell.

sion of a phagosome or autosome with a primary lysosome containing hydrolytic enzymes produces a secondary lysosome. Active enzymatic digestion within the secondary lysosome breaks down the contents into small molecules that pass back across the lysosomal membrane into the cytoplasm. Some material may be indigestible and the secondary lysosome, now inactive, then is termed a *residual body*. Morphologically, residual bodies are identified by a content of whorls of membranous material, and they tend to accumulate lipid, which may later become oxidized to a pigmented material called lipofuscin. This pigment accumulates with age and is found in nerve cells and cardiac muscle particularly.

Morphologically, lysosomes present a variety of appearances, as indicated above. All, of course, are membrane-bound. The primary lysosome has generally a finely granular or nearly homogeneous content and usually is spherical and 25 to 50 nm in diameter, with a limiting membrane of 6 to 7 nm thickness. Some are ellipsoidal in shape, for example, in neutrophil leukocytes, and they occasionally contain more dense material in irregular crystalline arrays. Secondary lysosomes vary in size up to 0.4 μm or more in diameter and the contents are pleomorphic.

Lysosomal enzymes may be released by exocytosis into the extracellular space, for example, in osteoclasts, cells found in bone and involved in bone resorption. In some secretory cells when secretion is diminished or ceases, newly formed secretory granules may be passed directly into the lysosomal pathway to prevent over-accumulation of secretory material, this process being termed *crinophagy*. It occurs, for example, in the mammary gland and some endocrine cells. One interesting and incompletely understood phenomenon is the integrity of the lysosomal membrane that obviously resists the degradative action of its own enzymes. This may be due, in part at least, to a protecting coating on the inner membrane surface of highly charged glycoproteins.

Lysosomes thus play an essential role in cellular defense mechanisms, being the site for destruction of foreign bodies such as bacteria and fungi, and they also function in the normal replacement of cellular components and organelles. In cells which are damaged, the membranes bounding lysosomes may rupture or become permeable, thus exposing the general cytoplasm to the action of hydrolytic enzymes, resulting in lysis of the cell and cell death. Such a process occurs in neutrophil leukocytes during infections, when the cells are killed during phagocytosis of bacteria, and a similar process probably occurs during growth and remodeling of tissues.

Mitochondria

Mitochondria are present in all animal cells, are membrane-bound organelles, and lie free within the cytoplasm. They are of great importance in energy metabolism as the major source of adenosine triphosphate (ATP) and are the site of many metabolic reactions. While not visible in routine H and E preparations, they can be demonstrated by iron hematoxylin and after supravital staining with dyes such as Janus green B by which they convert the colorless, reduced form of the dye to a colored

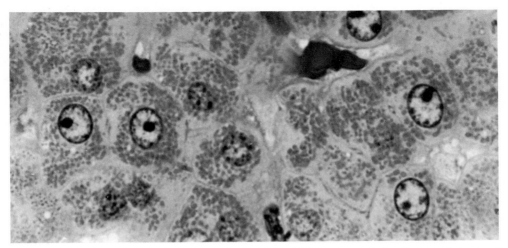

Figure 1–21. Photomicrograph to show mitochondria which appear as dark spheres and short rods within the cytoplasm of rat liver cells. × 1100.

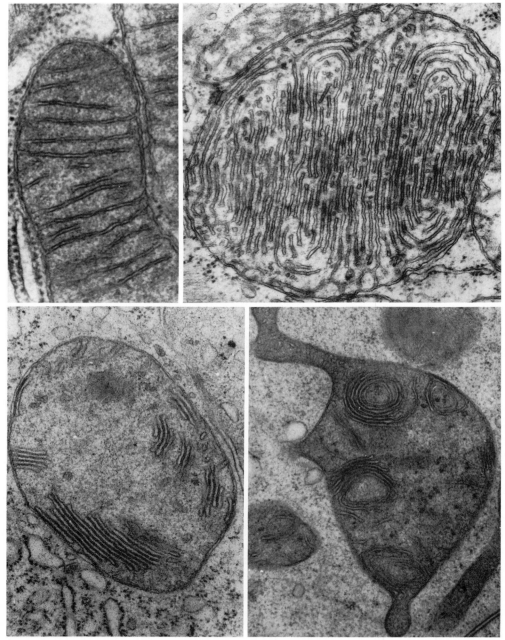

Figure 1–22.   Electron micrographs of mitochondria showing different morphological types. *Top left: From pancreatic acinar cell. Top right:* From cardiac muscle. *Bottom left and right:* From interstitial cells of the human testis. All × 40,000.

oxidized state. By phase contrast microscopy of living cells, they appear as spheres, rods, ovoids, or threadlike bodies that move, change shape and size, divide, and fuse. They vary greatly in size and shape from 0.1 to 0.5 μm wide with lengths up to 10 μm, but usually they are of similar size and shape in any single cell type. They vary in number with cell activity, with few, for example, in lymphocytes, but large numbers in cells of high metabolic activity, e.g., parietal (acid-secreting) cells of the stomach, kidney tubule cells, and adrenal cortex. In hepatic parenchymal cells there may be more than 1000 in each cell.

By electron microscopy, they show a basic form. All are bounded by two smooth-surfaced membranes of 6 nm thickness, each showing the trilaminar unit membrane structure, with an electron-lucent space of 8 nm between the membranes. The inner membrane "inflects" or infolds to form *cristae mitochondriales,* which vary from transverse membranous plates to tubular or vesicular forms. Thus, two compartments are defined: the outer between the two membranes and the inner or *matrix* within the inner membrane. The matrix appears finely granular and contains a high concentration of proteins, includ-

ing enzymes, with a few electron-opaque intramitochondrial dense granules (30 to 40 nm diameter) consisting of divalent cations, some ribosomes (25 nm diameter), and fine strands of DNA, here lying as circular threads. Attached to the inner (matrix) surface of the inner membrane are closely packed particles of 8.5 nm diameter ("elementary" particles) that appear club-shaped, with a short stem of 5 nm length and 3 nm width attaching them to the cristal membrane. These contain an enzyme, the F1 coupling factor (ATPase), and are visible only after treatment by special techniques.

The outer bounding mitochondrial membrane is permeable to water and ions, the inner membrane (bounding

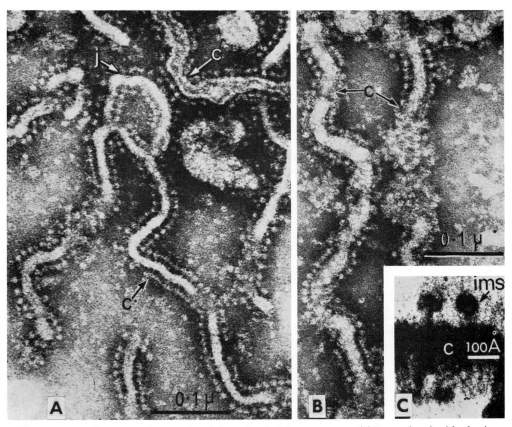

Figure 1–23. Electron micrograph of the subunit (elementary particle) associated with the inner mitochondrial membranes or cristae of mouse liver: *A,* A few cristae (c) consisting of long filaments which sometimes branch (j). The surfaces of the cristae are covered with projecting subunits. × 192,000. *B,* Similar cristae with subunits. × 192,000. *C,* Higher magnification showing a few subunits (ims) with spherical heads having a diameter of approximately 90 Å and stems 30 to 35 Å wide and 45 to 50 Å long. The center to center spacing is 100 Å. Reversed print, × 770,000. (Preparation courtesy of Dr. D. F. Parsons and reproduced by permission from Science, *140*:985, 1963.)

the matrix) is not, so that transport across this membrane requires active carrier mechanisms.

Mitochondria show a change in conformation, the appearance as described above being the *orthodox* form. This is typical of mitochondria when inactive in oxidative phosphorylation with a low level of ADP and when the outer compartment comprises a small fraction of the volume. In the *condensed* form, water moves from the inner to the outer compartment, with increase in volume of the outer compartment and reduction in volume of the matrix.

Within cells, mitochondria vary in location with functional requirements. For example, in muscle cells they lie adjacent to contractile elements; in protein-secreting cells they are found near the ribosomes and granular reticulum; and in kidney tubule cells they lie basally in the cytoplasm to provide energy for active transport mechanisms.

The functions of mitochondria are localized precisely within the organelle, although most of the activity occurs in the inner compartment via enzymes located either in the matrix (citric acid cycle) or on the inner mitochondrial membrane (electron transport and oxidative phosphorylation). As indicated, mitochondria are the major energy source of cells. Additionally, they concentrate calcium and maintain a general calcium environment within the cytoplasm.

Peroxisomes

Peroxisomes or microbodies are similar to lysosomes in structure but do not contain lysosomal hydrolases. They are membrane-bound bodies, 0.3 to 1.5 μm in diameter, usually with a finely granular homogeneous content but sometimes containing a crystalline body or nucleoid. They are numerous in hepatic parenchymal cells and proximal convoluted tubule cells of the kidney, but are widely distributed in other cell types.

Peroxisomes are formed in the granular endoplasmic reticulum and contain several enzymes involved in the production (urate oxidase and other oxidases) or destruction (catalase) of hydrogen peroxide. The function of these bodies remains obscure. However, hydrogen peroxide is highly toxic to cells and, presumably, it is advantageous to limit reactions that would produce it to an organelle where it can be broken down as soon as it is formed.

Microtubules

Microtubules are slender, hollow, cylindrical, unbranched structures of 25 nm diameter and indeterminate length. They run a straight course in the cytoplasm, and this implies that they have some degree of stiffness. They show a central, electron-lucent core with a wall formed by 13 globular subunits, 5 nm in diameter, composed of the protein tubulin. The subunits are arranged linearly to form protofilaments that spiral along the wall of the microtubule in a left-handed helix. In a very few specific locations, microtubules may be of smaller overall diameter, with only 12 protofilaments in the wall, or larger, with 15 protofilaments. Microtubules are present in nearly all cells and often occur as single elements randomly scattered in the cytoplasm, in groups in parallel array, or partially fused in two's and three's to form doublets and triplets. The adjacent microtubules at the areas of fusion in doublets and triplets share three or four subunits. This is discussed later in reference to centrioles and cilia.

Microtubules probably have several functions. Their relation to cilia (motile cell processes) as both structural and force-generating elements and to centrioles and the process of mitosis is discussed below. Here they have specific arrangements and are relatively static. In most other locations, microtubules are believed to have a cytoskeletal function in the sense of development of cell shape. They are, for example, numerous in nerve cell processes (where the microtubules are called neurotubules) and here they may also function in intracellular transport mechanisms. Microtubules as skeletal elements are particularly prominent as bundles at the cell periphery in blood platelets, for example, where they maintain the dis-

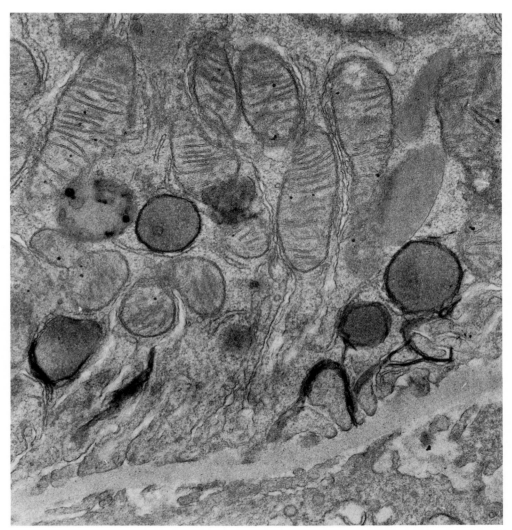

Figure 1–24. Electron micrograph of the basal region of a kidney tubule cell showing mitochondria with transverse cristae, several microbodies (peroxisomes), and a lysosome. This is a special preparation in which the benzidine reaction product is localized at the periphery of the peroxisomes. The lysosome (left edge) shows a few dense granules. × 22,000. (Preparation courtesy of Drs. S. Goldfischer and E. Essner.)

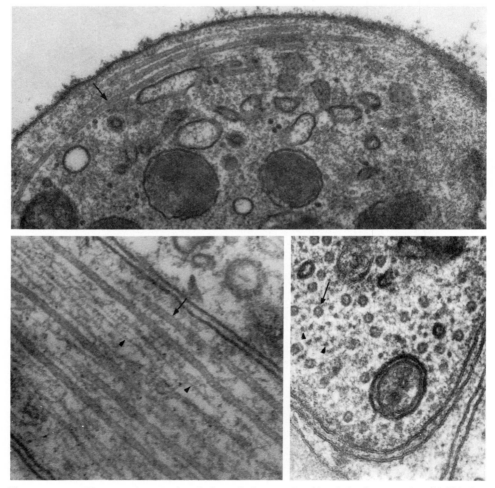

Figure 1–25. Electron micrographs of microtubules. *Top:* In a blood platelet (arrow). × 76,000. *Bottom:* In a nerve axon, in longitudinal (*left*) and transverse (*right*) sections. Here microtubules (neurotubules) are found with microfilaments (neurofilaments, arrowheads). Left, × 76,000; right, × 88,000.

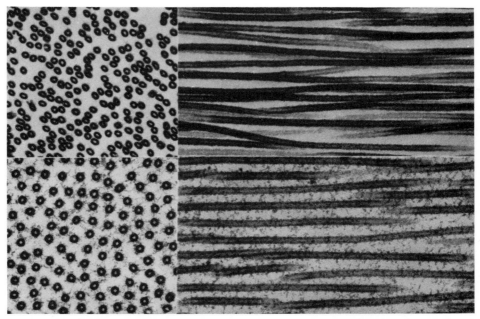

Figure 1–26. Transverse and longitudinal sections of *in vitro*–assembled flagellar microtubules; *above,* in the absence of brain MAPs (microtubule associated protein) and, *below,* in the presence of brain MAPs. × 75,000. (Courtesy of Dr. Joel L. Rosenbaum and reproduced by permission of the Editor, The Journal of Cell Biology.)

coid shape. The relation of microtubules to cell movement is less well established. In all probability, they do not generate motile forces but interact with other cellular components, such as filaments, to determine a direction of cytoplasmic movement. For example, cells in tissue culture exhibit motility that after the addition of colchicine (which destroys microtubules) is changed in character but not stopped. Additionally, movements within the cytoplasm of organelles such as lysosomes and of inclusions, e.g., pigment granules, tend to be oriented parallel to bundles of microtubules (long saltatory movement), and these can be abolished by treatment with colchicine.

It should be emphasized that the cytoplasmic microtubules that participate in cell motility or in the development of cell shape are plastic in the sense that they can be formed and can increase in length, or, alternatively, can be dispersed. The formed or polymerized microtubule is, then, in equilibrium with a pool of unpolymerized tubulin lying in the cytoplasm. Colchicine interferes with this equilibrium by binding to free tubulin subunits and, by changing that equilibrium, causes breakdown of microtubules.

Centrioles

Centrioles appear by light microscopy as short rods or granules located near the nucleus, and in most interphase or nondividing cells there are two, called a *diplosome.* Often the pair lies adjacent to the Golgi apparatus in a specialized area of cytoplasm called the *centrosome* or cell center. By electron microscopy, each centriole appears as a short cylinder 0.3 to 0.5 μm long and about 0.15 μm in diameter, with one "end" open and the other closed by dense material. When seen in transverse section, the wall of the cylinder is composed of nine triplets, i.e., sets of three fused microtubules. The triplets are arranged somewhat tangential to the circumference of the centriole at an angle of about 30 degrees, and in each triplet the microtubules are called subfibers A, B, and C,

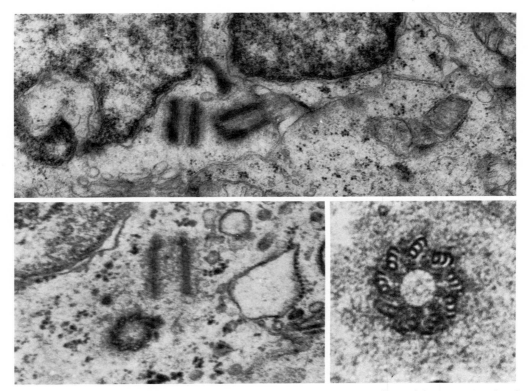

Figure 1–27. Electron micrographs to demonstrate the appearance of centrioles. *Top:* A pair of centrioles near the nucleus (top left) of a supporting (Sertoli) cell of the testis. Both are cut longitudinally, but oriented approximately at right angles to each other. × 35,000. *Bottom left:* A similar pair, but one centriole is cut in cross section and shows nine subunits in its wall. × 42,000. *Bottom right:* A centriole in cross section to show that each of the nine subunits is composed of triple microtubular elements. × 110,000.

with A being the most central or innermost. In the diplosome, the two centrioles usually lie at right angles to each other, and attached more or less directly to them are microtubules that radiate from them and from associated clumps of dense material called pericentriolar satellites.

Centrioles are microtubule-organizing centers and are important in mitosis. They are self-replicating and double in number immediately before cell division, the two separating and a new centriole developing in relation to each pre-existing centriole from a ring-like condensation of granular material called a *procentriole*. Later, microtubules develop in the procentriole to form a daughter centriole. Centrioles also may replicate, pass to the cell surface, and form basal bodies (kinetosomes) from which cilia develop. Flagella arise in a similar fashion. Little is known as yet

about the way in which centrioles and kinetosomes cause the formation of microtubules.

Cilia and Flagella

Cilia and flagella are motile processes protruding from cell surfaces. Cilia are eyelash or hairlike processes and are very numerous in epithelial cells of the upper respiratory tract, parts of the male and female reproductive tracts, and the ependyma lining the cavities of the central nervous system. There may be 250 or more cilia on the surface of a ciliated cell, arranged in regular rows. A single cilium is found in many cell types. All cilia are about 0.2 μm in diameter and vary in length from about 5 to 10 μm. A flagellum is a whiplike process similar in structure to a cilium but considerably longer, being up to 15 to 30

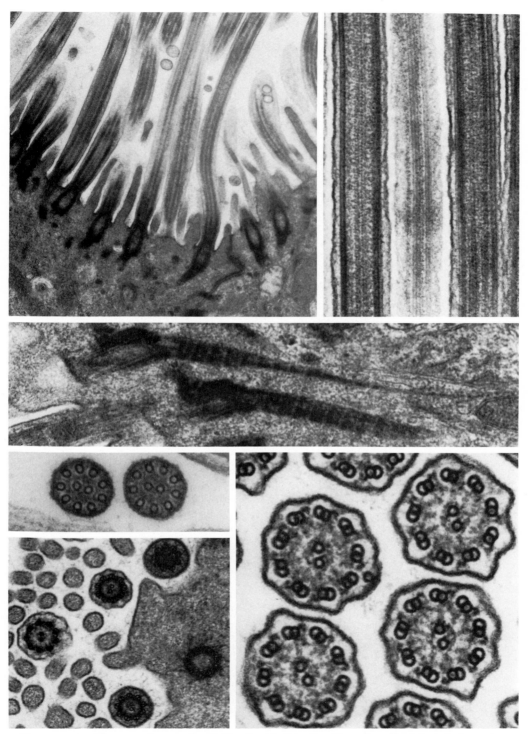

Figure 1–28. Electron micrographs of cilia of epithelial cells of bronchus. *Top left:* Apical cytoplasm with cilia and microvilli in longitudinal section. × 19,500. *Top right:* Cilia in longitudinal section showing peripheral and central microtubules. × 60,000. *Center:* Two cilia at their bases showing striated rootlets in apical cytoplasm. × 60,000. *Left insert:* Two cilia in transverse section at their tips showing nine peripheral singlets and two central microtubules. × 88,000. *Lower left:* Cilia in transverse section at their bases. Note the lack of central tubules, and peripheral triplets in the profile within apical cytoplasm. × 42,000. *Lower right:* Cilial shafts in transverse section. × 88,000.

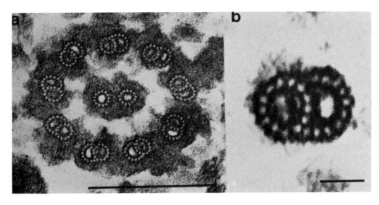

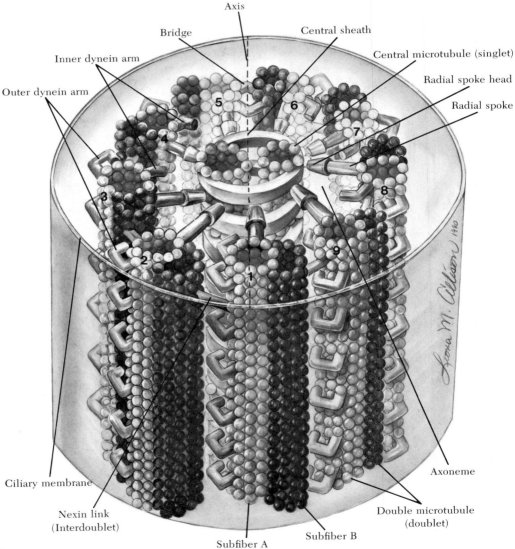

Figure 1–29. *Top:* Electron micrograph of the axoneme (*a*) of a cilium showing nine outer doublets and two central singlet microtubules and (*b*) one outer doublet demonstrating the A subfiber with 13 protofilaments and the B subfiber (C-shaped) with 11 protofilaments in its wall. a, × 165,000; b, × 360,000. (Courtesy of Dr. Joel L. Rosenbaum and reproduced by permission of the Editor, The Journal of Cell Biology.) *Bottom:* Three-dimensional diagram of a cilium showing relationships of the major components.

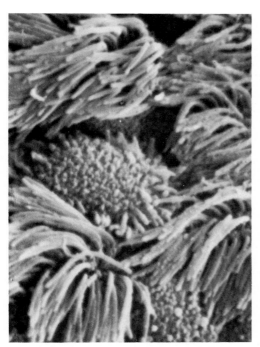

Figure 1–30. Scanning electron micrograph of cilia of tracheal epithelium. × 6000. (Courtesy of Dr. W. Krause.)

μm in length, and usually there are only one or two associated with each cell.

Each cilium is covered by an extension of the plasmalemma and consists of a long cylindrical shaft, a tapering tip, and a basal body or *kineotosome* located in apical cytoplasm. By light microscopy, the basal body is visible as a dense granule at the base of the cilium. In the shaft and visible only by electron microscopy is a characteristic arrangement of microtubules called the *axoneme* consisting of nine peripheral doublets (pairs) and two central singlets or single microtubules. In each of the peripheral doublets, one microtubule (subfiber A) is complete with 13 protofilaments in its wall and the outer (subfiber B) is incomplete with 11 protofilaments and fused to subfiber A, thus closing the "defect" in its wall. From each subfiber A, extending toward the subfiber B of the adjacent doublet, are pairs of armlike processes regularly arranged along the length of the A subfiber. These are formed by the protein dynein, a high molecular weight ATPase. Also present are "links" attaching each A subfiber to the B subfiber of the adjacent doublet similarly arranged at periodic intervals along the length of the subfiber (and believed to be composed of an elastic material called nexin) and a complex arrangement of radial spokes extending to the peripheral doublets from the central sheath that lies around the central pair of microtubules. At the base of a cilium, the central pair of single microtubules terminates and each of the peripheral doublets is continuous with a triplet of the kinetosome, a subfiber C being "added" to the doublet. With nine peripheral triplets, the kinetosome resembles a centriole and, as in a centriole, the triplets lie tangential to the surface. In many cases, strands of fibrous material extend from the basal body into apical cytoplasm (the "striated rootlets") and other fibrous material may extend to the adjacent plasmalemma. These structures are presumed to anchor the cilium firmly in apical cytoplasm.

In living cells, cilia beat in a rhythmical, wavelike manner, moving materials such as mucus over the cell surface. Analysis of the movement shows a stiffening of cilia on the rapid effective stroke and a slower recovery stroke with the cilia more flexible. In transverse section, the axoneme has a bilateral symmetry formed by the central pair of microtubules, with the peripheral doublet lying at right angles to the axis between the central pair designated 1 and doublets 5 and 6 opposite. A cilium bends along the axis by a type of sliding filament mechanism between microtubules similar to that seen between myofilaments in striated muscle fibers; the dynein arms extending between the A subfiber of one doublet and the B subfiber of an adjacent doublet undergo a cyclic break and reattachment cycle, with the effect that doublets slide past each other and cause bending of the cilium. This process requires ATP and calcium ions. Relaxation is believed to be passive and perhaps due to elasticity of the nexin links and the enveloping plasmalemma.

Flagella structurally are similar to cilia but are longer, show a somewhat different, undulating wave type of movement, and are much fewer per cell. The motile tail of a spermatozoon is a flagellum and may be 70 μm or more in length. They are found elsewhere in some epithelia, e.g., of the kidney and rete testis, where their function is uncertain. Single cilial projections are also found associated with some sensory epithelial cells, e.g., the rods and cones of the retina and hair cells of the inner ear. Usually, they are nonmotile and lack the central pair of single microtubules.

Microfilaments and Filamentous Material

The terminology concerning filamentous material is confusing. It is necessary to distinguish between fibrils that are within the cytoplasm (intracellular) and those lying outside and between cells (extracellular), the latter being discussed as part of connective tissue. Also, different terms are used for different sizes. Generally, *filaments* or *microfilaments* are about 4 to 15 nm in diameter and can be seen only with the electron microscope; a *fibril* is composed of a bundle of filaments, is about 0.2 to 1 μm diameter, and is seen by oil immersion light microscopy; and a *fiber* is formed of bundles of fibrils and is visible with low power microscopy or even the naked eye. The term *fiber* also is used to describe an elongated cell (e.g., muscle) or part of a cell (e.g., nerve).

Microfilaments are found in nearly all nonmuscle cell types, often closely related to microtubules. In muscle cells, two main types of filament are present, the thin filament about 6 to 7 nm in diameter and containing actin, and the thick filament about 15 nm in diameter, containing myosin. These are contractile proteins. A third group of filaments is about 10 nm in diameter and is termed "intermediate." This type of filament is present also in muscle cells, where it apparently forms a type of cytoskeleton or framework and appears to contain the protein desmin (the name desmin indicating a linking or bonding function). In nonmuscle cells, the basis of movement in many cellular processes (e.g., locomotion, cell division, pinocytosis, phagocytosis) appears to be contractile mechanisms, and it recently has become clear that the filamentous material involved in these processes is the same as that present in muscle cells. In the cores of microvilli of the brush border of epithelial cells of the intestine, there are bundles of 5- to 7-nm filaments that contain actin. These filaments are attached at the apex and pass from the base of the microvillus into apical cytoplasm to blend with the filamentous components of the "terminal web" (see page 96), a web that probably also contains thick myosin filaments and 10 nm intermediate filaments, the latter passing into the web from junctional complexes at lateral cell interfaces. Contraction of this filamentous network probably results in bending and shortening of microvilli. In addition, in many cells near the cell surface, i.e., in ectoplasm, there is a network of 5- to 7-nm filaments that function in local movements of the surface membrane. Such movements, e.g., in phagocytosis, are inhibited by cytochalasin B, a metabolite that interferes directly with actin-containing microfilaments.

Intermediate or 10-nm filaments are widely distributed in nonmuscle cells and often are a prominent feature. For example, in squamous and other epithelial cells they are called *tonofilaments,* are found as large bundles or tonofibrils inserting into desmosomes, and are chemically similar to the desmin-containing intermediate filaments of muscle. In nerve cells and their processes, 10-nm filaments are numerous and in these cells are called *neurofilaments.* Neurofilaments, however, are different chemically from tonofilaments and their function is unknown. Indeed, the term "intermediate filament" probably includes filaments of several different chemical compositions.

In summary, microfilaments of basically three sizes are widely distributed in nonmuscle as well as muscle cells; they are concerned with movements in cellular processes and probably also perform a cytoskeletal function.

Annulate Lamellae

This organelle is visible only with the electron microscope, the lamellae being flat, membranous, parallel cisternae with numerous pores or annuli. The organelle apparently is related to rough endoplasmic reticulum and the nuclear envelope and, indeed, in structure it closely resembles the latter. The membranes of the lamellae are 7 to 9 nm thick, enclose a space 30 to 50 nm wide, and have pores 40 to 50 nm in diameter. Generally the pores are spaced regularly at intervals of 100 to 200 nm. The pores appear to be closed by a single dense membrane and, like those of the nuclear envelope (see page 59), they have eight globular subunits around their peripheries with a small central granule in the membrane closing the pore. Lamellae occur singly and in parallel stacks in the cytoplasm and in a few cells are present within the nucleus. They are found in rapidly growing cells such as germ cells, embryonic and tumor cells, and in other cell types where they may be transitory during the life cycle. They are thought to be derived from the nuclear envelope and, while their significance is uncertain, they may convey material from the nucleus to the cytoplasm, functioning in nucleocytoplasmic interactions. They often show direct connections to the endoplasmic reticulum.

Cytoplasmic Vitality

Very few, if any, cell types are static. Structurally and functionally they constantly undergo changes. The probable

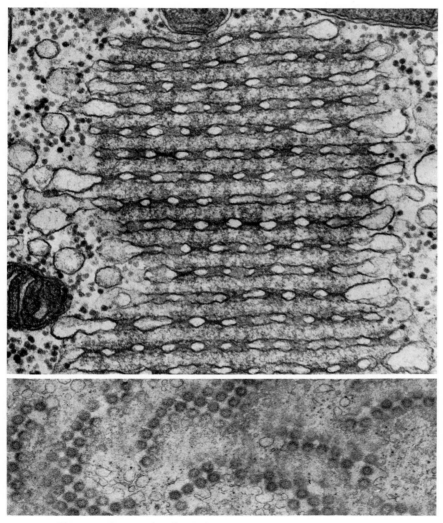

Figure 1–31.   Electron micrographs of annulate lamellae from a frog oocyte, sectioned in different planes. Top, × 50,000; bottom, 25,500. (Courtesy of Dr. R. G. Kessel.)

constant breakdown and re-formation of microtubules is one example of this. By way of a further example and to emphasize the dynamic aspect of cells, the exchanges which occur between cytomembranes and their turnover is very interesting. For example, while the rat parenchymal liver cell probably lives for a period of six months, the life-span of its cytomembranes is in the order of days. Membrane constantly is re-formed within a cell, and formed membranes can and do move from one site to another. Examples of such transfers have been indicated in the previous descriptions of cell organelles. They include the transfer of nuclear envelope in annulate lamellae formation, movement of endoplasmic reticulum membrane as transfer vesicles, membrane movement from the Golgi apparatus to the plasmalemma and to lysosomes, endocytotic vesicle and vacuole formation from the plasmalemma, and the formation of multivesicular bodies and phagosomes. However, it must be remembered also that the cytomembranes vary in structure and function and perhaps particularly in associated enzymes. So membrane transfer implies a change in structure and function. Study of tissue sections and electron micrographs tends to give the false impression that cells and their components are static. The student can dispel this impression only by attempting constantly to correlate structure and function.

Inclusions

While inclusions previously were considered nonliving accumulations of metabolites, cell products resulting from synthesis, or materials from outside taken into (i.e., included in) the cell, many of them in fact are now known to participate in the normal functioning of the cell. The term inclusion covers materials such as stored foods, pigments, and some crystalline materials. Bodies such as secretory granules or droplets were formerly considered inclusions, but these are membrane-bound packets of enzymes and have been discussed in relation to granular endoplasmic reticulum and the Golgi apparatus.

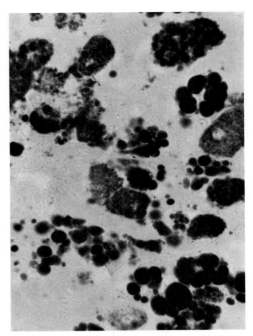

Figure 1–32. Photomicrograph of lipid inclusions in liver cells, showing a marked difference in the content of lipid material from cell to cell. Osmic acid. × 450.

Stored Foods

Fat. Although fat is stored mainly in connective tissue cells which, if present in large numbers, together form adipose tissue, it is present in many other cell types, e.g., liver and muscle cells and cells of the adrenal cortex. Fat is segregated in the cytoplasm as membrane-bound vacuoles and droplets containing neutral fats (triglycerides), fatty acids, cholesterol, and cholesterol esters. In usual preparations, fat is dissolved, leaving clear, spherical, smooth deficiencies; however, it can be preserved, e.g., by osmium tetroxide fixation, when it appears as dark brown or black droplets. It can be stained in frozen sections by Sudan black or Scharlach red. Fat droplets appear to rise in the Golgi apparatus or in relation to agranular endoplasmic reticulum and are bounded by a membrane 60 to 70 Å (6 to 7 nm) thick.

Carbohydrate. Carbohydrate as a food material is absorbed from the intestine mainly as glucose, which is then polymerized to glycogen for storage, particularly in the liver. Glycogen is water-soluble and in ordinary preparations is removed, leaving a characteristic appearance of irregular, ragged spaces between strands of cytoplasm and thus giving a "moth-eaten" appearance to the cytoplasm. In special preparations, glycogen can be stained by the periodic acid–Schiff reagent, which imparts a brilliant red color to the glycogen. On electron microscopy, glycogen appears as free cytoplasmic particles, often lying between tubular profiles of the agranular endoplasmic reticulum. Commonly, two types of glycogen particle are seen. The beta particle is an irregular, spherical body about 300 Å (30 nm) in diameter. The alpha particle is about 900 to 950 Å (90 to 95 nm) in diameter and is a complex of several smaller particles, which are clumped together in rosettes.

Pigments. Pigments are materials with natural color; i.e., they do not require staining by dyes as do other cell components. Pigments are classified into two types: *exogenous* pigments are formed outside the body and later taken into it, and *endogenous* pigments are formed within the body. Exogenous pigments include carotenes, yellowish-red pigments of vegetables which are fat-soluble (lipochromes); dusts, e.g., carbon, which is particularly prominent in cells in the lung; and minerals, such as lead and silver. Also grouped as exogenous pigments are those used in tattooing, a process whereby pigments are introduced into the deeper layers of the skin.

Endogenous pigments are mainly of two types: (1) melanin and (2) hemoglobin and its breakdown products, such as hemosiderin, which contains iron, and bilirubin (hematoidin) which does not. Both are yellowish-brown in color. Melanin, the dark brown or black pigment found in the skin and the eye, is the pigment of sun tan and is found in large amounts in the epidermis of the Negroid races. Lipofuscin occurs in many cells as yellowish-brown granules, particularly in older individuals, and is contained within residual bodies. It has been described previously in the section on lysosomes.

Crystals. Crystals and crystalloids, probably proteinaceous, occur in a few cell types, e.g., Sertoli (sustentacular) and interstitial cells of the testis, where the materials occur free in the cytoplasm, not bounded by a membrane. Crystalloids occur in other situations, e.g., the granules of eosinophilic leukocytes, which are to be classified as lyso-

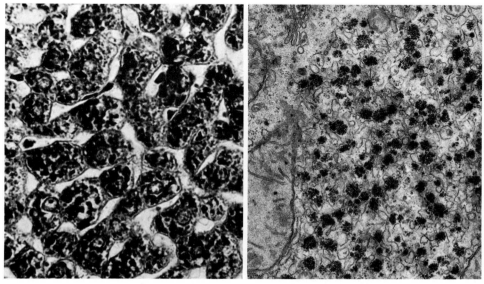

Figure 1–33. *Left:* Photomicrograph of a section of the liver to show glycogen. Best's carmine, × 350. *Right:* Electron micrograph of particulate glycogen in a liver cell. × 24,000. (Courtesy of J. Steiner.)

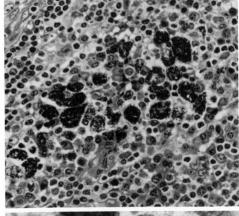

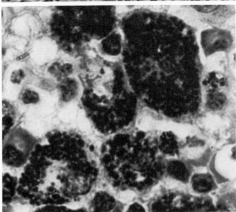

Figure 1–34. Photomicrograph of carbon, an exogenous pigment, in a lymph node from the lung. Top, × 300; bottom, × 1250.

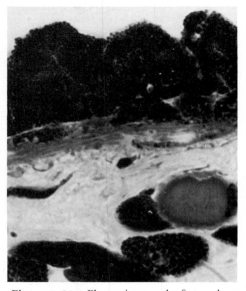

Figure 1–35. Photomicrograph of an endogenous pigment, melanin, in the iris. Melanin granules are present in cells at the surface (above) and in connective tissue (below). × 1100.

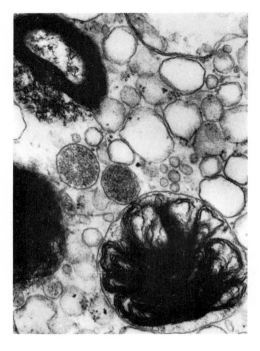

Figure 1–36. Electron micrograph of pigment (fuchsin) granules from the pigment epithelium of the rat retina. × 40,000.

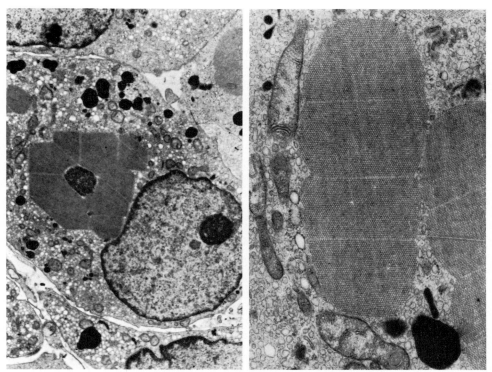

Figure 1–37. *Left:* Survey electron micrograph of an interstitial cell of the human testis. Contained in the cytoplasm near the nucleus is a large crystalloid (gray) and several lipid inclusions (black). × 4200. *Right:* A higher magnification of a crystalloid from a similar cell. The crystalloid shows a regular lattice pattern. There also is a lipid inclusion (bottom right). × 28,000.

somes, some microbodies (peroxisomes), and occasionally within mitochondria associated with the cristae.

NUCLEUS

A nucleus (or nuclei if multiple) is found in all cells except mature erythrocytes and platelets of the blood. The shape varies with cell shape, but the nucleus usually is spherical or ovoid; it may be cup-shaped or show indentations, and in a few cells, it is lobated. The nucleus usually is in the range of 3 to 14 microns (μm) in diameter, although it can be 25 microns (μm) or more in the ovum and some large ganglion cells. The nucleus is usually single, but cells such as parenchymal liver cells and cardiac muscle may be binucleate, while skeletal muscle cells and osteoclasts are multinucleate. Characteristically, the nucleus stains blue, i.e., it is basophilic, because of its content of nucleic acids and basic proteins (histones), but it also contains some acidic proteins. Its content of deoxyribonucleic acid (DNA) accounts for its strongly positive reaction when stained with the Feulgen technique. The volume of the nucleus is related to its DNA content and, therefore, the number of chromosomes, and there is evidence that the volume increases with synthetic activities of the cell. The nucleus contains the genetic material of the cell and has a direct influence on the metabolic activities of the cytoplasm. It is essential for the life of the cell, and if removed experimentally, protein synthesis in the cytoplasm ceases and the cell soon dies. Those cells that lack a nucleus, e.g., erythrocytes, are incapable of protein synthesis, cannot undergo cell division, and have limited metabolic activity. There is a constant exchange of material between the nucleus and the cytoplasm.

The nucleus of an interphase or rest-

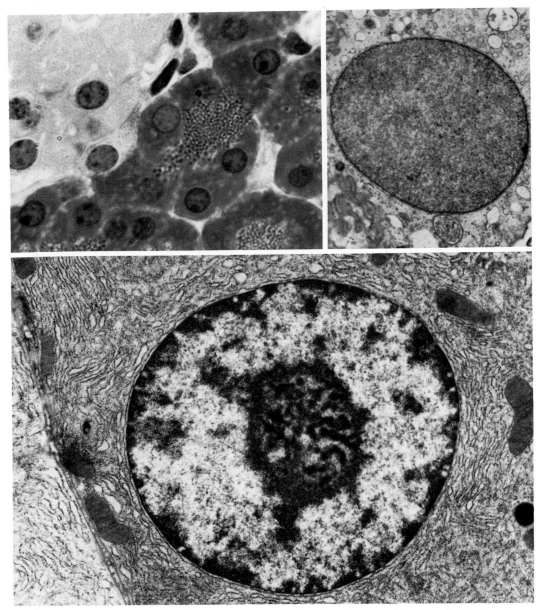

Figure 1–38. Interphase nuclei. *Top left:* Photomicrograph of pancreas showing nuclei of various types. In the exocrine basophilic cells, they are vesicular, spherical with prominent nucleoli. In islet (endocrine) cells, they are spherical and speckled chromatin (top left), and two ovoid heterochromatic nuclei of connective tissue cells are seen at top center. × 1100. *Top right:* Electron micrograph of the euchromatic nucleus of a kidney tubule cell. No nucleolus or chromatin material is seen, but there is some increased density at the nuclear envelope which represents the fibrous lamina. × 7000. *Bottom:* Electron micrograph of the nucleus of a pancreatic exocrine cell. It is spherical and contains a large central nucleolus with chromatin masses (heterochromatin) dispersed mainly on the internal aspect of the nuclear envelope. The clear channels in the peripheral chromatin are at the sites of pores in the nuclear envelope. × 10,500.

ing cell (i.e., nondividing) is bounded by a nuclear envelope or nuclear membrane, is filled with nuclear sap or karyoplasm, and contains nuclear chromatin and a nucleolus.

Nuclear Envelope

A thin, darkly staining membrane surrounds the nucleus and separates it from the cytoplasm. This nuclear envelope is only 40 nm thick but associated with its inner surface is chromatin and some fibrous material that accounts for its visibility on light microscopy. On electron microscopy, the envelope is composed of two 7-nm membranes, an inner and an outer, enclosing a perinuclear space or cistern of about 25 nm width. The outer membrane bears ribosomes on its cytoplasmic surface and often shows continuity with the membranes of the endoplasmic reticulum; the perinuclear space communicates with cisternae of the reticulum. Both the perinuclear space and cisternae of the reticulum may contain in their lumina dense secretory material. On the inner, karyoplasmic surface of the envelope there is in some cell types a thin layer formed by fine filamentous material, the fibrous lamina, to which clumps of nuclear chromatin apparently are attached firmly. This lamina may provide some mechanical support for the envelope and affect its permeability, but its functional significance remains in question.

Characteristically, the nuclear envelope shows the presence of nuclear pores or annuli that may occupy up to 20 per cent of the surface. Each pore is 40 to 100 nm in diameter and the pore-to-pore distance may be as little as 130 nm. At the rim of each pore, inner and outer membranes are in continuity, and the pore appears to be closed by a thin membrane or diaphragm in which there is a small, dense central granule. High resolution studies indicate that each annulus contains a "pore complex," a short cylinder formed by eight regular subunits and containing a central granule, the whole lying in and part of the fibrous lamina. It is believed that pore complexes have a role in the transfer of material between nucleus and cytoplasm. Apparently, the permeability of

nuclear pores shows some variation with the functional state of the cell, and it is known also that the number of pores varies with changes in nuclear activity.

Karyoplasm

Nuclear sap or karyoplasm is a term which describes the clear or apparently empty areas of the nucleus, i.e., those areas not occupied by nucleolus or chromatin. The karyoplasm is relatively electron-lucent on electron microscopy, although it contains dispersed chromatin, some small granules, and protein. Karyoplasm is a semifluid, colloidal solution in which the chromatin material and the nucleolus are suspended and serves as a medium for the diffusion of metabolites and larger macromolecules.

Nuclear Chromatin

Chromosomes in a dividing cell are simply threads of chromatin that are tightly coiled or "condensed" along their entire lengths and thus visible by light microscopy. Chromosomes in the interphase nucleus are not visible but in fact remain intact. Chromatin is nuclear material that contains DNA (deoxyribonucleic acid) and proteins and is the structural manifestation of chromosomes in interphase. It is basophilic and stains Feulgen positive owing to its DNA content. In the interphase nucleus, chromatin is dispersed in the nucleus in an uneven manner, with two types distinguished. *Euchromatin,* or dispersed chromatin, is loosely packed and thus only lightly basophilic, with a very light or nonapparent Feulgen staining. It is metabolically active with regard to RNA (ribonucleic acid) synthesis. *Heterochromatin* or condensed chromatin is tightly packed and thus is intensely basophilic and stains strongly with the Feulgen reaction. It is relatively inactive metabolically. Thus, condensed regions of chromosomes that persist in interphase are seen as heterochromatin; coiled or dispersed parts are represented as euchromatin. The proportion or amount of euchromatin, usually associated with a large nucleolus (or nucleoli), can be

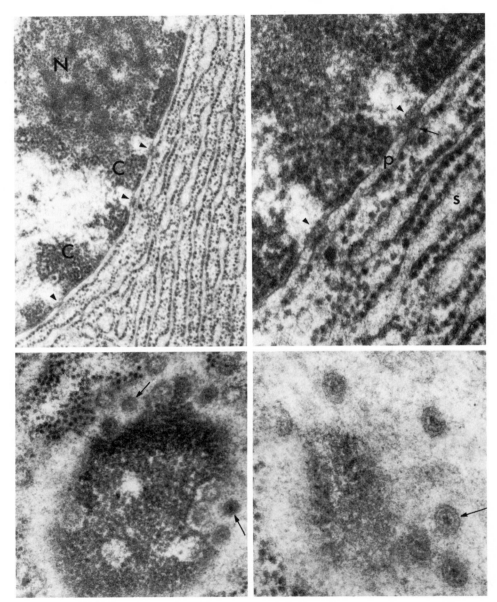

Figure 1–39.   Electron micrographs to show the nuclear envelope and nuclear pores. *Top left:* Three pores (arrowheads) are seen. N is the nucleolus and C is chromatin. × 26,000. *Top right:* A higher magnification of two of the pores seen in the top left figure. Some fibrous material appears to traverse the pores, the upper of which shows a central dense granule (arrow). Note some flocculent material both with intracisternal spaces (s) of granular reticulum and in the perinuclear space (p) of the nuclear envelope. × 45,000. *Bottom left:* Tangential section of the nucleus illustrating close spacing of the pores, seen as circular profiles, some with a central dense granule (arrows). × 30,000. *Bottom right:* A higher magnification of the pores. × 45,000.

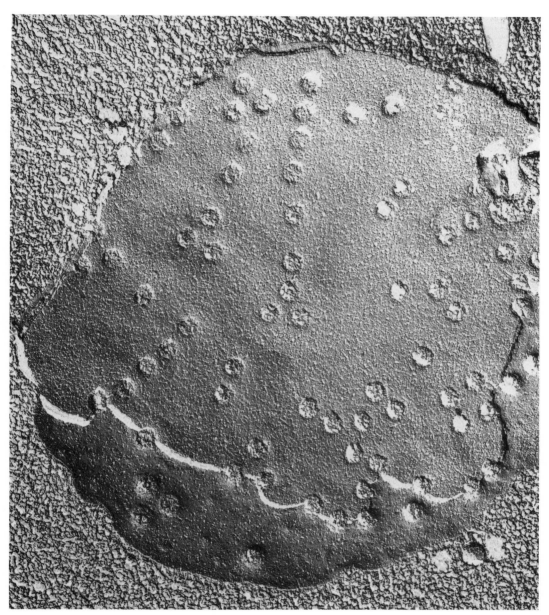

Figure 1–40. Freeze-etch preparation of a portion of an isolated rat liver nucleus to show the nuclear envelope, its outer (lower edge) and inner membrane, and nuclear pores. × 60,000. (Courtesy of Dr. G. G. Maul.)

used as an indication of the metabolic activity of a specific cell or cell type, because euchromatin usually is active in RNA synthesis, this RNA being used in protein synthesis in the cytoplasm. Conversely, a high proportion of heterochromatin indicates a cell with low metabolic activity. Nuclei themselves are basically of two types: (1) small, darkly staining nuclei with much stainable chromatin, e.g., of fibrocytes and some blood cells, are called condensed or hyperchromatic nuclei, while (2) the larger, paler-staining nuclei, e.g., of nerve cells and liver cells, are referred to as vesicular (bladder-like) nuclei. In cells that are dying, the heterochromatin is extremely dense and the nuclei of such cells are called *pyknotic*. Heterochromatin can transform into euchromatin, and vice versa, for example, in lymphocytes that normally show heterochromatic or hyperchromatic nuclei but when active become euchromatic (vesicular), also with an increase in size of the nucleolus.

Electron microscopy shows that chromatin consists of a mass of fine fibrils of 8 to 20 nm in diameter, the fibrils more closely packed in heterochromatin. There may be associated granules. Chromatin contains DNA and proteins, including histones, but the organization of these molecules in the chromatin fibrils is not known. The DNA double helix itself is only 2 nm in diameter, and so in the chromatin fibril the DNA and associated proteins may form a superhelix or perhaps the chromatin fibrils are multistranded. In special preparations, isolated chromatin appears as fine threads with 10-nm particles called nucleosomes attached to the threads, both the threads and particles containing DNA, with histones also in the particles. It is believed that, in interphase, chromosomes maintain their positions in the nucleus. Several chromatin fibrils appear to attach to sites on the nuclear envelope and, perhaps, particular regions of chromosomes attach to the envelope. The significance is unknown.

Nucleolus

Each interphase nucleus contains one to four nucleoli, although in a nucleus of the condensed type the nucleolus may be obscured. The number and size (up to 1 μm in diameter or more) of the nucleolus is constant for any particular cell type. They are prominent and usually multiple in cells actively engaged in protein synthesis. They disperse and disappear during cell division and are re-formed in the nuclei of the two daughter cells.

Nucleoli are discrete, darkly staining spherical or ovoid bodies, not delineated by a membrane, and lie either free within the karyoplasm or attached to the inner aspect of the nuclear envelope. They are larger, more dense, and more regular in outline than masses of heterochromatin. They consist of 5 to 10 per cent ribonucleic acid (RNA) with the rest protein and a small amount of deoxyribonucleic acid (DNA) and often are surrounded by a rim of condensed chromatin termed the *nucleolus-associated chromatin*. Staining varies with the relative proportions of RNA and basic protein but usually they are basophilic due to the RNA content, may stain metachromatically with dyes such as toluidine blue, and usually are Feulgen-negative, although the rim of nucleolar-associated chromatin is strongly Feulgen-positive. With some silver staining techniques, the nucleolus may show a coiled, threadlike structure termed the *nucleolonema*. By electron microscopy, the morphology shows some variation but there are four basic components: these are granules of 12 to 15 nm diameter composed of RNA and protein; fibrils of 5 nm diameter also composed of ribonucleoprotein and often closely packed; chromatin both as peripheral, nucleolar-associated chromatin and as fine loops of chromatin passing from the peripheral rim into the interior; and a proteinaceous, amorphous material usually occurring in aggregations. The components may form a compact mass or may occur as a core of fibrils surrounded by masses of granules, but often the fibrils and granules together form a thick, anastomosing cord, the nucleolonema, with patches along the cord formed either by granules or by fibrils.

Nucleoli lie at certain specific sites on certain chromosomes (the nucleolar organizing sites) where there are gene

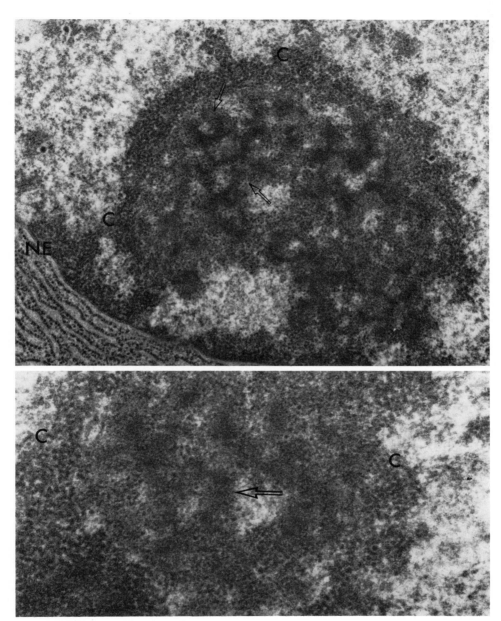

Figure 1–41. Electron micrographs of the nucleolus (see also Figure 1–38, *bottom*). *Top:* Here lying adjacent to the nuclear envelope (NE), the nucleolus is spongelike and consists of granules and fibrils arranged in a coiled cord (the nucleolonema) with areas of densely packed fibrils (the fibrillar centers, arrows) around less dense material. Surrounding the nucleolus is nucleolus-associated chromatin (C). × 34,000. *Bottom:* A higher magnification. × 48,000.

sequences or cistrons that encode genetic information for the synthesis of ribosomes. At these sites, ribosomal RNA is transcribed basically as subunits, although the final assembly of discrete ribosomes from the two complete subunits occurs only when the various components have been passed from the nucleus into the cytoplasm. Additionally,

the role of the nucleolus in the processing of messenger RNA (see page 74) has yet to be defined clearly.

CELL CYCLE

In a cell population which constantly is being renewed, e.g., in the epithelium lining the intestinal tract, individual cells divide periodically. This process of mitosis and interphase (the period between cell divisions) is termed the cell cycle. The duration of this cycle for any particular cell type now can be estimated accurately. Toward the end of interphase, DNA is synthesized. This stage is called the DNA duplication or the S (synthesis) stage. After the S stage, prior to mitosis, the cell enters a relatively quiescent period called the post-duplication or G2 stage, and then passes through prophase, metaphase, anaphase, and telophase (see page 68). At the termination of mitosis, the daughter cells enter the preduplication or G1 stage of interphase, which lasts until DNA duplication occurs prior to the succeeding mitosis. Obviously the length of the cell cycle varies with the cell type, for example, being short in the case of the epithelium lining the gut and much longer in liver cells.

CHROMOSOMES

Fine Structure of Chromosomes

As described above, the chromosomes during interphase are present partly as euchromatin, where they (or parts of them) are greatly dispersed or uncoiled, and partly as heterochromatin, where they (or parts of them) are tightly coiled and stain densely. Early in cell division and after synthesis and DNA replication, the chromosomal threads become highly coiled and visible as darkly staining rodlike structures. Each chromosome consists of a pair of chromatids, each of which is a fully replicated chromosome. The chromatin of these chromosomes on electron microscopy is a mixture or meshwork of fibrils of about 30 nm in diameter. These fibrils probably represent a supercoiling or superhelix of a beaded strand of only 2 nm in diameter with chromatin subunits or *nucleosomes* as small beads of 7 to 10 nm diameter placed at intervals along the strand. This strands represents the linear double helix of DNA (see following discussion). The nucleosomes probably contain about 140 to 200 base pairs of

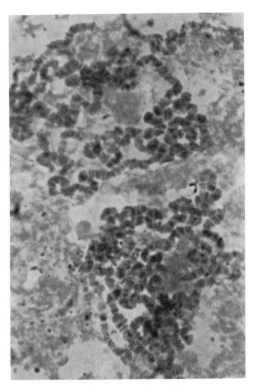

Figure 1–42. Photomicrograph of a giant chromosome from a salivary gland of the fruit fly *(Drosophila)*. A smear preparation. × 850.

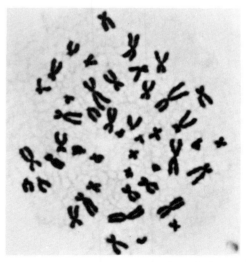

Figure 1–43. Photomicrograph of human (male) chromosomes from a squash preparation. Notice the various positions of the centromeres. × 1250. (Courtesy of Dr. M. L. Barr.)

DNA and the flexible strand between the particles or beads contains 30 to 60 base pairs.

DNA Structure and Replication

The DNA molecule is formed by two parallel strands of molecular chains twisted into a spiral to form a double helix. Each of the parallel chains is formed by alternating phosphoric acid and pentose sugar (deoxyribose) groups with side chains passing from the pentose groups to one of four nitrogenous bases. The bases of the two chains are connected by cross links (like the steps in a ladder). The four bases are adenine, guanine, cytosine, and thymine, and the pair bonding occurs always between adenine and thymine or between cytosine and guanine. During mitosis, if each daughter cell is to have an identical DNA content to the parent cell, the DNA content must be doubled before division. This process is called DNA replication or duplication and corresponds to the S stage of the cell cycle. To achieve this conservation of genetic information during cell division, the DNA double helix unwinds and each strand becomes a template for the assembly of a new molecular chain, an adenine of the new chain pairing always with a thymine of the old strand and a cytosine of the new chain pairing with a guanine of the old strand. Each new strand thus is complementary to an old strand. Each daughter double helix therefore is composed of one strand or chain from the parent and one new strand and the linear array of genes is copied exactly.

A *gene* is a triplet, i.e., three bases in a row, and this corresponds to a single amino acid in the protein that is formed. A single polypeptide (a chain of amino acids) is encoded by a sequence of several triplets, this sequence being called a *cistron*.

Chromosome Numbers

Human male somatic (body or nongerm) cells have 46 chromosomes arranged in 23 pairs; 22 pairs are called *autosomes,* and one pair is formed by the X and Y or *sex chromosomes.* In females there are 22 pairs of autosomes plus two X chromosomes, and in males there are 22 pairs of autosomes plus one X and one Y chromosome. This number, i.e., 46, is called the *diploid* or double number. In the gonads, the sex cells (ova or spermatozoa) contain one-half this number, or 23 chromosomes. This is called the *haploid* number and involves a special type of cell division called meiosis or reduction division. Thus, each ovum or female sex cell contains 22 autosomes and one X chromosome, and each spermatozoon or male sex cell contains 22 autosomes and one X or Y chromosome. After fertilization, i.e., after union of the sex cells, the fertilized ovum or gamete will contain either 44 autosomes plus two X chromosomes (a combination that develops into a female) or 44 autosomes plus one X and one Y chromosome (a combination that develops into a male).

In some cases, human somatic cells may not have the correct number of chromosomes. *Polyploidy* is a condition

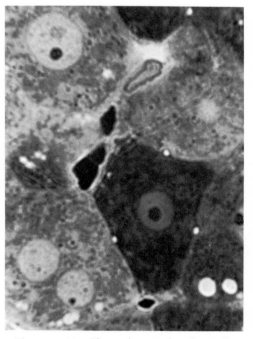

Figure 1–44. Photomicrograph of rat liver showing polyploidy. The cell at top left has a single, large polyploid nucleus; a cell at bottom left has two nuclei. Plastic section. × 1200.

in which cells contain a multiple of the haploid number, e.g., a tetraploidy, in which four times the number of haploid chromosomes are present (double the diploid number), or 92. Polyploidy is quite common in liver cells, and is characterized by a very large nucleus. It results, of course, from an abnormal mitosis. *Aneuploidy* is a condition in which a cell contains either less than the normal diploid number of chromosomes or a greater number that is not a multiple of it. Such a variation may result in an individual with a disease condition, such as a congenital condition called Down's syndrome (mongolism) in which children are mentally retarded; in this case the somatic cells contain one extra chromosome. Chromosome abnormalities of the aneuploid type also quite commonly involve the sex chromosomes and are associated with varying degrees of abnormality of the sex organs, e.g., Klinefelter's syndrome.

nucleus in a smear preparation. It is not seen in normal male somatic cells.

If both X chromosomes in a female cell were active, a double dose of identical genetic activity would result. Thus, one of the X chromosomes is extended (uncoiled) and invisible in the female interphase nucleus, and the second remains inactive and tightly coiled; the latter is visible as the heterochromatic Barr body. Therefore, a Barr body indicates that a cell contains a second X chromosome, and generally, this means that the cell is from a female. However, there are genetic abnormalities that confuse the picture: in Turner's syndrome, the female somatic cells contain only one X chromosome and so no Barr bodies are seen although the individual is female; in Klinefelter's syndrome, the cells contain one Y and two (or more) X chromosomes and, although the individual is male, Barr bodies are present in somatic cells. In some cases, as shown in Figure 1–45, the cells may contain

Sex Chromatin (Barr Body)

As described above, chromosomes may show irregular densities of staining along their lengths, those darkly staining or heterochromatic parts being regions in which the chromosomal threads are tightly coiled. In the normal female, with a chromosome content including two X chromosomes, one X chromosome is extremely heterochromatic and forms a visible mass in the interphase nucleus. This small visible mass is the *Barr body*. The Barr body, or sex chromatin, is about 1 micron (μm) in diameter, and commonly occurs lying against the inner aspect of the nuclear envelope in a planoconvex form (epithelial cell nuclei). In some cells (neutrophil granular leukocytes) it is seen as a "drumstick" or slender protrusion of the nucleus, or as a small body associated with the nucleolus (nucleolar satellite, in nerve cells). Occasionally it lies free within the karyoplasm as a discrete mass. It is seen particularly well in the nuclei of squamous epithelial cells scraped from the inside of the cheek, but only 20 to 70 per cent of female somatic cells will show it because of the plane of sectioning or position of the

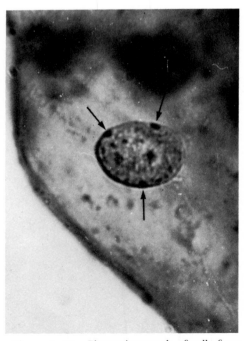

Figure 1–45. Photomicrograph of cells from the buccal smear of a 2-month-old, mentally retarded child. The somatic cells of this child, presumably a Klinefelter syndrome patient, contain 22 times 2 autosomes plus XXXXY. The nucleus illustrated contains three female sex chromatin, or Barr bodies. × 1200. (Courtesy of Dr. B. Smith.)

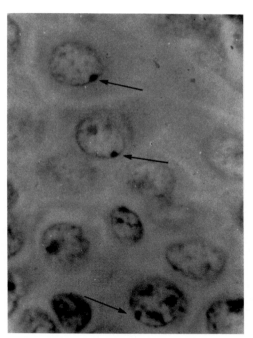

Figure 1–46. Photomicrograph of sex chromatin (arrows) or Barr bodies, in epidermal nuclei from the cheek of a human female. × 1800.

four X chromosomes plus one Y chromosome and in such a case the cells show three Barr bodies in the nuclei.

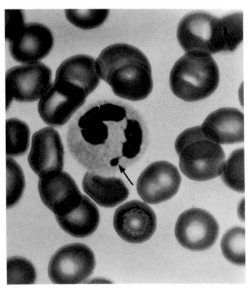

Figure 1–47. Photomicrograph of a polymorph (white blood cell) from a human female. The sex chromatin, or Barr body, appears as a nuclear "drumstick" (arrow), × 1600. (Courtesy of Dr. M. L. Barr.)

The presence, then, of a Barr body within the nucleus of a somatic cell merely indicates that the nucleus contains two X chromosomes. Sex actually is determined by the Y chromosome.

CELL DIVISION

Cell division is related to the demand for growth and replacement in tissues, and basically there are three types of cell populations in this respect. Some cell populations are static and do not undergo DNA synthesis and cell division, e.g., neurons of the adult nervous system. Many others are expanding in the sense that a small proportion of the cells undergo DNA synthesis and cell division to permit growth, e.g., liver, kidney, and some glands. The third type occurs in cells that show a definite lifetime and in these renewing populations there is needed a continuous cell division to replace dying cells, e.g., in bone marrow (forming blood cells), in the epithelium of the intestinal tract, and in epidermis.

Cell division involves both division of the cytoplasm (cytokinesis) and division of the nucleus (karyokinesis), both usually occurring together, although karyokinesis can occur without cytokinesis, resulting in the formation of a cell that is binucleate (or multinucleate after several karyokineses). This occurs in, for example, liver cells, megakaryocytes, and perhaps osteoclasts. In somatic cells, division of the nucleus occurs by *mitosis* and, as indicated above, is preceded in the S stage of the cell cycle by DNA replication to ensure that each daughter cell has a DNA genetic content identical to that of the parent cell. In the formation of sex cells or gametes (ova and spermatozoa), karyokinesis involves a *meiosis*, whereby a haploid chromosome number results so that, after fertilization, the resulting fertilized ovum regains the diploid number of chromosomes present in somatic cells.

Mitosis

As indicated above, mitosis is the process whereby a somatic cell divides to form two daughter cells identical to each other and to the parent cell. It involves a doubling of the DNA content and the subsequent equal distribution of this genetic material between the two daughter cells. Although a cell in the G2 or postduplication stage has a doubled DNA content, this is not visible and the chromosome number remains 46, i.e., diploid, the new DNA being located in separate chromatin strands within the old chromosomes. For descriptive purposes, mitosis is divided into four stages but it must be emphasized that all four are part of a continuous process. These stages are based on a series of structural changes.

Prophase. In prophase, four main structural changes occur relatively simultaneously. First, the chromatin threads become condensed (shortened and thickened) so that the chromosomes become visible as short, dark, rodlike structures. Each chromosome is split longitudinally in half, and the two halves are attached at some point along their lengths at a small region called the *centromere.* Each half is a *chromatid.* In fact, due to DNA duplication which occurred prior to mitosis, each chromatid is a completely replicated chromosome, although it is not so called at this stage. Second, the pair of centrioles, usually adjacent to the nucleus of the interphase cell, start to duplicate, a daughter centriole forming adjacent to each, and the pairs of centrioles then start to move away from each other to take up positions at opposite poles or ends of the cell. As this occurs, microtubules start to form between the separating pairs of centrioles. Some are arranged around each pair as *astral fibers* or *rays,* which are not very prominent in human cells, and the whole complex of astral fibers and centrioles is termed the *aster.* Other, longer microtubules develop between the asters as *spindle fibers.* Some of these eventually will extend from aster to aster as continuous microtubules, but these are complete only after disappearance of the nuclear envelope. Third, the nucleolus gradually disappears, its content being attached to some of the chromatids. Finally, the nuclear envelope starts to disintegrate.

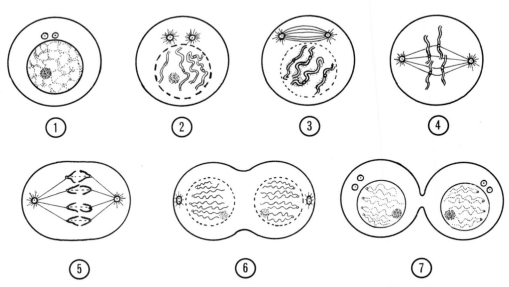

Figure 1–48. Diagram of the stages of mitosis. (1) Interphase: Nuclear envelope, nucleolus, chromatin, and a pair of centrioles are illustrated. (2) Early prophase: Two centrioles are forming asters, nuclear envelope and nucleous are dispersing, and chromosomes are becoming visible. (3) Late prophase: A spindle is formed between the two centrioles. Nuclear envelope has virtually disappeared and the nucleolus is broken up and dispersed over the chromosomes, four of which are illustrated, each split into two chromatids, and each joined only at a centromere. (4) Metaphase: The chromosomes (pairs of chromatids) are arranged at the equator of the spindle. (5) Anaphase: The chromosomes have split, and the chromatid of each pair is moving toward one pole of the cell. (6) Early telophase: The chromatids (now chromosomes) of each daughter cell are becoming uncoiled: a nuclear envelope and nucleolus are re-forming and the centriole is duplicating. (7) Late telophase: The plasma membrane is constricting, and two new daughter cells are formed.

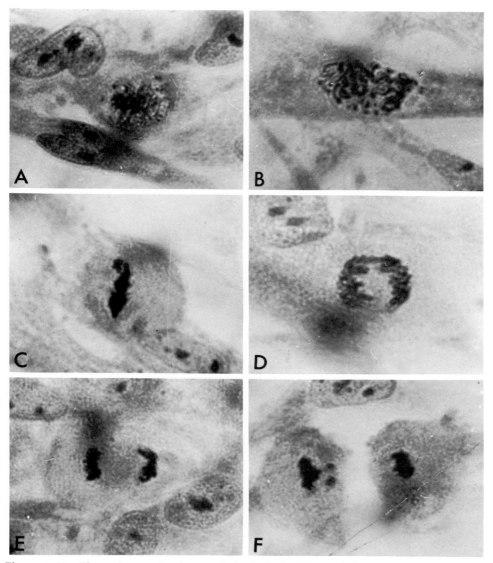

Figure 1–49. Photomicrographs of stages of mitosis obtained from cells in tissue culture. *A,* Interphase and early prophase. *B,* Late prophase. *C,* Metaphase. *D,* Anaphase. *E,* Early telophase. *F,* Late telophase. × 950.

It becomes less obvious and thinner as a result of movement of chromatin material away from its inner surface, and then it breaks down into small vesicles indistinguishable from elements of the granular endoplasmic reticulum. In sections, early stages of prophase are difficult to detect, but a late prophase is quite obvious.

Metaphase. At metaphase, all the chromosomes (pairs of chromatids) move to the center of the cell in relation to the spindle and are arranged at the equatorial plate, i.e., at right angles to the long axis of the spindle and parallel to the axis along which cytokinesis will occur. At this stage, the two chromatids of a chromosome are attached at the paler-staining centromere with the "arms," i.e., chromatids, extending outward. Viewed from either pole of the cell, the chromosomes are arranged as a starlike ring. Further development of the microtubules of the spindle also

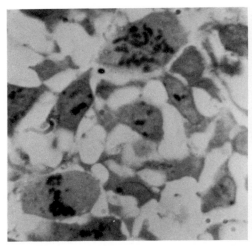 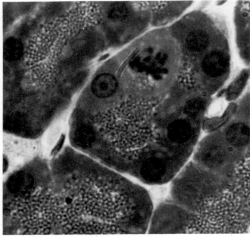

Figure 1–50. Photomicrographs to illustrate mitosis in tissue sections. *Left:* Two cells in embryonic mesenchyme. *Right:* In adult pancreas. Both ×900.

occurs in that spindle fibers from each pair of centrioles, having met in the region of the equatorial plate to form continuous microtubules, continue to elongate and thus move the pairs of centrioles further apart. At the equatorial plate, these continuous microtubules pass between the chromosomes. Also, the centromere of each chromosome contains two small disclike bodies which can be seen only with the electron microscope. These bodies, or *kinetochores,* one for each chromatid, organize the formation of more microtubules, the so-called chromosomal microtubules, which extend toward the two poles of the cell, one set associated with each kinetochore and thus with each chromatid. One set of chromosomal microtubules thus extends from the kinetochore of one chromatid to one pole of the cell. Finally, at the end of metaphase a total split of the two chromatids of each chromosome occurs at the centromere, the kinetochores separating. At this stage, the chromatids are daughter chromosomes and thus the metaphase cell has a tetraploid number (92) of chromosomes, i.e., two complete sets.

Anaphase. After complete splitting of the chromosomes at their centromeres, daughter chromosomes move to opposite poles of the cell, one diploid set (46) to each end. The actual mechanism of chromosome movement is poorly un-

derstood but is believed to involve a sliding interaction between the continuous (spindle) microtubules and the chromosomal microtubules. This apparently results in each set of chromosomal microtubules moving toward their pole of the cell, "dragging" behind them the daughter chromosomes which are attached by kinetochores to these microtubules. It is accompanied by a detachment from the two asters of the continuous microtubules and their movement to, and accumulation in, the center of the cell near the region of ultimate cytokinesis. Here, the massing of microtubules forms a dense mass called the *midbody.* Toward the end of anaphase and extending into telophase, a bandlike constriction occurs around the cell (the cleavage furrow) in the region of the midbody, and mitochondria and other cytoplasmic components are distributed evenly around the cell periphery.

Telophase. At each pole of the cell, the chromosomes detach from chromosomal microtubules and the microtubules disintegrate. The chromosomes start to elongate or disperse, become less distinct, and eventually only portions of them remain tightly coiled as heterochromatin, the dispersed regions being euchromatin. The nucleoli of each nucleus reappear in association with specific chromosomes, and the nuclear envelopes re-form from cytoplas-

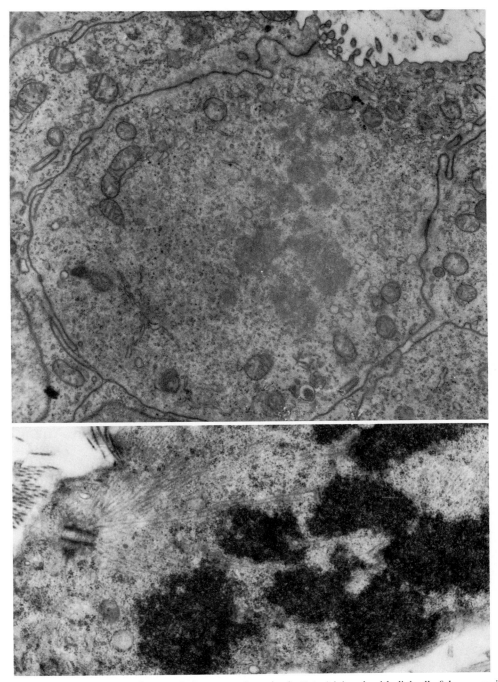

Figure 1–51. Electron micrograph demonstrating mitosis. *Top:* A jejunal epithelial cell of the mouse in late prophase. The cell has rounded up, chromosomes are apparent, and the nuclear envelope has disappeared. × 8500. *Bottom:* A fibroblast in metaphase with spindle fibers (microtubules) extending from the centriole (left) to chromosomes (chromosomal microtubules) and between them to the other pole of the cell (spindle fibers or continuous microtubules). × 19,000.

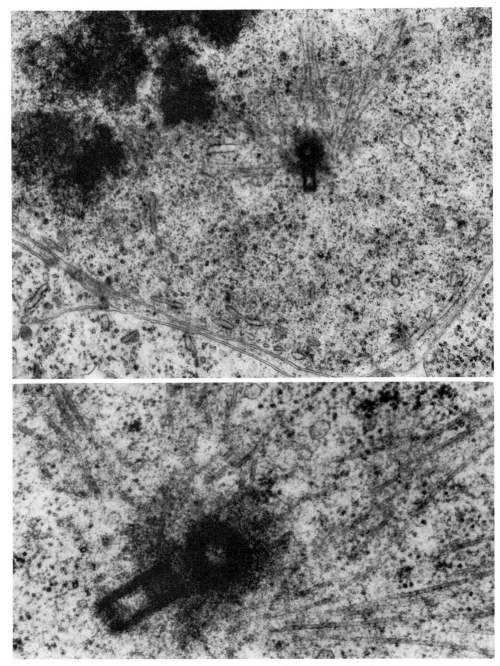

Figure 1–52. Electron micrographs illustrating anaphase in an epithelial cell, the lower picture at higher magnification showing a pair of centrioles with radiating microtubules. Top, × 19,000; bottom, × 60,000.

mic membranous vesicles, probably originating from granular endoplasmic reticulum. These events continue until each nucleus is interphase in appearance. At the same time, the cleavage furrow deepens around the midbody. In many cell types, a subsurface ring of microfilaments has been described in the cleavage furrow, and contraction of these probably is responsible for the deepening of the cleavage furrow until it is closely apposed to the midbody. At this stage, only a slender bridge of cytoplasm remains between the two daughter cells, and finally this bridge breaks and two discrete daughter cells are formed. Cytoplasmic components are distributed equally between the two, and microtubules, formerly in the midbody, disintegrate or disperse.

In sections, cells undergoing division are recognized by the presence of *mitotic figures,* this term referring to any cell undergoing mitosis. Usually, the chromatin material, being more condensed, stains more densely than in an interphase nucleus, and of course, other features may be apparent, as described. In many cases, a cell changes its shape and moves its position when undergoing mitosis. For example, in simple epithelia, the cell becomes rounded and apparently moves toward the surface, losing its connection with the basal lamina.

Effect of Colchicine and Vinblastine on Mitosis. Colchicine, some derivatives of colchicine, and vinblastine block the assembly of microtubules as described earlier. In mitosis, therefore, spindle microtubule formation does not occur. If these drugs are administered to an experimental animal, any cell undergoing cell division will be arrested at the metaphase stage. This has proved to be a valuable technique for studying cell turnover rates and for cytogenetic studies, since the chromosomes are most easily studied in the metaphase stage.

Meiosis

All somatic cells contain a diploid number of chromosomes (46, or 23 homologous pairs) but the gametes possess the haploid number (23), containing only one member of each pair of chro-

mosomes. This is achieved by a special form of cell division called *meiosis* which consists of two successive nuclear divisions without an intervening period of DNA replication. In the first division, only one chromosome (pair of chromatids) from each homologous pair passes to each daughter cell, this halving the number of chromosomes to 23. In the second division, the two chromatids of each chromosome are separated, thus producing finally four nuclei each with a haploid number of chromosomes. When male and female gametes unite, the diploid number is regained. In meiosis, also, genetic variation can occur by the exchange of segments of homologous chromosomes and the completely random selection of one of the two homologous chromosomes during the reduction division.

First Meiotic Division. Prophase is extremely prolonged and divided into four stages. In leptotene, chromosomes become visible as long, thin threads and, later, homologous chromosomes move together and pair with corresponding sites on the two in register. This is termed zygotene, and the pairings are referred to as synapses. (Note that originally, one member of each pair came from the father, the other from the mother.) In pachytene, chromosomes coil and appear shorter and thicker and it becomes apparent that each homologous pair or bivalent consists of four chromatids, each chromosome being split longitudinally into two chromatids. The centromere does not split. In diplotene, the chromosomes start to separate but this separation is incomplete and at certain points along their lengths they contact each other at sites of crossing called chiasmata and exchange segments. This separation proceeds and at this stage (diakinesis) the nuclear envelope starts to disappear and the nucleolus fragments and disappears. In metaphase, the bivalents arrange themselves at the equator of the now formed spindle. In anaphase, the kinetochores or centromeres of the bivalents do not divide, with the result that whole chromosomes (or two chromatids) separate and move to opposite poles of the cell. Telophase follows.

Second Meiotic Division. This commences with prophase after a brief interval (interkinesis). A spindle forms, the nuclear envelope breaks down, and chromosomes move to the equator to form a metaphase plate. Kinetochores divide and chromatids (of each chromosome) become free of each other, diverge to opposite poles in anaphase, and in telophase form daughter nuclei and daughter cells. The entire process results in four daughter cells with haploid nuclei.

In meiosis of male germ cells, cytokinesis results in equal distribution of cytoplasm and, of the four cells, two will be 22 +X in chromosome content and two will have 22 +Y. In the female, all four are 22 +X, but cytoplasmic division is unequal and only one, containing most of the cytoplasm, is a viable oocyte.

CELL DIFFERENTIATION

In development of the embryo, a single cell, the fertilized ovum, divides eventually to form all cells of the body. This process of cell proliferation leads also to cell differentiation, with various types of cells being specialized for different functions. There is strong evidence that all differentiated cell nuclei possess identical and complete chromosome — and therefore gene — sets (the genome). Why then do they not all synthesize the same proteins and perform identical functions? It is evident that most of the genome in the highly differentiated cells is repressed; i.e., most of the genes do not express themselves. This may occur because the means whereby a gene can express itself are not present in the cell and, certainly, some control over cellular synthetic mechanisms resides in the cytoplasm. However, while identification of the components mainly responsible for gene regulation and gene repression have not been identified, repression undoubtedly is controlled mainly by the activities of the genetic material, i.e., the DNA together with nucleoproteins and nucleic acids that form the chromatin of the interphase nucleus. As cells develop, some regions of the genome become active, others become inactive.

PROTEIN SECRETION AND TRANSCRIPTION OF DNA

While the preceding description of the cell is mainly morphological in emphasis, it must not be forgotten that the cell is a living, dynamic entity. One example of cell function is protein synthesis and secretion. Cells specialized for protein secretion show the presence of one or more large nucleoli, a mass of granular endoplasmic reticulum, and usually a prominent Golgi apparatus. The type of protein secreted, i.e., the sequence of amino acids in its peptide chain, is determined by the DNA of the nucleus, the nucleotide sequence in the DNA molecule comprising a chemical code which the cell then interprets as amino acid sequences of the protein. This direction of secretion by the DNA is a complicated process. It involves transcription or decoding of the DNA code into a disposable molecule of messenger RNA (mRNA). The mRNA then moves to the cytoplasm where its information is translated into protein production by ribosomes (rRNA). This process of correct assembly of amino acids also requires the participation of transfer RNA (tRNA).

Transcription of DNA. This involves local separation of the two helical strands of the DNA molecule at a specific site where a molecule of RNA polymerase attaches. This separation exposes a particular *cistron* or structural gene on one of the strands, the master strand, the other strand being the complementary strand. Upon this exposed template a strand of RNA is constructed, the RNA polymerase moving along the master strand of DNA and, like a zipper, exposing further triplets, thus permitting the strand of RNA to grow in length. The RNA strand is similar to that of DNA, and the process of formation of the RNA strand is similar to that of DNA replication, but there are three differences: (1) the RNA strand is single and not double as in DNA, (2) it contains ribose and not deoxyribose groups, and (3) the base uracil replaces thymine, the other three bases being adenine, cytosine, and guanine. As in DNA, base pairing occurs between cyto-

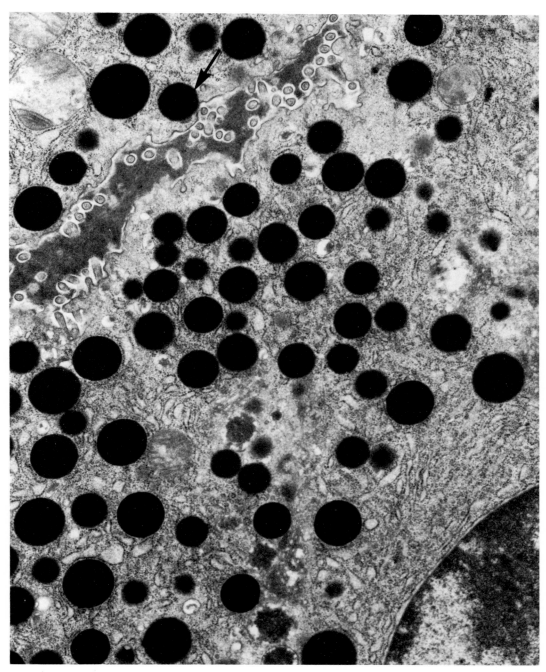

Figure 1–53. Electron micrograph of the apical portion of a pancreatic acinar cell to demonstrate the dynamic process of protein secretion (see text). Part of the nucleus limited by the nuclear envelope lies at bottom right, with part of the nucleolus at the internal aspect of the nuclear envelope. In apical cytoplasm is a mass of granular endoplasmic reticulum with some mitochondria, portions of Golgi apparatus at lower center and near the right edge of the micrograph just above the center, condensing vacuoles or prezymogen granules in relation to the Golgi apparatus, and zymogen granules. The last are very dense, spherical and membrane-bound. At top left is part of the lumen of the acinus with microvilli in transverse and longitudinal section. The lumen contains discharged, electron-dense secretory material. The zymogen granule or droplet at arrows is in the process of fusing with the apical plasmalemma and discharging its contents (exocytosis). × 18,000.

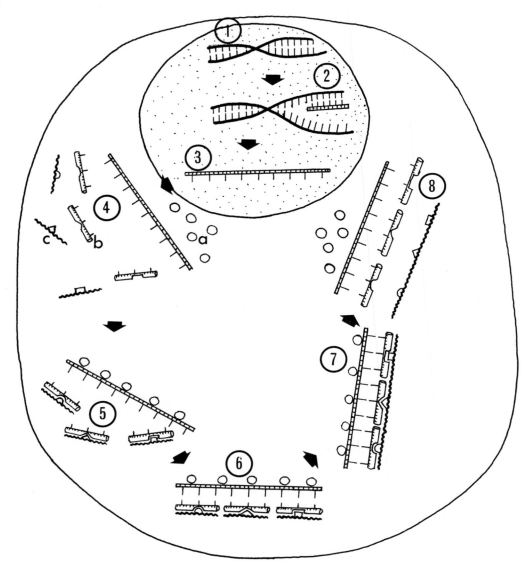

Figure 1–54. Diagrammatic representation of the steps involved in the synthesis of a three–amino acid protein. 1. DNA molecule. 2. Synthesis of a messenger RNA molecule from the DNA. 3. Release of the messenger RNA molecule and its transfer from nucleus to cytoplasm. 4. Messenger RNA molecule in the cytoplasm and its association with (a) ribosomes, (b) three transfer RNA molecules, and (c) three amino acids. 5. Linkage of amino acids to transfer RNA molecules and association of ribosomes with the messenger RNA molecule. 6. Transfer of amino acids by transfer RNA to messenger RNA and correct alignment. 7. Linkage of amino acids to form a polypeptide. 8. Release of the polypeptide and dissociation of ribosomes from messenger RNA. The newly synthesized protein (polypeptide) then is transported in the channels of the endoplasmic reticulum to the Golgi region where it is membrane-wrapped and either stored or transported to the cell surface for release.

sine and guanine, but in RNA, uracil instead of thymine pairs with adenine. The DNA triplets are thus transcribed into complementary triplets or *codons* of RNA. The completed RNA molecule and the polymerase molecule then are released from the DNA strand and the RNA molecule moves from the nucleus into the cytoplasm as mRNA.

Protein Synthesis. In the cytoplasm, the mRNA molecule attaches to ribosomes. The ribosomes function as essential sites on which amino acids are linked in a definite order dictated by the codons of the mRNA. However, the ribosomes are nonspecific in the sense that they simply form any protein (or polypeptide chain) on "orders" from the mRNA. Usually, several ribosomes attach to the mRNA strand, seen as the 150 Å (15 nm) filament connecting ribosomes to form a polysome. Protein formation involves a "carrier" in the form of tRNA. Each small molecule of tRNA has, as it were, two sides. One side is specific for a particular amino acid, to which it attaches. The other side, by complementary base pairing using the adenine, cytosine, guanine, uracil code, "mates" with a triplet on the mRNA strand. Thus, amino acids are carried by tRNA to specific sites on the mRNA strand: there are in the cytoplasm a large number of tRNA molecules, each recognizing a particular triplet of mRNA and a specific amino acid.

At the ribosome, as the mRNA molecule moves along it and passes through its "reading head," amino acids carried by tRNA are brought together in a definite order prescribed by the code words or triplets of the mRNA and are linked together into a polypeptide chain. The tRNA molecule detaches both from the amino acid (now linked in the polypeptide chain) and from the mRNA strand and is available then to pick up another amino acid of the same kind for a further cycle. The mRNA molecule, having transmitted its information, may remain to form further protein of the same type or may be degraded. When the decoding is complete, the ribosome detaches from the mRNA strand and is available for further protein synthesis.

Ribosomal RNA and transfer RNA both are also transcribed in the nucleus from the DNA template and then pass to the cytoplasm.

In summary, the ribosomes are nonspecific as to which type of protein they synthesize. They are, as it were, for hire. Specificity is determined by mRNA, carrying the message directly from DNA of the nucleus; tRNA acts simply as a carrier of amino acids.

If destined for secretion, the newly formed protein passes into canals of the endoplasmic reticulum and thence by transfer vesicles to the Golgi apparatus. Here it is concentrated, a carbohydrate moiety may be added, and it then leaves the Golgi apparatus as a condensing vacuole which progresses to a secretory granule. Such granules are stored in the apical cytoplasm until released by the cell.

THE FOUR PRIMARY TISSUES

As explained previously, the body is composed of only three basic elements, i.e., cells, intercellular substances, and body fluids. During development, the embryo consists of three cellular layers (ectoderm, mesoderm, and endoderm), each specialized in respect of function, future development, and differentiation. All adult tissues develop from these and, in the adult, only four primary tissues are present. A primary or basic tissue may be defined as a group of similar cells specialized in a common direction and able to perform a common function. The four primary tissues are epithelium, connective tissue, muscle, and nervous tissue.

In turn, organs are formed from these tissues and, usually, all four types are present in a single organ. The student who has learned to recognize these four basic tissues will have taken a large step toward the understanding of histology and the identification of tissues. A section that at first appears complex and confusing when seen under the microscope is, in fact, composed only of the four basic tissues. A few characteristics usually will prove adequate for identification.

Epithelium. The cells are closely apposed with very little cementing substance between, and they are arranged as sheets covering or lining surfaces or as masses of cells in glands.

Connective Tissue. The cells usually are widely separated by a relatively large amount of intercellular substance. This group includes certain specialized tissues such as blood and blood-forming tissues, bone, and cartilage.

Muscle. There are three types; cells are elongated, contained cytoplasmic filaments, are relatively closely associated, and are separated by fine, vascular connective tissue.

Nervous Tissue. This consists of cells, some of which are very large, and their elongated processes, which are usually grouped as relatively isolated masses or bundles.

The subdivisions and varieties of these four primary tissues can be classified according to structure and function (Table 1–1).

TABLE 1–1. Classification of Tissues

Epithelium

Covering external body surface or limiting internal surface

Simple
- Squamous ——— Bowman's capsule (kidney), endothelium, mesothelium, (the last two derived from mesoderm)
- Cuboidal ——— Collecting tubule (kidney), small ducts
- Columnar ——— Gallbladder (nonciliated), uterine tube (ciliated)

Pseudostratified columnar ——— Male urethra (nonciliated), trachea (ciliated)

Stratified
- Squamous ——— Cornea (without connective tissue papillae), skin (keratinizing, with connective tissue papillae), vagina (nonkeratinizing, with connective tissue papillae)
- Cuboidal ——— Sweat gland ducts
- Columnar ——— Male urethra
- Transitional ——— Urinary tract

Glands, multicellular

Exocrine
- Simple ——— Gastric, sweat
- Compound ——— Salivary, pancreas

Endocrine
- Cord and clump ——— Hypophysis
- Follicle ——— Thyroid

TABLE 1–1. Classification of Tissues (*Continued*)

Muscle

Smooth (involuntary)	Intestinal tract, blood vessels
Striated (voluntary)	Skeletal muscle
Cardiac (striated involuntary)	Heart

Connective Tissue

General	Loose	Mesenchyme	Mainly restricted to embryo and fetus
		Mucoid	Wharton's jelly (umbilical cord)
		Areolar	"Loose packing" in most organs and tissues
		Adipose	Subcutaneous tissue (hypodermis)
		Reticular	Bone marrow, lymph node
	Dense	Irregular	Dermis, capsules of organs
		Regular	Tendon, stroma of cornea
Special	Cartilage	Hyaline	Costal cartilage, trachea
		Fibrous	Intervertebral disc
		Elastic	External ear, epiglottis
	Bone	Cancellous	Center of long bone
		Compact	Shaft of long bone
	Hemopoietic	Myeloid	Bone marrow
		Lymphoid	Spleen, lymph node
	Blood		
	Lymph		

Nervous Tissue

Central nervous system	Gray matter	Brain, spinal cord
	White matter	Brain, spinal cord
Peripheral nervous system	Nerves	Peripheral nerves
	Ganglia	Sensory, autonomic
	Nerve endings	Naked, encapsulated
Special receptors		Eye, ear, nose

REFERENCES

Barr, M. L.: Sex chromatin and phenotype in man. Science, *130*:679, 1959.

Bennett, G., Leblond, C. P., and Haddad, A.: Migration of glycoprotein from the Golgi apparatus to the surface of various cell types as shown by radioautography after labeled fucose injection into rats. J. Cell Biol., *60*:258, 1974.

Binder, L. I., and Rosenbaum, J. L.: The in vitro assembly of flagellar outer doublet tubulin. J. Cell Biol., *79*:500, 1978.

Brökelmann, J.: On the fine structure of polyribosomes. Cell Tiss. Res., *179*:531, 1977.

Cardell, R. R.: Smooth endoplasmic reticulum in rat hepatocytes during glycogen deposition and depletion. Int. Rev. Cytol., *48*:221, 1977.

Cohen, A. H., and Sundeen, J. R.: The nuclear fibrous lamina in human cells: Studies on its appearance and distribution. Anat. Rec., *186*:471, 1976.

Dustin, P.: Microtubules. Berlin, Springer-Verlag, 1978.

Dyson, R. D.: Cell Biology. A Molecular Approach. Boston, Allyn and Bacon, Inc., 1978.

Erickson, H. P.: Microtubule surface lattice and subunit structure and observations on reassembly. J. Cell Biol., *60*:153, 1974.

Fawcett, D. W.: The Cell: Its Organelles and Inclusions. Philadelphia, W. B. Saunders Co., 1966.

Flickinger, C. J., Brown, J. C., Kutchai, H. C., and Ogilvie, J. W.: Medical Cell Biology. Philadelphia, W. B. Saunders Co., 1979.

Ghosh, S.: The nucleolar structure. Int. Rev. Cytol., *44*:1, 1976.

Giese, A. C.: Cell Physiology, ed. 5. Philadelphia, W. B. Saunders Co., 1979.

Gilbert, D.: 10 nm filaments. Nature, *272*:577, 1978.

Goldfischer, S.: Further observations on the peroxidative activities of microbodies (peroxisomes). J. Histochem. Cytochem., *17*:681, 1969.

Hopkins, C. R.: Structure and Function of Cells. Philadelphia, W. B. Saunders Co., 1978.

Ito, S.: The enteric surface coat on cat intestinal microvilli. J. Cell Biol., *27*:475, 1965.

Kessel, R. G.: Fine structure of annulate lamellae. J. Cell Biol., *36*:658, 1968.

Kessel, R. G., and Kardon, R. H.: Tissues and Organs: A Text-Atlas of Scanning Electron Microscopy. San Francisco, W. H. Freeman and Company, 1979.

Kornberg, R. D.: Structure of chromatin. Ann. Rev. Biochem., *46*:931, 1977.

Margolis, R. L., Wilson, L., and Keifer, B. I.: Mitotic mechanism based on intrinsic microtubule behaviour. Nature, *272*:450, 1978.

Maul, G. G.: On the octagonality of the nuclear pore complex. J. Cell Biol., *51*:558, 1971.

Palade, G.: Intracellular aspects of the process of protein secretion. Science, *189*:347, 1975.

Parsons, D. S. (editor): Biological Membranes. Oxford, Clarendon Press, 1975.

Parsons, D. F., and Subjeck, J. R.: The morphology of the polysaccharide coat of mammalian cells. Biochim. Biophys. Acta, *265*:85, 1972.

Reinert, J., and Ursprung, H.: Origin and Continuity of Cell Organelles. New York, Springer-Verlag, 1971.

Singer, S. J., and Nicolson, G. L.: The fluid mosaic model of the structure of cell membranes. Science, *175*:720, 1972.

Skerrow, C. J., and Matoltsy, A. G.: Isolation of epidermal desmosomes. J. Cell Biol., *63*:515, 1974.

Sjöstrand, F. S.: The structure of mitochondrial membranes: A new concept. J. Ultrastr. Res., *64*:217, 1978.

Sorokin, S. P.: Reconstructions of centriole formation and ciliogenesis in mammalian lungs. J. Cell Sci., *3*:207, 1968.

Warner, F. D., and Satir, P.: The structural basis of ciliary bend formation: radial spoke positional changes accompanying microtubule sliding. J. Cell Biol., *63*:35, 1974.

Young, R. W.: The role of the Golgi complex in sulfate metabolism. J. Cell Biol., *57*:175, 1973.

EPITHELIUM

Epithelial tissues are formed by closely apposed cells, with little or no intercellular material between cells, and occur as *membranes* and as *glands*. Membranes are formed by sheets of cells and cover an external surface or line an internal surface. Glands develop from epithelial surfaces by downgrowths into underlying connective tissue and, usually, the connection to the surface remains as the duct of the gland. Such are *exocrine* glands, the secretion passing externally to the surface, but in some cases the surface connection is lost and the gland secretes internally into the vascular system, these being *endocrine* glands.

All epithelia lie upon or are surrounded by a *basal lamina* (see page 117) that separates the epithelium from subjacent connective tissue, blood vessels, and nerves lying in that connective tissue. Functionally, epithelia form the coverings or linings of surfaces, provide secretions from both membranes and glands, and are involved in the process of absorption. A few specialized epithelial cells are contractile (myoepithelial cells) and a few are sensory (neuroepithelia).

MEMBRANES

Most epithelial cells, being packed closely together, are polygonal in outline although they may be highly irregular. In membranes, basically epithelial cells take three forms: *squamous* cells are very flat, with height much less than width, and in profile show a thickening centrally at the site of the nucleus; *cuboidal* cells are boxlike, with height and width approximately equal; and *columnar* cells are much greater in height than in width. Membranes are classified on just two factors: the cell shape and the arrangement into one or more layers. *Simple* epithelia are those with cells in a single layer, all cells contacting the basal lamina and reaching the surface. *Stratified* or compound epithelia are composed of two or more layers of cells, only cells in the deepest layer contacting the basal lamina. *Pseudostratified* epithelia are those in which all cells contact the basal lamina but not all reach the surface. Basically they are formed by a single layer of cells but with several cell types present and, usually, with nuclei at different levels giving the false appearance of several layers. Further classification depends upon cell shape and, in the case of stratified epithelia, this applies only to the surface layer of cells. Thus, there are, for example, simple squamous, simple cuboidal, and simple columnar epithelia and similarly with stratified epithelia; e.g., a stratified squamous epithelium is one formed by several layers of cells, the surface layer of squamous cells. Further subclassification depends on cell type and thus, for example, pseudostratified columnar epithelia may be ciliated or nonciliated. It is not feasible to classify epithelia on the basis of embryological origin, as all three layers — ectoderm, endoderm, and mesoderm — give rise to epithelia.

As cells lie in epithelial membranes, for descriptive purposes the surface adjacent to the lumen is termed the apical surface or pole, that toward the basal lamina the basal surface, and those surfaces between adjacent cells as lateral cell surfaces. There are no blood or

81

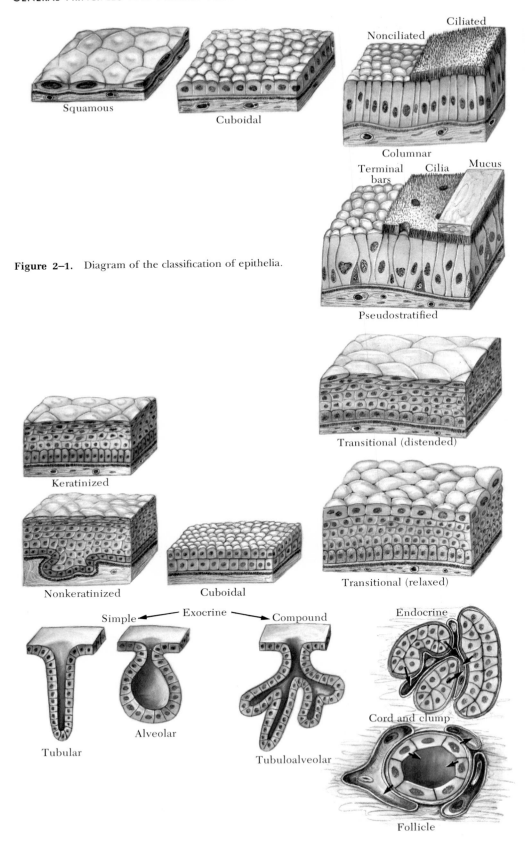

Figure 2–1. Diagram of the classification of epithelia.

lymph vessels in epithelium, nutrition occurring by diffusion of tissue fluid from vessels in the underlying connective tissue. Epithelial cells thus are kept moist mainly by fluid from beneath, although in many cases an epithelial membrane lines a moist cavity, e.g., the digestive tract. Numerous small nerve fibers are located in the connective tissue beneath epithelial membranes, and fine terminal branchings from them may penetrate the basal lamina to run between epithelial cells.

SIMPLE EPITHELIA

Simple Squamous Epithelium

Simple squamous epithelium is composed of very thin, flat cells of irregular outline fitted closely together to form a continuous sheet. From the surface, this epithelium has the appearance of a tiled floor, but with grossly irregular outlines, whereas in section the cells show attenuated cytoplasm with local protuberances where the cytoplasm contains the nuclei. Structurally, this description also includes endothelium lining blood and lymph vessels and mesothelium lining the serous cavities (pleura, pericardium, and peritoneum), these being derived from mesoderm. Other examples of simple squamous epithelium are found

in the parietal layer of Bowman's capsule and the loop of Henle in the kidney, lining pulmonary alveoli, and in the inner and middle ear.

Simple Cuboidal (Cubical) Epithelium

Simple cuboidal (cubical) epithelium is so termed because of its appearance in sections at right angles to the surface of the membrane, each cell appearing box- or cubelike. From the surface, the cells appear as polygons. Such an epithelium is found in many glands, both in secreting units and ducts, and, for example, covering the surface of the ovary.

Simple Columnar Epithelium

Simple nonciliated columnar epithelium has a similar appearance in surface view to the simple cuboidal type, but in perpendicular sections is seen to be composed of tall cells, the nuclei of which usually are all approximately at the same level and situated nearer to the basal than to the apical (luminal) surface. Such an epithelium usually is associated with secretion or absorption and thus is found lining much of the digestive system and the larger ducts of many glands. In such sites, there may be more

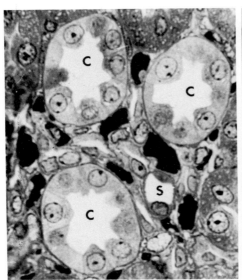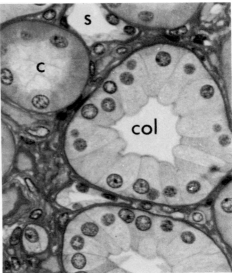

Figure 2–2. Photomicrographs of kidney, plastic sections, showing tubules lined by simple squamous (s), simple cuboidal (c) and simple columnar (col) epithelium. × 550.

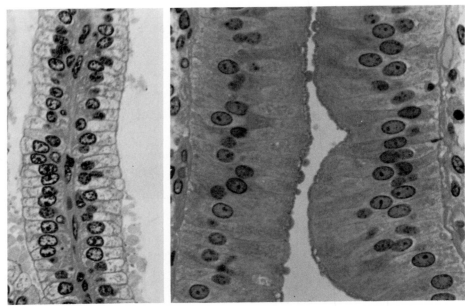

Figure 2–3.   Photomicrographs to illustrate simple columnar epithelium of the seminal vesicle *(left)* and of the gallbladder *(right)*. Plastic sections, both × 400.

than one cell type present; e.g., interspersed among the columnar cells often are mucus-secreting cells which are goblet-shaped. Each "goblet" cell is regarded as a unicellular gland and will be discussed in more detail later.

Simple ciliated columnar epithelium has an appearance identical to simple nonciliated columnar epithelium on low power, but high magnification shows that the free surface of the cells is covered with cilia (see page 97). This type of epithelium lines the uterus and uterine tubes, the ductuli efferentes of the testis, small intrapulmonary bronchi, and the central canal in the spinal cord.

PSEUDOSTRATIFIED EPITHELIA

Pseudostratified columnar epithelium is composed of more than one type of cell with the cell nuclei lying at different levels in a perpendicular section, thus giving the impression that the membrane is composed of more than one layer of cells. Some of the cells may not reach the lumen, although all are adja-

cent to the basal lamina. Such an epithelium lines the larger excretory ducts of many glands and parts of the male urethra. This type of epithelium may be ciliated, usually in association with gob-

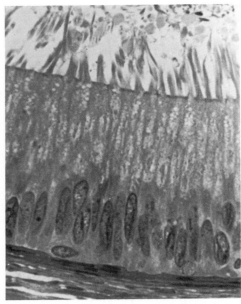

Figure 2–4.   Photomicrograph of pseudostratified epithelium with apical stereocilia, from ductus epididymidis. Plastic section, × 600.

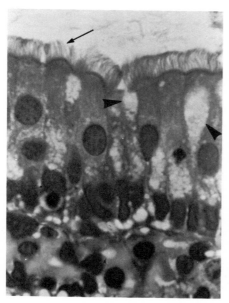

Figure 2–5. Photomicrograph of pseudostratified ciliated columnar epithelium lining the trachea. Nuclei are at various levels, cilia are seen at the apical (luminal) surface (arrow), and parts of goblet (mucous) cells are seen (arrowheads), these being unicellular glands. Plastic section, × 1000.

let cells, and is found lining the larger respiratory passages and some of the excretory ducts of the male reproductive system.

STRATIFIED EPITHELIA

All stratified epithelia can withstand more trauma than the simple types and thus are located in sites where they are subjected to friction and shearing forces, but because of their thickness they are not membranes through which absorption can occur readily.

Stratified Squamous Epithelium

Stratified squamous epithelium is a thick membrane, only the more superficial cells being flat. The deeper layers of cells vary from cuboidal to columnar, and often the basal layer, i.e., that adjacent to the basal lamina, shows considerable irregularity. That covering the cor-

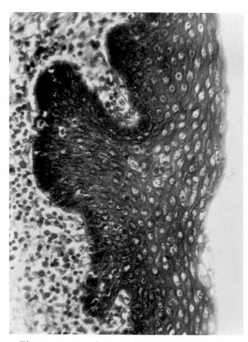
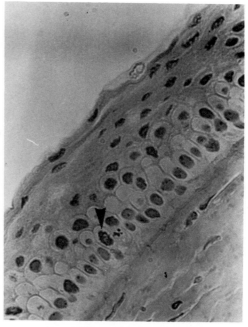

Figure 2–6. Photomicrographs of stratified squamous nonkeratinizing epithelium from the tongue *(left)* and the cornea *(right)*. The underlying connective tissue is irregular and raised into papillae in the tongue but shows a smooth surface in the cornea. Note also the mitotic figure (arrowhead). Left, × 450; right, plastic section, × 800.

nea of the eye lies upon connective tissue with a smooth, regular surface, but in other locations the underlying connective tissue is raised into ridges and folds which appear as finger-like processes (papillae) in perpendicular section. Such an arrangement is found in, for example, the vagina, the esophagus, and the skin. In the vagina and esophagus, the surface of the epithelium is moist, and here the epithelium is nonkeratinized, whereas in the skin the surface is dry, and the surface cells undergo a transformation into a tough, resistant, nonliving layer of material called keratin. Hence the name of stratified squamous keratinizing epithelium. Keratin will be discussed in detail later (see Chapter 10), but it is important to appreciate that this material is resistant to friction, is relatively impervious to bacterial invasion, and is waterproof.

Stratified Cuboidal Epithelium

Stratified cuboidal epithelium is found only in the ducts of sweat glands in the adult and consists of two layers of cuboidal cells. As this type lines a tube, it is obvious that the cells of the superficial layer or layers are smaller as seen in cross section than those of the basal layer.

Stratified Columnar Epithelium

Stratified columnar epithelium also is relatively rare, and usually the basal layer or layers consist of relatively low, irregularly polyhedral cells and only the cells of the superficial layer are of the tall columnar type. Such an epithelium lines part of the male urethra and is found also in some larger excretory ducts.

Transitional Epithelium

Transitional epithelium is so termed because originally it was believed to represent a transition between the stratified squamous nonkeratinizing and stratified columnar types. It is found lining the urinary system from the renal pelvis down to the urethra, sites where it is subject to considerable variations in internal pressure and capacity. Hence

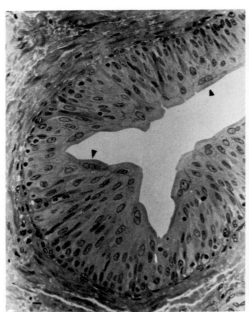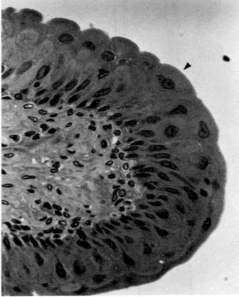

Figure 2–7. Photomicrographs of transitional epithelium lining the uteter *(left)* and the bladder *(right)*. Note convex border of luminal cells, often more darkly staining, and occasional binucleate cells (arrowheads). Plastic sections. Left, × 150; right, × 350.

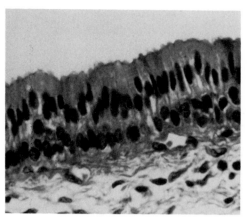

Figure 2–8. Photomicrograph of stratified columnar epithelium from a large lactiferous duct of the mammary gland. × 450.

its appearance varies with the degree of distention. The basal layer is cuboidal or even columnar in type, the intermediate levels are cuboidal and polyhedral, and the superficial layers vary from cuboidal to squamous depending upon the degree of distention. The superficial cells lining a nondistended organ characteristically have a convex free border and are often binucleate; i.e., they exhibit polyploidy.

ENDOTHELIUM, MESOTHELIUM

Endothelium lines all blood and lymph channels and mesothelium is the

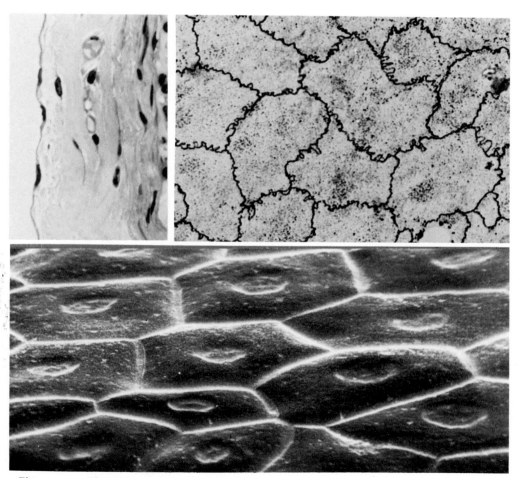

Figure 2–9. Photomicrographs of mesothelium (peritoneum) lining the abdominal cavity. The section *(top left)* shows parts of three cells with their dark flattened nuclei. *Top right:* A surface view with cell outlines made visible by treatment with silver. Left, × 350; right, × 400. *Bottom:* Scanning electron micrograph of simple squamous epithelium. (See also Figure 2–2.) (Courtesy of W. J. Krause.) × 800.

lining of the serous body cavities (pericardial, pleural, and peritoneal). Structurally, both are simple squamous epithelia but they differ in their origin and potentialities, being capable of many functions not shown by ordinary simple squamous epithelium. For example, endothelial and mesothelial cells are actively phagocytic, can form fibroblasts by cell division, and are responsible for a variety of interesting tumors. They formerly were called false epithelia or pseudoepithelia.

CELL ADHESION IN EPITHELIAL MEMBRANES

Within an epithelial membrane and other tissues, there is cell-to-cell adhesion that can resist considerable mechanical forces tending to separate the cells, e.g., in the stratified squamous nonkeratinizing epithelium lining the oral cavity and esophagus where relatively hard food material passes over the surface. As indicated already, spaces between adjacent epithelial cells are narrow, on the order of 15 to 20 nm (150 to 200 Å), and this space is occupied by the glycocalyx of adjacent cells. The binding action of the exposed carbohydrates of these glycoproteins provides some adhesion. The material also contains cations, particularly calcium, which also are important in cell adhesion. In many instances also, plasma membranes of two adjacent cells do not run in parallel fashion but show reciprocal tongues and grooves. These are termed "zipper" or "jigsaw" interlockings. In addition, there are several specializations of the cell surface or junctional specializations. These are found also in tissues other than epithelium, although they are perhaps developed maximally in epithelium, and are concerned not only with cell adhesion but also permit cells to interrelate functionally in several ways.

Cell Junctions

Several different terminologies have been used to describe the various types of specialized junctional regions between cells. In describing them, usually two factors are taken into account: the shape and extent, and the nature or relative closeness of the cell contact. A junction can take the form of a spot of punctate area of limited extent called a *macula,* or it can pass around the entire cell in a belt or corona-like manner called a *zonula* or as a sheet or striplike area called *fascia.* With regard to closeness of contact, if the intercellular space is virtually obliterated with the outer surfaces of the two membranes apparently in contact or even fused, the term *occludens* is used. If the intercellular space is apparent, usually 20 to 25 nm wide, and with dense material both within the space and associated with the cytoplasmic surfaces of the opposed membranes, the term *adherens* or *adhaerens* is used. However, terms other than those described above are in common usage and three main types of junctional specialization will be described.

Tight or Occluding Junction. These usually are in the form of a belt encircling a cell near its terminal or apical border and apparently with fusion of the outer leaflets of the opposed plasma membranes. Thus, a tight junction also may be termed a *zonula occludens.* Often on electron microscopy, a pentalaminar structure is seen, i.e., three dense lines separated by two electron-lucent lines. In fact, the outer leaflets are fused at a series of points only, and freeze-etch material shows a network of linear ridges and complementary grooves, each ridge formed by a double row of particles that are 3 to 4 nm in diameter. These particles probably are integral membrane proteins, one row arising from each adjacent membrane and making contact in an arrangement similar to that of a zipper. Indeed, the ridges appear to extend across the width of both membranes, effectively obliterating the intercellular space. The particles thus form lines of attachment or sealing strands that physically bar the passage of molecules. There is a considerable variation in the number and complexity of sealing strands from tissue to tissue, the more impermeable junctions usually having more strands. Thus, tight junctions reduce or prevent intercellular transport through the intercellular space.

Adhering Junctions. Adherent

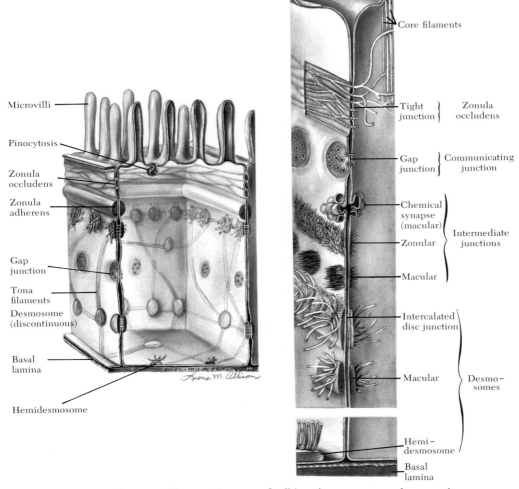

Figure 2–10. Diagram to illustrate the types of cell junctions as seen on electron microscopy.

junctions are concerned with cell attachment, permitting groups of similar cells to function as a structural unit. Two different types are recognized on their form and the associated filamentous material.

The first type forms a band around epithelial cells just to the basal side of a tight junction and is referred to as a *belt desmosome* or *zonula adherens*. Here, the opposed plasma membranes are parallel and the intercellular gap is 15 to 20 nm wide and is filled with fine filamentous material. On the cytoplasmic surfaces of the plasma membranes are filaments running both along the membrane and passing from the junction into the cytoplasm as a flat horizontal band contin-

uous with the terminal web (see later). These filaments are 7 nm in diameter and appear to contain actin, a contractile protein. Zonulae adherentes of epithelia and other tissues, e.g., cardiac muscle, function in mechanical attachment of cells and perhaps, because of their association with actin, transmit forces generated within cells. The suggestion has been made that they close gaps in epithelial membranes that result from death and loss of cells.

The second type of adhering junction is the *spot desmosome* or *macula adherens*. These are small, discoid structures about 410 nm long by 250 nm wide, their long axes perpendicular to the basal lamina in epithelial membranes

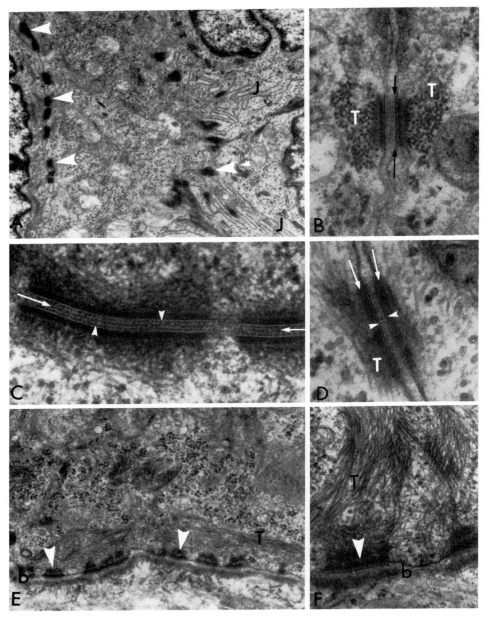

Figure 2–11.   Electron micrographs of spot desmosomes and hemidesmosomes. *A,* In stratum spinosum of epidermis. Note desmosomes (arrowheads) and complex cell interfaces (jig-saw interlocking, J). × 5,000. *B,* Note central stratum (arrows) and associated tonofilaments in transverse section (T). × 88,000. *C,* Extensive desmosome with central stratum (arrows) and thin transmembrane linkers (arrowheads) passing between plasmalemmae. × 100,000. *D,* Desmosome showing transmembrane linkers (arrowheads), dense cytoplasmic plaques (arrows), and associated tonofilaments (T). × 100,000. *E* and *F,* Hemidesmosomes (arrowheads) at base of epidermis in relation to the basal lamina (b). Note associated tonofilaments (T). E, × 20,000; F, × 80,000.

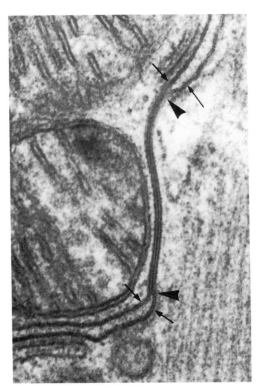

Figure 2–12. Electron micrograph of a gap junction or nexus between two cardiac muscle cells of the rat atrium. Plasmalemmae of adjacent cells (arrows) form an extensive nexus extending between the arrowheads. × 80,000.

the particles probably representing filaments that were broken in the fracturing process. Spot desmosomes are numerous in cells subject to mechanical stress, an indication of their function in cell adhesion.

Hemi- or *half desmosomes* occur on basal surfaces of epithelial cells where mechanical stress occurs, e.g., in cervical epithelium and epidermis. They are morphologically half a spot desmosome joining epithelial cells to the underlying basal lamina and connective tissue. Tonofilament bundles anchor in the hemidesmosomes as they do in normal desmosomes.

Gap Junctions. Gap junctions are concerned with cell-to-cell communication. Here, adjacent plasma membranes are separated by a space of only 2 to 3 nm and in tangential or grazing sections show a hexagonal array of particles of 7 to 9 nm diameter, each particle cylindrical in shape with a central channel. Freeze-etch preparations show that gap junctions vary from discoid, macula-like structures to more extensive beltlike regions. Each plasma membrane contains closely packed particles, each with a central channel, and with the particles in register and meeting in the intercellular space so that the central channels within them are confluent. There is evidence that each particle is composed of 6 subunits, the resulting cylindrical structure being about 7 nm in diameter with a central channel of about 1.5 nm. Since the cylindrical particles, to be compared to short pipes, meet within the intercellular space, it is believed that the channels within them provide a direct route for exchange between cells of molecules such as ions, sugars, amino acids, vitamins, and some hormones. In some tissues, gap junctions transmit electrical impulses, e.g., in the heart and in smooth muscle of the intestine (where they also are referred to as *"nexuses"*). The speed of conduction is virtually instantaneous, which permits synchronization of activity between cells so coupled.

Terminal bars are found on lateral epithelial cell interfaces near the free (luminal) surface and are seen particularly well on light microscopy after staining with iron hematoxylin. In grazing sections near the cell surface or in whole

and found at various levels on lateral cell interfaces. At the desmosome, adjacent plasma membranes are parallel, with an intercellular space of 20 to 30 nm filled with filamentous material and bisected by a linear density termed the "central stratum." Each plasma membrane on its cytoplasmic surface shows a dense plaque into which pass cytoplasmic filaments of 10 nm diameter. These tonofilaments are noncontractile and form a cytoskeleton. Some of them arise deeply in the cytoplasm and loop through the dense plaques of the desmosome; others pass through the plaque but are parallel to the junction. Thinner filaments extend from the adjacent cells into the intercellular space to the central stratum as "transmembrane linkers" to provide a direct mechanical linking between the tonofilament networks of adjacent cells. The freeze-etch technique shows that spot desmosomes are disc shaped and contain particles,

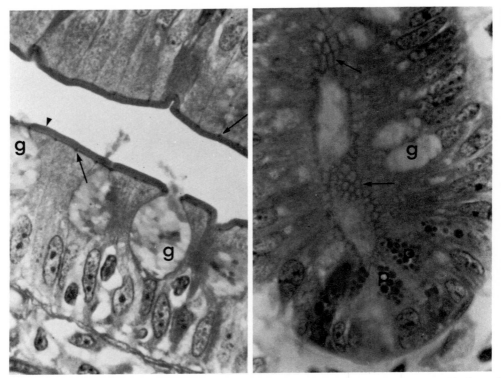

Figure 2–13. Photomicrographs to show terminal bars (arrows) in the simple columnar epithelium of the small intestine, in vertical *(left)* and oblique *(right)* sections. Note also the brush or striated border (arrowhead), goblet (mucous) cells (g), and Paneth cells (p). Plastic sections, both × 1000.

mounts, terminal bars outline cells in a hexagonal pattern (Figure 2–13, right) and are seen as dense dots near the luminal surface in perpendicular sections (Figure 2–13, left). By electron microscopy, the terminal bar shows two of the cell junction specializations. The whole complex usually is referred to as the *junctional complex*. Immediately beneath the free surface, on the lateral interface, is a tight junction or zonula occludens, and, more basally, a zonula adherens, both extending around the entire cell perimeter like a crown. The whole complex covers a depth of up to 0.5 micron (μm). Deep to the zonula adherens, i.e., lying on the lateral cell interfaces closer to the base of the cell, are scattered desmosomes or maculae adherentes, but these are limited in extent and are not part of the junctional complex.

SPECIALIZATIONS OF THE CELL SURFACE IN EPITHELIA

Many of these specializations have been described briefly in Chapter 1. Such specializations are developed to different degrees in different sites, and these will be indicated later during description of the organ systems.

Microvilli

Microvilli are small, slender, finger-like projections of the apical cell surface consisting of tubelike evaginations of the plasma membrane of the apical surface containing a core of cytoplasm. Individually, they are too small to be seen with the light microscope. In many

Text continued on page 96

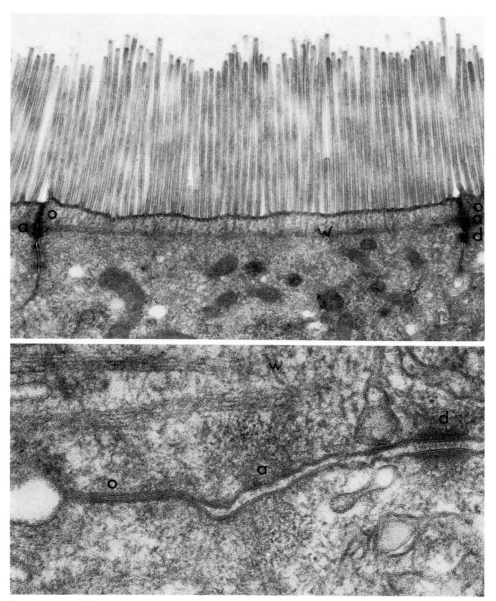

Figure 2–14. Electron micrographs to illustrate the junctional complex in intestinal epithelial cells. *Top:* The apical region of one cell is seen with junctional complexes at right and left borders showing zonula occludens (o) and zonula adherens (a), with a spot desmosome (d). Note apical microvilli of the brush border with cores of filaments passing to the terminal web (w) that continues into zonulae adherentes at the cell periphery. × 17,000. *Bottom:* A higher magnification of a junctional complex. × 110,000. (Courtesy of Dr. B. E. Hull and reproduced by permission of the Editor, The Journal of Cell Biology.)

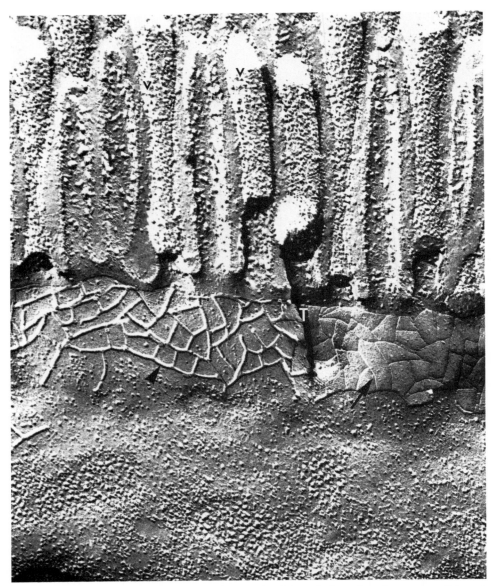

Figure 2–15. A freeze-fracture electron micrograph of the apical portion of mouse small intestinal epithelial cells showing microvilli (v) with a tight junction or zonula occludens below. The fracture shows a fracture face transition (T) and has exposed both faces of the junction: on the left (P face) there is a network of ridges (arrowhead), on the right (E face) a network of furrows (arrow). Direction of shadowing from below. × 108,000. (Courtesy of Dr. S. Bullivant.) (See also Figure 2–14.)

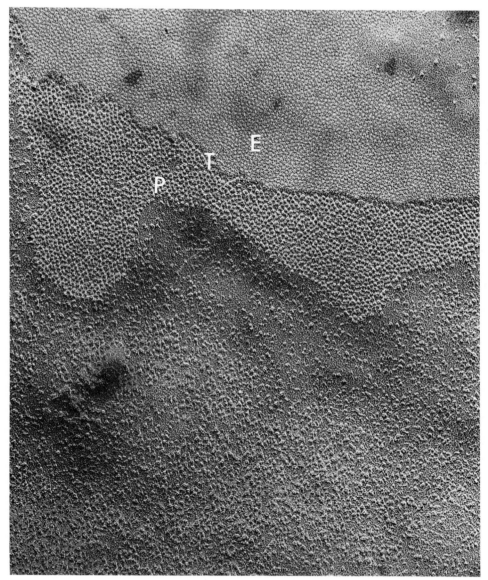

Figure 2–16. A freeze-fracture electron micrograph of an extensive gap junction between mouse liver cells. The polygonal arrangement of pits of the gap junction is seen above (E, or E face), and below a fracture face transition (T) is an area of closely packed particles of the gap junction (P, or P face). The rest of the P face (bottom) is nonjunctional. Direction of shadowing from below. × 108,000. (Courtesy of Dr. S. Bullivant.) (See also Figure 2–12.)

epithelia, particularly high cuboidal and columnar types, they are numerous and of regular dimensions and form a brush or striated border, visible by light microscopy. In such cells there often is a condensation of fibrillar material in the apical cytoplasm extending into the cores of the microvilli and continuous at the circumference of the cell with the fibrillar material of the terminal bar.

This network of fibrils is called the "terminal web." It is evident, for example, in the columnar epithelium of the intestine after staining with the tannic acid, phosphomolybdic acid, and amido black technique.

In epithelial cells lining part of the male generative tract, the so-called *stereocilia* are present on the apical surface (see Figure 2–4). By light microsco-

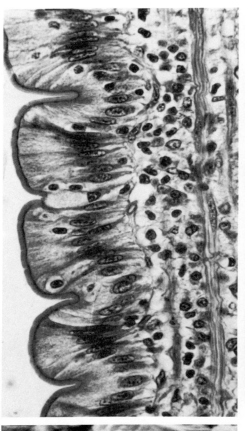

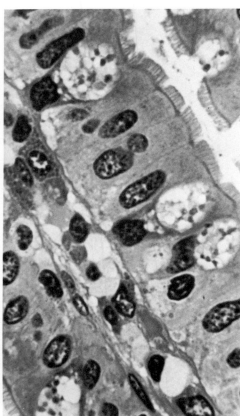

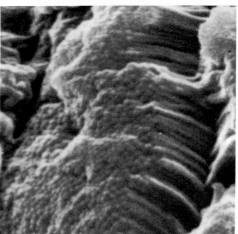

Figure 2–17. Photomicrographs to illustrate the brush or striated border of simple columnar epithelium. The upper sections are both of an intestinal villus with goblet cells (unicellular glands). *Left,* Paraffin section, × 400; *right,* plastic section, × 600. The lower figure shows closely packed microvilli of the brush border of duodenal epithelium as seen on scanning electron microscopy. × 17,000. (Courtesy of W. J. Krause.)

py they appear as long, slender, sometimes branching, processes which are nonmotile. By electron microscopy, it can be demonstrated that stereocilia bear no resemblance to true cilia but are composed of groups of extremely long, slender, often branching microvilli.

Basal Infoldings

At the basal surface of epithelial cells the plasma membrane may show numerous infoldings, thus forming "pockets" of basal cytoplasm. These infoldings are one method of increasing the surface area at the base of a cell, functioning in this respect similarly to microvilli which increase the apical surface area. Indeed, in many epithelial cells, both of these specializations are present, as, for example, in the convoluted tubules of the kidney. Such epithelia show rapid absorption and/or secretion of fluid.

Cilia

Cilia have been described previously (page 48). They project from the free apical surfaces of some epithelial cells and may be very numerous. For example, there are some 270 cilia on each ciliated cell lining the trachea. In movement, each cilium undergoes a rapid forward beat with a slower recovery stroke, the beat appearing as a wave of movement in a ciliated epithelial membrane, transporting material (e.g., mucus) in one direction along the surface of the membrane. The mechanism of cilial beat is not clear, but its direction is associated with the orientation of cilial filaments.

Cilia occur also in the maculae and cristae of the inner ear and in a modified form as retinal rods of the eye; in such sites they appear to be nerve receptors. In other sites single cilia have been considered chemoreceptors. The single flagellum of spermatozoa is of similar structure and, of course, is motile.

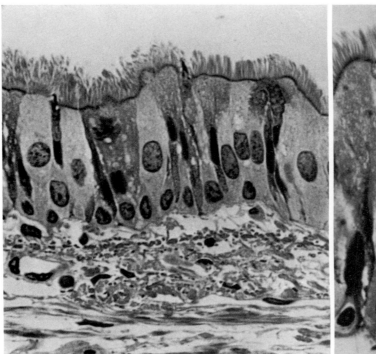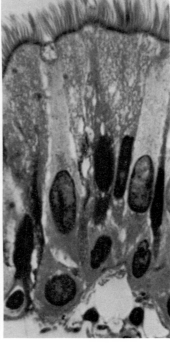

Figure 2–18. Photomicrographs to show pseudostratified, ciliated columnar epithelium of trachea. Plastic sections. Left, × 500; right, × 750.

GLAND EPITHELIUM

As has been noted previously, cells of epithelial membranes in many instances secrete materials in addition to their other functions such as protection and absorption. However, this function of secretion is often of secondary importance in that a cell highly specialized for protection or absorption cannot also be highly specialized for secretion. In addition, the epithelial surfaces of the body are of inadequate surface area to accommodate the numbers of secretory cells required. Thus, a system of multicellular glands is present, each composed of masses of epithelial cells highly specialized for secretion. The secretory product of these cells is passed into a system of tubes or ducts which then transport it to a surface. The glandular secretion consists of an aqueous fluid containing the secretory product, e.g., a hormone, an enzyme, or mucin. This process of synthesis involves interaction of cell organelles and the expenditure of energy.

Classification of Glands

Glands usually are divided into two main groups, exocrine and endocrine. A gland of the exocrine type passes its secretion to a duct system and thus to a body surface; i.e., there is an external secretion. An endocrine gland passes its secretion directly into the blood or into the lymph; i.e., it is an internal secretion or hormone, which is transported throughout the body and thus to the target organ or organs where its actions are performed. Both types of glands develop in the embryo in a similar fashion by an invagination of epithelial cells into the connective tissue underlying an epithelial membrane. In exocrine glands the site of the original invagination persists as the duct system, whereas connection with the epithelial membrane is lost in endocrine glands, the secretion then passing into the vascular system.

In some glands the secretion characteristically contains intact, living cells, e.g., the sex glands, which secrete living germ cells. Three other types of secretory cells are described according to the manner in which their secretory product is elaborated. In some glands the entire secretory cell, having formed and accumulated secretory products within its cytoplasm, dies, disintegrates, and is discharged from the gland as the secretion. Such a gland, where the entire cell is secreted, is called *holocrine*, and obviously cell division in such a gland must be rapid to replace cells lost in secretion. Examples of this type are sebaceous and tarsal glands. In *apocrine* glands the secretory product accumulates in the apical portion of the cell, which is then pinched off, the cell losing some of its apical cytoplasm together with the specific secretory product. The cell then passes through another secretory cycle after a short recovery period. An example of an apocrine gland is the mammary gland. However, in general, electron microscopy studies have failed to demonstrate loss of apical cytoplasm in apocrine glands. Nevertheless, the term is retained. The great majority of glands are of the *merocrine* type whose secretory product is formed in and discharged from the cell without the loss of any cytoplasm. Examples of this type are the salivary glands and pancreas.

Unicellular Glands

Unicellular glands, in which a single cell forms a gland, are represented by mucous or goblet cells, mentioned previously in relation to epithelial membranes. These cells, for example, in the epithelia lining the trachea and the large and small intestines, characteristically resemble a goblet or wine glass in shape, the dilated, oval apical portion being filled with a mass of mucigen droplets which are pale staining in an H and E preparation but which can be stained specifically by other methods. The mucin which is secreted by these cells is a protein-polysaccharide complex that forms mucus in water, mucus being a slimy, lubricating fluid. It should be emphasized that not all mucin-secreting cells are goblet cells. The stomach epithelium, for example, contains three different types of columnar, mucin-secreting cells, none of which is goblet-shaped, and each of which is a little different from the others

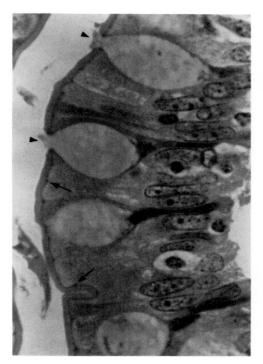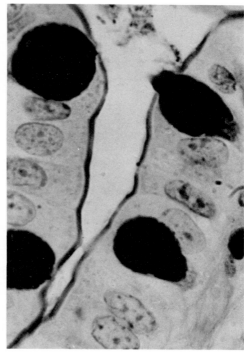

Figure 2–19. Photomicrographs to show unicellular glands (goblet cells) in the simple columnar epithelium lining the intestinal tract. In the right photomicrograph, the brush border and the goblet cells stain positively with the periodic acid–Schiff technique; in the left, note goblet cells discharging mucus at the surface (arrowheads), the brush border, and terminal bars (arrows). Plastic sections. Both × 600.

both in structure and in chemical composition of the mucin secreted.

Multicellular Glands

Multicellular glands are represented most simply by an epithelial sheet composed of secretory cells, but the majority arise as an invagination of an epithelial sheet into underlying connective tissue. Thus, a gland consists of epithelial elements lining its duct system, epithelial elements of the secretory units, and the supporting fibroconnective tissue. The latter contains an extensive network of blood vessels and nerve terminals of the autonomic nervous system. In exocrine glands the epithelial cells of the secretory elements are supported by a basal lamina which separates them from the blood capillaries, but a basal lamina usually is not demonstrable in endocrine glands, e.g., the thyroid.

Exocrine Glands

The various types of multicellular exocrine glands are classified according to whether the duct branches and according to the shape of the secretory unit (tubular, alveolar, or mixed). As indicated in Figure 2–1, the duct may be unbranched or branched, and this distinction provides two large groups of *simple* and *compound* glands. In simple glands the duct may be straight or coiled. The secretory unit situated at the termination of a duct, or a small branch of a duct in a compound gland, may be tubular or flask-shaped, the latter being called alveolar or acinar (like a hollow vessel or like a berry). In many glands the secretory units are mixed and the gland is then termed tubuloalveolar. The nature of the secretion may be either mucous or serous, the latter being a clear, watery fluid usually containing enzymes. The cells responsible for the production of these two types of secretion differ greatly in their appearance. Often both serous and mucous alveoli or acini are found in the same gland, which then is called a mixed gland. An acinus which contains cells of both types is called a mixed acinus. It is by these three characteristics that exocrine glands are classified; thus we describe, for example, simple tubular serous glands and compound alveolar mucous glands.

Connective Tissue Elements. During development of both exocrine and endocrine glands, invagination of cells from an epithelial membrane extends into the connective tissue (mesenchyme) underlying that membrane. This connective tissue forms the fibroconnective tissue capsule and supporting framework of the gland. The amount of such tissue varies, being, for example, relatively profuse and dense in salivary glands but much thinner and finer in the pancreas. From the capsule, septa of connective tissue extend into the center of the gland but are never complete in

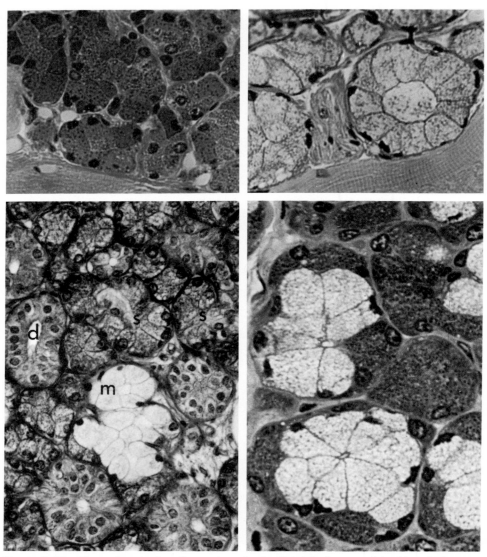

Figure 2–20. Photomicrographs of exocrine glands. *Top left:* Serous acini with apical secretory granules. Plastic section, × 500. *Top right:* Mucous acini with nuclei dark and flattened at the bases of cells. Plastic section, × 500. *Lower left:* A "mixed" gland with serous (s) and mucous (m) acini, and ducts (d). × 500. *Lower right:* "Mixed" acini, i.e., mucous acini with serous crescents or demilunes. Plastic section, × 600.

Myoepithelial cells

Acinus

Intercalated
duct

Intralobular
duct

Interlobular
duct

Lobar duct

Main duct

Lobule

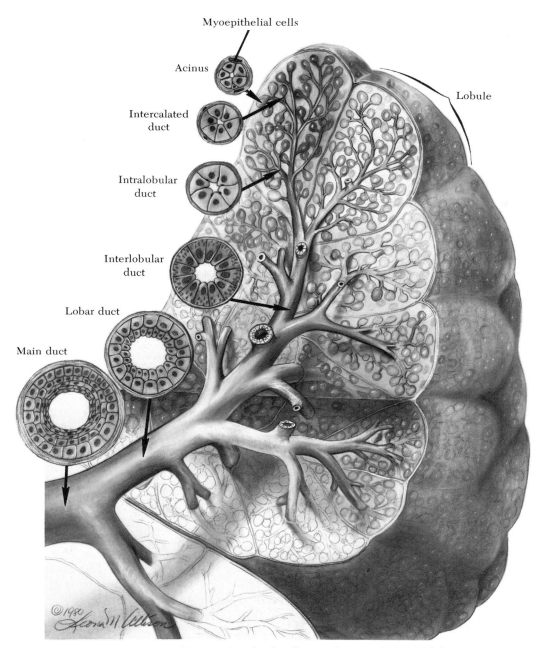

©1980 *Leonard M Allison*

Figure 2–21. Diagram of an exocrine gland to illustrate its organization and duct system.

that they are pierced by blood vessels. The major septa subdivide the glands into lobes, and each lobe is subdivided by finer connective tissue into lobules. The supporting tissue of the lobule is fine reticular connective tissue, containing within its mesh the secretory units and ducts, and connected at the periphery of the lobule to the more substantial fibroconnective tissue surrounding the lobule.

Blood vessels, lymphatics, and nerves are carried in the connective tissue of the gland, entering the gland through its capsule and then being distributed along interlobar and interlobular septa, the small arteries passing from interlobular septa into the lobule where they break up into a capillary network in the intralobular reticular tissue between secretory units.

Epithelial Duct Elements. Usually one major duct supported and surrounded by connective tissue leaves a gland, and, to use an analogy, this is like the trunk of a tree whose branches and twigs are the smaller ducts and whose leaves are the secretory units. The smallest ducts are the intercalary or intercalated ducts, the term indicating that they are inserted between (and therefore connect) secretory units and intralobular ducts. The intralobular ducts are supported by fine reticular connective tissue and are lined by small cuboidal cells, the nuclei of which resemble a necklace of beads when the duct is cut in cross section. Several of these intralobular ducts join to form a larger lobular duct, this also lying between acini, and in turn, several lobular ducts unite to form an interlobular duct which is situated in the fibroconnective tissue of an interlobular septum. At the apex of a lobe, the interlobular ducts of that lobe unite to form a lobar duct, this being surrounded by relatively dense fibroconnective tissue. Finally, the lobar ducts unite to form the (usually) single duct which drains the entire gland and terminates by opening onto a surface.

The epithelium lining the duct system varies from the squamous or low cuboidal type of the intercalated duct through cuboidal and columnar to, usually, stratified columnar or stratified squamous in the main duct. Although the duct epithelium mainly functions as a passive lining of the drainage system of a gland, there is evidence that in many glands it can modify the nature and concentration of the secretion. In passing from smaller to larger ducts (i.e., from twigs to branches of the tree) not only does the lining epithelium become more robust, but the supporting elements of the duct change from fine reticular to fibroconnective tissue, usually with an outer smooth muscle coat, the muscle cells often being arranged in inner circular and outer longitudinal layers.

Glandular Units. As indicated previously, exocrine glands generally are classified into serous, mucous, or mixed glands, each being identified on a histological slide by the appearance of its secretory units. In all instances, the units of a lobule will be cut in different planes, some showing a lumen and occasionally continuity with an intercalated duct, and others appearing as a solid clump of cells, the plane of section having missed the lumen. The following features should serve to distinguish the types of exocrine glands.

Serous Glands. Usually the cytoplasm is darkly staining, being pink or pinkish purple with H and E stain, and somewhat darker toward the cell base. Cell membranes often are not easily defined. Nuclei are regularly spherical or ovoid and situated near, but not at, the base of the cell. In the apical cytoplasm, zymogen (secretory) granules or droplets are present and may be stained specifically. The lumen of the acinus is usually definite and smaller in diameter than that of a mucous acinus. By electron microscopy, an extensive granular endoplasmic reticulum is present in the basal cytoplasm with quite numerous mitochondria scattered throughout the cell. The Golgi apparatus is well developed and situated on the apical side of the nucleus. Zymogen granules of varying density, each surrounded by a single membrane, are present in the apical cytoplasm. In serous cells it is easy to visualize the cycle of secretion as outlined on page 77.

Mucous Glands. The cytoplasm stains much lighter in an H and E preparation and may have a foamy, "motheaten" appearance. Specific stains for mucoprotein, e.g., alcian blue, mucicarmine, and the PAS stain, demonstrate mucous acini well. The nuclei are usually small, dark, and thin and are flattened against the basal plasma membrane of the cells. Normally the lumen is small and irregular. By electron microscopy the cytoplasm usually is seen to be filled with large "mucigen" droplets between which are strands of cytoplasm containing sparse organelles.

Mixed Glands. As explained previously, a mixed gland is one in which both mucous and serous acini are present or one in which component acini contain both mucous and serous cells. In a mixed acinus the majority of cells are the mucous type but to one side is a collection of serous cells arranged in a

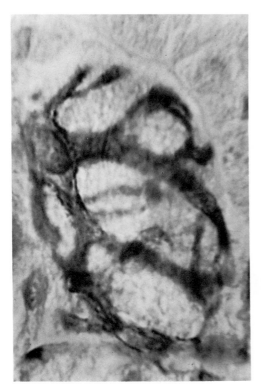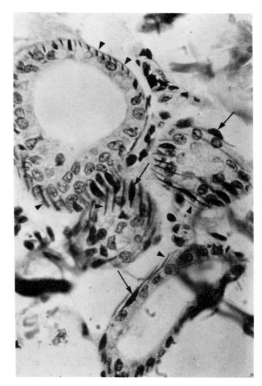

Figure 2–22. Photomicrographs of myoepithelial or "basket" cells. *Left:* A single cell with its nucleus (top left) and cytoplasmic "arms" surrounding a glandular acinus. This cell lies *within* the basal lamina of the acinus. Alkaline phosphatase technique. × 1500. *Right:* Slips or "arms" of cytoplasm (arrowheads) and nuclei (arrows) of myoepithelial cells in relation to ducts of labial mucous glands. × 350.

crescent or half-moon fashion. The cells of these serous demilunes pass their secretion into tiny intercellular canals between adjacent mucous cells and thus into the lumen of the acinus.

Myoepithelial Cells. Each acinus, of whatever type, is surrounded by a fine extracellular basal lamina. Surrounding the acinar cells are the myoepithelial or basket cells, which usually are seen as small dark nuclei surrounded by a small amount of cytoplasm lying just within the basal lamina. From the central mass of cytoplasm containing the nucleus, long thin arms of cytoplasm extend around the cells of the acinus to grasp it rather in the fashion of an octopus or in the form of a basket. These cells, although epithelial in origin, contain fibrillar cytoplasmic elements and show many of the features of smooth muscle cells. They can be clearly demonstrated by the alkaline phosphatase technique.

They are thought to be contractile and thus to aid in expelling secretion from the gland. Myoepithelial cells can be demonstrated also in relation to the smaller ducts of mucous, serous, and mixed glands — for example, around the secretory units of sweat glands.

Endocrine Glands

These will be discussed in detail in a later chapter, but they are much simpler histologically than exocrine glands. Usually they are surrounded by a thin connective tissue capsule from which incomplete septa extend into the glands to divide them into lobes. The main supporting tissue, however, is composed of very fine reticular (connective tissue) fibers associated with a very rich blood capillary or sinusoidal meshwork. Between the fine blood channels are

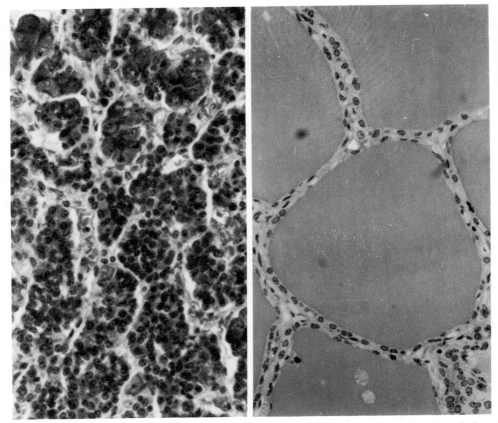

Figure 2–23. Photomicrographs of endocrine glands. *Left,* "Cord and clump" type (anterior pituitary). × 250. *Right,* "Follicle" type (thyroid). × 250.

clumps and cords of epithelial cells which elaborate the specific hormone or hormones of the gland, each cell closely associated with a fine blood vessel into which it passes its secretion. Storage of hormones is intracellular in most cases, but in some glands, the thyroid for example, a group of cells may pass their secretion centrally to form a vesicle or follicle surrounded by the secretory cells. When required, the hormone passes back peripherally through the cells and into blood capillaries situated between follicles.

Many glands are mixed, having both exocrine and endocrine functions. Liver cells not only formulate bile as an exocrine secretion, passing it into a duct system, but also secrete internal secretions directly into the blood system. In other mixed glands, i.e., pancreas, testis, and ovary, one group of cells secretes into a duct system and another group secretes directly into the blood system.

Polarization in Epithelial Cells

Because the majority of materials entering or leaving the body pass through epithelia, there often is within epithelial cells a specific arrangement or *polarization* of cytoplasmic organelles. Nuclei tend to be centrally located, often nearer the basal than the apical surface, with the Golgi apparatus and associated secretory material supranuclear or apical in position. The apical surface itself in many simple epithelia shows microvilli and cilia. Basally, as already indicated, basal infoldings with many mitochondria lying in the cytoplasmic "pockets" between the infoldings are seen commonly in epithelia, e.g., of kidney tubules, that actively pump ions across the epithelium. Granular endoplasmic reticulum is situated primarily in basal cytoplasm and is present as large masses in those cells concerned with protein secretion. In many types of epithelial cells, there exists a complex network of tonofilaments (10 nm filaments) forming a cytoskeleton that, as already explained, is connected to certain types of surface specializations. Apically, fine filaments lie in the cytoplasm and extend into the cores of microvilli, and many of these are of actin, which suggest that they are concerned with subtle changes in cell shape and, perhaps, with movement of the microvilli.

REFERENCES

Bennett, H. S.: Morphological aspects of extracellular polysaccharides. J. Histochem. Cytochem., *11*:2, 1963.

Campbell, R. D., and Campbell, J. H.: Origin and continuity of desmosomes. *In* Origin and Continuity of Cell Organelles, edited by J. Reinert and H. Ursprung. New York, Springer-Verlag, 1971, p. 261.

Claude, P., and Goodenough, D. A.: Fracture faces of zonulae occludentes from "tight" and "leaky" epithelia. J. Cell Biol., *58*:390, 1973.

Farquhar, M. G., and Palade, G. E. Junctional complexes in various epithelia. J. Cell Biol., *17*:375, 1963.

Fawcett, D. W.: Surface specializations of absorbing cells. J. Histochem. Cytochem., *13*:75, 1965.

Gabe, M., and Arvy, L.: Gland cells. *In* The Cell: Biochemistry, Physiology, Morphology, edited by J. Brachet and A. E. Mirsky. New York, Academic Press, 1961, Vol. 5, p. 1.

Hull, B. E., and Staehelin, L. A.: The terminal web. A re-evaluation of its structure and function. J. Cell Biol., *81*:67, 1979.

Leeson, C. R.: Localization of alkaline phosphatase in the submaxillary gland of the rat. Nature, *178*:858, 1956.

Puchtler, H., and Leblond, C. P.: Histochemical analysis of cell membranes and associated structures as seen in the intestinal epithelium. Am. J. Anat., *102*:1, 1958.

Revel, J. P., and Ito, S.: The surface components of cells. *In* The Specificity of Cell Surfaces, edited by B. D. Davis and L. Warren. Englewood Cliffs, N.J., Prentice-Hall, Inc., 1967, pp. 211–234.

Staehelin, L. A., and Hull, B. E.: Junctions between living cells. Sci. Am., *238*:140, 1978.

CHAPTER
3

CONNECTIVE TISSUE PROPER

Early during embryological development, the ectoderm and endoderm become separated by the third germ layer, the mesoderm. The tissue formed by the cells of this layer is known as *mesenchyme* (*mesos*, middle; *enchyma*, infusion), and it is from mesenchyme that the connective tissues of the body develop. These include the connective tissue proper, cartilage, bone, and blood.

Mesenchyme is typically a loose spongy tissue which in early embryonic life is found as packing between structures developing from other germ layers. It is composed of stellate and fusiform cells forming a network and of an amorphous intercellular sub-

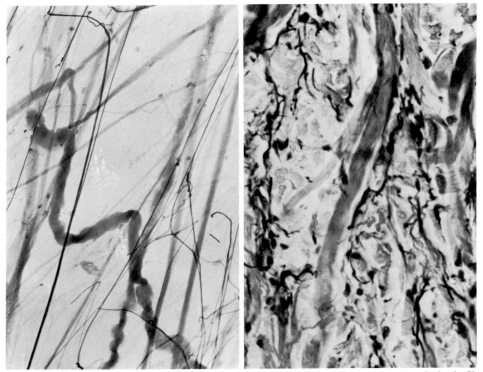

Figure 3–1. *Left:* Photomicrograph to illustrate collagenous fibers (lighter, wavy) and elastic fibers (darker, thinner, straight, and branching) in loose areolar connective tissue. This is a "spread" preparation, not a section, of rat mesentery. × 900. *Right:* Photomicrograph of a section of dense, irregular connective tissue showing elastic (black) and collagen (gray) fibers. × 900.

stance which contains a few scattered fibers.

Mesenchymal cells have multiple developmental potentialities. They are able to differentiate along several different lines to produce many different kinds of connective tissue cells. Thus the tissues which have a common origin from mesenchyme are known as *mesenchymal tissues* or the *connective tissues*.

Connective tissues differ from epithelium by the presence of abundant intercellular material or matrix. Matrix is composed of fibers and an amorphous ground substance. The student should be cognizant of the fact that some authors apply the term "matrix" to ground substance alone. Throughout this text, however, we shall use the term to include both fibers and ground substance, i.e., all intercellular (or extracellular) material. The proportions of cells and intercellular substance show considerable variation and form the basis of classification. The classification is inexact since various types are linked by transitional forms.

In any type of connective tissue there are three elements to consider: the cells, the fibers, and the amorphous ground substance. The elements are bathed in tissue fluid. These elements will be discussed in detail before consideration is given to the features of the various types of connective tissue.

TISSUE FLUID

It is the blood vascular system which is responsible for transporting oxygen and food materials to, and removing waste products from, the cells but it must be appreciated that the great majority of cells are situated external to and some distance removed from blood vessels. Thus it is necessary for oxygen and nutritive materials to leave the blood, pass through the thin walls of small blood vessels called capillaries, and enter the intercellular spaces to reach the cells. Waste materials follow a similar route in the reverse direction. The capillaries have walls which permit the ready passage through them of a watery fluid containing crystalloids, dissolved oxygen, and food materials. This fluid is called *tissue fluid*. The capillary wall, however, permits passage of colloid materials, e.g., protein, less readily or not at all. This filtrate of the blood, the tissue fluid, is formed by simple *diffusion* and occurs at the arterial end of a capillary, i.e., toward the heart. The drainage of tissue fluid back into a capillary is accomplished by *osmosis*, the thin endothelial lining of the blood capillary functioning as a living semipermeable membrane.

In the intercellular spaces, tissue fluid is related to the intercellular substances, and this relationship varies with the type of intercellular material. In tissues where the amorphous type of intercellular substance is in the form of a sol, and fluid or semifluid in nature, it is the tissue fluid which functions as the dispersion medium. In sites where intercellular substance is present in the form of a rigid or semirigid gel, there is a high content of bound water which is obtained from tissue fluid at the time of formation of the intercellular substance. Such a gel is readily permeable because diffusion can occur through the bound water. In sites where the intercellular substance not only is gelled but becomes impermeable because of impregnation with calcium and other salts, e.g., in bone matrix, tiny channels exist in the matrix to permit passage of tissue fluid. Thus cellular metabolism, although dependent on the blood vascular system, occurs by the exchange of material with tissue fluid. Tissue fluid sometimes is called "extracellular fluid" or "intercellular fluid," as opposed to "intracellular fluid" within the cells.

Composition of Tissue Fluid

Tissue fluid contains those constituents of the blood that can diffuse readily through capillary walls. Blood consists of a fluid component, the *plasma*, which is a fluid containing both crystalloids and colloids, and cellular elements. Only the crystalloid component of plasma can diffuse readily through the capillary walls to enter the tissue fluid, the cells and the great majority of the colloids remaining inside the blood vessels. The volume of tissue fluid varies from tissue to tissue and within any tissue there are physiological and pathological variations also. One common pathological condition, *edema*, occurs when there is an increase in the volume of tissue fluid.

Formation

As stated earlier, the capillary wall, consisting only of a single layer of very thin, attenuated, endothelial cells supported by a basal lamina, acts as a semipermeable membrane. If diffusion of tissue fluid through the capillary wall is to occur, there must be a powerful hydrostatic pressure inside the capillary. This pressure, of course, is derived from the heart and although the hydrostatic pressure is comparatively low in a capillary, it is of sufficient magnitude to cause diffusion of fluid through the capillary wall. In spite of the fact that hydrostatic pressure is much greater in the arteries, diffusion of fluid does not occur here due to the thickness of the arterial wall. It is important to appreciate also that hydrostatic pressure decreases along the length of the capillary from arterial to venous end, and thus the formation of tissue fluid occurs mainly at arterial ends of capillaries. In general, veins do not act as a source of tissue fluid because, although there is some hydrostatic pressure, the walls are too thick to allow production of tissue fluid.

Absorption

It is obvious that there must be some mechanism for the absorption of tissue fluid; otherwise, the tissues rapidly would become swollen with excess fluid. There are two mechanisms for absorption and together they balance the rate of formation of tissue fluid.

Capillary Absorption: Osmosis. Osmosis can be defined as the diffusion of water (or fluid) through a membrane in response to a concentration gradient. Crystalloids in solution give a relatively high osmotic pressure to the solution. This means that if such a fluid is separated from a weaker one (e.g., water) by a semipermeable membrane, then the crystalloid solution will exert an os-

motic or "suction" force and attract water through the membrane. Both blood and tissue fluid contain crystalloids and are separated by a semipermeable membrane, viz., the endothelium lining the blood capillary. However, they cause little flow of fluid because the osmotic pressures due to the crystalloid content are approximately equal on both sides and cancel out. Blood does contain, however, more colloids than tissue fluid. Although colloidal solutions have low osmotic pressures, those present in blood are in sufficient quantities to cause a concentration gradient, and tissue fluid will pass through the capillary endothelium into the blood, the endothelial lining permitting the passage of crystalloids but not colloids. The osmotic pressure of the blood colloids, then, attracts tissue fluid into the capillaries, but this force in part is canceled by the hydrostatic pressure of the capillaries which tends to force fluid out. At the arterial end of a capillary, the hydrostatic pressure is greater than the osmotic pressure of the blood, and fluid passes out through the capillary wall to become tissue fluid. At the venous end of a capillary, however, the osmotic pressure exceeds the hydrostatic pressure, and tissue fluid returns through the capillary wall to the blood. This results in a circulation of tissue fluid. The actual mechanism of fluid transport across endothelium lining blood capillaries is discussed in Chapter 8, page 264.

Transport of fluid occurs either between endothelial cells, i.e., at cell interfaces, or across endothelial cytoplasm by a process termed *pinocytosis*. Pinocytosis involves the formation of small pits or caveolae in the plasma membrane which then pinch off to form small vesicles (pinocytotic vesicles) containing fluid. These vesicles pass through the endothelial cytoplasm to reach the opposite cell surface where they fuse with the plasma membrane and release their fluid contents. It is possible that colloids may also be transported via pinocytosis.

Lymphatic Absorption. In most regions of the body there are capillaries which start blindly in the tissues and drain ultimately into the venous system. These are the lymphatic capillaries.

Tissue fluid can pass through the endothelial walls of these lymphatics and, once inside, is called *lymph* and not tissue fluid. These small vessels drain to larger ones which finally open into veins near the heart to return the contained lymph to the vascular system.

There probably is some slight leakage of blood colloids through the endothelium of blood capillaries into tissue spaces. It is important that this colloid be removed or obviously it would retain water in the tissues by its osmotic pressure, upsetting the mechanism of osmosis in capillary absorption described previously. The escaped colloid can pass through the endothelial lining of lymphatic capillaries, and thus is drained from the tissues. The lymphatic capillaries not only regulate the quantity of tissue fluid, but, by removing colloid, also regulate its quality.

Diffusion of fluid into lymphatic capillaries probably occurs both in pinocytosis and by passage of material through endothelial interfaces. The latter mechanism particularly is important in relation to lymphatics of the intestine where small fat particles (chylomicrons) move into lymphatics (called *lacteals*) by passing between endothelial cells (see page 368).

Demonstration of Tissue Fluid

In histological preparations, tissue fluid is removed and therefore cannot be seen as such under the microscope. However, in all organs there are small, empty spaces and slits, and although most of these are caused by shrinkage of tissues in preparation and therefore are artifactual, they do represent to some extent the tissue spaces which in life are occupied by tissue fluid.

INTERCELLULAR SUBSTANCES

These substances have greater strength than the colloidal protoplasm of cells and greater consistency than tissue fluid. They are nonliving and form the matrix or mold in which cells live. Intercellular substances, then, pro-vide the strength and support of tissues and act as a medium for the diffusion of tissue fluid between blood capillaries and cells to permit cellular metabolism. They also have an important role in tissue differentiation. From these functions listed, it is an obvious deduction that the intercellular substances are widely distributed throughout all tissues of the body.

There are two main types of intercellular substances, fibrous (formed) and amorphous (nonformed).

Fibrous Intercellular Substances

The function of providing strength and support for tissues is performed mainly by the fibrous intercellular substances, which include three types of fibers — collagenous, reticular, and elastic — distinguished by their appearance and chemical reactions. All are complex proteins formed by long chains of amino acids with peptide linkages, i.e., polypeptide chains, and all are comparatively insoluble in neutral solvents, which explains their ability to exist as formed fibers in the fluid internal environment of the body. The characteristics of each type of fiber will be considered in more detail later in this chapter.

Amorphous Intercellular Substances

Some of the amorphous intercellular substances are in the form of stiff gels and thus help to provide strength and support for tissues, but their main function is that of providing a medium through which tissue fluid containing nutrients and waste products can diffuse between cells and capillaries. Amorphous intercellular materials, in the form of sols and gels, permit such a diffusion from capillaries to cells and from cells to capillaries much more readily than do the fibrous kinds, which are embedded in the amorphous materials. Usually two kinds of amorphous material are recognized: *ground substance*, which is relatively soft, and *cement substance*, which is firmer. These materials are formed by connective tissue cells and contain some protein, including collagen in molecular dispersion, glycoproteins, mucopolysaccharides, carbohydrates, lipid, and water. Glycoproteins are polysaccharide-protein complexes, and mucopolysaccharides* are polysaccharides with one or more amino-sugar moieties, such as hyaluronic acid and chondroitin sulfuric acid. Many of these molecules are long, branching polymers which form branching, three-dimensional networks for strength and support and have many hydrophilic groups which account for the water-binding properties of amorphous intercellular substance. In addition, they may function as selective barriers to the diffusion of inorganic ions and charged molecules.

Hyaluronic acid is a viscous, fluidlike mucopolysaccharide found in the connective tissue of most organs, Wharton's jelly of the umbilical cord, synovial fluid, and humors of the eye. It readily binds water, i.e., becomes hydrated, and is responsible for changes in the viscosity and permeability of ground substance, thus having an important influence on the exchange of material between tissue cells and blood plasma. The enzyme hyaluronidase hydrolyzes it, reducing its viscosity, and thus increases permeability of the tissue. Chondroitin sulfuric acid is found in cartilage and bone matrix, in the aorta and heart valves, in the cornea of the eye and in the umbilical cord, and, as mentioned previously, is sulfated.

Amorphous intercellular substance has the same refractive index as water and thus is invisible in fresh preparations but can be seen in tissue spreads mounted in a medium of different refractive index, e.g., serum or a sugar solution. Generally, the ground substances, particularly chondroitin sulfuric acid, stain more readily, if somewhat erratically, with hematoxylin. Both types of mucopolysaccharide stain

metachromatically, for example, with a dilute solution of toluidine blue.

Fibrous Intercellular Substances

Collagenous Fibers. Collagenic or collagenous fibers are found in all types of connective tissue and consist of the protein collagen. They are extremely tough and in bulk in the fresh state (e.g., in tendons) appear white, and hence also are termed "white" fibers.

Collagenous fibers vary from 1 to 12 microns (μm) in diameter, although several fibers may be collected together to form a bundle of greater size. Within a bundle, fibers are held together by a small amount of amorphous cement substance (mucoprotein). The fibers have a straight or slightly wavy course, are of indeterminate length, and may be loosely or densely packed, depending upon location and functional need. In the fresh state, collagenous fibers are soft and flexible, relatively inelastic, and of high tensile strength. The fibers are transparent and homogeneous but show a faint longitudinal striation. In tissue sections, collagenous fibers are eosinophil and are stained red by Van Gieson's picrofuchsin, blue-purple by the aniline blue of Mallory's connective tissue stain, and green by Masson's trichrome. They are birefringent under polarized light, indicating a longitudinal orientation of subunits or *fibrils*. The fibers may branch and recombine owing to the interchange of clusters of fibrils between one fiber and another.

The finest strand of collagen visible by light microscopy is the *fibril*, about 0.3 to 0.5 micron (μm) thick. As indicated above, a fiber is composed of the parallel aggregation of several fibrils. In turn, a fibril is composed of still smaller units of a diameter from 450 to 1000 Å (45 to 100 nm), averaging 650 Å (65 nm). These are the *microfibrils* or *unit fibers* of collagen. Newly formed microfibrils are only about 200 Å (20 nm) in diameter, and there is evidence that they increase in size with age, although in certain areas of the body the microfibrils show a uniform diameter throughout life. The microfibrils are visible only with the electron micro-

---

Mucopolysaccharides is a term that has been used widely and rather loosely in the past and at present is being replaced by the more precise term *glycosaminoglycans* (polysaccharides that contain amino sugars). Students should be aware that they may encounter both terminologies in their reading of the literature.

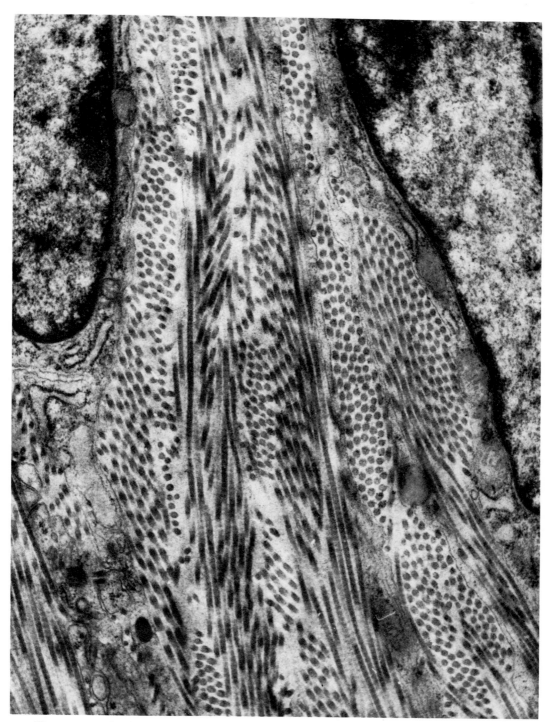

Figure 3–2. Electron micrograph of portions of two fibroblasts and collagenous fibrils in the dense connective tissue of the epididymis. × 40,000.

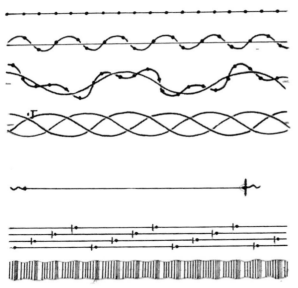

Molecular chain of aminoacids

Single chain molecular helix

Single chain coiled helix

Triple chain coiled helix

forming a

Tropocollagen molecule

Tropocollagen molecules

forming a

Collagen microfibril

(Unit fiber)

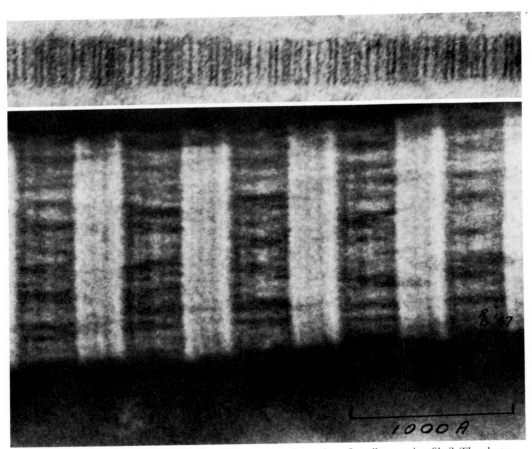

Figure 3–3. The diagrams (after Gross) illustrate the formation of a collagen microfibril. The electron micrograph *(center)* is of a single collagen microfibril stained positively with uranyl acetate. × 185,000. The lowest micrograph is a single microfibril stained negatively by phosphotungstic acid. × 430,000. (Photograph courtesy of Dr. R. Borasky.)

scope and show a characteristic cross-banding with a major periodicity of 640 Å (64 nm). Between the major bands are several finer bands.

Collagenous material in boiling water becomes hydrated and softens, forming gelatin. The fibers can be digested by pepsin in acid solution and by the enzyme collagenase. After treatment with salts of heavy metals or tannic acid, collagen forms an insoluble product, this being the basis of the "tanning" process in the preparation of animal hides (leather) which consist chiefly of collagen.

After treatment with dilute acids and alkalis, collagen fibrils swell and disintegrate into fibrillar units or macromolecules of *tropocollagen*,* each 14 Å (1.4 nm) wide and 2800 Å (280 nm) long. The tropocollagen molecule in turn is composed of three polypeptide chains, twisted around each other to form a right-handed superhelix. Each individual polypeptide chain is formed by about a thousand amino acids linked together and twisted into a left-handed helix or spiral. Collagen is rich in proline, glycine, hydroxyproline, and hydroxylysine, the latter also forming strong cross-links between adjacent tropocollagen molecules within a microfibril. In a microfibril, tropocollagen molecules lie end to end in parallel chains or rows, all molecules facing the same direction, and between rows there is an overlap of one-quarter of the length of the tropocollagen molecule. The 640 Å major periodicity is caused by this 25 per cent overlap (four times 640 is 2560, approximately the length of a tropocollagen molecule).

In connective tissues, collagen is formed and maintained by cells called *fibroblasts* (see page 118), although other cells also form it, e.g., chrondroblasts, osteoblasts, and odontoblasts. Amino acids and polypeptides of the tropocollagen molecule are formed and assembled on ribosomes, passed into cisternae of the endoplasmic reticulum and then to the Golgi apparatus where glycoprotein probably is added. The material then moves to the cell surface where tropocollagen units are released

and polymerized into fine threads of 40 × 7000 Å (4 × 700 nm). These filaments show nodules at intervals of 640 Å (64 nm).

The filaments act as templates for the further polymerization of tropocollagen and by aggregation become immature or thin microfibrils and then adult microfibrils with the characteristic periodicity and size.

In summary, the tropocollagen molecule, consisting of three polypeptide chains arranged in a superhelix, is synthesized within the fibroblast and is released at the cell surface where tropocollagen molecules polymerize to form procollagen filaments. With the addition of more tropocollagen molecules, the procollagen filament grows in length and diameter to form the microfibril, visible only on electron microscopy. Parallel aggregation of microfibrils forms fibrils, visible by light microscopy, and fibrils aggregate in bundles to form fibers.

Recent detailed studies on the molecular organization of collagen have shown that the polypeptide chains of tropocollagen can be separated into two classes, alpha-1 and alpha-2, which differ in their amino acid sequences. Additionally, several types of alpha-1 chains, differing slightly in their amino acid composition, are known to exist in different locations in the body. In most regions, including tendon and skin, the tropocollagen molecule consists of two alpha-1 type I chains and one alpha-2 chain. In cartilage, however, each tropocollagen molecule is composed of three alpha-1 type II chains.

In addition to the microfibril with the periodicity of 640 Å (64 nm) characteristic of native collagen, collagen can exist also in a long-spacing form with a periodicity of about 2400 Å (240 nm). There are two varieties of this: the fibrous long-spacing (FLS) form found in the trabecular meshwork of the eye and aging cartilage, and the segment long-spacing (SLS) type. Each type can be dissolved readily and reprecipitated into either of the other two forms. FLS collagen is formed by rows of tropocollagen units lying end-to-end in parallel-antiparallel array without overlap, and SLS collagen is formed by lateral and lengthwise aggregation of similar units.

---

*Tropocollagen is a term derived from the Greek *tropos*, turning, i.e., turning into collagen.

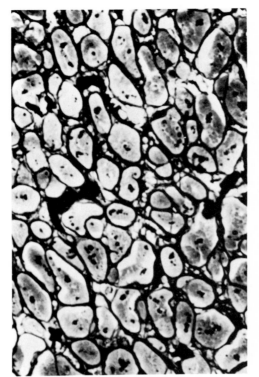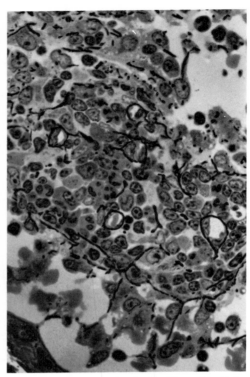

Figure 3–4. Silver staining of reticular fibers. *Left:* photomicrograph of reticular fibers (black) in cardiac muscle (unstained). Each muscle fiber is surrounded by a close network of reticular fibers. ×450. *Right:* section of a portion of a lymph node. Delicate reticular fibers form a loose network in relation to lymphoid cells. Plastic section. × 400.

Reticular Fibers. Reticular fibers are of small diameter and branch to form a netlike supporting framework or reticulum. They occur as fine networks around small blood vessels, muscle fibers, nerve fibers, and fat cells, in the fine partitions of the lung and, particularly, at boundaries between connective tissue and other types of tissue. Beneath epithelial membranes, for example, reticular fibers form dense networks as components of basal laminae. They also are found in myeloid and lymphoid tissues in association with reticular cells (see page 176). Reticular fibers are continuous with collagenous fibers, and there appears to be a gradual transition from one to the other. They are not seen easily in H and E sections but can be demonstrated by silver impregnation methods, e.g., Bielschowsky's method, when they become visible as thin dark lines, collagenous fibers being colored yellow or brown. The coloration of reti- cular fibers by silver impregnation has led to the term "argyrophil." They stain more darkly with the PAS technique (see below) than do collagenous fibers, and are not birefringent, but on elec- tron microscopy show the periodicity of 640 Å (64 nm) characteristic of collagen- ous fibers. The staining differences be- tween the two types may be due to physical size, for reticular fibers usually are of smaller diameter, or may be de- pendent upon differences in the amor- phous intercellular material that sur- rounds individual fibers.

Elastic Fibers. Elastic fibers are present in loose fibrous connective tis- sue and are seen as long, thin, highly refractile, cylindrical threads or flat rib- bons, ranging in size from less than a micron to 4 microns (μm) in diameter, although in some elastic ligaments they may reach a diameter of 10 to 12 mi- crons (μm). In contrast to collagenous fibers, by light microscopy they appear

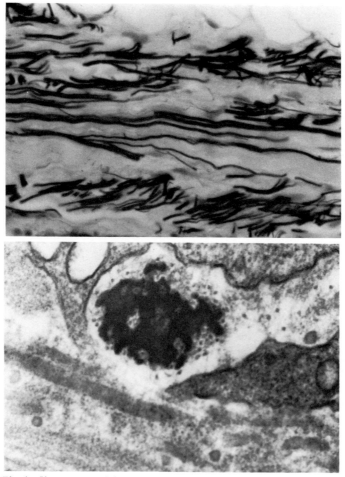

Figure 3–5. Elastic fibers. *Top:* Light photomicrograph of elastic fibers in loose connective tissue. Weigert's stain. × 250. *Bottom:* Electron micrograph of transverse section of an elastic fiber, showing the amorphous central component surrounded by groups of microfibrils. × 55,000.

homogeneous and not fibrillar in nature. They may form extensive, perforated sheets, e.g., around blood vessels. In the fresh state adult elastic tissue in bulk has a yellowish color. Elastic fibers stain erratically with eosin but can be stained selectively with orcein (brown) and resorcin-fuchsin (dark blue-purple). If fresh tissue is treated with dilute acid solutions, collagen fibers swell and become transparent, but elastic fibers become visible as highly refractile, homogeneous, shining threads.

Elastic fibers are composed of the albuminoid elastin which shows a remarkable resistance to most agents. It is not affected by hot or cold water or by dilute solutions of acids or alkalis but is digested enzymatically by pancreatin. As indicated by the name, elastic fibers yield easily to stretching and return to their former length when tension is released.

On electron microscopy, elastic fibers show two components. The *microfibrils* are 130 Å (13 nm) in diameter and tubular with a light central core. They may show an indistinct segmentation and usually are found in parallel array. The *amorphous component* usually lies centrally in a mass of elastic material and is surrounded by groups of micro-

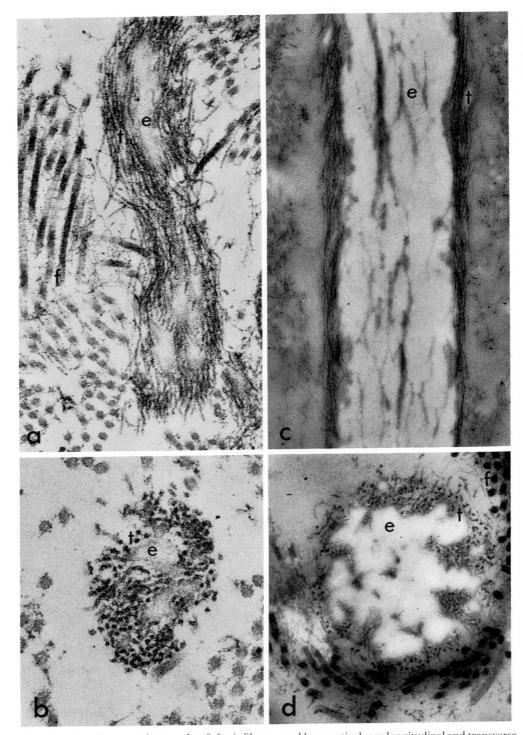

Figure 3–6.   Electron micrographs of elastic fibers; *a* and *b* respectively are longitudinal and transverse sections from the ligamentum nuchae of a three-month fetal calf, and *c* and *d* from a calf at term (nine months). Note the tubular fibrils (t) surrounding a core of amorphous material (e). With increasing age the amorphous component increases in amount. There is evidence that the central amorphous component is elastin, the tubular fibrils being an as yet unidentified protein. Unit fibrils of collagen (f) also are present. *a,* × 50,000; *b,* × 80,000; *c,* × 25,000; *d,* × 45,000. (Courtesy of Russell Ross.)

fibrils. In embryonic tissues, the microfibrils appear first, synthesized by fibroblasts and smooth muscle cells, and later small clumps of amorphous material are formed within the groups of microfibrils. With age, the microfibrils are reduced in number and the amorphous component increases. The amorphous component chemically is elastin, while the microfibrils consist of a connective tissue protein that is neither collagen nor elastin, being rich in hydroxyproline.

The Periodic Acid–Schiff Reaction in Connective Tissue. Collagenous and elastic fibers in general are colored only faintly by the PAS technique, whereas reticular fibers are strongly positive. The Schiff reagent, as explained in the Introduction, is basic fuchsin which has been bleached with sulfurous acid. In the presence of free aldehyde, the magenta (pink-purple) color of unbleached basic fuchsin is produced. Periodic acid is an oxidizing agent and can be used on tissue sections to produce aldehydes from polysaccharides. In the PAS technique, tissue sections are exposed to periodic acid which forms aldehydes from polysaccharides, and the sections then are treated with the Schiff reagent which colors the sites

of aldehyde production magenta. The PAS technique is a good method for the demonstration of the polysaccharide glycogen, and it might be expected that all connective tissue mucopolysaccharides also would give a positive reaction. However, recent studies have indicated that both pure hyaluronic acid and purified chondroitin sulfate are PAS negative. The positive reaction of reticular fibers presumably is due to the presence of sugars intimately associated with the fibers.

Basal Laminae. Basal laminae are sheets of extracellular material present under the basal surface of epithelial cells, around muscles, nerves, capillaries, and fat cells, and situated between these elements and the underlying or surrounding connective tissue. Thus, they are distributed widely, and in many organs, the connective tissue elements virtually are limited by basal laminae.

Basal laminae vary in thickness, are rich in mucopolysaccharides, and have a high content of collagen. They stain intensely with the PAS and silver techniques but are poorly demonstrated in H and E preparations. On electron microscopy, the basal lamina appears as a dense layer composed of fine fibrillar

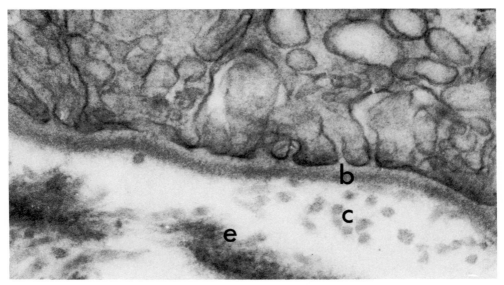

Figure 3–7. Electron micrograph showing the bases of epithelial cells above, beneath which is the basal lamina (b), microfibrils of collagen (reticular fibers) (c), and some elastin (e). × 80,000.

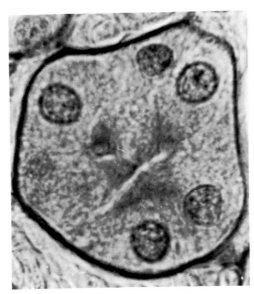

Figure 3–8. Photomicrograph of a cross section of a renal tubule lined by low columnar epithelium to illustrate the homogeneous basement membrane (dark) surrounding the tubule. PAS stain. × 1500.

material 40 Å (4 nm) in diameter arranged in a feltwork, usually 300 to 700 Å thick, but extending in certain regions to 3000 Å or more. On its external, or connective tissue space, side, it blends with fine reticular fibers and microfibrils of collagen, often also with some elastic material. On the other, cellular, side, there usually is a thin, electron-lucid zone separating the lamina from the cellular elements, and this is occupied by the glycocalyx or cell coat (glycoprotein) of the cell. All three elements — basal lamina, reticular fibers, and ground substance — constitute the *basement membrane* seen with the light microscope. Although the terms lamina and basement membrane commonly are used synonymously, this practice does not distinguish between these two different structures. Further, the use of the latter term leads to confusion with membranes that are components of cells. Principally for these reasons, the term basement membrane is used less frequently today.

The PAS technique probably stains the basal lamina itself, the glycolcalyx (cellular) zone, and reticular fibers on the connective tissue surface. The fine fibrillar material probably is collagen.

Basal laminae are synthesized by the related cells and act as diffusion barriers to rapid ion exchanges, selectively changing molecular and ionic diffusion rates. They also provide for a strong connection between epithelia and underlying connective tissue, and between muscle and connective tissue, by the intermingling of fibrillar elements between basal laminae and connective tissue.

CONNECTIVE TISSUE CELLS

The description of the cells is based upon their appearance in areolar (loose) connective tissue, which is the chief "packing" material in the adult, and which may be considered as the prototype of the connective tissues. It must be appreciated that some of the cell types present in connective tissue are also found in the circulating blood and lymph since there is a dynamic equilibrium between connective tissue proper and these specialized connective tissues.

Fibroblasts

These are one of the two most numerous cells of areolar connective tissue, the other being *macrophages* (or *histiocytes*). Fibroblasts, as their name suggests, are considered to be responsible for the formation of the fibers and also are thought to elaborate most, if not all, of the amorphous component of the matrix. They are large, flat, branching cells which appear fusiform or spindle-shaped in profile. The branching processes are slender. The nucleus is oval or elongated and has a delicate nuclear membrane, one or two distinct nucleoli, and a small amount of finely granular chromatin. In connective tissue spreads the nucleus appears pale, but in sectioned material it usually appears shrunken and deeply stained with basic dyes. In most histological preparations the outlines of the cells are indistinct, and the nuclear characteristics are of considerable value in identification. In young fibroblasts, which are actively engaged in protein synthesis for the production of intercellular substance, the cytoplasm ap-

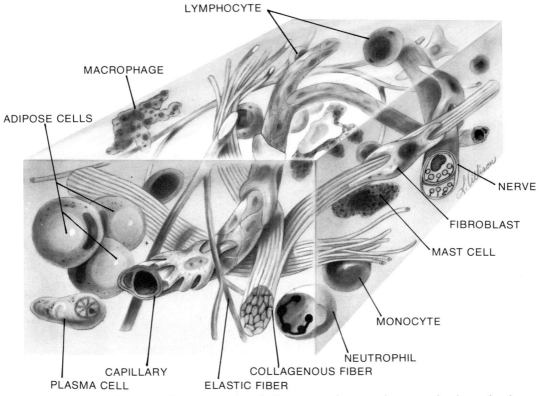

LYMPHOCYTE

MACROPHAGE

ADIPOSE CELLS

NERVE

FIBROBLAST

MAST CELL

MONOCYTE

NEUTROPHIL

CAPILLARY

COLLAGENOUS FIBER

PLASMA CELL

ELASTIC FIBER

Figure 3–9. A diagrammatic representation of subcutaneous, loose areolar connective tissue, showing the characteristic cell and fiber types.

pears relatively homogeneous and is basophilic because of the high concentration of granular endoplasmic reticulum. After suitable staining, mitochondria appear as slender rods and are most numerous near the nucleus, where the Golgi apparatus also is located. In old and relatively inactive fibroblasts, the cytoplasm is sparse and only weakly basophilic since the endoplasmic reticulum is scanty. Such mature and relatively inactive fibroblasts are sometimes called *fibrocytes*.

Fibroblasts are regarded as fixed cells of connective tissue but they retain throughout adult life a capacity for growth and regeneration, and when stimulated, as on the periphery of healing wounds or in inflamed tissues, they are capable of a slow gliding movement. The increased number of fibroblasts that are present in a wound may be due to the fact that fibroblasts themselves are capable of acting as stem cells. Some authors, however, believe

that in such situations, although fibroblasts are of local origin, they arise from cells somewhat less differentiated than themselves.

Undifferentiated Mesenchymal Cells

Some embryonic cells are thought to persist in the adult. They are difficult to distinguish from active fibroblasts but in general are smaller. Whereas fibroblasts are seen usually in close association with collagen fibers, undifferentiated mesenchymal cells often are located along the walls of blood vessels, particularly capillaries, where they are referred to as *perivascular cells.* Their recognition comes not with the microscope but from numerous observations of their responses to certain stimuli, when they are capable of differentiation either into the normal cell types found within loose connective tissue or

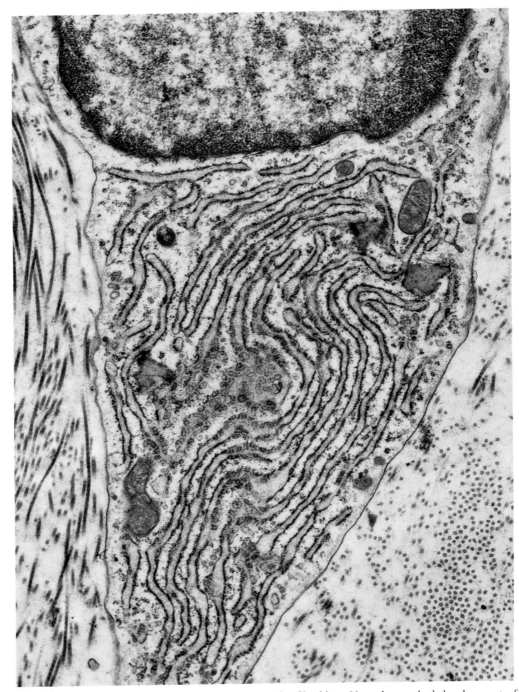

Figure 3–10.   Electron micrograph of a portion of a fibroblast. Note the marked development of granular endoplasmic reticulum within the cytoplasm and the close association of collagenous fibrils with the cell membrane. × 35,000. (Courtesy of Russell Ross.)

into other cell types such as smooth muscle cells following injury to blood vessels. Many investigators consider these cells, rather than fibroblasts, to be the precursors of adipose cells. Probably they should be considered pluripotential cells, similar in many respects to the primitive reticular cells of blood-forming tissue (see Chapter 5).

Macrophages

Often termed histiocytes, macrophages are almost as numerous as fibroblasts in loose connective tissue and are most abundant in richly vascularized areas. They may be either attached to the fibers of the matrix ("fixed" or "resting" macrophages) or free within the matrix (free wandering cells). Generally they are irregularly shaped cells with processes which usually are short and blunt. Occasionally they may exhibit long, slender branching processes. When stimulated, macrophages are capable of ameboid movement and in this phase they are very irregular in outline with pseudopodia extending in numerous directions. The nucleus is ovoid, sometimes indented, and smaller and more heterochromatic than that of the fibroblast. Nucleoli are not conspicuous. The cytoplasm stains darkly and may contain a few small vacuoles which stain supravitally with neutral red. These cells, when they are activated, can be distinguished readily from fibroblasts, owing to their ability to ingest particulate matter. Then the cells appear much larger and the cytoplasm is filled with granules and vacuoles containing ingested material. Sections of tissue from animals which have received injections vitally of colloidal carbon or of colloidal dyes such as trypan blue show macrophages with accumulations of the dye within vacuoles in the cytoplasm. Fibroblasts contain little or none of the dye.

Macrophages are important agents of defense. Because of their mobility and phagocytic activity, they are able to act as scavengers, engulfing extravasated blood cells, dead cells, bacteria, and foreign bodies. During phagocytosis, there is an uptake of particulate matter

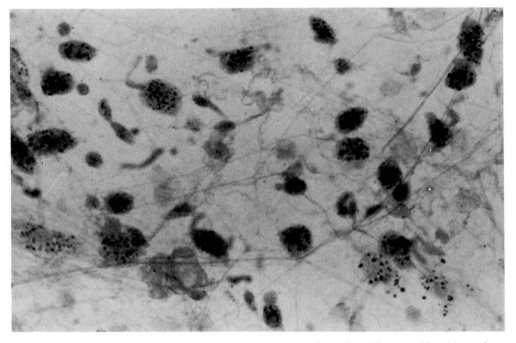

Figure 3–11. A spread preparation of rat omentum after vital staining with trypan blue. Macrophages contain numerous particles of ingested dye. × 425.

by an invagination of the cell membrane. Once the phagocytosed particle, enclosed within the invaginated cell membrane, becomes detached and moves away from the cell surface into the cytoplasm, it is referred to as a *phagosome*. Ingested organic material is destroyed by the action of intracellular proteolytic enzymes, derived from primary lysosomes. The latter fuse with phagosomes to form secondary lysosomes which later, as lysis proceeds, become *residual bodies*. Inert foreign matter which resists digestion may remain in the cytoplasm indefinitely. An example of the latter is the inhaled carbon particles which accumulate within macrophages of the lung.

Macrophages also contribute to the immunological reactions of the body. They ingest, process, and store antigens and pass specific information to neighboring immunologically competent cells (lymphocytes and plasma cells). They are a component of the macrophage system, which will be discussed in more detail on page 134. When macrophages encounter large foreign bodies, they eventually fuse together to form *multinucleated foreign body giant cells*.

Fat Cells

These conspicuous cells are a normal component of areolar tissue. They occur singly or in clumps along small blood vessels. If they accumulate in large numbers, the tissue is transformed into *adipose tissue*. In fresh tissue they appear as glistening droplets of oil surrounded by an exceedingly thin rim of cytoplasm. Each fat cell contains a single large droplet of oil, and the thin rim of cytoplasm contains in one area the flattened nucleus. In fresh or formalin-fixed tissue the fat droplet can be stained with osmic acid or with Sudan dyes, but in most histological preparations the lipid has been extracted, leaving only the delicate protoplasmic envelope. Individual cells are surrounded by a fine network of reticular (argyrophil) fibers.

Fat cells are fully differentiated cells and are incapable of mitotic division. New fat cells therefore, which may de-

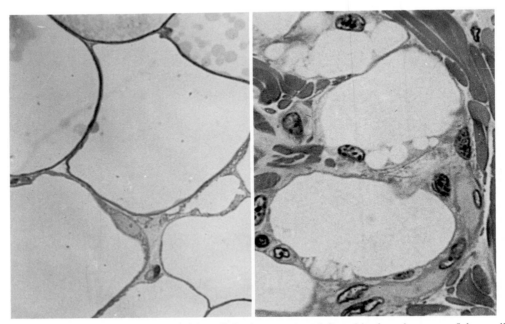

Figure 3–12. Photomicrographs of fat cells in the omentum *(left)* and in the submucosa of the small intenstine *(right)*. In the left figure, note the nucleus and the thin rim of cytoplasm surrounding the large fat globule, which has been dissolved in preparation. In the right figure, fat cells appear less mature in that each contains a few small droplets which have yet to coalesce with the single large droplet. Plastic sections. Left, × 650; right, × 600.

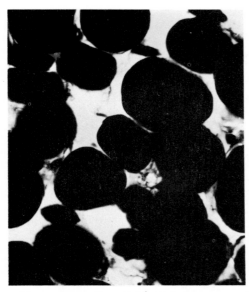

Figure 3–13. Fat cells in which the content of fat has been preserved. Osmic acid. × 350.

velop at any time within connective tissue, arise as a result of differentiation of more primitive cells. Although fat cells, before they store fat, resemble fibroblasts, it is likely that they arise directly from undifferentiated mesenchymal cells present within the body. Initially small droplets of fat make their appearance within the cytoplasm. The droplets increase in size and finally coalesce to form a single large droplet, and the cytoplasm is reduced to a thin encompassing layer. The nucleus is compressed and flattened.

When fat is utilized it leaves the cell as soluble components (the same form in which it enters), and the cell takes on a wrinkled appearance.

Mast Cells

These elements are widely distributed in connective tissues but tend to occur in small groups in relation to blood vessels. They are particularly common in connective tissue of rodents. Mast cells are identified easily by their content of cytoplasmic granules. They are irregularly oval in outline and occasionally have short pseudopodia, an indication of their slow mobility. The nucleus is small and inconspicuous, often masked by the crowded granules. In most preparations many mast cells are ruptured and their granules escape into the surrounding tissue. The granules are refractile and water soluble and stain with basic dyes. Neutral red stains them supravitally a dark red-brown, and they exhibit metachromasia with basic aniline dyes such as methylene blue or azure A. The granules also show a positive staining reaction with the periodic acid–Schiff reagent. In electron micrographs, the granules average 0.5 micron (0.5 μm) in diameter and are bounded by a unit membrane. They have a heterogeneous content that varies with the species; in man the dense osmiophilic material commonly is in the form of membranous whorls.

Mast cells appear to be involved in the normal functional relationship between blood vessels and the intercellular compartment. They produce an *anticoagulant* similar to, if not identical with, *heparin*. Chemically, heparin is a sulfated polysaccharide, which gives a metachromatic staining reaction with basic aniline dyes, as do mast cell granules. Quantitative studies have shown that tissues and organs in which mast cells are most numerous contain more heparin-like substance than do structures containing few mast cells. Mast cell tumors possess a heparin-like content many times greater than that of liver, which is used as a commercial source of the anticoagulant. Similar evidence has demonstrated that mast cells also con-

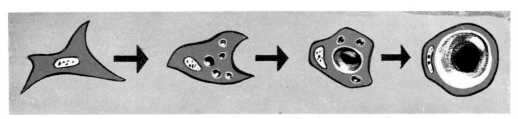

Figure 3–14. Diagram to illustrate the development of a fat cell.

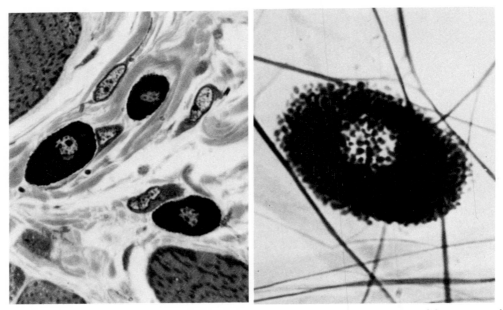

Figure 3–15.   Photomicrograph of mast cells in relation to skeletal muscle fibers *(left)* of the tongue and in loose connective tissue *(right)*. Toluidine blue stain. Plastic sections. Left, × 600; right, × 1100.

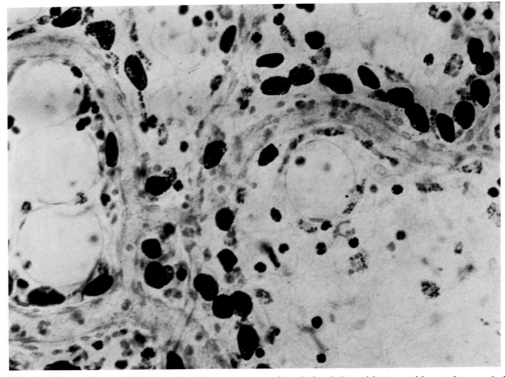

Figure 3–16.   A spread preparation of rat omentum after vital staining with trypan blue and supravital staining with neutral red. A small quantity of vital dye was injected, with the result that macrophages contain only a small quantity of the dye (compare with Figure 3–11). Mast cells are stained densely with neutral red and are aligned along the capillary network. Unstained fat cells are present also. × 425.

tain and secrete histamine, which causes vasodilation and increases the permeability of capillaries and small venules. The precise role of mast cells in relation to anaphylactic shock and to antigen-antibody complexes is currently under active investigation. The mast cell granules of some species, but not those of man, also contain serotonin, a vasoconstrictor.

Blood Leukocytes

Although leukocytes are transported by the blood stream, they perform their chief functions extravascularly, and thus it is not surprising that they are encountered within connective tissue. A brief description of these cells follows; they are discussed in more detail in Chapter 5.

Lymphocytes

Lymphocytes are the smallest of the free cells of connective tissue, the majority being only 7 to 8 microns (μm) in diameter. They have a spherical, darkly staining nucleus which occupies most of the cell. Around the nucleus is a thin rim of homogeneous cytoplasm which is basophil. Lymphocytes are not seen in large numbers in connective tissue generally but are numerous in the connective tissue which supports the epithelial lining of the respiratory and alimentary tracts. They accumulate in sites of chronic inflammation, and it is thought by some authorities that they are concerned with antibody production. The majority of lymphocytes present in the loose connective tissue are thought to emigrate there from the blood stream. In tissue cultures lymphocytes appear to be actively ameboid; it is thought that they egress from the circulation between lining cells of the blood vessels. Some lymphocytes originate in the connective tissue and they remain there. They may, however, enter or re-enter the circulation at any time.

Recent radioautographic studies have indicated that there are two distinct populations of lymphocytes, one with a brief life span and the other living for months or years. It is the latter group which is migratory in the connective tissues. Functionally, at least two types are recognized: T lymphocytes, which are long-lived and responsible for initiating cell-mediated immune responses, and B lymphocytes. The latter are short-lived cells which, when stimulated by an antigen, are capable of transforming into large immature cells, some of which further differentiate into plasma cells that synthesize antibodies against the stimulating antigen.

Eosinophil Cells

Eosinophil cells also may emigrate from the blood stream into the connective tissue. They are not numerous in human connective tissue generally but are plentiful in connective tissue of the lactating breast and of the respiratory and alimentary tracts. They are a marked feature of the loose connective tissue of rat, mouse, and guinea pig. The nucleus is usually reniform or bilobed, and the cytoplasm contains spherical granules which are highly refractile and stain with acid dyes. Eosinophils accumulate in the blood and in the tissues in certain allergic and subacute inflammatory conditions, and the suggestion has been made that they may be related in some way to the phenomenon of hypersensitivity. It is believed that eosinophils also contain histamine, although the amount is small in comparison with the histamine content of mast cells. In addition, evidence is accumulating that eosinophils are attracted to antigen-antibody complexes, which they later phagocytose.

Other white blood cells which may be found in connective tissue are *neutrophils,* but generally these escape into the connective tissue from capillaries only in regions of inflammation. They may be recognized by the multilobation of the nucleus. *Monocytes* are seen rarely.

Plasma Cells

These cells bear a resemblance to lymphocytes. They possess more cytoplasm which, like that of the lymphocytes, is basophil, and a nucleus which

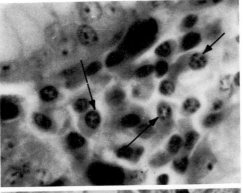

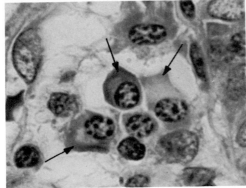

Figure 3–17. Sections of the lining of the fundus of the stomach, in which numerous plasma cells are present (arrows). The nuclei of these cells show the typical peripheral condensations of chromatin, and in the lower illustration, the basophilic cytoplasm shows a clear area in the location of the centrosphere and the Golgi apparatus. Upper, × 600; lower, × 1200.

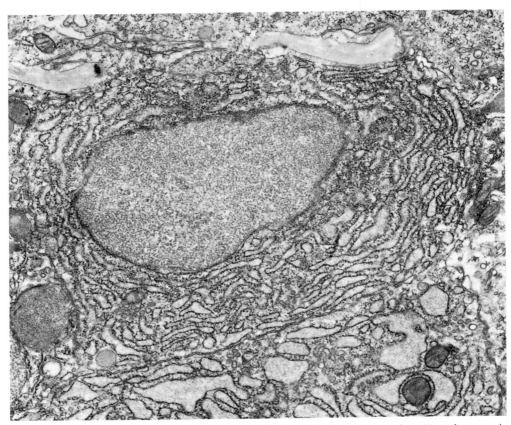

Figure 3–18. Electron micrograph of a plasma cell in the red pulp of mouse spleen. Note the extensive development of granular endoplasmic reticulum. × 12,500. (Courtesy of T. K. Shnitka.)

usually is eccentric in position. Within the nucleus, chromatin occurs in coarse clumps peripherally and often is arranged in a pattern suggestive of the spokes of a wheel or the hours on a clock. Accordingly, the nucleus is described as having a cartwheel or clock-face appearance. The cytoplasm contains a clear, rounded area which is the site of the centrosphere and the Golgi apparatus. An extensive endoplasmic reticulum with associated ribosomes is a fine structural feature of the cytoplasm.

Plasma cells are rare in connective tissues generally but are found frequently in serous membranes and lymphoid tissue and are plentiful in sites of chronic inflammation. They probably represent a special differentiation of the lymphocyte, and their principal function is the production of antibodies, which are synthesized within the granular endoplasmic reticulum. These may be released locally or into the circulation, or they may be stored temporarily within cytoplasmic vesicles.

Occasionally acidophil inclusions called *Russell bodies* are present in the cytoplasm of plasma cells. Some authors consider these bodies to be the sites of large accumulations of secretory material, but other observers are of the opinion that they are indicative either of an aberrant state or of cellular aging and degeneration.

The plasma cell precursor, or proplasmocyte, has a basophil cytoplasm that stains readily with the red basic dye pyronin and with hematoxylin or azure II. As mentioned previously, it is thought that the proplasmocyte is derived from the B lymphocyte following stimulation by antigen.

Pigment Cells

Cells containing pigment (chromatophores) are rare in loose connective tissue but are found commonly in the dense connective tissue of the skin, in pia mater, and in the choroid coat of the eye. Some pigment cells, the *melanocytes*, are derived from embryonic neural crest, however, and do not arise directly from mesenchyme. Typically such cells have irregular cytoplasmic processes which, like the general cytoplasm, contain small granules of pigment, the *melanosomes*. These are membrane-bound ovoid bodies, and the pigment that they contain, *melanin*, has a role in the absorption of light rays. In addition to melanocytes, the dermis of the skin may also contain *melanophores*, which are macrophages that have phagocytosed melanosomes from disintegrating or aging melanocytes.

TYPES OF CONNECTIVE TISSUE PROPER

The character of connective tissue varies greatly in different parts of the body. The appearance depends upon the relative proportions and arrangement of the cellular, fibrous, and amorphous components. The major subdivision in the classification of connective tissues is determined by the concentration of fibers. The connective tissues which are characterized by a loose arrangement of fibers are referred to as *loose connective tissues.* In *dense connective tissues* there is an abundance of compactly arranged fibers. A further division of loose connective tissues into those which are present only in the embryo and those which are found in the adult can be made.

Loose Connective Tissues

Mesenchyme. Mesenchyme, as mentioned in the introduction to this chapter, is the typical, unspecialized connective tissue of the early weeks of embryonic life. Subsequently it disappears as such when component cells undergo differentiation. It is composed of mesenchymal cells, whose branching processes appear to join although they do not form a true syncytium, and of a ground substance which is a coagulable fluid in the earliest stages but later contains fine fibrils.

Mucous Connective Tissue. This is a transient type of tissue which appears in the normal development and differentiation of the connective tissues. It occurs also as *Wharton's jelly* in the umbilical cord, where it does not differentiate further.

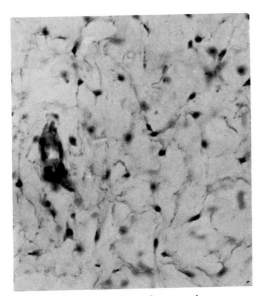

Figure 3–19. Section of mesenchyme, containing a small blood vessel, from subcutaneous tissue of a 10-mm pig embryo. × 425.

Component cells are large, stellate fibroblasts whose processes often appear to fuse with those of neighboring cells. A few macrophages and wandering lymphocytes are encountered occasionally. The ground substance is soft and jelly-like, gives a mucin reaction, and stains metachromatically with toluidine blue. It contains a delicate meshwork of fine collagenous fibers.

Loose (Areolar) Connective Tissue. Loose connective tissue is formed by the direct differentiation of mesenchyme. It is a loosely arranged, fibroelastic connective tissue, which is encountered in almost every microscopic section of the body, since it is the packing and anchoring material and is the embedding medium of many structures, including blood vessels and nerves. It binds other tissues, organ components, and organs together and allows, owing to its flexibility, a considerable degree of mobility between such parts.

All the structural elements, cells, fibers, and ground substance, previously described, are present within it. The two commonest cell types are fibroblasts and macrophages. Collagenous fibers are most prominent; elastic fibers, which form a continuous branching network, are relatively in-

conspicuous. Reticular fibers are represented also but are abundant only where areolar tissue borders upon other structures. The ground substance is relatively fluid-like and occupies many little areas (*areolas*) in which no structure ordinarily can be seen.

Areolar connective tissue is studied usually in two different types of preparation. It can be found in most sectioned material and can be examined also in spread preparations of subcutaneous tissue and of mesentery. The distinction between these two types of preparation is important. Study of sectioned material alone, although it reveals many cytological details, does not easily demonstrate the three-dimensional organization of areolar connective tissue. In spread preparations, unlike sectioned material, whole cells are viewed and the pattern of the fiber networks can be discerned.

Adipose Tissue. Fat cells are scattered in areolar connective tissue. When fat cells form large aggregations and are the principal cell type, the tissue is designated adipose tissue. Each fat cell is surrounded by a web of fine reticular fibers; in the spaces between are fibroblasts, lymphoid cells, eosinophils, and some mast cells. The closely packed fat cells form *lobules*, separated by fibrous septa. There is a rich network of blood capillaries in and be-

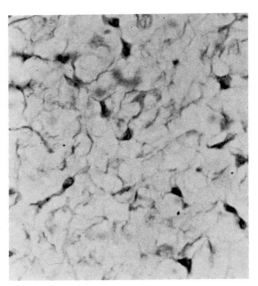

Figure 3–20. Section of mucous connective tissue of the umbilical cord. × 425.

the tissue normally are crowded with other cell types, principally lymphocytes and other blood cells.

Dense Connective Tissues

Dense connective tissues are characterized by the close packing of their fibers. Cells are proportionally fewer than in loose connective tissues and there is less amorphous ground substance. In areas where tensions are exerted in all directions, the fiber bundles are interwoven and without regular orientation and the tissues are termed *irregularly arranged*. In structures subject to tension in one direction, the fibers have an orderly parallel arrangement and the tissues are designated *regularly arranged*. In most regions collagenous fibers are the main component, but in a few ligaments elastic fibers predominate

Irregularly Arranged. This tissue occurs in sheets, its fibers interlacing to form a coarse, tough feltwork. Although coarse collagenous fibers are the main component, elastic and reticular fibers are present also in small numbers. Dense irregularly arranged connective tissue forms the basis of most fascias, the dermis of the skin, the fibrous capsules of some organs, including testis, liver, and lymph nodes, and the fibrous sheaths of bone (periosteum) and cartilage (perichondrium).

Regularly Arranged. This tissue contains fibers which are densely packed and lie parallel to each other forming structures of great tensile strength. This group includes tendons, ligaments, and aponeuroses. The latter two are less regularly arranged than tendons but in general have a similar organization.

In *tendons*, the collagenous fibers, or *primary tendon bundles*, run parallel courses. Each fiber or bundle is composed of a large number of fibrils. Fibroblasts, or *tendon cells*, are the only cell type present and in longitudinal

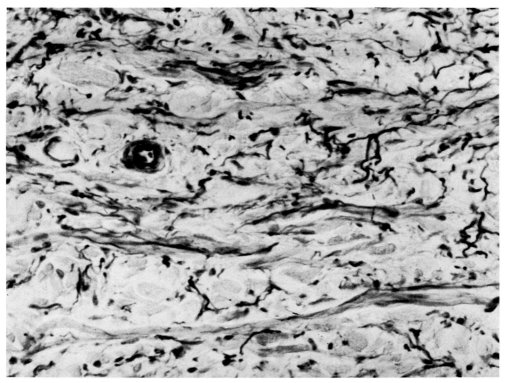

Figure 3–23. Section of dense irregular connective tissue of human scalp. Elastic fibers are stained darkly, collagenous fibers more lightly. Note the relative lack of cells. Weigert's elastin stain and hematoxylin and eosin. × 425.

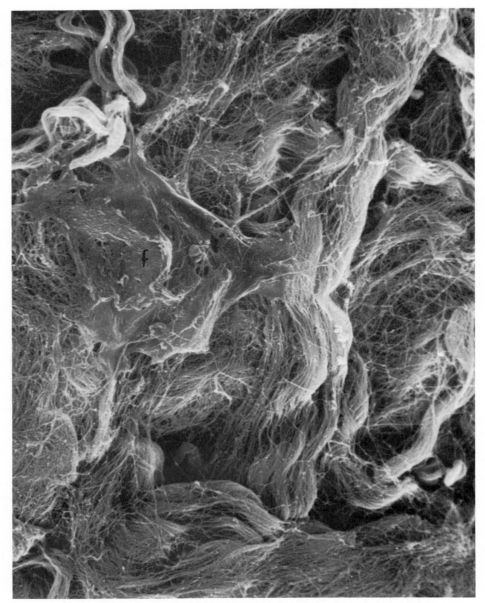

Figure 3–24. A scanning electron micrograph of dense, irregularly arranged connective tissue. Note the network of delicate fibrils and coarse collagenous fibers in association with a fibroblast (f). × 1500. (Courtesy of Dr. P. M. Andrews.)

sections of tendon they are aligned in rows between the collagenous fibers. Cytoplasm of the cells is often indistinct. In cross sections, the cells appear stellate in shape with cytoplasmic processes extending between the collagenous bundles. Each primary bundle is covered by a small amount of loose areolar (fibroelastic) connective tissue, termed the *endotendineum*. Generally, several primary bundles are grouped together into secondary bundles or fascicles bounded by a coarser type of connective tissue, the *peritendineum*. The tendon, composed of a number of fascicles, is ensheathed by thick connective

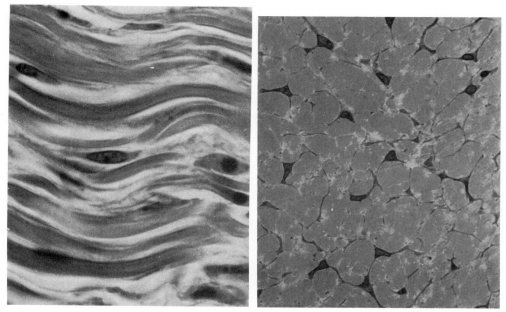

Figure 3–25. Sections of dense, irregularly arranged connective tissue. Note the coarse collagenous fibers, sectioned longitudinally *(left)* and transversely *(right),* and the relative paucity of cells, principally fibroblasts. Plastic sections. Left, × 500; right, × 450.

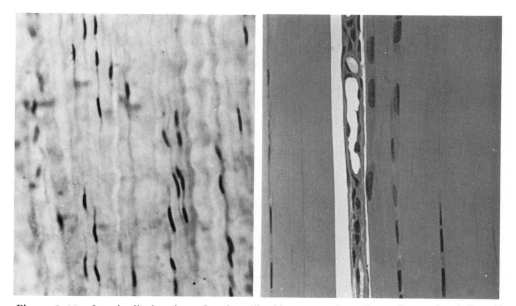

Figure 3–26. Longitudinal sections of tendon. Fibroblasts, or tendon cells, are flattened and aligned in rows between the bundles of collagenous fibers. In the right figure, a portion of the peritendineum, containing small blood vessels, is present (center) between secondary bundles. Left, × 350; right, plastic section, × 300.

tissue called the *epitendineum.** Nerves and blood vessels course in the major connective tissue septa but do not invade the fascicles.

Aponeuroses have the same composition as tendons but are broad and flat. Generally, the fibers are arranged in multiple sheets or layers, with those of one layer running at an angle to those of neighboring layers. The layers often interweave, and an isolation of the layers is seldom possible. Most ligaments have a similar composition but a few are composed almost entirely of elastic fibers.

In *yellow elastic ligaments,* coarse parallel fibers of elastic tissue are bound together by a small amount of delicate connective tissue, in which typical fibroblasts are present. The elastic fibers branch frequently and fuse with one another. Individual fibers are surrounded by a network of reticular fibers. Yellow elastic ligaments show numerous oval or elongated nuclei of fibroblasts between the parallel elastic fibers. This is one feature of elastic liga-

---

*Note on terminology: The prefixes "endo-," "peri-," and "epi-" indicate a progression in size. They are also used in reference to muscle with the word stem "-mysium," and to nerve with the word stem "-neurium."

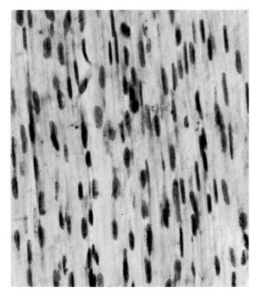

Figure 3–27. Longitudinal section from ligamentum nuchae of ox. Fibroblast nuclei are present between the elastic fibers. Compare with Figure 3–26. × 425.

ments which distinguishes them histologically from tendons and collagenous ligaments, in which fibroblasts are sparse and their nuclei markedly flattened. The most typical form of yellow elastic ligament is found in the ligamentum nuchae of quadrupeds. In the human, examples are found in the ligamenta flava of the vertebrae, the suspensory ligament of the penis, and the true vocal cords.

THE MACROPHAGE (RETICULOENDOTHELIAL) SYSTEM

The use of the word "system" here is somewhat unfortunate since it refers to physiological and pathological considerations rather than to a discrete anatomical entity. It is a collective term for a widespread system of highly phagocytic cells. They are present in large numbers in the body in certain situations. They possess no morphological characteristics that distinguish them with certainty from other cells. They are identified by their marked affinity for nontoxic colloidal dyes and for inert particulate matter. The macrophages take up the dye or inert particles and segregate them into vacuoles, and thus can be identified easily. True endothelial cells, fibroblasts, lymphocytes, and certain other cells may phagocytose small amounts of the dye but can be distinguished from cells of the macrophage system by a marked quantitative difference.

Cells of the macrophage system are found in the following situations: (1) In connective tissues, where they correspond to the macrophages or histiocytes just described. They occur in large numbers in relation to small blood vessels and lymphatics of the subserous connective tissue of the pleura and peritoneum. Here, often they are aggregated into small patches known as *milky spots.* (2) In the blood, where they are represented by the monocytes. (3) In the liver, lining the sinusoids, where they are known as *Kupffer's cells.* (4) Perivascular macrophages of sinusoids of the spleen, lymph nodes, and bone marrow. (5) In the *microglia* of the central nervous system, which are phagocytic and of mesodermal origin. The source of these cells has been the subject of much investigation in recent years. Numerous studies, principally involving radioactively labeled cells, have indicated that most, if not all, of these phagocytic cells are derived from promonocytes, mononuclear cells of bone marrow origin. Hence the most appropriate name for this system is the mononuclear phagocyte system, or, more simply, the macrophage system.

The functional importance of the macrophages is considerable. On account of their phagocytic and ameboid properties, they are active in the defense of the body against microorganisms. They are also intimately involved, along with other cells, in the antigen-antibody response. In the spleen and liver they phagocytose broken down erythrocytes and store iron-containing pigment within their cytoplasm. Foreign particulate matter in the blood stream is removed by the macrophages of the spleen, liver, and bone marrow, and foreign particulate matter in lymph is removed by macrophages of the lymph nodes.

REFERENCES

Alpert, E. N.: Developing elastic tissue. Am. J. Pathol., *69*:89, 1972.

Asboe-Hansen, G. (editor): Connective Tissue in Health and Disease. Copenhagen, E. Munksgaard, 1954.

Barnard, T.: The ultrastructural differentiation of brown adipose tissue in the rat. J. Ultrastruct. Res., *29*:311, 1969.

Briggaman, R. A., Dalldorf, F. G., and Wheeler, C. E., Jr.: Formation and origin of basal lamina and anchoring fibrils in adult human skin. J. Cell Biol., *51*:384–394, 1971.

Burwen, S. J., and Satir, B. H.: Plasma membrane folds on the mast cell surface and their relationship to secretory activity. J. Cell Biol., *74*:690–697, 1977.

Cohn, Z. A., Fedorko, M. E., and Hirsch, J. G.: The in vitro differentiation of mononuclear phagocytes. 4. The ultrastructure of macrophage differentiation in the peritoneal cavity and in culture. 5. The formation of macrophage lysosomes. J. Exp. Med., *123*:747, 1966.

Collet, A. J., and Des Biens, G.: Evolution of mesenchymal cells in fetal rat lung. Anat. Embryol., *147*:273–292, 1975.

Cotta-Pereira, G., Guerra, R. F., and Bittencourt-Sampaio, S.: Oxytalan, elaunin, and elastic fibers in the human skin. J. Invest. Dermatol., *66*:143, 1976.

Davies, D. V.: Specificity of staining methods for mucopolysaccharides of the hyaluronic acid type. Stain. Techn., *27*:65, 1952.

de Petris, S., Karlsbad, G., and Pernis, B.: Localization of antibodies in plasma cells by electron microscopy. J. Exper. Med., *117*:849, 1963.

Edds, M. V., Jr.: Origin and structure of intercellular matrix. *In* The Chemical Basis of Development, edited by W. C. McElroy and B. Glass. Baltimore, Johns Hopkins Press, 1958.

Fawcett, D. W.: A comparison of the histological organization and cytochemical reactions of brown and white adipose tissues. J. Morphol., *90*:363, 1952.

Fawcett, D. W., and Jones, I. C.: The effects of hypophysectomy, adrenalectomy and of thiouracil feeding on the cytology of brown adipose tissue. Endocrinology, *45*:609–621, 1949.

Furth, R. van, Cohn, Z. A., Hirsch, J. G., Humphrey, J. H., Spector, W. G., and Langevoort, H. L.: The mononuclear phagocyte system: A new classification of macrophages, monocytes and their precursor cells. Bull. World Health Org., *46*:845–852, 1972.

Gersh, I., and Catchpole, H. R.: The organization of ground substance and basement membrane and its significance in tissue injury, disease and growth. Am. J. Anat., *85*:457, 1949.

Greenlee, T. K., Jr., Ross, R., and Hartman, J. L.: The fine structure of elastic fibers. J. Cell Biol., *30*:59, 1966.

Gross, J.: The collagen fibril and its building block, tropocollagen. J. Biophys. Biochem. Cytol., *2*:261, 1956.

Hodge, A. J., and Schmitt, F. O.: The tropocollagen macromolecule and its properties of ordered interaction. *In* Macromolecular Complexes, edited by M. V. Edds, Jr. New York, Ronald Press, 1961.

Jackson, S. F.: Connective tissue cells. *In* The Cell: Biochemistry, Physiology, Morphology, edited by J. Brachet and A. E. Mirsky. New York, Academic Press, 1964, Vol. 6, p. 387.

Jacoby, F.: Macrophages, *In* Cells and Tissues in Culture, edited by E. N. Willmer. London, Academic Press, 1967.

Kefalides, N. A.: Chemical properties of basement membranes. Intern. Rev. Exp. Pathol., *10*:1–39, 1971.

Kewley, M. A., Steven, F. S., and Williams, G.: The presence of fine elastin fibrils within the elastin fibre observed by scanning electron microscopy. J. Anat., *123*:129–134, 1977.

Kobayasi, T., Midtgard, K., and Asboe-Hansen, G.: Ultrastructure of human mast cell granules. J. Ultrastruct. Res., *23*:153, 1968.

Leduc, E. H., Scott, G. B., and Avrameas, S.: Ultrastructural localization of intercellular immune globulins in plasma cells and lymphoblasts by enzyme-labeled antibodies. J. Histochem. Cytochem., *17*:211–224, 1969.

Maximow, A. A.: The macrophages or histiocytes. *In* Special Cytology, ed. 2, edited by E. V.

Cowdry. New York, Paul B. Hoeber, 1932, Vol. 2, p. 709.

Morse, D. E., and Low, F. N.: The fine structure of developing unit collagenous fibrils in the chick. Am. J. Anat., *140*:237–262, 1974.

Papadimitriou, J. M., and Archer, M.: The morphology of foreign body multinucleate giant cells. J. Ultrastruct. Res., *49*:372–386, 1974.

Porter, K. R.: Cell fine structure and biosynthesis of intercellular macromolecules. Biophys. J., *4*:167, 1964.

Porter, K. R.: Morphogenesis of connective tissue. *In* Cellular Concepts in Rheumatoid Arthritis, edited by C. A. L. Stephens and A. B. Stanfield. Springfield, Ill., Charles C Thomas, 1966.

Robert, A. M., Robert, B., and Robert, L.: Chemical and physical properties of structural glycoproteins. *In* Chemistry and Molecular Biology of the Intercellular Matrix, edited by E. A. Balars. New York, Academic Press, 1970, Vol. 1, p. 237.

Ross, R.: The elastic fiber. A Review. J. Histochem. Cytochem., *21*:199, 1973.

Ross, R., and Bornstein, P.: The elastic fiber. I. The separation and partial characterization of its macromolecular components. J. Cell. Biol., *40*:366–381, 1969.

Ross, R., and Bornstein, P.: Elastic fibers in the body. Sci. Am., *224*:44–59, 1971.

Slavin, B. G.: The cytophysiology of mammalian adipose cells. Int. Rev. Cytol., *33*:297, 1972.

Smith, R. E., and Horwitz, B. A.: Brown fat and thermogenesis. Physiol. Rev., *49*:330, 1969.

Spicer, S. S., Horn, R. G., and Leppi, T. J.: Histochemistry of connective tissue mucopolysaccharides. *In* The Connective Tissue, edited by B. M. Wagner and D. E. Smith. Baltimore, Williams & Wilkins, 1967, pp. 251–303.

Sutton, J. S., and Weiss, L. V.: Transformation of monocytes in tissue cultures into macrophages, epithelioid cells and multinucleated giant cells: An electron microscope study. J. Cell Biol., *28*:303, 1966.

Ten Cate, A. R.: Morphological studies of fibrocytes in connective tissues undergoing rapid remodeling. J. Anat., *112*:401, 1972.

Vracko, R.: Basal lamina scaffold — anatomy and significance for maintenance of orderly tissue structure. Am. J. Pathol., *77*:314–346, 1974.

Wislocki, G. B., Buntin, H., and Dempsey, E. W.: Metachromasia in mammalian tissues and its relationship to mucopolysaccharides. Am. J. Anat., *81*:1, 1947.

Wisse, E.: Kupffer cell reactions in rat liver under various conditions as observed in the electron microscope. J. Ultrastruct. Res., *46*:499–520, 1974.

SPECIALIZED CONNECTIVE TISSUE: CARTILAGE AND BONE

Cartilage and bone, the skeletal tissues, are specialized connective tissues and, like all connective tissues, are composed of three elements: cells, fibers, and ground substance, the latter two constituting the intercellular substance or matrix. They differ from the connective tissues discussed previously in the rigidity of their matrices. In cartilage the ground substance is composed principally of chondromucoids which are rich in chondroitin sulfates. In bone the ground substance is impregnated with certain inorganic salts, principally calcium phosphate.

CARTILAGE

In early fetal life, cartilage temporarily forms most of the skeleton and it persists in adult mammals over the articular surfaces of bones and as the sole skeletal support in the respiratory passages and parts of the ear. The matrix contains collagenous or elastic fibers that increase the tensile strength and the elasticity respectively and adapt the tissue to the mechanical requirements of the different regions of the body. The differences in the kind and abundance of fibers incorporated within the matrix form the basis of classification. There are three common types: *hyaline cartilage*, *elastic cartilage*, and *fibrocartilage*. Of these, hyaline cartilage is the most

widely distributed and the most characteristic.

Development and Growth of Cartilage. Cartilage, like other connective tissues, develops from mesenchyme. In an area where cartilage will develop, mesenchymal cells round up and become closely packed, and collagenous fibrils are deposited within the intercellular substance. These cells, now re-

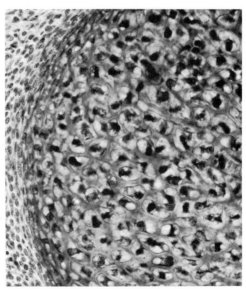

Figure 4–1. Fetal hyaline cartilage from developing human ilium. The primitive perichondrium lies to the left of the figure. × 300. (Courtesy of R. D. Laurenson.)

137

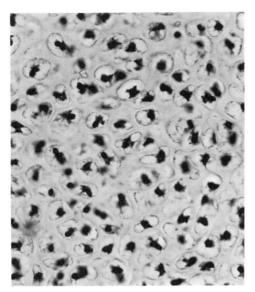

Figure 4–2. Fetal hyaline cartilage from developing human ilium. This specimen was from a fetus older than that demonstrated in Figure 4–1 and shows a greater development of ground substance. × 300. (Courtesy of R. D. Laurenson.)

ferred to as *chondroblasts*, elaborate ground substance, and the collagenous fibrils become masked. As the cells differentiate further and gradually be-

come more separated, due to the elaboration of matrix around them, they acquire the characteristics of mature cartilage cells or *chondrocytes* (see page 139). They accumulate vacuoles, lipid, and glycogen. Mesenchyme surrounding the enlarging mass of cartilage is compressed and forms a fibrous envelope, the *perichondrium*. This merges gradually into the cartilage on one side and into the surrounding connective tissue on the other.

Continued growth of cartilage occurs by two methods. Young chondrocytes, which retain the ability to divide, proliferate and lay down new matrix. This expansion of cartilage from within, called *interstitial* (or *endogenous*) *growth*, occurs only in relatively young cartilage which is malleable enough to allow expansion. The cell groups or cell nests seen in mature cartilage are an indication of the condition that existed when interstitial growth ceased. The second method by which cartilage increases in size, known as *appositional* (or *exogenous*) *growth*, is a process in which new layers of cartilage are added to one surface. It results from activity within the inner layer of the perichondrium. Fibroblasts

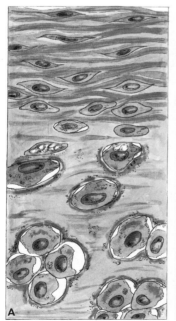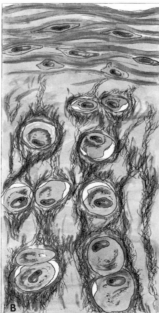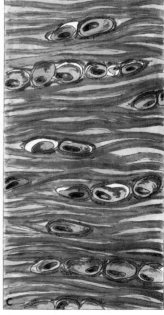

Figure 4–3. Diagram of the three types of cartilage. The diagrams of hyaline (*A*) and elastic cartilage (*B*) show perichondrium above. Note that intercellular elastic and collagenous fibers are prominent respectively in elastic (*B*) and fibrocartilage (*C*). *A* also illustrates both appositional (above) and interstitial (below) forms of growth.

in the perichondrium multiply by division and some transform into cartilage cells and surround themselves with intercellular substance. These in time become overlaid by still newer cells and matrix added from the perichondrium.

Hyaline Cartilage

The word "hyaline" is derived from the Greek *hyalos*, meaning glass. Hyaline cartilage appears as a translucent, bluish-white mass in the fresh condition. It forms the articular surfaces of bones within joints, the costal cartilages, and the cartilages of the nose, larynx, trachea, and bronchi. In the fetus nearly all the skeleton is first laid down as hyaline cartilage, which is replaced later by bone.

The Cells. The *cartilage cells* or *chondrocytes* occupy small cavities or lacunae within the matrix. The cells usually are ovoid or spherical, and each contains a large, spherical, centrally placed nucleus with one or more nucleoli. The surface of each cell is irregular and has short processes that extend into depressions within the matrix. This structural feature increases the surface area and is thought to aid in maintaining nutrition of the cell by permitting greater exchange with the extracellular fluid. The cytoplasm is finely granular and moderately basophil, due to the presence of abundant free ribosomes and of a relatively well-developed granular endoplasmic reticulum; in addition, it contains large mitochondria, vacuoles, fat droplets, and some glycogen. In living cartilage the chondrocytes completely fill their lacunae, but, owing to shrinkage resulting from fixation and dehydration, cartilage cells in paraffin sections show marked distortion and seldom conform to the shape of their lacunae. In the center of a mass of cartilage in the adult, the cells may be arranged in groups, each group representing the offspring of a single parent chondrocyte. Such a group of cells within a single lacuna is referred to as a *cell nest* or isogenous group. Toward the periphery of a mass of cartilage the cells are elliptical and flattened parallel to the surface. In fetal cartilage the cells often are flattened and cell nests are seen rarely.

The Matrix (Intercellular Substance). Although the matrix appears homogeneous in the fresh condition and after ordinary fixation, it contains considerable quantities of both formed and amorphous kinds of intercellular substance. The formed kind is represented by collagenous fibers, which are

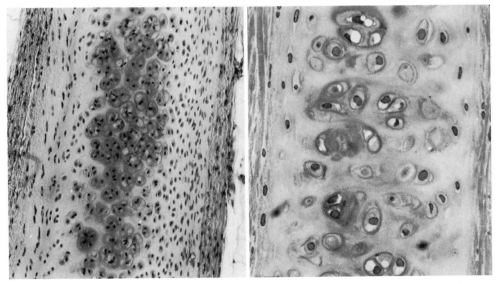

Figure 4–4. Hyaline cartilage from human trachea. The chondrocytes increase in size from the perichondrium to the interior of the cartilage. Left, × 125; right, plastic section, × 250.

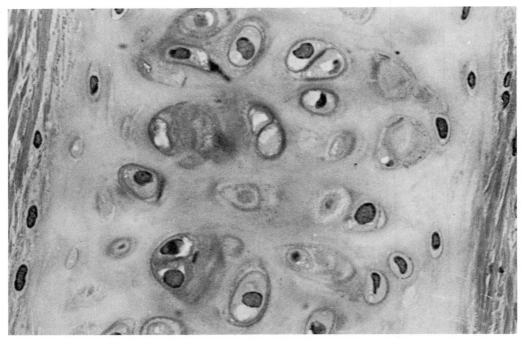

Figure 4–5.   Hyaline cartilage from the same preparation as Figure 4–4 (right). Cell nests and cartilage capsules are evident within the interior of the cartilage. The large vacuoles within the cytoplasm of many chondrocytes represent the sites of fat droplets, lost during preparation. Perichondrium is present at both surfaces of the cartilage. Plastic section, × 500.

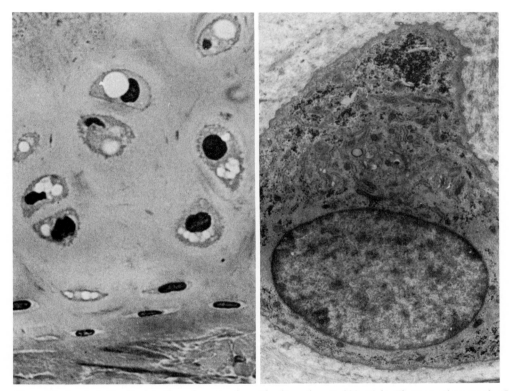

Figure 4–6. *Left:* Hyaline cartilage from trachea. Plastic section. × 600. *Right:* Electron micrograph of chondrocyte from tracheal cartilage. The dark granular mass in the cytoplasm (above) is glycogen. × 5800.

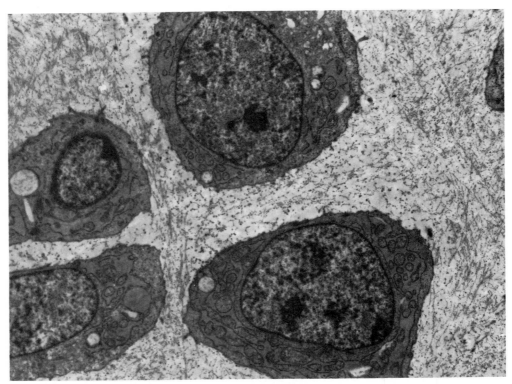

Figure 4–7. Electron micrograph of hyaline cartilage from developing trachea. Chondrocytes generally appear spherical in shape and their cytoplasm contains small fat droplets, mitochondria, and granular endoplasmic reticulum. Collagenous fibrils form a fine feltwork within the surrounding ground substance. × 5500.

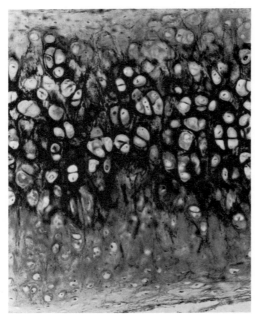

Figure 4–8. Elastic cartilage from human external ear, with perichondrium above and below. Elastic fibers within the ground substance have been stained with orcein. × 150.

not apparent in fresh material since they have approximately the same refractive index as that of the surrounding ground substance. Collagenous fibers can be detected in thin sections examined with the polarizing microscope, and they can be demonstrated after digestion with trypsin or dilute alkalis. They can be seen readily in electron micrographs. They rarely occur in definite bundles but form a fine feltwork. As noted in Chapter 3, the collagen of cartilage differs from that of tendon and skin in that it has three alpha-1 type II chains.

The ground substance of cartilage is markedly basophil owing to its content of *chondromucoids*, which are *glycosaminoglycan complexes* containing *chondroitin 4-sulfate, chondroitin 6-sulfate,* and some *keratin sulfate.* The latter is small in amount at birth but increases with age. Chondromucoids are abundant throughout the matrix of embryonic cartilage, but in mature cartilage they are unevenly distributed. The region around cells and cell groups is often more basophil than the general matrix and is referred to as *territorial matrix* (or the *cartilage capsules*). The ground substance stains metachromatically with toluidine blue and gives a positive reaction with the periodic acid–Schiff reaction (PAS). Since pure chondroitin sulfate is not PAS positive, the response is thought to be due to some undetermined carbohydrate component present within the matrix. Radioautographic studies have shown that the chondrocytes are responsible for the formation of collagenous fibrils and the ground substance. Amino acids, such as proline and glycine, are synthesized into peptide chains in the region of the granular endoplasmic reticulum and are transported to the Golgi complex. Here they are combined with polysaccharides that themselves are synthesized in the Golgi complex to form the chondromucoids which later are secreted by the cells.

Perichondrium. Except over articular surfaces, cartilage is enclosed by a tough layer of dense connective tissue, the *perichondrium.* This is composed of spindle-shaped cells, indistinguishable from fibroblasts, and of elastic and collagenous fibers. Next to the cartilage, the perichondrium is more cellular and merges by a smooth transition into cartilage. This is due to the fact that cells in the inner zone of the perichondrium have the potentiality of being able to surround themselves with matrix and become incorporated into the cartilage as typical chondrocytes.

Nutrition. In general, cartilage is devoid of blood vessels, lymphatics, and nerves. Consequently, chondrocytes are nourished by substances diffusing through the intercellular substance from blood vessels of the perichondrium.

Some cartilages are penetrated by small branching canals, each containing a small artery or arteriole. The significance of these *cartilage canals* is poorly understood. In the past, many authors have assumed that they are merely passing to another destination. More recently, other authors have concluded that their primary role is the provision of stem cells for interstitial growth in the cartilage and that secondarily they may provide an additional source of nourishment, particularly for the deeply placed cells within expanding masses of cartilage. However, the main source of nourishment undoubtedly is diffusion from perichondrial vessels, which generally is adequate since the requirements of cartilage are modest.

Retrogressive Changes. With old age, cartilage loses its translucency and becomes less cellular, and the matrix shows less basophilia owing to a loss of chondromucoids and an increase in noncollagenous proteins.

The most important retrogressive change within cartilage is *calcification.* Calcification also occurs as a temporary strengthening expedient during the replacement of cartilage by bone. Minute granules of calcium phosphate and calcium carbonate are deposited in the intercellular substance, initially in the vicinity of the cells and later in the general matrix. The granules enlarge and merge, and the cartilage becomes hard and brittle. When the intercellular substance becomes calcified in this manner, it no longer permits ready diffusion of nutrients and the cells die. With their death, the calcified matrix undergoes a slow process of resorption.

Regeneration. The ability to regenerate an area of cartilage that has been lost or damaged is low. Injuries are repaired by a slow process which occurs primarily as a result of activity of the perichondrium. Tissue from the perichondrium proliferates and fills in the defect. This vascularized connective tissue gradually may be converted to cartilage in a manner similar to appositional growth. A fracture of mature cartilage may be repaired not by cartilage but by dense fibrous tissue which itself later may be replaced by bone.

Elastic Cartilage

This type of cartilage occurs in locations where support with flexibility is required, as in the external ear, auditory tube, epiglottis, and certain cartilages of the larynx. It is yellow in color, owing to the preponderance of elastic fibers, and is more opaque than hyaline cartilage, of which it is a modification. Component cells show less accumula-

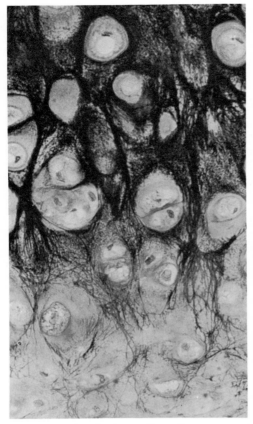

Figure 4–9. Elastic cartilage from external ear. A preparation similar to that in Figure 4–8. There is a profusion of elastic fibers within the ground substance (above). Fewer elastic fibers surround chondrocytes close to the perichondrium (below). × 500.

tion of fat and glycogen than do those of hyaline cartilage. The matrix contains masked collagenous fibers and, in addition, extensive networks of elastic fibers. These vary in thickness and abundance and in general are larger and more densely packed in the interior of a cartilage. The cartilage is surrounded by a perichondrium and growth occurs both interstitially and by apposition from the perichondrium. Elastic cartilage is less likely to undergo retrogressive changes, principally calcification, than hyaline cartilage.

Fibrocartilage

This type of cartilage occurs where a tough support or tensile strength is required. It occurs in the intervertebral discs, in the symphysis pubis, and in the intra-articular discs of certain other joints. It is also present in the cartilage that borders the shoulder and hip joints and where some tendons and ligaments are attached to bone. It never occurs alone, but merges gradually into neighboring hyaline cartilage or with dense fibrous tissue. Unlike elastic cartilage, it cannot be considered a modification of hyaline cartilage. It is composed of dense collagenous connective tissue between bundles of which there are small regions of hyaline cartilaginous matrix containing lacunae with enclosed cells. These may occur singly or in groups, but commonly are in short rows. Fibrocartilage lacks a perichondrium. It is found closely associated with the dense connective tissue of ligaments and joint capsules and should be considered a transitional form between cartilage and dense connective tissue. It develops in a manner similar to that of ordinary connective tissue, and initially only fibroblasts, separated by considerable amounts of fibrillar material, are present. Later the cells become transformed into chon-

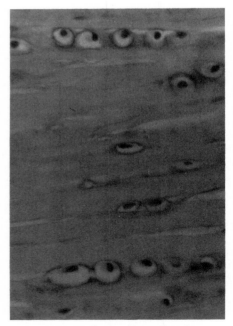

Figure 4–10. Fibrocartilage taken from a tendon close to its insertion into bone. Note that the cartilage cells lie within definite lacunae. × 450.

drocytes and surround themselves with a thin layer of cartilaginous matrix.

BONE

Bone, or *osseous tissue*, is a rigid form of connective tissue that constitutes most of the skeleton of higher vertebrates. It consists of cells and of an intercellular matrix. The matrix contains an organic component, chiefly collagenous fibers, and an inorganic component which accounts for approximately two-thirds of the weight of bone. The inorganic salts which are responsible for the hardness and rigidity of bone include calcium phosphate (about 85 per cent), calcium carbonate (10 per cent), and small amounts of calcium fluoride and magnesium fluoride. Collagenous fibers contribute greatly to the strength and resilience of bone.

Macroscopically, two types of bone may be distinguished: the *spongy* (*cancellous*) and the *compact* (*dense*). Spongy bone consists of slender, irregular trabeculae or bars which branch and unite with one another to form a meshwork, the intercommunicating spaces of which are filled with bone marrow. Compact bone appears solid, except for microscopic spaces. No sharp boundary may be drawn between the two types of osseous tissue,

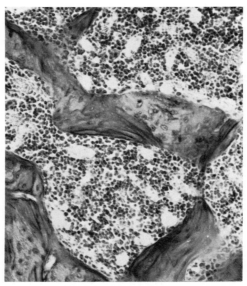

Figure 4–12. Spongy bone of the tibia. Bone marrow lies between the bony trabeculae. × 150.

and the differences between them depend merely upon the relative amount of solid matter and the size and number of spaces in each. They both contain the same histological elements. With few exceptions, both spongy and compact types are present in every bone, but the amount and distribution of each vary considerably. In typical long bones, the shaft (*diaphysis*) is chiefly compact bone surrounding a *medullary* (or bone marrow) *cavity*. Each end (*epiphysis*) consists of spongy bone covered by a thin shell of compact bone. The cavities of the spongy bone are continuous with the bone marrow cavity of the diaphysis. In flat bones, two plates of compact bone enclose a middle layer of spongy bone (diploë). Most irregular bones consist of spongy bone covered by a thin shell of compact bone.

Each bone, except over its articular surfaces, is enveloped by a specialized connective tissue coat, the *periosteum*. A similar, but less well developed, connective tissue layer, the *endosteum*, lines the marrow cavity and marrow spaces.

Microscopically, the most characteristic feature of bone is its lamellar structure, the calcified intercellular substance, or *bone matrix*, being organized into layers or *lamellae* arranged in various ways. Within the interstitial substance there are small

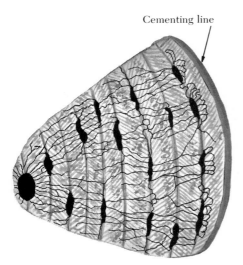

Cementing line

Figure 4–11. Diagram of a segment of a Haversian system in cross section to illustrate the arrangement of osteocytes, canaliculi, and lamellae.

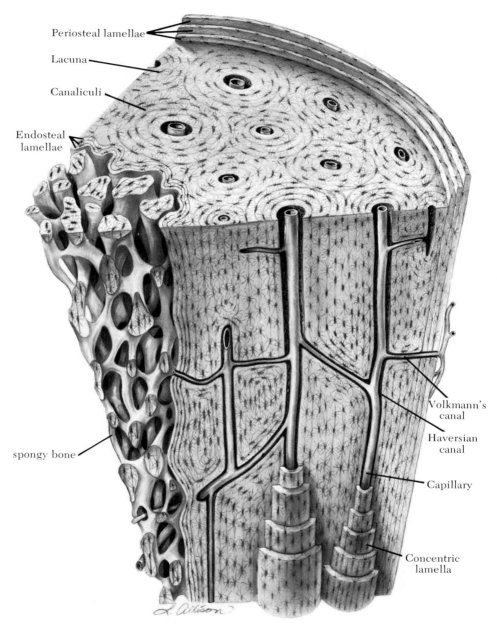

Periosteal lamellae

Lacuna

Canaliculi

Endosteal
lamellae

spongy bone

Volkmann's
canal

Haversian
canal

Capillary

Concentric
lamella

L. Allison

Figure 4–13.   A diagrammatic representation of a small portion of compact bone.

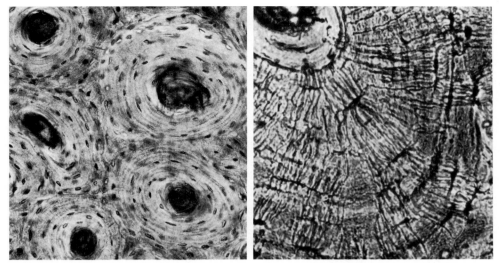

Figure 4–14. Photomicrographs of ground compact bone. *Left:* Portions of five Haversian systems, showing Haversian canals, lacunae, and the lamellar arrangement of bone matrix. *Right:* A segment of one Haversian system, with the Haversian canal (top left). An extensive canalicular system connects lacunae with the Haversian canal. Left, × 150; right, × 500.

cavities, or *lacunae,* which contain the bone cells (*osteocytes*). Radiating from each lacuna are numerous narrow channels, termed *canaliculi,* which penetrate adjacent lamellae to join with canaliculi of neighboring lacunae. Thus all lacunae are interconnected by a system of minute channels.

Structural Elements

In a histological study of bone, it must be borne in mind that, owing to its inorganic component, bone cannot be examined in routine histological preparations. Two special methods of preparation are employed commonly. In one the cellular and organic components of bone are preserved and the inorganic component is removed by *decalcification* in an acid solution. After decalcification bone can be embedded and sectioned in the normal manner. Cells in decalcified bone tend to be shrunken, and details of the matrix are blurred owing to swelling of osteocollagenous fibers by the reagents used. In *ground bone* sections, which are prepared by taking a thin piece of bone and grinding it down with abrasives until a section thin enough to be viewed

under the microscope is obtained, details of matrix structure are well preserved. However, bone cells are removed by this method and lacunae appear empty.

Bone Cells

Three cell types peculiar to bone are recognized: *osteoblasts, osteocytes,* and *osteoclasts.* They are closely interrelated, and transformation from one to another is thought to occur readily.

Osteoblasts. Osteoblasts are associated with bone formation and are found in relation to the surface of bone where osseous matrix is being deposited. They vary in shape, some being cuboidal and others pyramidal, and are present frequently in a continuous layer suggestive of an epithelial arrangement. The nucleus is large and usually has a single prominent nucleolus. The cytoplasm exhibits marked basophilia, suggesting the presence of ribose nucleoprotein, which is concerned probably with the synthesis of protein components of the bone matrix. Fine granules are present in the cytoplasm of osteoblasts closely associated with sites of active deposition of matrix. Osteoblasts contain the enzyme

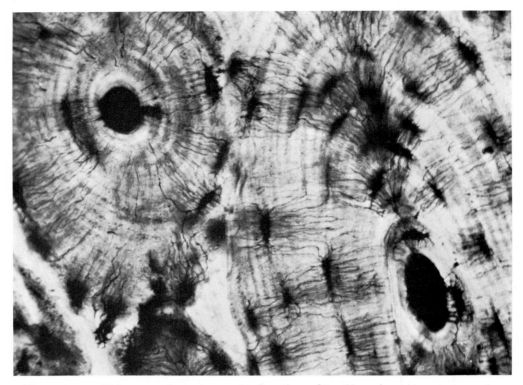

Figure 4–15. High-power photomicrograph of portions of two Haversian systems transversely sectioned. Note the arrangement of lacunae and canaliculi. × 500.

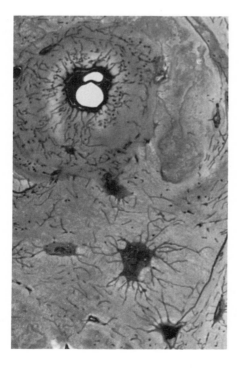

alkaline phosphatase, which would suggest that they are concerned not only with the elaboration of matrix but also with its calcification.

Osteocytes. The osteocyte, or bone cell, is an osteoblast which has become imprisoned within bone matrix. It has a faintly basophil cytoplasm which can be shown to contain fat droplets, some glycogen, and fine granules similar to those present within osteoblasts. The nucleus is darkly staining. Osteocytes are often somewhat shrunken in preparation, but their normal configuration can be inferred from the shape of the lacunae which they occupy. A la-

Figure 4–16. A portion of one Haversian system obliquely sectioned. One osteocyte, which fills its lacuna, shows numerous branching processes that lie within canaliculi. Note also the Haversian canal (top left) and a portion of a cement line (top right). Undecalcified plastic section. × 550.

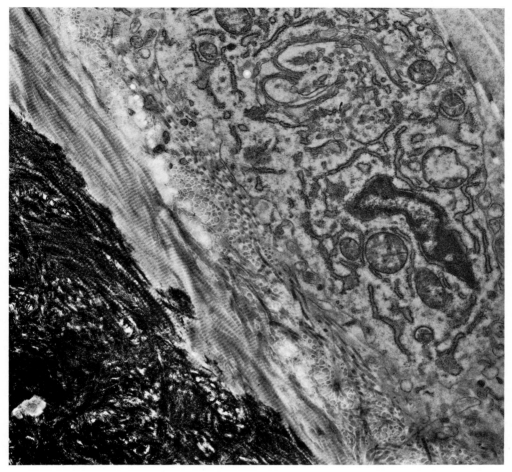

Figure 4–17. Electron micrograph of a portion of an osteoblast with abundant rough-surfaced endoplasmic reticulum. Note the unmineralized matrix, containing collagen fibrils, running obliquely across the center of the figure, and mineralized matrix at left. × 18,400. (Courtesy of R. R. Cooper.)

cuna is irregularly oval on the flat and biconvex on edge. Fine cytoplasmic processes of osteocytes extend for some distance into the canaliculi which radiate out from the lacunae. In developing bone the processes of osteocytes extend even further so that there is direct contiguity (but not continuity) between neighboring osteocytes. In mature bone the processes are withdrawn almost completely, but the canaliculi remain to provide an avenue for the exchange of metabolites between the blood stream and the osteocytes. Electron microscopy has shown that osteocytes and their processes are not opposed directly to the surrounding matrix but are separated from the walls of the lacunae and canaliculi by a narrow amorphous

zone. This zone probably acts as an additional medium for the exchange of metabolites.

Osteoclasts. Osteoclasts are multinucleated giant cells which vary greatly in size and in the number of nuclei they possess. They are found in close association with the surface of bone, often in shallow excavations known as *Howship's lacunae.* The cytoplasm, which appears faintly basophil and granular, contains characteristic vacuoles, some of which are lysosomal in nature. Electron micrographs show that the surface of the osteoclast facing the matrix has numerous cytoplasmic projections and microvilli, described as a *ruffled border.* Osteoclasts are thought to arise by fusion either of uninucleate, osteopro-

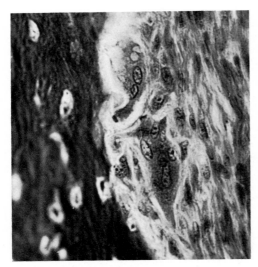

Figure 4–18. A portion of spongy bone, in immediate relationship to which are two osteoclasts. × 350.

genitor cells or of mononuclear cells emigrating from the blood, presumably monocytes. The neighboring bone surface in relation to osteoclasts often is partly demineralized, and it is probable that these cells are involved in the resorption of bone, although the mechanism of this activity remains unclear. Once the resorption process is complete, the osteoclasts disappear probably either by degeneration or by reversion to their parent cell type.

Bone Matrix

Although the intercellular substance of bone is apparently homogeneous, it has a well-ordered structure. The organic portion, comprising about 35 per cent, is chiefly *osteocollagenous fibers* similar to the collagenous fibers of loose connective tissue. The fibers are difficult to see in ordinary preparations but can be revealed by special methods. They are united by a special *cementing substance* which consists mainly of glycosaminoglycans (protein-polysaccharides). In the amorphous ground substance, the amount of sulfated polysaccharides (chondroitin sulfates) is much less than in cartilage. Thus, the bone matrix generally is acidophil, unlike cartilage matrix which is basophil and metachromatic. The inor-

ganic component is located solely in the cement between fibers and accounts for 65 per cent of the weight of a bone. The minerals are present principally as crystals of calcium phosphate with an *apatite* pattern or structure. X-ray diffraction studies have shown that more specifically the pattern is that of *hydroxyapatites.* The minerals are deposited as dense particles aligned in relation to the osteocollagenous fibers. Lacunae and canaliculi are bordered by a layer of special organic cement which differs from the rest of the intercellular substance in that it lacks fibrils.

Bone matrix is arranged characteristically in layers or lamellae 3 to 7 microns (μm) thick. The lamellae result from the rhythmical manner in which matrix is deposited. The fibers in any lamella are roughly parallel to each other and take a spiral or helical course. The pitch of the spiral changes in adjacent lamellae in such a manner that fibers in one make an angle of nearly 90 degrees with the fibers in the next. This alternating arrangement in fiber direction explains why lamellae appear to be so distinct, one from another. In one lamella, collagenous fibers will appear elongated on section; in the next, the fibers are sectioned transversely and appear granular.

Architecture of Bone

Spongy bone is simple in structure and consists of trabeculae or plates forming a network, the pattern of which is determined by the mechanical functions of individual bones. The trabeculae comprise a varying number of lamellae in which are lacunae containing osteocytes and a system of intercommunicating canaliculi. In prenatal spongy bone, the lamellae are indistinct, since the osteocollagenous fibers form an irregular network. This is characteristic of rapid bone development and is referred to as *woven bone.* Isolated patches of such bone occur in the adult and during repair of fractures.

In compact bone the lamellae are regularly arranged in a manner determined by the distribution of blood vessels which nourish the bone. The bone is traversed by longitudinal channels, the *Haversian canals*, which anastomose freely with each other by transverse and oblique connections. From the periosteal and endosteal surfaces, *Volkmann's canals* (or nutrient canals) enter the bone at right angles to its long axis and communicate with the Haversian canals. Thus there is a continuous and complex system of canals which contains the blood vessels and nerves of the bone.

Each Haversian canal is surrounded by a varying number (8 to 15) of concentric lamellae. The lamellae of bone matrix, the cells, and the central canal constitute the *Haversian system*, or *osteone*, the unit of structure of compact bone. Canaliculi that border upon a Haversian canal communicate with its cavity and thus bring all lacunae of a system into continuity with the canal. Canaliculi at the periphery of a Haversian system generally do not communicate with those of neighboring systems: they form loops and return to their own lacunae. Since Haversian systems are oriented mainly in the long axis of the bone, in cross section the canals appear as round openings surrounded by ring-shaped concentric lamellae and in longitudinal sections the canals are long slits bordered by columns of lamellae. The intervals between Haversian systems are filled with the *interstitial lamellae,* which are the remnants of Haversian systems partly destroyed during the internal reconstruction of the bone (see page 159). At the periphery and on the internal surface in relation to the marrow cavity lamellae run parallel with the surface and are oriented circumferentially with respect to the axis of the bone. These are the outer (periosteal) and inner (endosteal) *circumferential* or *general* lamellae. Canaliculi within these lamellae open freely onto periosteal and endosteal surfaces. Adjacent lamellar systems are delimited by a thin layer of refractile, modified matrix *(cement line, cement membrane)*.

In addition to the osteocollagenous fibers contained within lamellae, coarse collagenous bundles, or *Sharpey's fibers*, are found in the outer layers of the bone. They are fibers which pass from the periosteum into the outer circumferential and interstitial lamellae and are not found in Haversian systems or in the internal circumferential lamellae. They are surrounded by a narrow zone of uncalcified or only partially calcified matrix. Sharpey's fibers serve to anchor the periosteum firmly to bone and are particularly numerous at points of insertion of ligaments and tendons.

Periosteum.   This fibrous sheath envelops bone, except on articular surfaces. Its close connection with bone depends upon the presence of Sharpey's fibers. It consists of two layers, al-

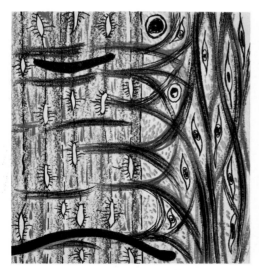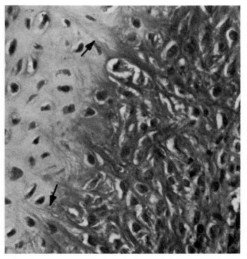

Figure 4–19.   *Left:* Diagram of Sharpey's fibers extending into compact bone as direct continuations of fibers of the periosteum. *Right:* Photomicrograph of Sharpey's fibers. Collagenous (Sharpey's) fibers (arrows) pass from the periosteum, here sectioned close to a joint capsule, into the bone matrix (left). × 250.

though these are not sharply defined. The outer layer is dense fibrous connective tissue and contains a network of blood vessels. The inner layer is composed of more loosely arranged connective tissue, some component collagenous fibers of which enter the bone as Sharpey's fibers. In the adult, the inner layer contains numerous spindle-shaped connective tissue cells (osteoprogenitor cells) which on stimulation (e.g., by fracture) become activated.

Endosteum. This delicate layer lines the marrow cavities and extends as a lining into the canal system of compact bone. It consists of a condensed reticular tissue which has both osteogenic and hemopoietic potencies.

Development and Growth of Bone

Bone has certain unique qualities which must be borne in mind when consideration is given to the methods whereby a bone develops and increases in size. First, bone has a canalicular system, the tiny canals of which extend from one lacuna to another and to bony surfaces, where they open into tissue spaces. Tissue fluid in these spaces becomes continuous with fluid within the canalicular system and thus allows for exchange of metabolites between the blood stream and the osteocytes. By this mechanism cells of bone remain alive even though surrounded by an intercellular substance that is calcified. Second, bone is vascular. The canalicular system cannot operate effectively if it is more than about 0.5 mm removed from a capillary. Hence bone is richly supplied with capillaries which are carried in Haversian and Volkmann's canals. Third, bone can grow only by an appositional mechanism. Interstitial growth, as in cartilage, is impossible in bone because the presence of lime salts in the matrix prevents expansion within the interior. Finally, bone architecture is not static. Bone is destroyed locally and re-formed repeatedly. There is thus a continuous process of reconstruction to consider.

According to the embryological origin there are two types of bone development, *intramembranous* and *endochon-*dral (or *intracartilaginous*). In the former bone develops directly on or within membrane, whereas in the latter it develops within cartilage which must be removed before ossification can occur. Some of the cartilage matrix may remain as a framework upon which bone is laid down. It must be realized, however, that the actual process of bone deposition is the same in both cases. The first bone formed is woven, or immature bone, in which lamellae are indistinct. Soon this is replaced by the mature, lamellar variety of spongy bone, which later may become compact, owing to internal reconstruction.

Intramembranous Bone Formation. This process can be studied best in the flat bones of the skull. In the area where bone is to develop, the mesenchyme consists of primitive connective tissue cells connected to one another by their processes, but without cytoplasmic continuity, and of a semifluid intercellular substance containing delicate collagenous fibers. This mesenchymal sheet or membrane becomes richly vascularized, and consequently some of the cells differentiate into osteogenic or osteoprogenitor cells. They enlarge and assume a polyhedral form, and their cytoplasm becomes more basophil. They now can be identified as osteoblasts. Between such cells thin bars of dense intercellular substance appear. They mask the connective tissue fibers already present within the matrix. The bars of dense matrix increase in size and the cells become surrounded by them. At this stage the matrix is not calcified and constitutes the organic component of bone matrix, termed *osteoid*.

Later the matrix becomes calcifiable through some transformation, supposedly the result of activity by osteoblasts. The minerals are deposited in an orderly fashion as minute crystals in close association with the collagenous fibers. There often is a delay in the deposition of mineral salts in osteoid, and thus matrix at the periphery of growing bone stains less densely than the fully mineralized matrix at the center. As calcified matrix is deposited around osteoblasts and their processes, lacunae and canaliculi are formed, and since processes of adjoining cells are in contact with one another, canaliculi of

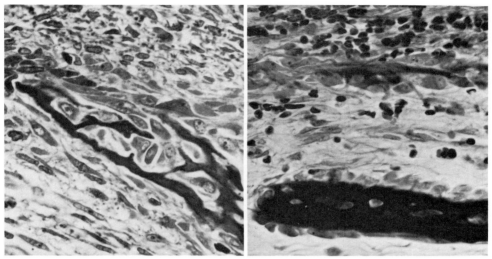

Figure 4–20. Photomicrographs of intramembranous bone formation. *Left:* A section through a newly formed spicule of bone of the developing skull of a human embryo. Note that osteoblasts, which have differentiated from surrounding mesenchymal cells, lie in close relationship to the spicule. *Right:* A later stage of development. The large bony spicule (below) contains osteocytes within lacunae and is surrounded by osteoblasts. A smaller spicule (above) also is present within the vascular mesenchyme. Left, × 550; right, × 350.

adjoining lacunae connect with each other. After the initial stages of bone formation, a layer of osteoblasts appears on the surface of the developing bone. Through the activity of the osteoblasts the bone increases in

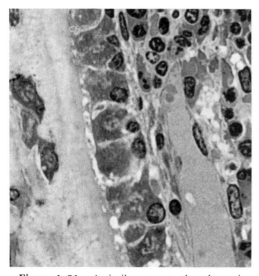

Figure 4–21. A similar stage to that shown in Figure 4–20 (right). Bony matrix, with contained osteocytes, lies to the left. A row of osteoblasts, with densely staining (basophilic) cytoplasm, is associated with the surface of the bone, and the primary marrow cavity (right) contains myeloid tissue. Plastic section, × 600.

thickness. Successive layers of matrix are added by apposition, and osteoblasts, which lie on the surface of bone initially, become included within it as osteocytes. The number of osteoblasts on the surface is maintained by mitosis and by formation of osteoblasts from osteogenic cells within the surrounding connective tissue.

As growth continues at several foci of bone formation, initially the bone consists of spicules and trabeculae, and it is spongy and of the woven type. Later some of this spongy bone is replaced by compact bone as the areas between trabeculae are filled with concentric lamellar bone, thus creating inner and outer plates. Between the plates, spongy bone remains (as the diploë) and the spaces within it, the *primary marrow cavities*, are filled with richly vascularized connective tissue which gradually becomes transformed into myeloid, or *hemopoietic*, tissue. The connective tissue which surrounds a growing mass of bone gives rise to the periosteum.

Endochondral (Intracartilaginous) Bone Formation. This type of ossification, involving the replacement of a cartilage model by bone, is best observed in a long bone. The shape of the

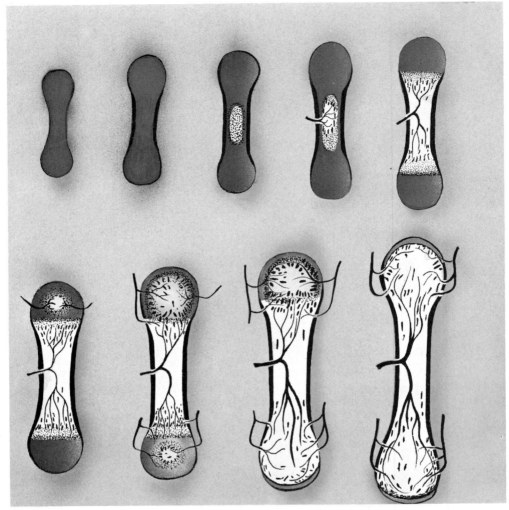

Figure 4–22. Diagram of stages in endochondral ossification. See text for description of stages, beginning on page 153.

cartilage model corresponds closely to that of the future bone, although, of course, it is much smaller in size. During development the cartilage is replaced by bone except at the joint surfaces, but this is a slow process which is not achieved until the bone has reached its full size and growth has ceased. Externally the cartilage is covered by a perichondrium which shows marked cellularity owing to the presence of numerous embryonic connective tissue cells.

The early cartilage model continues to grow by both interstitial and appositional growth. Increase in length follows interstitial growth, whereas in-crease in thickness, although partly due to interstitial growth, principally results from appositional growth.

Bone formation is initiated within a band-shaped area of perichondrium surrounding the center of the diaphysis. The perichondrium here assumes an osteogenic function. Cells of the perichondrium adjoining the cartilage hypertrophy and become osteoblasts. They begin to form bone of the intramembranous type. This is the *periosteal bone ring* or *collar* which surrounds the middle of the diaphyseal region of the cartilage. The perichondrium around this area becomes a periosteum.

Simultaneously with the appearance of the bony collar, changes become apparent in the cartilage itself. In the center of the diaphysis, the cartilage cells hypertrophy and the matrix between the lacunae becomes reduced in amount and calcified. Through apertures in the bony collar, connective tissue sprouts, together with blood vessels, grow into the region of the changed cartilage matrix. These are the *periosteal buds*, which penetrate the partitions between the enlarged cartilage cells and open up cavities. The cavities thus formed are the *primary marrow spaces*, which contain thin-walled blood vessels and embryonic connective tissue cells. Some of the embryonic cells become osteoblasts and enclose the calcified cartilage matrix, first with osteoid and then with calcified bone, just as in intramembranous bone formation. The fate of the cartilage cells in this region is not known, but many undoubtedly die. It is believed by some investigators that some may survive and become osteogenic. The deposition of bone in the center of the diaphysis constitutes the *primary ossification center*.

The zone of endochondral ossification extends toward both ends of the

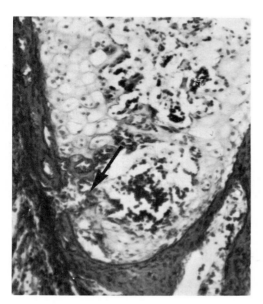

Figure 4–23. Ossification of the human ilium. The periosteal cuff of bone is well developed and a periosteal bud (arrow), comprising bone forming and vascular elements, has entered the cartilage model. × 160. (Courtesy of R. D. Laurenson.)

cartilage by a sequence of changes similar to that which took place in the establishment of the primary ossification center. At the same time the periosteal bone collar becomes thicker and widens toward the epiphyses. It assists in maintaining the strength of the shaft, which otherwise would be weakened by the dissolution of cartilage within the diaphysis. Thus the periosteal bone collar acts as a buttress to support the central zone of resorbing cartilage prior to its replacement by bone.

With the continued growth of cartilage in the epiphyses, the entire cartilage model increases in size. As a result of this and of the extension of the primary ossification center, definite zones become apparent within the cartilage. Of course, each zone changes character as ossification advances toward it. Beginning at the ends of the cartilage and passing toward the ossification center, the following zones, which illustrate the continuing process of endochondral bone formation, can be recognized:

Quiescent or Reserve Zone. This zone, composed of primitive hyaline cartilage, is present nearest to the ends of the bone. Initially it is a relatively long zone but shortens progressively as ossification encroaches upon it. It is a zone which shows slow growth in all directions.

Zone of Proliferation. This is an active zone showing numerous mitoses. Cells of the quiescent zone divide and produce daughter cells which align themselves in distinct rows or columns parallel with the long axis of the cartilage model. Each row consists of a number of cells which are crowded, flattened, and separated by little matrix. A row grows principally by the addition of cells at the distal, free end in relation to the quiescent zone. By this mechanism the cartilage increases in length more than in breadth.

Maturation Zone. Mitoses no longer occur and the cells and lacunae enlarge, becoming cuboidal in shape. This enlargement adds further to the length of the cartilage in this region. The cytoplasm of the cells accumulates considerable amounts of glycogen.

Zone of Calcification. In this zone the matrix surrounding the enlarged

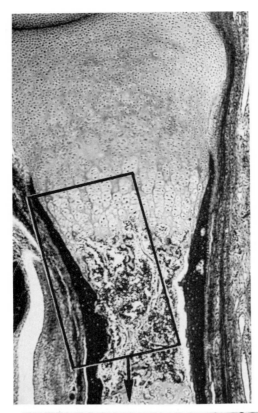

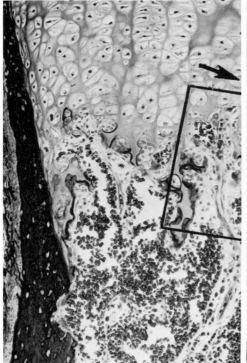

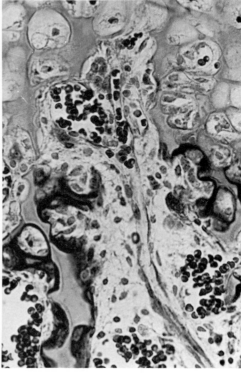

Figure 4–24. Endochondral ossification in the phalanx of a finger. At this stage, the primary center of ossification and the periosteal collar of bone are well developed. The cartilage of the epiphysis shows definite zones of activity, and resorption of bone within the center of the diaphysis has led to the development of the secondary marrow cavity. Top, × 50; lower left, × 125; lower right, × 300.

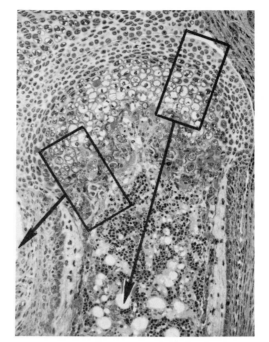

Figure 4–25. An earlier stage of endochondral bone formation than that seen in Figure 4–24. The different zones of cells within the epiphysis are shown in the lower two figures. Plastic sections. Top, × 100; bottom left and right, × 400.

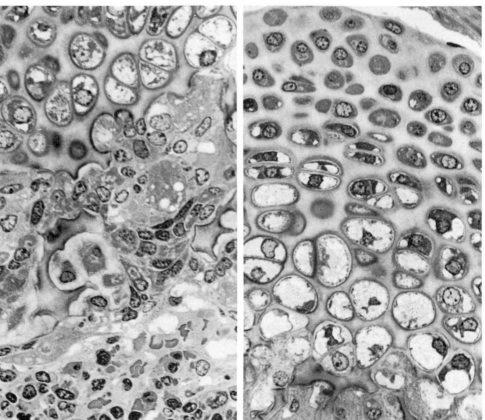

lacunae stains deeply basophil owing to the deposition of minerals within it.

Zone of Retrogression. The cartilage cells die and undergo dissolution as does the matrix between cells. The thicker plates of matrix between rows of cells remain virtually intact. Thus this zone on cross section has the appearance of a honeycomb. Vascular primary marrow extends into the spaces resulting from the destruction of cells and matrix.

Zone of Ossification. Here osteoblasts differentiate from mesenchymal cells of the marrow tissue and gather on the exposed plates of calcified cartilage, where they commence to lay down bone. The remnants of calcified cartilage form a supporting framework.

Zone of Resorption. As ossification advances toward the ends of the cartilage, the marrow cavity increases in size, owing to resorption of bone in the center of the diaphysis. As a result, the length of spongy bone remains nearly constant. The cavity which forms is the *secondary marrow cavity.*

While all these changes are taking place, there is further activity in the periosteum. The periosteal collar of bone thickens and extends at each end. The increase in extent of the periosteal collar compensates for the loss, by resorption, of endochondral bone centrally. The zone of reserve cartilage is maintained by cell division, but it becomes reduced in length as ossification of the diaphysis proceeds.

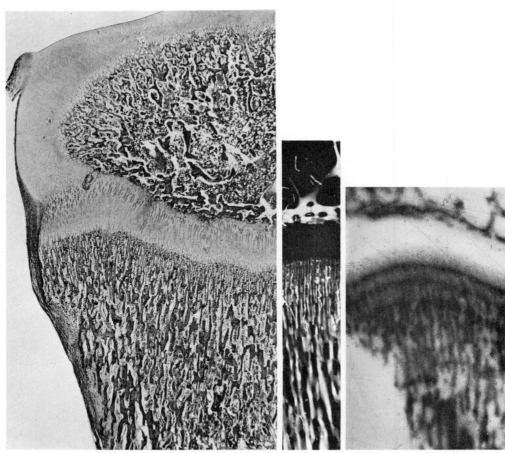

Figure 4–26. *Left:* Upper tibial epiphysis of two-week-old rabbit, showing secondary center of ossification and epiphyseal disc. Undecalcified section. × 12. *Center:* Contact microradiograph of a thin slice of upper tibial epiphysis in which the arterial system was injected with Micropaque. The epiphyseal bony plate, cartilage, and metaphysis are set at the same levels as adjacent figures. *Right:* Radioautograph to illustrate growth of epiphysis. Radioactive calcium injected, 9, 8, 3, 2, and 1 day prior to sacrifice. (Courtesy of F. W. Fyfe.)

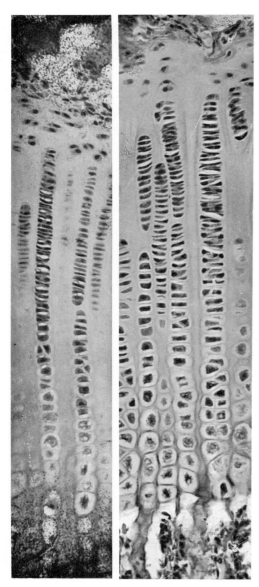

Figure 4–27. Sections of growth cartilages of upper end of tibias of two-month-old *(left)* and three-month-old *(right)* rabbits. Radioactive calcium was injected 30 hours before sacrifice, and the undecalcified sections were dipped in photographic emulsion and developed after several weeks. Silver grains overlie the secondary ossification center (above) and the calcifying ends of the cartilage columns (below), in continuity with the primary bony trabeculae. × 250. (Courtesy of F. W. Fyfe.)

At about the time of birth, *secondary centers of ossification (epiphyseal centers)* appear in both ends of most long bones. The sequence of changes in the cartilage of these centers is identical with that observed in the diaphysis. Cartilage

cells proliferate and hypertrophy, and vascular osteogenic buds enter from the periphery or through tunnels from the diaphysis. Cartilage removal and bone deposition follow. Ossification spreads peripherally in all directions until there is replacement of cartilage by bone except in two regions. Cartilage remains over the free end as articular cartilage and as a plate between the epiphysis and the diaphysis. This is the *epiphyseal plate* or *disc*.

The epiphyseal disc continues to form new cartilage at the proximal surface facing the diaphysis. The formation of cartilage columns, the calcification of cartilage, and the deposition of bone continue here as earlier in the shaft. These processes cause an increase principally in the length of the bone. Proliferation of cartilage and bony replacement occur at about the same rate so that the thickness of the epiphyseal disc remains constant. When growth ceases, there is no further proliferation of cartilage and the epiphyseal disc is replaced by bone. The epiphysis and diaphysis are united by bone, a union which is visible in the adult since the bone formed here is particularly dense. This is the *epiphyseal line*. Henceforth increase in length is impossible.

Increase in diameter of long bones occurs by the deposition of new periosteal bone, which forms intramembranously by appositional growth. The thickness of bone does not increase at the same rate since, as bone is added progressively to the periosteal surface, bone in lesser amounts is resorbed from the endosteal surface. Thus the secondary marrow cavity increases in extent.

Remodeling and Reconstruction of Bone

As a bone enlarges in size, its structure is complicated by internal reconstruction and by remodeling. Remodeling results from resorption in certain areas and deposition of new bone elsewhere. Resorption is associated with the appearance of osteoclasts. At the interface between osteoclasts and bone there is evidence of surface activity in the form of cytoplasmic striations. On electron microscopy they appear as irregular, deep infoldings of the cell membrane. Any reconstruction of bone occurs in response to local mechanical stresses to which the bone is subjected.

In growth of bone, we have been concerned so far with the deposition of spongy bone. In certain areas this is replaced by compact bone. In this process osteoblasts produce layer after layer of bone inward on the surface of longitudinal cavities within spongy bone until the cavities are reduced to narrow canals containing the blood vessels. The system of concentric lamellae with its canal and blood vessels is called a *primitive Haversian system.*

The majority of Haversian systems develop in compact bone by a more complicated process. Bone substance may be dissolved by vascular buds from endosteal or periosteal surfaces. Recent evidence suggests that the normal mechanism of internal bone resorption may occur under the influence of mature osteocytes. This process is referred to as *osteolysis.* The cells responsible for this activity are able to produce both alkaline phosphatase and protease. They are surrounded by a matrix which has a low concentration of both salts and organic matter. The lytic process, which is hormonally controlled (see page 161), results in the formation of wide cylindrical cavities containing blood vessels and embryonic marrow tissue. The tunnel resulting from the erosion process becomes lined by osteoblasts which differentiate from the primitive cells present within the marrow. Successive lamellae of bone are deposited progressively inward until the tunnel is reduced to a narrow canal around the blood vessels. The reconstruction of bone does not terminate, however, with the replacement of primary bone by secondary bone, but continues throughout life. Resorption cavities appear continuously and are replaced by third, fourth, and higher orders of Haversian systems. In this process portions of former Haversian systems may escape destruction and become interstitial lamellae which fill in between new systems. As growth nears completion, the periosteum and endosteum lay down successive layers of basic

or circumferential lamellae, which persist as concentric lamellae.

In a mature bone, therefore, the majority of the matrix is of intramembranous origin. Bone of endochondral origin persists only as narrow trabeculae in the diaphysis and the metaphyses and as the central spongy bone of the epiphyses.

Development of Irregular Bones. The foregoing description is based upon conditions in a typical long bone. Irregular bones develop in a manner similar to the epiphyses of long bones. Ossification begins in the center and extends out in all directions. Cartilage at the periphery serves as a proliferative zone until growth within it ceases, when it is replaced by bone. Further bone may be added by apposition from the periosteum.

Repair of Bone

After a fracture there is hemorrhage from torn vessels and clotting. Proliferating fibroblasts and capillaries invade the clot and form granulation tissue, the *procallus.* The granulation tissue becomes dense fibrous tissue and later transforms into a mass of cartilage. This is the *temporary callus* that unites the fractured bones. Osteoblasts develop from the periosteum and endosteum and lay down spongy bone which progressively replaces the cartilage of the temporary callus in a manner similar to endochondral ossification. Bony union of the fracture is achieved. The bony callus, initially spongy, undergoes reorganization into compact bone and excess bone is resorbed.

The sequence of callus formation after bony injury illustrates the multipotentiality of cells of the periosteum and of the endosteum. After injury the nature of cell differentiation is dependent upon the blood supply. Initially the blood supply to the area is poor, and differentiation of cells is in the direction of fibroblasts and of chondroblasts. After the ingrowth of blood vessels, osteoblasts make their appearance.

Histophysiology of Bone

Both vitamins and hormones play an important role in ossification and the maintenance of bone. In vitamin D deficiency there is a faulty absorption of calcium from foods and a diminished concentration of phosphate in the blood plasma. In children this results in *rickets.* The cartilage matrix and the osteoid tissue fail to calcify completely, and the epiphyseal discs become thick and irregular. In adults the deficiency causes a diminution in calcium content of the bones, a condition known as *osteomalacia.* Vitamin C deficiency results in a condition known as *scurvy,* which is characterized by an inability of tissues of mesenchymal origin to produce and maintain fibers and ground substance. This causes a destruction of osteocollagenous fibers and a diminished production of organic matrix in bones. In vitamin A deficiency osteoblasts do not synthesize bone matrix normally. There is a diminution in the rate of growth of the skeleton and interference with the process of remodeling and with the balance between bone deposition and erosion.

Hormones profoundly influence the growth and maintenance of bones. The *growth hormone* of the anterior pituitary is essential for normal bone growth. Lack of growth hormone results in *dwarfism;* excessive production leads to *gigantism.* Parathyroid hormone regulates the resorption of bone and controls the release of calcium to the blood. The action of parathyroid hormone appears to be in direct opposition to that of thyrocalcitonin, which inhibits resorptive activity and calcium mobilization. Thus there is a balance between release and deposition of calcium to maintain the level of calcium in the blood. The appearance and closure of epiphyseal centers of ossification are related to the production of sex hormones by the gonads.

THE JOINTS

The sites where two or more components of the skeleton, whether bone or cartilage, meet are referred to as joints or *articulations.* They may be either *temporary* or *permanent.* Temporary joints occur during the period of growth: for example, the epiphysis of a long bone is united to the bone of the shaft by hyaline cartilage of the epiphyseal disc. Such a joint disappears when growth ceases and the epiphysis fuses with the shaft. Most joints, however, are permanent, and they may be classified on the basis of their structural features into three main types: fibrous, cartilaginous, and synovial. The first two types frequently are termed synarthroses (*syn,* together; *arthron,* joint), joints which are immovable or only slightly movable. Synovial joints, which allow considerable freedom of movement, are referred to as diarthroses (*di.* apart).

Fibrous Joints. These are joints that are held together by dense fibrous tissue. If the union is extremely tight, the joint is termed a *suture.* Sutures occur only in the skull, and strictly speaking, they are not permanent since the uniting fibrous tissue may be replaced by bone in later life. The resulting bony union is known as a *synostosis.* Joints in which the participating bones are held together by a considerably greater amount of fibrous tissue than in a suture are called *syndesmoses.* Such joints, examples of which are the radioulnar and tibiofibular articulations, allow a certain degree of movement. The third type of fibrous joint, the *gomphosis,* is a specialized articulation restricted to the fixation of teeth in the maxilla and mandible, where the uniting fibrous tissue constitutes the periodontal membrane (see page 339).

Cartilaginous Joints. These joints, often termed secondary cartilaginous to distinguish them from primary joints, are best exemplified by the joints between the bodies of adjacent vertebrae. The surfaces of the opposed bones are covered with sheets of hyaline cartilage, and these in turn are united firmly by a plate of fibrocartilage. *Symphyses,* such as the pubic and manubriosternal joints, are further examples of secondary cartilaginous joints. They differ from the intervertebral discs in that the center of the uniting fibrocartilaginous plate usually contains a small cavity. However, this joint cavity lacks the specializations of a synovial joint.

Synovial Joints. In synovial joints, the participating bones are held together by an articular capsule and their opposed surfaces, covered with articular cartilage, are separated by a narrow interval containing synovial fluid.

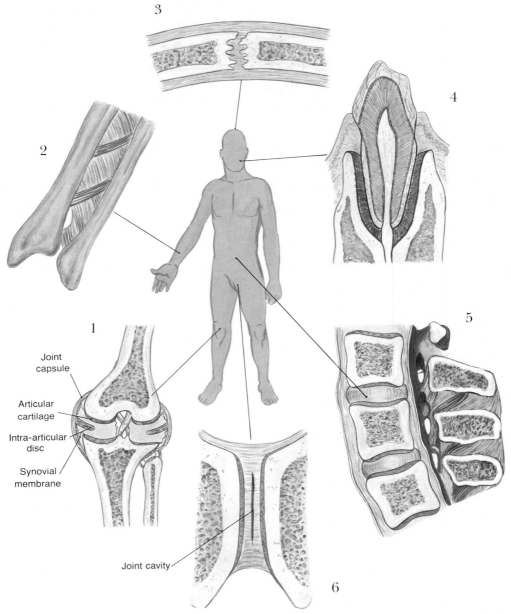

Joint
capsule

Articular
cartilage

Intra-articular
disc

Synovial
membrane

Joint cavity

Figure 4–28. Types of joints. 1, Synovial joint. Fibrous joints; 2, Syndesmosis. 3, Suture. 4, Gomphosis. Secondary cartilaginous joints: 5, Intervertebral disc. 6, Symphysis. (From Leeson, C. R., and Leeson, T. S.: Human Structure: A Companion to Anatomical Studies. Phiadelphia, W. B. Saunders Company, 1972, p. 26.)

Articular cartilage usually is hyaline in type, although the matrix does contain abundant collagenous fibers. In some situations, such as the margins of the glenoid fossa of the shoulder joint and of the acetabulum of hip joint, the cartilage is frankly fibrous in nature. The deepest layer of the articular carti-

lage is calcified and firmly adherent to the underlying bone. Articular cartilage possesses no nerve fibers or blood vessels, and it is not covered with perichondrium.

A *joint capsule* unites the bones. The outer layer of the capsule is dense fibrous tissue that is continuous with the

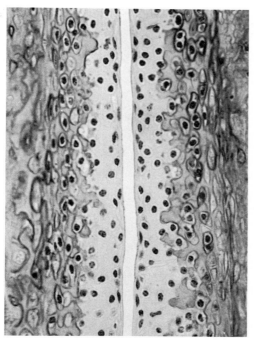

Figure 4–29. Photomicrograph of incudostapedial joint of the middle ear, a typical synovial joint. The joint cavity (center) is bounded by the opposed articular cartilages, the deepest layers of which are calcified and merge into bone. × 250.

margins of the articular cartilages and is surfaced by flattened fibroblasts, held together by junctional complexes. Two types of fibroblasts, or *synovial cells*, are described although they may represent only different functional states of the same cell type. Type A fibroblasts (or M cells), which predominate, contain within their cytoplasm numerous mitochondria and micropinocytotic vesicles, lysosomes, and a prominent Golgi apparatus. These cells are actively phagocytic. In type B synovial cells (or F cells), these organelles are poorly developed, but in contrast, the cells contain an extensive system of granular endoplasmic reticulum. The synovial membrane frequently projects into the joint cavity as coarse folds (*synovial villi*) and may evaginate through the outer layer of the capsule, between neighboring tendons and muscles, to form pockets known as *bursae*.

The synovial membrane is responsible for the production of *synovial fluid*. This viscous fluid is thought to arise principally as a dialysate of the blood plasma and lymph. The mucopolysaccharide fraction of the fluid, mainly hyaluronic acid, probably is synthesized by the synovial cells. This fluid acts as a lubricant and contributes to the nutrition of the articular cartilage.

The joint cavity sometimes is partially or completely subdivided by *intra-articular discs,* composed of fibrocartilage. At their periphery, the discs are connected to the fibrous layer of the capsule.

periosteum over the bones and is thickened in various places to form the ligaments of the joint. The inner layer of the capsule, the *synovial membrane*, lines the joint cavity, except over articular cartilage and, when present, intra-articular discs. The synovial membrane is a thin vascular membrane, rich in fat cells, that is attached around the

REFERENCES

Anderson, H. C.: Calcium-accumulating vesicles in the intercellular matrix of bone. *In* Hard Tissue Growth, Repair and Remineralization. Ciba Foundation Symposium II. Amsterdam, ASP (Elsevier, North Holland), 1973, p. 213.

Bernard, G. W., and Pease, D. C.: An electron microscopic study of initial intramembranous osteogenesis. Am. J. Anat., *125*:271, 1969.

Bonucci, E.: The organic-inorganic relationships in bone matrix undergoing osteoclastic resorption. Calcif. Tissue Res., *16*:13, 1974.

Brookes, M.: Cortical vascularization and growth in foetal trabecular bones. J. Anat., *97*:597, 1963.

Clark, E. R., and Clark, E. L.: Microscopic observations on new formation of cartilage and bone in the living mammal. Am. J. Anat., *70*:167, 1942.

Clarke, I. C.: Articular cartilage: a review and scanning electron microscope study. II. The territorial fibrillar achitecture. J. Anat., *118*:261, 1974.

Cooper, R. R., Milgram, J. W., and Robinson, R. A.: Morphology of the osteon. J. Bone Joint Surg., *48*:1239, 1966.

Davies, D. V.: The structure and functions of synovial membrane. Br. Med. J., *1*:92, 1950.

Goel, S. C.: Electron microscopic studies on developing cartilage. 1. The membrane system related to the synthesis and secretion of extracellular materials. J. Embryol. Exp. Morphol., *23*:169, 1970.

Gomori, G.: Calcification and phosphatase. Am. J. Pathol., *19*:197, 1943.

Haines, R. W.: The histology of epiphyseal union in mammals. J. Anat., *120*:1, 1975.

Hall, B. K.: The origin and fate of osteoclasts. Anat. Rec., *183*:1, 1975.

Ham, A. W., and Harris, W. R.: Repair and transplantation of bone. *In* the Biochemistry and Physiology of Bone, edited by G. H. Bourne. New York, Academic Press, 1971, Vol. 3, p. 338.

Hancox, N. M.: Biology of Bone. New York, Cambridge University Press, 1972.

Horowitz, A. L., and Dorfman, A.: Subcellular sites for synthesis of chondromucoprotein of cartilage. J. Cell Biol., *38*:358, 1968.

Jande, S. S.: Fine structural study of osteocytes and their surrounding bone matrix with respect to their age in young chicks. J. Ultrastruc. Res. *37*:279, 1971.

Jowsey, J.: Studies of Haversian systems in man and some animals. J. Anat. *100*:857, 1966.

Kallio, D. M., Garant, R. P., and Minkin, C.: Evidence of coated membranes in the ruffled border of the osteoclast. J. Ultrastruct. Res., *37*:169, 1971.

Lacroix, P.: Bone and cartilage. *In* The Cell: Biochemistry, Physiology, Morphology, edited by J. Brachet and A. E. Mirsky. New York, Academic Press, 1961, Vol. 5, p. 219.

Lutfi, A. M.: Mode of growth, fate and functions of cartilage canals. J. Anat., *106*:135, 1970.

Minor, R. R.: Somite chondrogenesis. A structural study. J. Cell Biol., *56*:27, 1973.

Owen, M.: The origin of bone cells. Int. Rev. Cytol., *28*:213, 1970.

Owen, M., and MacPherson, S.: Cell population kinetics of an osteogenic tissue. II. J. Cell Biol., *19*:33, 1963.

Palfrey, A. J., and Davies, D. V.: The fine structure of chondrocytes. J. Anat., *100*:213, 1966.

Pritchard, J. J.: General anatomy and histology of bone. *In* The Biochemistry and Physiology of Bone, edited by G. H. Bourne. New York, Academic Press, 1956, p. 1.

Sanzone, C. F., and Reith, E. J.: The development of the elastic cartilage of the mouse pinna. Am. J. Anat., *146*:31, 1976.

Schenk, R. K., Spiro, D., and Wiener, J.: Cartilage resorption in the tibial epiphyseal plate of growing rats. J. Cell Biol., *34*:275, 1967.

Silverberg, R., Silverberg, M., and Feir, D.: Life cycle of articular cartilage cells: An electron microscope study of the hip joint of the mouse. Am. J. Anat., *114*:17, 1964.

Streeter, G. L.: Developmental horizons in human embryos (fourth issue): A review of the histogenesis of cartilage and bone. Contributions to Embryology No. 220, Carnegie Institution of Washington Publ. No. 583, *33*:149, 1949.

Vaes, G.: On the mechanisms of bone resorption. The action of parathyroid hormone on the excretion and synthesis of lysosomal enzymes and on the extracellular release of acid by bone cells. J. Cell Biol., *39*:676, 1968.

Vaughan, J. M.: The Physiology of Bone. London, Oxford University Press, 1970.

SPECIALIZED CONNECTIVE TISSUE: BLOOD

Blood is a specialized form of connective tissue consisting of formed elements, or blood cells, and a fluid intercellular substance, the *blood plasma*. The volume of blood in the healthy adult human is about 5 liters, and quantitatively blood constitutes about 8 per cent of the body weight. Because of the fluidity of plasma, blood cells have no definite spatial relationship. Cells of blood are designated according to their appearance in the fresh, unstained condition and are of two main types: red *(erythrocytes)* and white *(leukocytes)*. Other formed elements present in blood are the *blood platelets*.

The examination of the formed elements of blood is of clinical importance, since the morphology, numbers, and proportions of the different cell types are indicators of many pathological changes in the body. Although some features of the formed elements are visible in fresh blood, many others are seen only after fixation and staining. The Romanovsky methods of staining, of which the Giemsa and Leishman stains are examples, are used extensively in histological and clinical laboratories. They involve staining in solutions that are mixtures of methylene blue and eosin. Additionally it should be noted that the figures given for cell dimensions and numbers are approximate ranges only and that, with the exception of red blood cells, the dimensions of cells when measured in the fresh state are smaller than when

measured in a dried and fixed smear of blood.

ERYTHROCYTES

The erythrocytes, or *red blood corpuscles*, are highly differentiated cells which functionally are specialized for the transportation of oxygen. In mammals the erythrocyte is a cell which has lost its nucleus and its cytoplasmic organelles during development. Each cell is shaped like a biconcave disc and when observed on the flat has a circular outline. In certain diseases human erythrocytes of altered shape are found in the circulation. The corpuscles are elastic and are capable of considerable distortion as is evident in their ability to pass through capillaries of small caliber. They average about 7.6 microns or μm in diameter and 1.9 microns or μm in greatest thickness in dried smears. The living undehydrated corpuscle has a diameter larger than this (about 8.5 microns or μm), and in sectioned material the diameter is smaller (about 7 microns or μm). (These figures, which show remarkable uniformity, should be remembered since they form a convenient means of estimating the size of adjacent cells in blood smears or in sections.)

The erythrocytes are much more numerous than any of the other formed elements of blood. In human males there are 5,000,000 to 5,500,000 erythrocytes per cubic millimeter; in

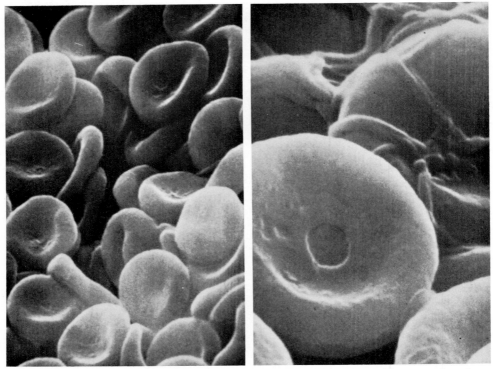

Figure 5–1. Human erythrocytes in a plasma clot. This picture, taken with a scanning electron microscope, illustrates well that the cells are biconcave discs. The strands visible at higher magnification *(right)* are of fibrin. Left, × 4000; right, × 13,000. (Courtesy of T. L. Hayes.)

females, 4,500,000 to 5,000,000. Prolonged residence at high altitude is accompanied by an increase in the number of erythrocytes. The figure for the total surface area of all the red blood corpuscles in the human body is impressive. It amounts to about 3500 square meters. This enormous area is available for exchange between the corpuscles on the one hand and the plasma and air on the other.

A single, fresh erythrocyte is pale greenish yellow in color. In dense masses of red blood corpuscles the color turns red. In a dried smear of peripheral blood the erythrocytes stain red (i.e., are acidophil) with the Leishman or Giemsa stain. The cytoplasm appears homogeneous and no nucleus is present. Each erythrocyte is bounded by a delicate plasma membrane which is a lipoprotein complex (i.e., a typical "unit" membrane). Normally about 1 per cent of the corpuscles encountered in peripheral blood are not fully mature. These immature elements, the *re-ticulocytes*, representing a stage in red blood cell maturation, appear a little larger than the red blood cells, and exhibit a slight bluish tinge after Romanovsky staining because of the presence of remnants of the apparatus of protein synthesis (residual RNA). When stained supravitally with brilliant cresyl blue, this material appears as a delicate internal network, or reticulum.

Erythrocytes have a tendency to adhere to each other along their concave surfaces, thus forming columns or rows like piles of coins. This phenomenon is termed *rouleaux formation* and occurs spontaneously in a stagnant circulation or in blood removed from the circulation. Although the exact cause is not known, it is thought by many to be due to surface tension.

Chemically the content of the erythrocyte consists of a lipid and protein colloidal complex, principally *hemoglobin*, which is responsible for the color of red blood corpuscles and partly determines the shape of the erythrocytes.

In the genetic disease sickle cell anemia, for example, the sickling is said to result from a slight structural change in the chemical composition of the hemoglobin. Hemoglobin has the property of binding oxygen, which it does in the capillaries of the lung. In the tissues the oxygen is distributed in exchange for carbonic acid.

The contents of the corpuscle normally are in osmotic equilibrium with the plasma. If plasma is concentrated by evaporation or if hypertonic solutions are added to the blood, *crenation* of the corpuscles occurs. This is the result of the passage of water from the corpuscles into the plasma, causing shrinkage of the corpuscles and so producing a scalloped contour. On the other hand, if the plasma is diluted, water enters the corpuscles and they swell, becoming spherical in shape. If this continues, hemoglobin escapes into the plasma and the corpuscles lose their color, becoming *blood shadows* or *blood ghosts*. The outward passage of hemoglobin is called *hemolysis* or *laking*. Hemolysis is accomplished also by agents that damage the plasma membrane, and the substances which effect it are known as *hemolysins* or *hemolytic agents*.

Agglutination or clumping of corpuscles is induced by various agents. It may occur in the circulating blood in a variety of pathological conditions. *Agglutinins* present in the plasma of some individuals may cause agglutination of erythrocytes in others. The agglutinins form the basis for the four main blood groups.

In certain pathological conditions not only the number, but also the size, shape, and hemoglobin content of the erythrocytes may vary enormously. A variation in size, *anisocytosis*, may occur. Cells smaller than 6 microns (μm) in diameter are termed *microcytes* and cells larger than normal, found commonly in some types of anemia, are known as *macrocytes* or *megalocytes*. Distortions in shape are termed *poikilocytosis*. When the rate of red blood cell formation is greater than the rate of hemoglobin synthesis, red blood cells are produced which contain a concentration of hemoglobin less than the normal. Such cells appear paler *(hypochromic)* than the normal erythrocytes *(normochromic)*.

LEUKOCYTES

Leukocytes, or *white blood corpuscles*, are cells that contain nuclei. There is an

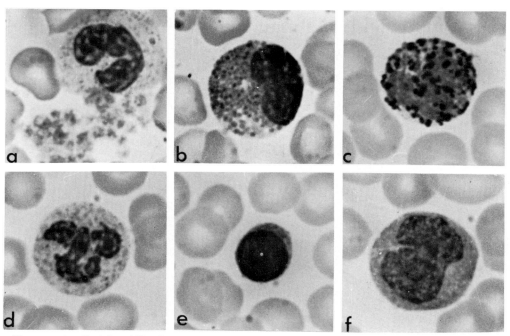

Figure 5–2. Peripheral blood smear. *a,* Platelets and neutrophil leukocyte. *b,* Acidophil leukocyte. *c,* Basophil leukocyte. *d,* Neutrophil leukocyte. *e,* Small lymphocyte. *f,* Monocyte, Wright's stain. All × 1350.

average of 5000 to 9000 leukocytes per cubic millimeter in normal human blood. The count in children is much higher and marked variations from the normal number occur pathologically. If the number is increased above 12,000, the condition is referred to as *leukocytosis*; if decreased below 5000, it is called *leukopenia.*

Leukocytes are of two main types, *agranular* and *granular.* Agranular leukocytes have a cytoplasm which appears homogeneous and nuclei which are spherical to reniform in shape. Granular leukocytes contain abundant specific granules (which in life are semifluid droplets) within their cytoplasm and possess nuclei which exhibit considerable variation in shape. There are two types of agranular leukocytes: *lymphocytes,* which are small cells with a scanty cytoplasm, and *monocytes,* which are slightly larger cells containing somewhat greater amounts of cytoplasm. The granular leukocytes are of three types: *neutrophil, basophil,* and *acidophil* (or eosinophil), distinguished by the affinity of their respective granules for neutral, basic, and acid stains. Leukocytes generally are involved in the cellular and humoral defense of the organism against foreign materials and perform their functions within the connective tissues. They are capable of ameboid movement, which aids in their passage through the walls of blood vessels and in penetration of the connective tissues.

It must be appreciated that leukocytes seen in the living state or in routine histological sections appear quite different from the same cells seen in dried smears. In sectioned material the leukocytes appear rounded as they do within the circulation, but their diameters are less than in the living condition owing to shrinkage. In smear preparations cells flatten and appear larger than in life and many structural details are altered or distorted; for instance, the nucleolus of granular leukocytes is obscured. Thus the type of preparation must be borne in mind when consideration is given to the histological appearances of the various cells.

Agranular Leukocytes

Lymphocytes. In human blood the lymphocytes are spherical cells which vary from 6 to 8 microns or μm in diameter, although a few may be larger. Most are only a little larger than erythrocytes. They constitute from 20 to 35 per cent of the leukocytes of normal blood. The most striking feature of the small lymphocyte is that it has a relatively large nucleus surrounded by a narrow rim of cytoplasm. The nucleus appears spherical and generally shows a small indentation to one side. The densely packed chromatin of the nucleus stains intensely, and the nucleolus is invisible in stained dried smears. The cytoplasm stains basophil, owing to a concentration of ribosomes throughout the cytoplasm, as is evident on electron micrographs. Purplish, azurophil granules occasionally may be seen within the cytoplasm, but unlike the specific granules of the granular leukocytes, they are not a constant feature.

A few of the lymphocytes of normal circulating blood may be as large as 10 to 12 microns or μm. Their larger size is due chiefly to a greater amount of cytoplasm. These cells sometimes are referred to as *medium-sized lymphocytes.* Some of the larger cells may appear to be intermediate between lymphocytes and monocytes. None of these large cells should be confused with the *large lymphocytes* which reside in the lymph nodes and appear in the blood only in pathological conditions. The latter are distinguished by the presence of a vesicular nucleus with prominent nucleoli.

Lymphocytes of blood, although they appear morphologically similar, constitute a heterogeneous cell population and they may be classified on the basis of origin, fine structural appearances, surface markers, life cycle, and function. They also have the capacity to be transformed into other cell types, as mentioned briefly in Chapter 3. There are two major categories of lymphocytes, T and B, and these are discussed in more detail on page 171.

Monocytes. Monocytes are large cells which constitute only from 3 to 8 per cent of the leukocytes of normal blood. They measure 9 to 12 microns or μm in diameter but in dried smears may flatten out to achieve a diameter of 20 microns or μm, or more. The nucleus usually is eccentrically placed within the cell and is ovoid or kidney-shaped. It may show a deep depression or be horseshoe-shaped in older cells. The chromatin material within it is disposed in a delicate network, and thus the nucleus does not stain as deeply as that of the lymphocyte. The cytoplasm is relatively abundant and with Wright's stain is pale grayish-blue in color in dried smears. It often has a vacuolated or reticulated appearance and contains a population of azurophil granules which generally are more numerous but smaller than those in lymphocytes. The granules are primary lysosomes. The cytoplasm also contains some granular endoplasmic reticulum but fewer free ribosomes than are found in lymphocytes.

Rarely one may find intermediates between monocytes and medium-sized lymphocytes, and in such cases positive identification is difficult.

Granular Leukocytes

In contrast to lymphocytes and monocytes, granular leukocytes always contain specific granules. They are further characterized by the presence of a many-lobed (polymorphous) nucleus. For this reason sometimes they are referred to as *polymorphonuclear leukocytes.*

Neutrophils. The neutrophil, polymorphonuclear leukocytes are 7 to 9 microns or μm in diameter in the fresh condition and 10 to 12 microns or μm in dried smears. They are the most numerous of the leukocytes in human blood and constitute 65 to 75 per cent of the total. The nucleus is highly polymorphous and shows a variety of forms. It usually consists of from three to five irregularly ovoid lobes connected by fine threads of chromatin. The number of lobes increases with age. No nucleoli can be seen. In dried smears of the peripheral blood of human females one can see a small nuclear appendage attached to the remainder of the nucleus by a fine strand of chromatin in about 3 per cent of the neutrophils. This "drumstick," first noted by Davidson and Smith, probably represents the sex chromosome. Presumably it is

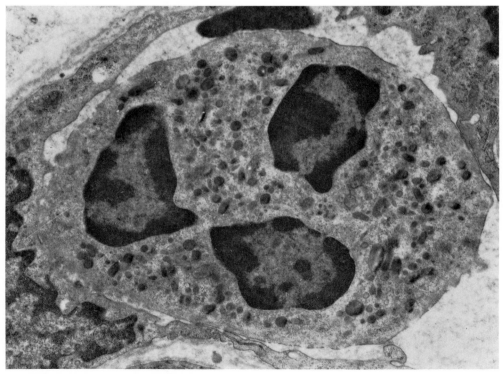

Figure 5–3. Electron micrograph of a neutrophil within a capillary. Three lobes of the nucleus may be seen. Numerous specific granules lie within the finely granular cytoplasm. × 14,500.

present in all the cells of females, but it is closely packed within one of the lobes of the nucleus in most cells and thus is obscured.

The abundant cytoplasm is filled with fine granules, the majority of which are neutrophil. In other mammals the granules have a variable size and staining reaction. In the rabbit and guinea pig the granules accept the acid stain, and thus in these animals the cells may be called *pseudoeosinophils*. Since the cells vary in their staining reactions in different species, sometimes they are called *heterophil* leukocytes rather than neutrophils. The granules mainly are a special type of lysosome which contains principally hydrolytic enzymes. The enzymes are liberated following ingestion by neutrophils of particles such as carbon, bacteria, and other microorganisms. In addition to the specific neutrophil granules, the cytoplasm contains azurophil granules. These appear relatively dense on electron micrographs and contain lysosomal enzymes and peroxidase. Both granule types are formed within the Golgi apparatus and are membrane bounded.

Eosinophils. The eosinophil, or acidophil, leukocytes are somewhat larger than the neutrophils and in the fresh condition are 9 to 10 microns or μm in diameter. In dried smears the size of the flattened cells varies from 12 to 14 microns or μm. They normally constitute about 2 to 4 per cent of the white blood cells. The nucleus is usually bilobed. The cytoplasm characteristically is filled with coarse, refractile granules of uniform size, which stain intensely with acid dyes. The specific granules have a striking appearance in electron micrographs: they appear banded because of the presence within them of dense cylindrical crystals. The granules have been shown to contain peroxidase as well as a number of hydrolytic enzymes. Thus, these granules, like those of neutrophils, are lysosomal in nature.

Basophils. These cells are difficult to find in human blood since they constitute only about 0.5 to 1 per cent of the total number of leukocytes. They are about the same size as neutrophils, 7 to 9 microns or μm in diameter in the fresh condition and 10 microns or μm or a little more in dried smears. The

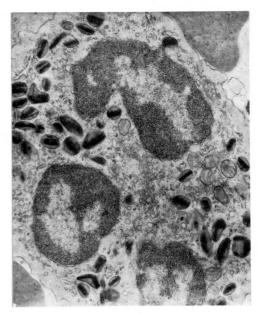

Figure 5–4. Electron micrograph of a portion of an eosinophil within a capillary. Three lobes of the nucleus may be seen. An element of the Golgi apparatus lies in the central region of cytoplasm. Note the large specific granules, each containing a dark, angular mass. × 13,500.

nucleus often is irregular in outline and partially constricted into two lobes. The cytoplasmic granules are spherical, coarse, and variable in size. Some characteristically overlie the nucleus and tend to obscure its outline. The granules are soluble in water and therefore are partly dissolved or absent in routine preparations. They are basophil and metachromatic and contain histamine, heparin, and serotonin. Unlike the granules in the other types of granular leukocytes, they are not considered to be lysosomes.

Functions of Leukocytes

Little is known about the functions of leukocytes while in the blood stream, where they appear to be largely inactive. They perform most of their functions outside the vascular system, where they show active movement and some exhibit phagocytosis. The movement they exhibit is a crawling or ameboid process on a substrate. Neutrophils are the most active, followed in order by monocytes and basophils. Lymphocytes generally appear the most sluggish but in certain conditions may become remarkably active. There is a constant migration of leukocytes out of the vessels into the tissues. Some cells may return into the blood or lymph vessels. Emigration is greatly increased toward the site of local injury or inflammation. This is a specific response to chemotactic stimulation. The first cells to respond to such a stimulus are granulocytes and later monocytes. Lymphocytes accumulate in the tissues at sites of chronic inflammation. Neutrophils constitute the first line of defense against invading organisms, but they are not equally effective against all types of bacteria. They possess the capacity to engulf bacteria by a process of endocytosis and form phagosomes. Membranes of the neutrophil and azurophil granules then fuse with the membranes of the phagosomes to form secondary lysosomes, and the enzymes present in the granules destroy the bacteria. After this activity, neutrophils become depleted of granules and eventually die.

Eosinophils, like neutrophils, possess granules that are lysosomal in nature, and they are thought to phagocytose antibody-antigen complexes. The number of eosinophils is greatly increased in certain allergic conditions and in parasitic infestations, and the number is decreased following the administration of adrenal corticosteroids. Basophils increase in number in relatively few pathological conditions. There is some evidence to support the view that they elaborate the heparin and histamine of circulating blood. These materials are aggregated in the granules and are discharged at the cell surface by exocytosis. Such features indicate that basophils have a close relationship to mast cells of the general connective tissues. It is possible that basophils, like mast cells, can release their granules in response to the action of certain antigens, but this is yet to be proved.

Monocytes migrate readily through vessel walls and are actively phagocytic. Once they leave the blood stream, they are indistinguishable from connective tissue macrophages (histiocytes), and it is generally considered that these two cell types are identical. In the tissues, they interact with the lymphocytes of the immune defense system.

In recent years, the functions of lymphocytes and the relationship of small, medium-sized, and large lymphocytes have received much attention. It is generally accepted that medium-sized lymphocytes represent either a step in the development of small lymphocytes from large lymphocytes or an intermediate stage in the differentiation of small lymphocytes into plasma cells. With regard to function, the majority of the evidence concerns small lymphocytes, which are known to play a major role in the initiation of the immune responses. It has been shown that small lymphocytes comprise at least two distinct populations of cells as determined by their site of formation, their life span, and their susceptibility to certain drugs. Some lymphocytes arise in the bone marrow and pass to the thymus, where they proliferate. These thymic-processed cells *(T lymphocytes)* then may re-enter the blood stream and return to the bone marrow or to peripheral lymphoid organs, where they may live for months or years. They are responsible for cell-mediated immune reactions, including foreign graft rejection. The exact manner in which T lymphocytes function in the latter instance is not fully understood. They surround the graft and produce factors that eventually destroy the graft. Other lymphocytes, the *B lymphocytes* (so called because they require the *bursa of Fabricius,* a lymphoid organ in the cloaca of birds or its unidentified equivalent in mammals for development) apparently do not pass through the thymus but move directly via the blood stream to the general lymphoid tissues. They are believed to survive for a matter of a few days only. When exposed to antigens in any unwanted or abnormal materials that are present within the body, B lymphocytes differentiate into plasma cells which synthesize antibodies that are released into the blood, lymph, and intercellular fluid. T lymphocytes and macrophages play an important role in this process by bringing antigens into contact with B lymphocytes. B lymphocytes also are the precursors of *memory cells,* which are lymphocytes that have been in contact with an antigen but have not differentiated into plasma cells. If such cells contact the same antigen again, they proliferate rapidly and differentiate into plasma cells that synthesize antibody against the antigen. This explains why a second injection of antigen results in a greater and faster production of antibody than the first injection.

Since lymphocytes play such an important role in cell-mediated immune reactions it is not surprising that they are particularly abundant in the connective tissues that underlie the epithelial lining of the respiratory and digestive tracts.

BLOOD PLATELETS

Blood platelets are small protoplasmic discs which are colorless in circulating blood. They are 2 to 4 microns or μm in diameter and their number varies considerably, but usually it is given as 200,000 to 300,000 per cubic millimeter of blood. Their number is

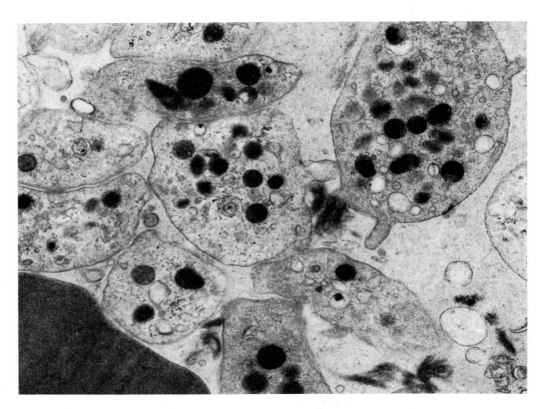

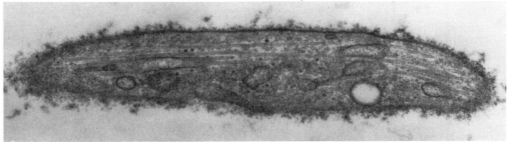

Figure 5–5. *Top:* Electron micrograph of a clump of platelets. Each contains a group of dense granules and microtubules, sectioned transversely, within the finely granular cytoplasm. A portion of an erythrocyte is also present *(lower left).* × 8,500. *Bottom:* A single platelet containing numerous microtubules, sectioned longitudinally. × 25,000.

extremely difficult to count since they adhere to each other and to all surfaces as soon as blood is removed from a vessel. Lower vertebrates lack platelets; instead they possess small nucleated cells, the *thrombocytes.*

Platelets are round or ovoid on the flat; when seen in profile they appear spindle- or rod-shaped. Blood stains demonstrate two regions of the platelet, a deeply basophil granular zone (the *granulomere*), usually centrally located, and a pale, homogeneous peripheral zone (the *hyalomere*). No nucleus is present. Electron micrographs of platelets reveal the presence of numerous microtubules and small granules within the cytoplasm, the majority of the latter being localized within the granulomere region. The fine structural appearance of the granules and recent biochemical evidence indicate that the granules contain a catecholamine.

Platelets arise as detached portions of peculiar giant cells of bone marrow, the *megakaryocytes.* Platelets play several roles in hemostasis. They adhere to injured regions of blood vessels, producing a *white thrombus* which covers injured surfaces and plugs deficiencies within the vessel walls. They are presumed to produce an enzyme, *thromboplastin*, which is of importance in the clotting mechanism. Thromboplastin aids in the transformation of *prothrombin* into *thrombin*, and thrombin in turn transforms *fibrinogen* into *fibrin.* Serotonin, an agent that causes contraction of smooth muscle in small blood vessels, also is present in platelets, probably located in small cytoplasmic granules.

A decrease in the number of circulating platelets is seen clinically in a condition known as *thrombocytopenia.*

PLASMA

Plasma is the fluid which transports all nutritive materials. In it are found the nutritive substances derived from the digestive system, the waste substances produced in the tissues, and the hormones. It constitutes 55 per cent of blood; cellular elements account for 45 per cent. Plasma is a homogeneous, slightly alkaline fluid which contains, in addition to the materials already mentioned, dissolved gases, inorganic salts, proteins, carbohydrates, lipids, and certain other organic substances. Suspended particles can be demonstrated within it by phase and by dark-field microscopy. These are *chylomicrons*, minute fat globules which are more numerous after a fatty meal.

When the circulation ceases, or when blood is exposed to air, one of the globulins of plasma (fibrinogen) precipitates as a network of fine filaments, the fibrin. The contraction of clotted blood or plasma (*syneresis*) expresses a clear, yellowish fluid, *serum.*

LYMPH

Lymph is the fluid which is collected from the tissues and returned to the blood stream. Its composition varies considerably. There are no cellular elements within the lymph of the smallest lymph vessels. Cells, the majority of them lymphocytes, are added to the lymph as it passes through the lymph nodes. The lymph nodes also add antibodies (immunoglobulins) to the lymph and, from there, to the blood stream. Lymph draining from the walls of the small intestine is milky because of the fat globules which it contains, and in this situation it is referred to as *chyle.* Lymph coagulates but the process occurs much more slowly than in blood and the clot is soft.

LIFE SPAN AND DISPOSAL OF BLOOD CELLS

In contrast to many cells, red and white blood cells live for only a relatively short period of time. The life span of the human erythrocyte is approximately 120 days. This may be determined by several methods. Differential agglutination, in which the length of time compatible donor cells survive in a recipient, is cumbersome and largely has been superseded by methods tagging red blood cells with isotopes. Of the latter, chromium tagging, utilizing ^{51}Cr, now is most commonly used. A small quantity of washed red blood cells simply is mixed with a solution of $Na_2[^{51}Cr]O_7$ and this is reinjected into the subject from whom the blood was removed. The life span is estimated by the persistence of radioactivity.

It is believed that the macrophages, particularly in the spleen and liver, remove most of the aging erythrocytes from the circulation. After destruction of red blood cells by the phagocytic cells, hemoglobin is broken down into an iron-containing portion (hematin) and an iron-free portion (globin). The hematin is further broken down into iron, which is reutilized or stored, and into bilirubin, which is transported to the liver and excreted in the bile.

The life span of the various types of white blood cells is difficult to determine since these cells leave the blood vascular system to enter the tissue spaces, but it appears to be quite variable. There is evidence that the white blood cells remain in the circulation only for about 24 hours. However, many lymphocytes undoubtedly return to the lymphoid organs and recirculate. How long white blood cells remain viable after leaving the circulation is unknown. Granulocytes appear to remain alive in the tissue spaces only a few days. Senile and dead cells are thought to be removed by phagocytes within the liver and spleen and locally within the connective tissues. There is a considerable loss of white blood cells owing to migration through the lining epithelia of mucous membranes, particularly into the lumina of the digestive and respiratory systems.

Platelets are believed to survive for four to five days in circulating blood. They are thought to be removed from the circulation similarly to erythrocytes, i.e., by phagocytic activity of macrophages in the spleen and liver.

HEMOPOIESIS

Formed elements of blood are short-lived and continuously are being destroyed. The number of formed elements within blood is kept at a constant number by the formation of new cells. The process by which blood cells are formed is called *hemopoiesis*, and this occurs in the *hemopoietic tissues*. The formed elements of blood are divided into two groups according to the major sites of their development and differentiation in the adult. Lymphocytes and monocytes are developed chiefly in the lymphoid tissues and are termed *lymphoid elements*. Erythrocytes and granulocytes normally are produced within the bone marrow (*myeloid tissue*) and are referred to as *myeloid elements*. This separation, however, is not absolute. There is now clear evidence, principally from radioautography and chromosome marker techniques, that monocytes and some lymphocytes arise from precursor cells within the bone marrow. Additionally, the separation is not seen in the fetus, where blood cells are formed in different sites at different ages and appear successively in the yolk sac, mesenchyme and blood vessels, liver, spleen, and lymph nodes. In the adult, in certain pathological conditions, myeloid elements may be formed again in the spleen, liver, and lymph nodes, a condition known as *extramedullary hemopoiesis*.

Hemopoiesis remains one of the greatest areas of controversy in the field of histology. The major point of disagreement concerns the nature of the stem cell or cells of the several lines of differentiation. One theory, the *unitarian* or *monophyletic* theory of hemopoiesis, holds that all blood cells, red and white, arise from a common stem cell, the *hemocytoblast*. The *dualistic* or *diphyletic theory* holds that lymphocytes and monocytes derive from one stem cell (called the *lymphoblast* by many authors) and granular leukocytes and erythrocytes from a separate cell (the *myeloblast*). At the other extreme, the complete polyphyletic theory maintains that there is a primitive stem cell for each type of blood cell. There has been considerable misunderstanding in the past with regard to these theories, and much of this has been the result of the use of different terminologies by proponents of the different theories. Today the unitarian theory appears to be accepted by the majority of hematologists. The following account is based upon this interpretation, and it should be emphasized that the controversies do not affect the factual descriptions of the

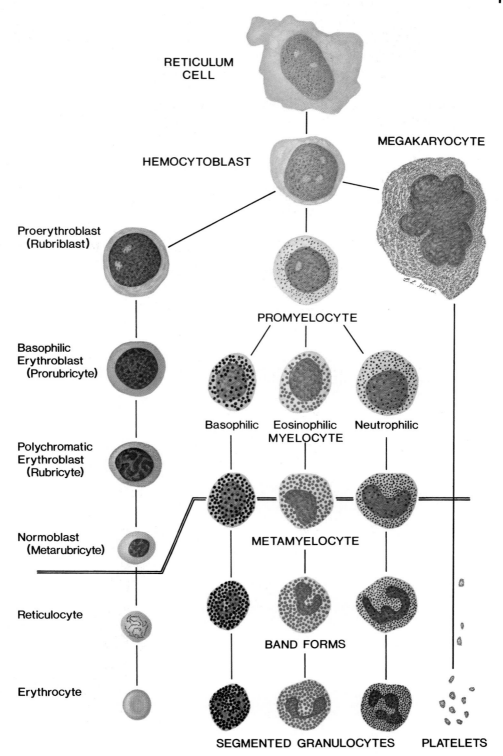

Figure 5–6. Development of myeloid elements. The double line separates the cells that are found in the bone marrow from the mature cells below the line seen normally in peripheral blood. Note that the myeloblast stage (between the hemocytoblast and the promyelocyte) has been omitted from this diagram. (Courtesy of J. H. Cutts.)

structural features of the cells of various developmental stages. The controversies essentially center around the relationships between cells of the earliest stages.

Development of Myeloid Elements

Myeloid tissue, under normal conditions, is confined to the marrow cavities of bone, where it is termed *bone marrow.* Bone marrow is the largest organ in the body, constituting about 4.5 per cent of the total body weight. In the adult there are two types of bone marrow, *red* and *yellow.* Red bone marrow is actively hemopoietic, whereas in yellow bone marrow most of the hemopoietic tissue has been replaced by fat. In the adult, red bone marrow occurs principally in the sternum, ribs, vertebrae, skull, and proximal epiphyses of some of the long bones.

Myeloid tissue consists of a framework or *stroma*, blood vessels, and the free cells lying within the meshwork of the stroma.

Stroma. The framework is a loose latticework of reticular (argyrophil) fibers in close association with primitive and phagocytic reticular cells. Fat cells are scattered singly within the stroma, unlike yellow bone marrow in which the fat cells are so concentrated as to exclude nearly all other elements.

Blood Vessels. The characteristic feature of the circulation of myeloid tissue is the presence of large, tortuous sinusoids, which differ from capillaries by their larger diameter and by their close association with adventitial reticular cells that are minimally phagocytic. The walls of the sinusoids possess wide fenestrations and the surrounding basal lamina is incomplete. The deficiencies within the walls allow newly formed blood cells ready entry into the circulation. Arterioles connect directly with the sinusoids, which themselves are drained by narrow, thin-walled veins that leave the bone marrow at numerous sites.

Free Cells. Cells lying free within the meshes of the stroma represent all stages in the maturation of red and white blood cells. Mature erythrocytes, the three types of granular leuko-cytes, and agranular leukocytes (lymphocytes, monocytes, and some plasma cells) are found between the immature elements.

The Stem Cell: The Hemocytoblast

The hemocytoblast is an ameboid cell of lymphoid nature. It is a relatively large cell, approximately 10 to 14 microns (μm) in diameter. The nucleus is relatively undifferentiated and contains one or two nucleoli. In dried smears the nucleus shows dense accumulations of chromatin material. In sectioned material of bone marrow the nucleus appears vesicular, with some peripheral condensation of heterochromatin, and the nucleoli are distinct. Azurophil granules are seen occasionally within the thin rim of basophil cytoplasm.

Hemocytoblasts arise chiefly by mitotic divisions of their own type. They are present in very small numbers in marrow and are thought to have a very slow turnover. They give rise to all myeloid elements and in addition, according to the unitarian theory of hemopoiesis, to lymphoid elements.

Erythrocytes

Although erythrocytes represent the majority of the formed elements of blood, developing and mature erythrocytes constitute only a minority of blood cells present within myeloid tissue. Two major reasons for this are that the development of a mature erythrocyte takes only about three days whereas a granular leukocyte requires 14 days or more for development, and the short life span of the latter. It should be borne in mind that the principal processes involved in the differentiation of erythrocytes are reduction in size, condensation of nuclear chromatin and eventually loss of the nucleus and of cellular organelles, and acquisition of hemoglobin.

For descriptive purposes, erythrocyte development is divided into a number of stages, but it must be emphasized that the process is a continuous one. The stages of erythrocyte development,

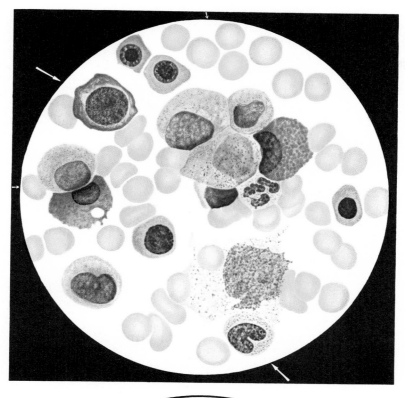

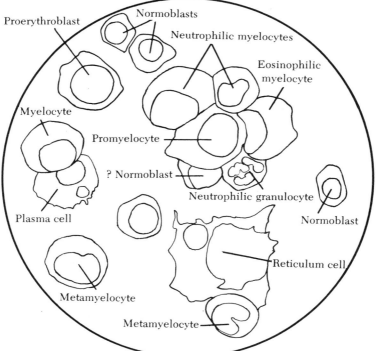

Figure 5–7. Normal marrow smear and diagram of a representative area. Leishman stain. (Plate from Heilmeyer, L., and Begemann, H.: Atlas der Klinischen Hamatologie und Cytologie. Berlin, Springer, 1955.)

in order of differentiation from the hemocytoblast, are *proerythroblast, basophil erythroblast, polychromatophil erythroblast, normoblast* (orthochromatic erythroblast), *reticulocyte*, and *erythrocyte*. The terminology used here has the advantage that it is descriptive of most of the stages, but the student should be aware of the fact that other terminologies do exist. A description of the stages follows, and the terms in parentheses represent those recommended by an International Committee on Nomenclature.

Proerythroblast (Rubriblast). This is the earliest recognizable cell of the erythrocyte series and is believed to differentiate from the hemocytoblast, or pluripotential stem cell, by way of a committed erythroid progenitor cell. The proerythroblast is the largest of the precursor cells, about 15 to 20 microns (μm) in diameter. The nucleus has a uniform chromatin pattern, more distinct than that of the hemocytoblast, and one or more prominent nucleoli. The amount of cytoplasm is greater than that of the hemocytoblast, and it is moderately basophil. A small amount of hemoglobin can be detected within the cytoplasm by special techniques but is obscured by the basophilia of the cytoplasm in stained preparations. After undergoing a number of mitotic divisions, the proerythroblast gives rise to the basophil erythroblast.

Basophil Erythroblast (Prorubricyte). The basophil erythroblast is a slightly smaller cell than the proerythroblast and averages 10 microns (μm) in diameter. The nucleus possesses a coarse network of dense heterochromatin, and the nucleolus usually is obscured. The sparse cytoplasm shows intense basophilia, indicative of a further increase in the numbers of free ribosomes and polyribosomes. Hemoglobin continues to be formed but is masked by the basophilia.

Polychromatophil Erythroblast (Rubricyte). Basophil erythroblasts undergo numerous mitotic divisions and produce cells that acquire sufficient hemoglobin for it to be observed in stained preparations. After staining with Leishman or Giemsa stain, the cytoplasm varies in color from a purplish-blue to a lilac or gray owing to the presence of varying amounts of pink-staining hemoglobin within the basophil cytoplasm of the erythroblasts. Thus they are *polychromatophil.* The nucleus of the polychromatophil erythroblast has a denser chromatin network than that of the basophil erythroblast and the cell is smaller.

Normoblast (Metarubricyte). The polychromatophil erythroblasts undergo a number of mitotic divisions. The basophilia of the cytoplasm decreases and the amount of hemoglobin increases to such an extent that the cytoplasm stains approximately as acidophil as that of the mature erythrocyte. Cells which exhibit this degree of acidophilia within their cytoplasm are referred to as normoblasts. The normoblast is smaller than the polychromatophil erythroblast and contains a smaller nucleus which stains densely basophil. Gradually the nucleus becomes pyknotic. There is no further mitotic activity. Finally the nucleus is extruded from the cell together with a thin rim of cytoplasm. Extruded nuclei are ingested by macrophages associated with the stroma of the bone marrow.

Reticulocyte. The reticulocyte, or immature erythrocyte, has been described previously (see page 166). It is thought that the majority of reticulocytes lose their reticular structure before leaving the bone marrow, since the reticulocyte count of peripheral blood normally is less than 1 per cent of the erythrocytes.

The stages just described in the process of *erythropoiesis* are, in the main, morphological manifestations of the synthesis of hemoglobin. The concentration of RNA in the ribosomal clusters (polyribosomes) that are synthesizing hemoglobin is responsible for the basophilia of the cytoplasm, most marked in the basophil erythroblast. The presence of RNA can be correlated with the active synthesis of nucleotides and hemoglobin.

The normal development of erythrocytes is dependent upon many different factors, including the presence of the parent substances (principally globin, heme, and iron) of hemoglobin. Additional factors, such as ascorbic acid, vitamin B_{12}, and the *intrinsic factor* (normally present in gastric juice), which function as coenzymes or as precursors of coenzymes in the synthetic process, also are necessary for the normal maturation of erythrocytes.

The most potent stimulus for development of erythrocytes is tissue hypoxia (oxygen deficiency), which induces formation of a humoral factor, *erythropoietin,* that travels in the plasma to the bone marrow, where it stimulates production of more erythrocytes. Erythropoietin is produced principally in the kidney and appears to act by stimulating committed erythroid progenitor cells to differentiate into proerythroblasts and erythroblasts. The rate of cell division also is increased, as is the rate of release of reticulocytes from the bone marrow. Thus the synthesis and release of erythropoietin is directly related to the availability of oxygen in the tissues and to the number of circulating erythrocytes carrying oxygen.

Granulocytes

The stages of granulocyte development, in order of differentiation from the hemocytoblast, are: *myeloblast, promyelocyte, myelocyte, metamyelocyte,* and granular leukocyte. Myelocytes of the three types (neutrophil, eosinophil, and basophil) contain their characteristic, specific granules and further differentiation involves a progressive (but modest) reduction in size, an increasing darkening and lobation of the nucleus, and a further accumulation of specific granules.

Myeloblasts. Myeloblasts are the most immature recognizable cells of the granulocyte series and are thought to arise from hemocytoblasts by way of an intermediate cell type. They are variable in size, ranging from 10 to 15 microns (μm) in diameter. The large spherical nucleus shows a delicate chromatin pattern and one or two nucleoli. Electron micrographs show that the cytoplasm, which is scanty and somewhat more basophil than that of the hemocytoblast, contains numerous mitochondria and free ribosomes, but few elements of granular endoplasmic reticulum.

Promyelocytes. These cells are somewhat larger than the myeloblast.

The nucleus is rounded or oval, with dense, peripheral heterochromatin and an indistinct nucleolus. Generally the cytoplasm is basophil, but it may show localized acidophil areas, and it is characterized by the presence of scattered, densely azurophil granules. These nonspecific, or primary, granules are thought to represent a special type of primary lysosome.

Myelocytes. Promyelocytes proliferate and differentiate into myelocytes. In the process of differentiation, the essential change is the appearance of specific granules which have the size, shape, and staining characteristics that allow one to recognize that they are neutrophils, eosinophils, or basophils. Since the primary, azurophil granules are produced only in the promyelocyte stage, their number in each cell is reduced with each myelocyte division. Myelocytes also show a reduction in size, averaging 10 microns (μm) in diameter, and decreased basophilia of the cytoplasm. There is an increased content of heterochromatin in the nucleus, and in late myelocytes, the nucleus indents and begins to assume a horseshoe shape.

Metamyelocytes. After repeated divisions of the myelocytes, the cells become smaller and cease dividing. The cells which are a product of the final division are metamyelocytes. They are juvenile forms of granular leukocytes and have a characteristic granular content. The nucleus, at first horseshoe-shaped, gradually indents further. At this stage, the late metamyelocyte is known as a *band cell.* As the cells age, the nucleus acquires its typical lobation, the number of lobes usually varying from three to five. The basophil metamyelocyte differs from the other two types of metamyelocytes in that its nucleus does not differentiate into distinct lobes. Thus it is difficult to distinguish basophil metamyelocytes from mature basophil leukocytes. The mature cells *(segmented granulocytes)* enter the sinusoids and thus reach the blood stream.

In each of the aforementioned myelocyte stages, the neutrophils far outnumber the eosinophils and basophils. The granular leukocyte precursors far outnumber the progenitors of the

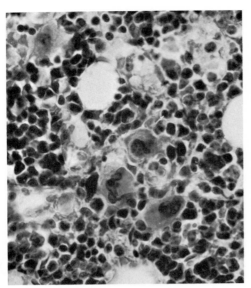

Figure 5–8. Section of active human bone marrow from the cranium. Three megakaryocytes and portions of three fat cells are present. × 400.

lationship can be explained partly by the fact that erythrocytes survive for a much longer time in the circulation than do the leukocytes.

Loss of leukocytes from circulating blood results in an increase in the rate of release of these cells from bone marrow, and a more severe loss induces an increased rate of differentiation of stem cells of the granulocyte series. This suggests that production of granulocytes is controlled by a humoral mechanism yet to be identified.

Megakaryocytes and Platelet Formation

The megakaryocytes are giant cells (30 to 100 microns or μm or more in diameter) which are thought to be derived from the hemocytoblast. They are characteristic of all adult mammalian bone marrow, and they may be found also in the hemopoietic tissues (liver, spleen) during embryonic development. The nucleus is complexly lobed, and individual lobes may be closely packed or connected by fine strands of chromatin material. The cy-

erythrocytes. This preponderance of early leukocyte forms over erythrocyte progenitors is in contrast to the opposite relationship in blood. As explained earlier, the difference in numerical re-

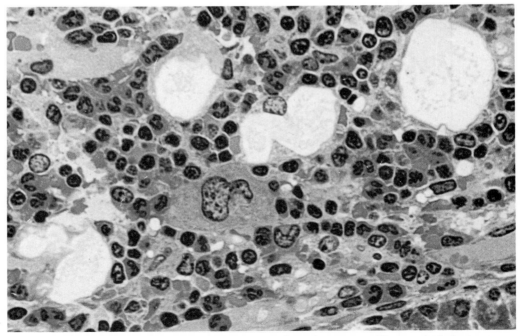

Figure 5–9. Section of active human bone marrow from the sternum. Note particularly the megakaryocyte (left center) and individual fat cells. Plastic section. × 600.

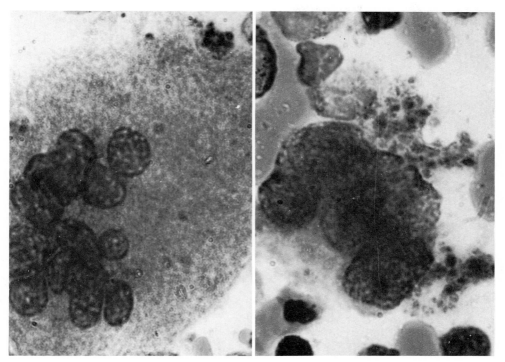

Figure 5–10. Bone marrow smears, showing megakaryocytes. Note the complexity of the nucleus and the granular cytoplasm *(left)*. In the right figure, the megakaryocyte exhibits active platelet formation and little of the peripheral cytoplasm remains. Left, × 500; right, × 450. (Courtesy of J. H. Cutts.)

toplasm contains numerous azurophil granules and exhibits a patchy basophilia. The cell outline often is indistinct since pseudopodial cytoplasmic processes extend through the walls of the sinusoids.

Megakaryocytes are said to arise from hemocytoblasts via an intermediate stage, the *megakaryoblast*. The latter cell is distinguished from a hemocytoblast by its nuclear characteristics: the nucleus is large, and often indented, and the peripheral heterochromatin is dense. The cytoplasm is homogeneous and basophil. Megakaryoblasts differentiate into megakaryocytes by a peculiar form of nuclear division in which the nucleus undergoes multiple mitotic divisions without cytoplasmic division. The number of mitoses is not known. After their formation, megakaryocytes extend cytoplasmic processes which become pinched off as platelets. Electron microscopic studies have revealed an extensive development of smooth-surfaced membranes within the cytoplasm, thus dividing it up into small compartments and delineating

the extent of future platelets. The azurophil cytoplasmic granules form the chromomeres of the future platelets. Following formation of *demarcation channels* by the membranes, the compartments readily separate to become free platelets. Megakaryocytes are short-lived and stages of degeneration are seen commonly. After the peripheral cytoplasm is shed as platelets, the megakaryocytes become shrunken and their nuclei fragment.

Development of Lymphoid Elements

The development of lymphocytes and monocytes occurs in the lymphoid tissues and, to some degree, in myeloid tissue as well. The process of differentiation of these cells, however, cannot be followed as readily as that of the myeloid elements. Morphological evidence of differentiation is not marked. The appearance of definitive characteristics such as nuclear disappearance or lobation, cytoplasmic granulation, and

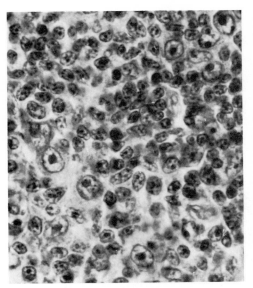

Figure 5–11. A small portion of a sectioned germinal center of a lymph nodule. A few large lymphocytes (lymphoblasts), distinguished by the presence of a large pale nucleus containing a distinct nucleolus, lie between the small lymphocytes. × 650.

lymphoblasts undergo differentiation, the nuclear chromatin becomes more dense and compact and azurophil granules appear within the cytoplasm. The cells are reduced in size and are termed *prolymphocytes* by some authorities. These cells give rise directly to the circulating lymphocytes.

In postnatal mammals most lymphocytes arise by proliferation of pre-existing lymphocytes within the lymphoid tissues, principally within lymph nodes and the spleen. Only when such a production is unable to supply the demand for lymphocytes is it likely that there is any marked differentiation from the stem cells that enter the circulation from bone marrow.

The development of small lymphocytes, principally in the lymph nodes and the spleen, generally represents a reaction to an invasion by foreign-body proteins. A further reaction to such a stimulus is the formation of *plasma cells*, which are responsible for the synthesis of antibodies. These cells may arise directly from hemocytoblasts (lymphoblasts) or from immunologically competent lymphocytes. In the latter process, small lymphocytes (B cells) pass through intermediate stages that are indistinguishable from large and medium-sized lymphocytes.

loss of cytoplasmic basophilia does not occur in lymphocytes and monocytes, which retain the cytoplasmic basophilia and generally primitive nuclear shape of the stem cell.

The stroma of lymphoid tissue, like that of myeloid tissue, contains a framework of reticular fibers closely associated with primitive reticular cells and fixed macrophages. The sinuses present within lymphoid tissue are lined by *littoral cells* of the macrophage system. The meshes of the stroma contain the free cells, megakaryocytes, and some fat cells.

Lymphocytes. The precursor cells of lymphocytes are the *lymphoblasts,* which are relatively large cells, spherical in shape. The nucleus is large and contains relatively condensed chromatin and prominent nucleoli. The cytoplasm is homogeneous and basophil. These immature lymphocytes resemble the hemocytoblasts of bone marrow and, according to the unitarian theory of development, they are the same cells in a different location. (Proponents of the dualistic theory claim that the lymphoblasts differ slightly from the hemocytoblasts and can differentiate only into lymphoid elements.) As

Monocytes. The monocyte is developed from a stem cell within the bone marrow. It is not possible to distinguish this stem cell, the *monoblast,* from the myeloblast. The monoblast gives rise to the *promonocyte,* which is about 15 microns (μm) in diameter. The nucleus is oval or indented and has a fine chromatin pattern with two or more nucleoli. The cytoplasm is basophil and contains a variable number of fine azurophil granules. This cell gives rise to the monocyte, which is present both in bone marrow and blood. It is slightly smaller than the promonocyte (10 to 12 microns or μm), and nucleoli are indistinct within the nucleus. The cytoplasm contains an abundance of fine azurophil granules that give a positive peroxidase reaction, unlike those of lymphocytes that show a negative peroxidase reaction. Monocytes leave the blood to enter the tissues, where their life span as macrophages may be as long as 70 days.

Embryonic Development of Blood Cells

There are three ill-defined phases of hemopoiesis during intrauterine development and in all the initiation of hemopoiesis is the same. It consists of a differentiation of mesenchymal cells into free cells whose cytoplasm acquires a definite basophil character. These cells, often termed hemocytoblasts, proliferate actively. Such a process occurs initially within the yolk sac during the third week of development. The hemocytoblasts become transformed into *primitive erythroblasts* by the elaboration and accumulation of hemoglobin within their cytoplasm. They differ from bone marrow–derived erythrocytes in that they are larger and retain their nuclei.

During the second phase, hemopoiesis occurs within the liver and spleen. It commences in the liver at about six weeks and continues actively until the middle of fetal life. Hemocytoblasts proliferate and differentiate into nucleated and non-nucleated red blood cells, leukocytes, and megakaryocytes. The formation of nucleated red blood cells gradually diminishes prior to the middle of fetal life and hemopoietic activity in the liver normally disappears at the time of birth. Hemopoiesis occurs within the spleen between the second and eighth months. Erythropoiesis ceases at or just after birth, although lymphocytes continue to be produced within the spleen postnatally. Additionally, during the second phase, the thymus commences to produce lymphocytes from the second month on.

The third phase involves the bone marrow and the lymph nodes. Myeloid tissue of bone marrow appears in the third fetal month when the cartilaginous primordia of the bones become invaded by mesenchyme during the process of ossification. Again mesenchymal cells round off and become hemocytoblasts, which give rise to erythroblasts, myelocytes, monocytes, lymphocytes, and megakaryocytes. With the appearance of bone marrow, production of nucleated red blood cells ceases. Lymph nodes develop relatively late during fetal life, and production of myeloid elements is never a marked feature within them. However, they continue to function throughout life, like the spleen, in the production of lymphocytes.

INTERRELATIONSHIPS BETWEEN CELLS OF BLOOD AND CONNECTIVE TISSUES: DEVELOPMENTAL POTENTIALITIES

Mesenchymal cells have great potentiality. They are able to differentiate along any one of several lines leading to the formation of many different kinds of cells in the connective tissues (Figure 5–13). The process of cellular differentiation implies the acquisition of a property or properties not possessed previously and leads to specialization.

It is important to realize that complete differentiation is not achieved by istics such as nuclear disappearance or

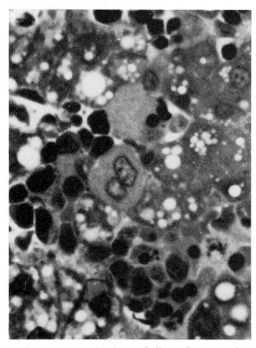

Figure 5–12. Section of liver from a six-month-old human fetus. At this stage, liver cells contain large amounts of lipid material within their cytoplasm and appear vacuolated owing to loss of lipid during tissue preparation. Note the presence of extramedullary hemopoiesis. Numerous myeloid elements, principally of the erythrocyte series, lie between the liver cells. Note the megakaryocyte. × 700.

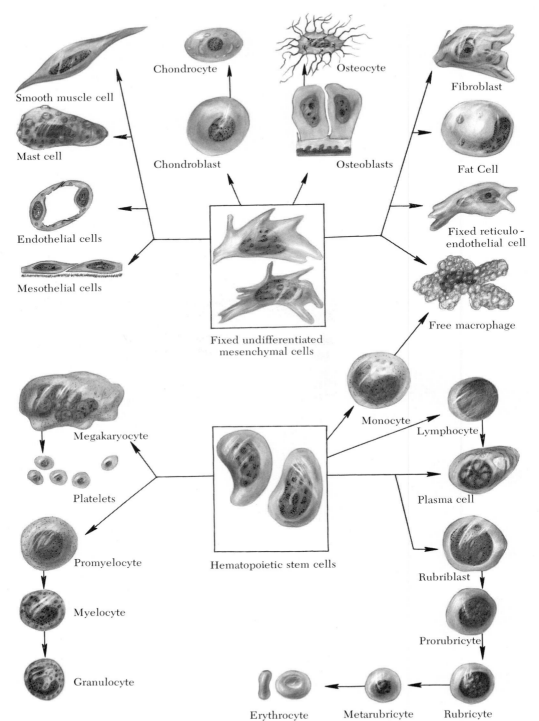

Smooth muscle cell

Chondrocyte

Osteocyte

Fibroblast

Mast cell

Chondroblast

Osteoblasts

Fat Cell

Endothelial cells

Fixed reticulo-
endothelial cell

Mesothelial cells

Fixed undifferentiated
mesenchymal cells

Free macrophage

Megakaryocyte

Monocyte

Lymphocyte

Platelets

Plasma cell

Promyelocyte

Hematopoietic stem cells

Rubriblast

Myelocyte

Prorubricyte

Granulocyte

Erythrocyte   Metarubricyte   Rubricyte

Figure 5–13. Diagram to illustrate the interrelationships between cells of blood and connective tissues.

all cells. Maximow originated the concept that in the development of any kind of adult connective tissue from mesenchyme some undifferentiated cells remain as a reservoir of multipotential cells. It should be appreciated that there is a tendency for the process of differentiation to be halted somewhere along the line of differentiation. Thus in any connective tissue there may be cells which are undifferentiated, cells which are partially differentiated, and cells which have achieved complete differentiation.

Two further concepts with regard to the process of cellular differentiation remain to be considered. In general, the more differentiated a cell becomes, the more restricted its developmental potencies. Once a cell has achieved a certain degree of differentiation along a particular line, further differentiation is possible only along the original line of differentiation. The second point is that once differentiation has been completed cellular proliferation becomes markedly restricted. Many specialized cells are incapable of division.

Metaplasia is a process which illustrates well the concepts of cellular differentiation just described. It occurs under certain pathological conditions when one specialized type of connective tissue appears to transform into another. This, in fact, is not the case since specialized cellular elements are unable to differentiate. Actually metaplasia represents a replacement of one type of connective tissue by another from undifferentiated cells present within the tissue. It occurs in response to altered environmental factors.

REFERENCES

Bainton, D. F.: Sequential degranulation of the two types of polymorphonuclear leukocyte granules during phagocytosis of microorganisms. J. Cell Biol., 58:249, 1973.

Bainton, D. F., and Farquhar, M. G.: Segregation and packaging of granule enzymes in eosinophilic leukocytes. J. Cell Biol., 45:54, 1970.

Barr, R. D., Whang-Peng, J., and Perry, S.: Hemopoietic stem cells in human peripheral blood. Science, 190:284, 1975.

Becker, R. P., and De Bruyn, P. P. H.: The transmural passage of blood cells into myeloid sinusoids and the entry of platelets into the sinusoidal circulation: a scanning electron microscopic investigation. Am. J. Anat., 145:183, 1976.

Bessis, M.: The blood cells and their formation. *In* The Cell: Biochemistry, Physiology, Morphology, edited by J. Brachet and A. E. Mirsky. New York, Academic Press, 1961, Vol. 5, p. 163.

Campbell, F. R.: Ultrastructural study of transmural migration of blood cells in the bone marrow of rats, mice, and guinea pigs. Am. J. Anat., 135:521, 1972.

Chao, F. C., Shepro, D., Tullis, J. L., Belamarich, F. A., and Curby, W. A.: Similarities between platelet contraction and cellular motility during mitosis: role of platelet microtubules in clot retraction. J. Cell Sci., 20:569, 1976.

Daems, W. Th.: On the fine structure of human neutrophilic leukocyte granules. J. Ultrastruct. Res., 24:343, 1968.

Davidson, W. M., and Smith, D. R.: A morphological sex difference in the polymorphonuclear leucocytes. Br. Med. J., 2:6, 1954.

Elves, M. W.: The Lymphocytes. London, Lloyd Luke Ltd., 1966.

Gutman, G. A., and Weissman, I. L.: Lymphoid tissue architecture: experimental analysis of the origin and distribution of T-cells and B-cells. Immunology, 23:465, 1972.

Hardin, J. H., and Spicer, S. S.: An ultrastructural study of human eosinophil granules: maturational stages and pyroantimonate reactive cation. Am. J. Anat., 128:283, 1970.

Jerne, N. K.: The immune system. Sci. Am., 229:52, 1973.

Lerner, R. A., and Dixon, F. J.: The human lymphocyte as an experimental animal. Sci. Am., 228:82, 1973.

McGregor, D. D.: The role of lymphocytes in antibody formation and delayed-type hypersensitivity. Anat. Rec., 165:117, 1969.

Miller, F., deHarven, E., and Palade, G. E.: The structure of eosinophil leukocyte granules in rodent and in man. J. Cell. Biol., 31:349, 1966.

Murphy, M. J. Bertles, J. R., and Gordon, A. S.: Identifying characteristics of the hematopoietic precursor cell. J. Cell Sci., 9:23, 1971.

Nelson, D. A.: Hematopoiesis. *In* Clinical Diagnosis and Management by Laboratory Methods, ed. 16, edited by J. B. Henry. Philadelphia, W. B. Saunders Co., 1979, p. 918.

Nichols, B. A., Bainton, D. F., and Farquhar, M. G.: Differentiation of monocytes. Origin, nature, and fate of their azurophilic granules. J. Cell Biol., 50:498, 1971.

Nowell, P. C., and Wilson, D. B.: Lymphocytes and hemic stem cells. Am. J. Pathol., 65:641, 1971.

Raff, M. C.: T and B lymphocytes and immune responses. Nature, 242:19, 1973.

Rebuck, J. W. (editor): The Lymphocyte and Lymphocytic Tissue. New York, Paul B. Hoeber, 1960.

Sabin, F. R.: Studies of living human blood cells. Bull. Johns Hopkins Hosp., 34:277, 1923.

Shaklai, M., and Tavassoli, M.: Demarcation membrane system in rat megakaryocyte and mechanism of platelet formation: a membrane reorganization process. J. Ultrastr. Res., 62:270, 1978.

Simpson, C. F., and Kling, J. M.: The mechanism of denucleation in circulating erythroblasts. J. Cell Biol., 35:237, 1967.

Skutelsky, E., and Danon, D.: An electron microscopic study of nuclear elimination from the late erythroblast. J. Cell Biol., 33:625, 1967.

Sorenson, G. D.: An electron microscopic study of hematopoiesis in the liver of the fetal rabbit. Am. J. Anat., 106:27, 1960.

Tanaka, Y., and Goodman, J. R.: Electron Micros-copy of Human Blood Cells. New York, Harper, 1972.

Tavassoli, M., and Crosby, W. H.: Fate of the nucleus of the marrow erythroblast. Science, 179:912, 1973.

Weiss, L.: The hematopoietic microenvironment of the bone marrow: an ultrastructural study of the stroma in rats. Anat. Rec., 186:161, 1976.

Whiteside, T. L., and Rowlands, D. T.: T-cell and B-cell identification in the diagnosis of lympho-proliferative disease. Am. J. Pathol., 88:754, 1977.

Yoffey, J. M., and Courtice, F. C.: Lymphatics, Lymph and Lymphoid Tissue. Cambridge, Harvard University Press, ed. 2, 1960.

MUSCLE

Muscle tissue is specialized for producing movement both of the body as a whole and of the many parts with respect to one another. Muscle cells show great development of the function of contractility and, to a lesser extent, of conductivity. This specialization involves elongation of the cells in the axis of contraction and because of this the cells often are referred to as muscle fibers.*

In muscle tissue, muscle cells or fibers usually are grouped into bundles, but muscle tissue consists of more than just muscle fibers. Muscle fibers, because they perform mechanical work, require a rich network of blood capillaries to provide food materials and oxygen and to eliminate toxic waste products. The blood vessels are carried in fibroconnective tissue which also serves to bind together the muscle fibers and to provide a harness for them so that their pull may be exerted usefully. Nerves also run in the connective tissue.

There are three types of muscle and these are classified on both a structural and a functional basis. Regular trans-verse bands along the length of the fibers are present in *striated* muscle and absent in *smooth* muscle. Functionally, muscle either is under the control of the will (*voluntary* muscle) or is not (*involuntary* muscle). The three types of muscle are smooth involuntary muscle, present chiefly in hollow organs; striated voluntary or skeletal muscle, attached to bones or fascia and constituting the flesh of the limbs and body wall; and striated involuntary or cardiac muscle, forming the wall of the heart and extending into the major veins opening into the heart.

For histological study of muscular tissue, sectioned material (for light and electron microscopy) is used mainly, but useful additional information may be obtained from *macerated tissue*. Small pieces of muscle are immersed in a solution of 10 per cent hydrochloric acid in physiological saline for 24 to 48 hours. After rinsing in water, individual muscle fibers can be teased out on a microscope slide using two mounted needles, covered with a glass coverslip, and examined under the microscope.

Striated muscle will be considered first.

---

*Note on terminology: There is a special terminology associated with muscle tissue: protoplasm is called sarcoplasm (*sarcos* = muscle) and the cell membrane complex is the sarcolemma. Other terms used are sarcoplasmic reticulum (endoplasmic reticulum), sarcosome (mitochondrion), and sarcomere (a linear unit); myofilaments and myofibrils are contractile elements.

STRIATED MUSCLE

Striated or skeletal muscle is that which the layman recognizes as muscle and comprises the flesh or meat of animals. In the fresh state, human striated muscle has a pink color owing partly to a pigment in the muscle fibers and partly to the rich vascularity of the tissue, but there is some variation in color and "red" and "white" muscles have been recognized. The individual striated muscle fiber or cell is long, cylindrical, and multinucleate, the ends tapering to a point or being somewhat rounded or notched at the junction of muscle and tendon. Each fiber is independent and may be of great length. In many muscles, however, individual fibers are shorter than the overall length of the muscle, one end being attached to tendon and the other to a connective tissue septum within the muscle. Variations in arrangement are described in textbooks of gross anatomy, but it is accepted generally that the power of a muscle is dependent not upon the length of the component muscle fibers but upon the total number of fibers present in the muscle. It is well known that muscles increase in size with exercise. This is due to an increase in the size of each individual muscle fiber (hypertrophy) and is not due to an increase in the number of fibers (hyperplasia). Striated muscle has a more rapid contraction than smooth muscle.

The individual, named muscle of gross anatomy is enveloped in a layer of relatively thick connective tissue called the *epimysium*, which appears as a white sheath to the naked eye. Within it are the muscle fibers arranged in fasciculi or bundles, each bundle surrounded by a sheath of thinner connective tissue, the *perimysium*. Within a fasciculus, individual muscle fibers are covered by delicate connective tissue, the *endomysium*.

In teased preparations of fresh or macerated muscle, individual fibers have a faint yellow coloration and are striated in both longitudinal and transverse directions. Fibers vary from 1 to 40 mm in length, and from 10 to 60 microns (μm) in diameter. Nuclei are numerous in each fiber, there being about 35 per mm of length. They are ovoid, situated peripherally in the fiber,

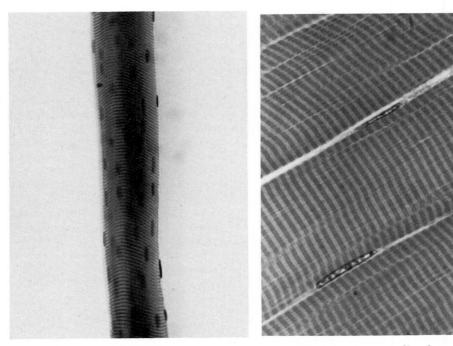

Figure 6–1. Photomicrographs of skeletal (striated) muscle. *Left:* A single teased fiber from the human gastrocnemius muscle. Note cross-banding and multiple, peripherally located nuclei. × 275. *Right:* Parts of several fibers from the diaphragm. Note that there are bundles of myofibrils in each fiber and that the cross-banding is in register across the myofibrils but that thin slips of sarcoplasm between myofibrils show no banding. Plastic section, × 650.

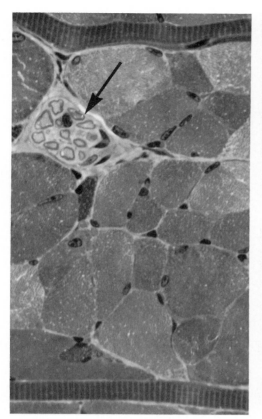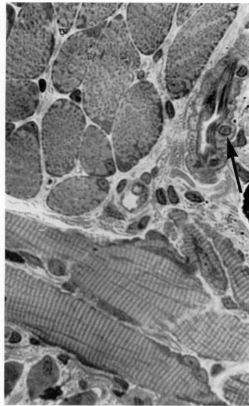

Figure 6–2. Photomicrographs of striated muscle fibers of the tongue cut in transverse and longitudinal sections. *Left:* A small peripheral nerve with myelinated nerve fibers is indicated (arrow). *Right:* Note smooth muscle fibers in the wall of an arteriole (arrow). Plastic section, both × 450.

and oriented lengthwise. An individual fiber is limited by a thin, structureless membrane, the sarcolemma, which is seen to advantage in regions where muscle fibers have been crushed with consequent retraction of sarcoplasm within the sarcolemma.

In routine light microscope preparations, the sarcoplasm is occupied mainly by longitudinal, parallel columns of myofibrils about 1 micron (μm) in diameter. In cross section these appear as dots, often grouped together with areas of clear sarcoplasm between the groups. These groups of myofibrils are termed the fields or areas of Cohnheim, but this appearance probably is artifactual. Nonfibrillar areas of the sarcoplasm occur between the myofibrils and adjacent to the nuclei and contain numerous mitochondria (sarco-

somes), often in rows between myofibrils, small Golgi apparatuses near nuclei, some lipid droplets, and glycogen.

Myofibrils and Striation

By light microscopy, the cytoplasm of each striated muscle fiber in longitudinal section shows alternating thin discs or bands of light and dark material, the dark bands being anisotropic (birefringent) and the light ones isotropic when seen with polarized light. Hence, the dark and light bands are called respectively "A" and "I" bands. The lighter I band is intersected by a thin dark line, the "Z" band. Although the A, I, and Z bands appear to cross the entire muscle fiber, in a good preparation all three are seen to be limited

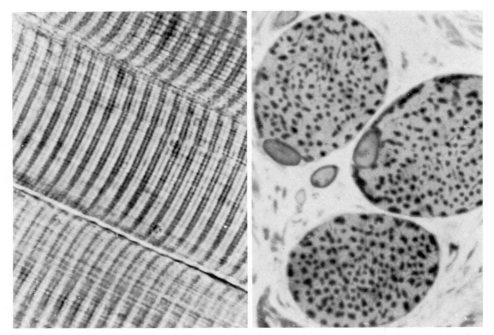

Figure 6–3.   *Left:* Photomicrograph of striated muscle fibers from human gastrocnemius in longitudinal section showing A, I, Z, and H bands. × 1250. *Right:* Striated muscle of rabbit tongue in transverse section. Note the numerous mitochondria. Plastic section. × 1000.

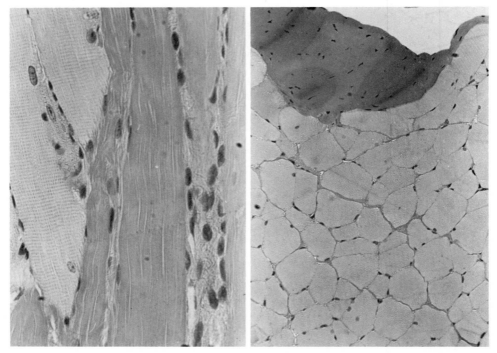

Figure 6–4.   Photomicrographs of striated muscle (gastrocnemius) and tendon of rat. *Left:* Longitudinal section, showing two muscle fibers (left) with endomysium around and between them inserting into tendon. Note that the tendon is organized into fiber (collagen) bundles with looser connective tissue between the bundles. Plastic section, × 450. *Right:* Transverse section with tendon above (collagen fibers and nuclei of fibroblasts) and muscle below, with endomysium between the muscle fibers. Plastic section, × 250.

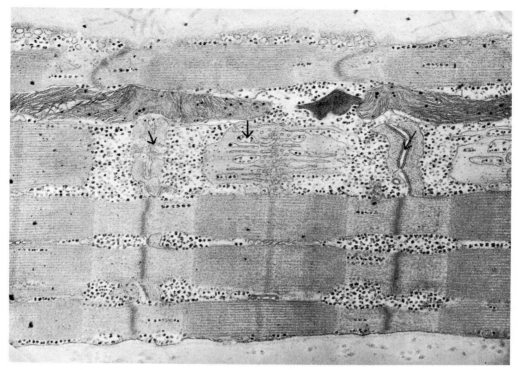

Figure 6–5. Electron micrograph of a longitudinal section of frog sartorius muscle. In the top center, a sheet of the sarcoplasmic reticulum (center arrow) at the level of the A band is grazed by the plane of section. Triads (left and right arrows) are visible at the level of the two Z lines. The dark granules between myofibrils are glycogen. Note also mitochondria and a lipid droplet (dark, angular mass). × 24,000. (Courtesy of Dr. H. E. Huxley.)

to the myofibrils and do not extend across the sarcoplasm lying between them. Other bands in the myofibril are visible occasionally. These are the pale, thin H bands bisecting the dark A band and, within this, a very fine, dark M or middle stripe.

In a cross section of a striated muscle fiber, the various bands are not seen. In longitudinal section, the cross bands are distinct in *relaxed* muscle, and it is customary to consider the muscle fibril as composed of structural units. Each unit extends between adjacent Z lines and is termed a *sarcomere*. The sarcomere, however, is not merely a structural unit, but is the basic contractile unit. In muscle fixed in a *contracted* state, the fibrils are thicker and the sarcomeres shorter, the distance between Z lines progressively shortening with the extent of contraction. As the I bands become shorter, the ends of the A bands approach the Z lines. Eventually A and I bands are indistinguishable, *but the*

length of the A band in contraction remains constant. The explanation for this is discussed later.

Fine Structure

The *sarcolemma* is too thin to be resolved clearly with the light microscope, but electron microscopy shows it to consist of the plasma membrane of the muscle cell covered by a fine extracellular basal lamina with which a few unit fibrils of collagen are associated. Fine slips of elastic tissue also are present between adjacent muscle fibers. Associated with the plasma membrane usually are some micropinocytotic vesicles.

In the sarcoplasm, the mitochondria or *sarcosomes* are numerous and large, each with closely packed cristae. This is to be expected in view of the high energy requirements for muscle contraction. Sarcosomes lie subjacent to the sarcolemma, concentrated near the poles of the elongated nuclei, and in parallel rows between the myofibrils: in all sites they lie with their long axes along the length of the fiber. Also in a paranuclear position is a small Golgi apparatus. Ribosomes and a few small elements of granular endoplasmic reticulum also are present, usually near the nucleus. A few lysosomes may be found in nonfibrillar sarcoplasm. Glycogen particles are numerous, scattered throughout muscle cells, but concentrations of the particles occur between myofibrils at the I bands. Lipid vacuoles normally are present also and increase with age.

Sarcoplasmic reticulum represents a special type of agranular (smooth) endoplasmic reticulum. It is extensive and comprises a continuous system of membrane-limited tubules and cisternae that form a sheath or collar around each myofibril, with connections between the collars of adjacent sarcomeres of neighboring myofibrils. In mammalian muscle, the sheath is formed mainly by longitudinally arranged tubular elements around the A band, with cross connections that are prominent in the region of the H band. At A-I junctions toward the ends of the sarcomere the tubules are connected to cisternae, called terminal cisternae, in the form of rings around myofibrils at A-I junctions. A similar network of tubules surrounds I bands with another terminal cisterna at each A-I junction, but they are separated by a more slender transverse or T tubule. This arrangement of two terminal cisternae of sarcoplasmic reticulum and a central T tubule is called a *triad,* and there are two triads to each sarcomere in mammalian muscle. (In amphibian muscle, a triad encircles each myofibril at the Z line; viz., triads lie between sarcomeres.)

Transverse (T) tubules are invaginations of the surface sarcolemma, their lumina being continuous with the extracellular space. They pass from the sarcolemma at regular intervals into the interior of the muscle fiber, undergo branching, and, as indicated above, lie between terminal cisternae of sarcoplasmic reticulum to form triads at the A-I junctions. At triads, the membranes of T tubules and sarcoplasmic reticulum form junctions or *couplings.* Their function in muscle contraction is discussed on page 195.

Myofibrils on light microscopy appear as long, parallel threads of 1 to 2 microns (μm) diameter. Each myofibril is a bundle of smaller units called *myofilaments* arranged in an orderly array, these filaments being of two sizes, thick and thin, and of different chemical composition. The cross banding of myofibrils seen on light microscopy is simply a reflection of the distribution of the two types of myofilaments. The thicker filaments contain myosin and are approximately 1.3 to 1.5 μm long and 12 to 15 nm diameter. They lie in the center of the sarcomere occupying the A band. The thin filaments contain actin, are only 5 nm in diameter and approximately 1.0 μm long, and are attached to each side of Z bands, with the free ends extending through the I band and part way into the A band, interdigitating there with thick filaments so that in a cross section of the A band each thick filament is surrounded by a group of six thin ones in hexagonal array. The H band is simply the central area of the A band free of thin filaments, its width determined by the state of contraction. Thus, in transverse sections, the I band contains only thin filaments, the extremities of the A band contain both thick and thin, and only thick filaments are present in the H band. At the M line in the center of the H band, thick filaments (at their centers) are interconnected by fine filaments composed of an unknown protein ("M protein") of only 4 nm diameter, with other slender filaments ("C protein") running parallel to the thick filaments. Also visible on electron microscopy is the presence of thin cross bridges passing from thick filaments to their neighboring thin filaments.

A *thick filament* is composed of a bundle of myosin molecules, each in the form of a golf club with a shaft and a head. Myosin molecules have two subunits, most of the shaft being formed by light meromyosin and the rest of the shaft and head by heavy meromyosin, the heads of the molecules protruding from the molecular bundle to extend as the cross bridges between thick and thin filaments. The center of the bundle, in the H band, is free of heads and the filaments are polarized in that the heads are directed away from the midpoint (the M line). Also, at the extremities of

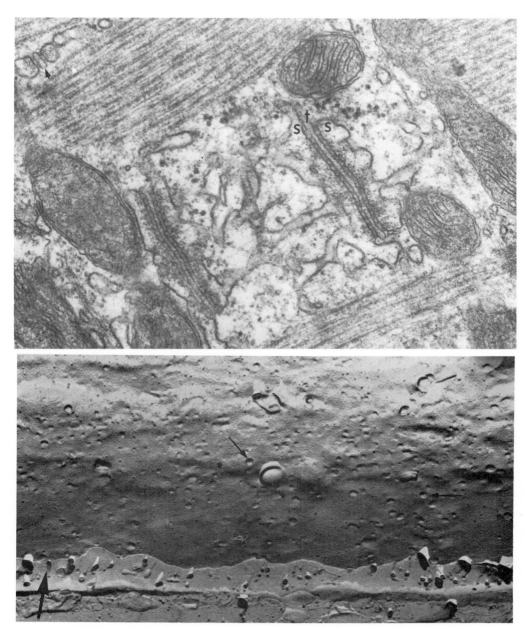

Figure 6–6. *Top:* Electron micrograph of rat striated muscle to demonstrate sarcoplasmic reticulum and transverse tubules. Above and below are myofilaments in a partially contracted fiber, centrally a meshwork of sarcoplasmic reticulum(s), forming in mammalian striated muscle two triads per sarcomere, located at A-I junctions. One of the two seen (right) in the center is labelled with a slender T tubule (t) lying between terminal cisternae of sarcoplasmic reticulum(s). A third triad is located at top left, in transverse section, the central T tubule indicated by an arrowhead. × 64,000. *Bottom:* Electron micrograph of a freeze-etch preparation of striated muscle. The fracture has exposed the outer surface of the plasma membrane in which numerous pits or depressions are visible (thin arrows); these represent apertures of transverse tubules or of caveolae. The direction of metal shadowing is indicated by the broad arrow. × 14,800. (Courtesy of Dr. D. G. Rayns.)

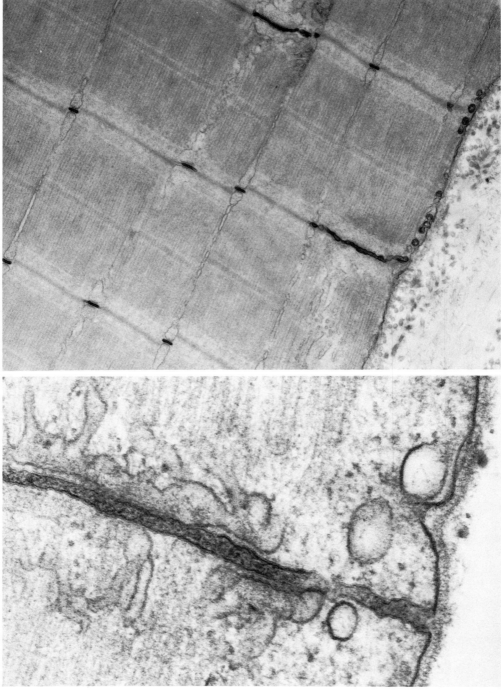

Figure 6–7.   Electron micrographs of frog sartorius muscle to illustrate transverse tubules, sarcoplasmic reticulum, and triads. In frog muscle, triads are located at Z lines and here *(top figure)* stain darkly. On each side, the T tubule is bordered by dilated cisternae of sarcoplasmic reticulum, seen best at top center in the upper figure. Subjacent to the sarcolemma are caveolae. In the lower figure, a T tubule is seen to be in continuity with the plasmalemma (right) passing into the fiber, i.e., to the left, where it is bordered on each side, above and below, by terminal cisternae of sarcoplasmic reticulum. Top, × 22,000; bottom, × 88,000.

the bundle, the heads protrude in a helical fashion in six longitudinal rows to connect with the six associated thin filaments. The head of the myosin molecule is flexible on the shaft.

A *thin filament* has as a major component F actin, a filamentous protein formed from globular subunits of G actin. In the thin filaments, there are two such strands arranged in a spiral or helix. F actin has a linear polarity, all filaments inserting into one side of a Z band being of the same polarity, all inserting into the other side (and those into the Z line at the other end of the same sarcomere) having the opposite polarity. Also present in thin filaments are the regulatory proteins tropomyosin and troponin. Tropomyosin molecules are of a long, slender form and lie end to end in the grooves of the F actin double helix with globular troponin molecules attached to tropomyosin molecules at regular intervals.

At the Z line, thin filaments of adjacent sarcomeres are not in register, and this gives a characteristic zigzag appearance to the Z line. Thin filaments are attached at the Z line by Z filaments. It has been reported that each thin filament of one sarcomere is linked to four thin filaments of the adjacent sarcomere by Z filaments. The Z line is known also to contain the proteins α actinin and desmin in the form of 10-nm filaments. When sectioned transversely, the Z line shows a lattice structure, apparently of variable form, which suggests that the Z line is a dynamic structure.

Bearing in mind that thin filaments are 1 μm long and thick filaments are about 1.5 μm long, it is obvious that thin filaments from adjacent Z lines will meet in the center of the A band when the sarcomere length is less than 2 μm and that further contraction will result in the ends of the thick filaments abutting against Z lines when the sarcomere length is less than 1.5 μm.

Mechanism of Contraction

In contraction, muscle fibers become shorter and broader. From phase contrast and interference microscopy, it is evident that in contraction the A band remains constant in length while the I band and the H band both diminish. This contraction occurs by a "sliding filament" mechanism that involves a change in relative position of the two sets of myofilaments, although neither thick nor thin filaments are altered in length. During contraction, thin filaments slide past thick filaments and are drawn inward in the sarcomere toward the centers of the thick filaments (the M line). This draws adjacent Z lines closer to each other, thus shortening the sarcomere, with decrease in width of the I band and H band and, eventually, their obliteration. In full contraction, the ends of the thick filaments approach Z lines. The mechanism involves the connection of thick myosin filaments by cross bridges or spines with active sites on neighboring actin thin filaments, the heads of the myosin molecules by virtue of their hinged shafts moving toward globular actin subunits of thin filaments. Contractile force is generated by a cycle of ratchet-like attachment, detachment, and reattachment of the myosin heads, thus sliding the filaments past each other and drawing the thin filaments inward in the manner of an animated cogwheel. This process requires energy that is derived from the breakdown of APT to ADP and phosphate, each myosin head acting as an ATPase. As the store of ATP is limited, the process relies on its continued replenishment by sarcosomes carrying the enzymes of the citric acid cycle.

On relaxation, all myosin heads become detached from the thin filaments, and the two sets of filaments slide back past each other to their original, relaxed position of partial overlap.

Contraction involves also the T system and the sarcoplasmic reticulum. Following stimulation of a muscle fiber, all myofibrils contract simultaneously and instantaneously. Contraction in a myofibril commences at the A-I junction, i.e., at the site of a triad, and it also is known that the regulation of contraction depends on the availability of calcium ions. Most of the calcium in a relaxed muscle fiber is concentrated in the sarcoplasmic reticulum. Following stimulation, a wave of membrane depolarization passes rapidly over the plasmalemma and spreads to the interior of the fiber by the T system. This induces a

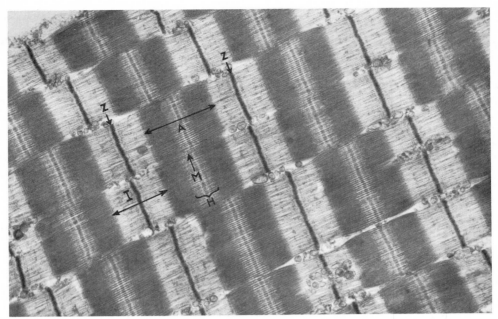

Figure 6–8. Electron micrograph, showing portions of seven myofibrils cut longitudinally from the noncontracted (i.e., relaxed) psoas muscle of a rabbit. The dark A (anisotropic) bands are bisected by the lighter H bands in which there is a thin, dark M band. The I (isotropic) bands are bisected by very dark Z lines. A single sarcomere extends from one Z line to the next Z line. × 13,000. (Courtesy of Dr. H. E. Huxley.)

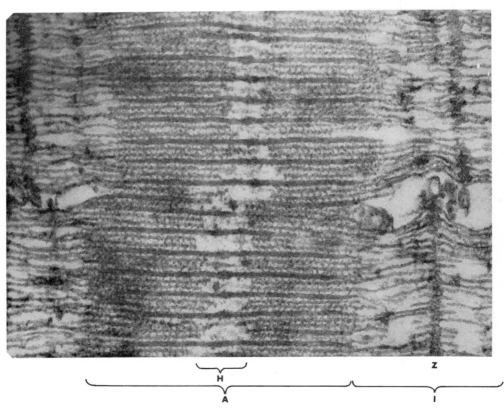

Figure 6–9. Electron micrograph of relaxed rabbit psoas muscle in longitudinal section. The thick myosin filaments extend throughout the length of the A band; the thin actin filaments are found in the I band and extend into the A band as far as the H band. There are two actin filaments between every two myosin filaments. Cross linkages between actin and myosin filaments are visible. × 74,000. (Courtesy of Dr. H. E. Huxley.)

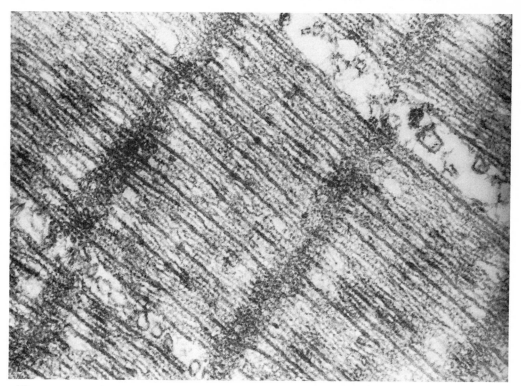

Figure 6–10. Electron micrograph of contracted rabbit psoas muscle in longitudinal section. Compare with Figure 6–9: The I and H bands have disappeared. × 74,000. (Courtesy of Dr. H. E. Huxley.)

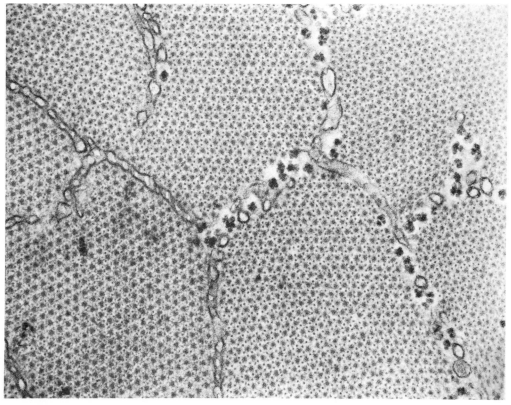

Figure 6–11. Electron micrograph of a cross section through the A band of skeletal muscle from the frog sartorius. The thin actin filaments have a hexagonal arrangement around the thicker myosin filaments. × 50,000. (Courtesy of Dr. H. E. Huxley.)

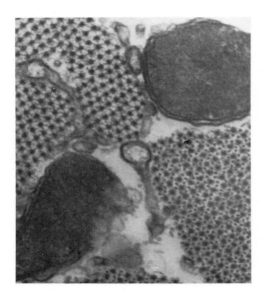

Figure 6–12. Electron micrograph of a transverse section of striated muscle showing myofibrils cut through the A band (lower right), with thin filaments interdigitating with thick filaments and through the M line (top left) where thick filaments are linked by fine interconnections. × 66,000.

Figure 6–13 *Below.* Three-dimensional diagram of part of a frog striated muscle fiber as seen by electron microscopy, demonstrating the various bands and sarcoplasmic reticulum and T tubules. Note that in mammalian muscle there are two triads per sarcomere, located at A–I junctions, whereas in the frog triads lie at Z lines, as shown here.

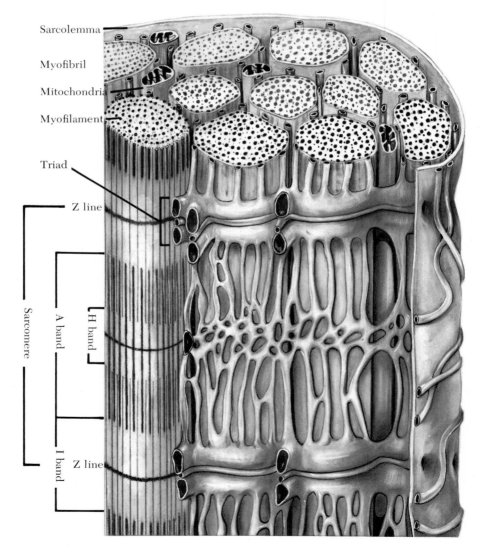

change in permeability of the adjacent terminal cisternae of the sarcoplasmic reticulum, with release of calcium from the sarcoplasmic reticulum to the sarcoplasm around myofibrils. This calcium binds to troponin of the thin filaments, which in turn allows tropomyosin to move, uncovering the myosin-binding sites on the actin filament. Thus, calcium "unlocks" the active myosin-binding sites on the thin filament and myosin heads swing on their flexible necks to attach to active actin sites and initiate the contraction mechanism. At the end of stimulation, the sequence is reversed, calcium returning to the sarcoplasmic reticulum and tropomyosin molecules returning to their former positions, preventing myosin-actin interaction.

In relaxed muscle, the troponin and tropomyosin molecules, in effect, form a molecular locking mechanism that prevents myosin-actin interaction. In contraction, calcium is the "key" that unlocks this mechanism and permits myosin heads to bind to active actin sites. It should be noted that a skeletal muscle cell cannot contract other than to maximum capacity — the "all-or-none law" — and that the power of contraction is varied by the number of muscle units that contract.

Types of Muscle Fiber

In most (named) muscles, the component fibers vary in appearance and function, some fibers contracting rapidly (fast or phasic, white fibers), some contracting more slowly (slow or tonic, red fibers), while some are intermediate between fast and slow. White fibers are of large diameter with numerous myofibrils, an extensive sarcoplasmic reticulum, and relatively little myoglobin and few mitochondria. Red fibers are of smaller diameter, and contain a large amount of myoglobin and numerous mitochondria. Intermediate fibers lie between the other two in appearance and function. In those muscles formed mainly by red fibers, contraction can be maintained for longer periods of time. Muscles composed mainly of white fibers contract more rapidly but fatigue comparatively quickly.

Organization of Striated Muscle Fibers into Muscles

In a muscle, muscle fibers lie in a parallel arrangement held together by fibroconnective tissue. As noted earlier, the entire muscle is wrapped in a substantial envelope of connective tissue, the *epimysium*. On cross section of a muscle, finer partitions of connective tissue, the *perimysium*, lie around bundles or fascicles of muscle fibers, and still finer connective tissue extends from the perimysium into a muscle bundle penetrating between individual muscle fibers. This tissue is the *endomysium*, and it consists of a network of reticular fibers carrying fine blood capillaries and a few connective tissue cells. The content of elastic fibers varies with the muscle but is prominent in the small muscles of the eye, face, and tongue. The total amount of fibroconnective tissue varies with the muscle. Some, e.g., gluteus maximus, have a large content and are coarse and relatively tough. Others, e.g., psoas major, have very little connective tissue and are tender: "filet mignon" is the psoas. Toughness of muscle thus is dependent on the amount of connective tissue and increases with age.

At the extremities of a muscle where it is attached to tendon, periosteum, aponeurosis, raphe, or dermis of the skin, the perimysium blends with, and is continuous with, the connective tissue of the attachment. Ends of muscle fibers are cone shaped and fit like fingers in a glove, the sarcolemmal sheaths being the material of the gloves in the analogy, and, further, the sarcolemma shows invaginations into which connective tissue extends and is firmly attached. At the extremities of a muscle fiber, the myofibrils are connected to the sarcolemma. Thus there are physical and mechanical forces attaching muscle fibers to the muscle origins and insertions so that the pull of contraction may be employed usefully and without separation of muscle from tendon. Indeed, from a clinical point of view, such a separation rarely occurs, and it is more usual for a tendon to pull off a flake of bone at its attachment after a too powerful contraction.

Blood and Lymph Supply

Arteries pierce the epimysium to reach the substance of the muscle and branch, and smaller vessels run in the perimysium, finally to terminate as capillaries which lie in the endomysium between individual muscle fibers. Most of these lie longitudinally along fibers but cross anastomoses are common, forming an extremely rich plexus. Lymphatic vessels, to drain tissue fluid, are quite numerous, but are not found in close association with fibers. They lie in epimysium and perimysium, but are not present in endomysium.

Nerve Supply

Each muscle receives one or more nerves of supply, the nerve piercing the epimysium at a point which is fairly constant—the so-called "motor point." The nerve contains motor fibers, sensory fibers to muscle spindles, neurotendinous sensory endings to fascia, and autonomic nerves supplying blood

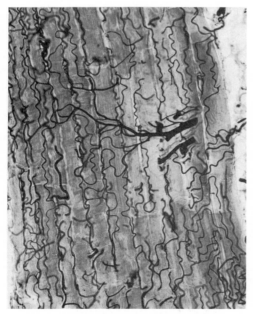

Figure 6–14. Photomicrograph of a thick section of human skeletal muscle after injection of the arterial supply with colored gelatin to demonstrate the capillary bed. Note that most capillaries are oriented longitudinally between muscle fibers but with numerous cross connections. × 150.

vessels. Functionally, muscles are composed of *motor units*, a unit being a single nerve and the muscle fibers it supplies. Where delicate movement is required, e.g., in eye muscles, a nerve fiber supplies each muscle fiber, but in trunk muscles, for example, a single nerve may supply 100 or more muscle fibers.

Motor End Plate. Each muscle fiber has a motor end plate or *myoneural junction,* the site at which a nerve axon terminates and is in close association with a muscle fiber. As the axon approaches the muscle, it loses its myelin sheath and branches to form either a platelike mass or a series of branches with terminal swellings like a bunch of grapes, each type lying in a gutter in the muscle fiber surface. These features can be demonstrated for light microscopy by silver impregnation techniques. Electron microscopy shows a series of small terminal swellings of the axon, the axon terminals, in a cluster covered externally by a thin sheath of Schwann cell cytoplasm. The terminals usually lie in depressions of the muscle fiber surface, separated by a gap called the synaptic cleft that is only 20 to 50 nm in width and contains basal lamina material. In the axon terminals are numerous small synaptic vesicles containing acetylcholine. The sarcolemma at the junction shows numerous invaginations called junctional folds, and the adjacent sarcoplasm usually contains numerous sarcosomes and, often, a nucleus or nuclei. Functionally, the synaptic cleft contains acetylcholinesterase, the enzyme that inactivates the neurotransmitter acetylcholine released at the endplate.

Motor end plates thus control muscle contraction, but coordination of muscle activity involves sensory endings discussed briefly in Chapter 17. In muscles, they are of two types. *Neuromuscular spindles* are fusiform in shape, lie longitudinally in muscle, and are formed by several small, slender muscle fibers, the intrafusal fibers, enclosed in a connective tissue capsule, associated with which is a nerve terminal. Intrafusal fibers are of two types: one, the nuclear bag fibers, are larger and fewer in number, with many nuclei concentrated in the centers of the cells; the other, nuclear chain fibers, are smaller, more numerous, and

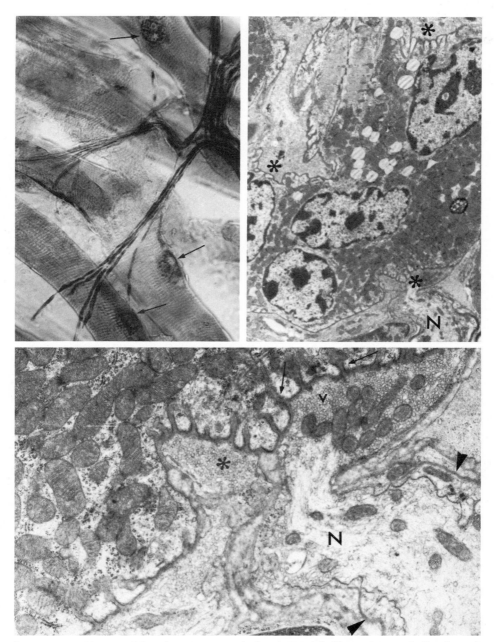

Figure 6–15. Myoneural junctions (motor end plates). *Top left:* Photomicrograph showing a large branching nerve (top right) with three myoneural junctions (arrows). Gold chloride preparation, × 250. *Top right:* Electron micrograph showing muscle fiber with parts of four nuclei and numerous mitochondria or sarcosomes, and a myelinated nerve fiber (N, lower right) and myoneural junctions (asterisks) around the periphery of the muscle fiber. × 5,500. *Bottom:* A higher magnification showing the terminal nerve fiber (N) with mitochondria and synaptic vesicles (v) and junctional folds (arrows) of the sarcolemma adjacent to the axon terminal. Myelin of the nerve fiber is indicated by arrowheads and a second terminal axon is also seen (asterisk). × 24,000.

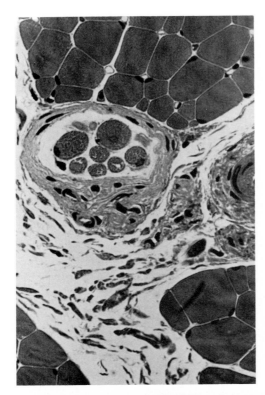

Figure 6–16. A transverse section of striated muscle with a muscle spindle (center) containing seven small muscle fibers ensheathed in connective tissue. Also seen are numerous capillary blood vessels between muscle fibers (above). Plastic section, × 350.

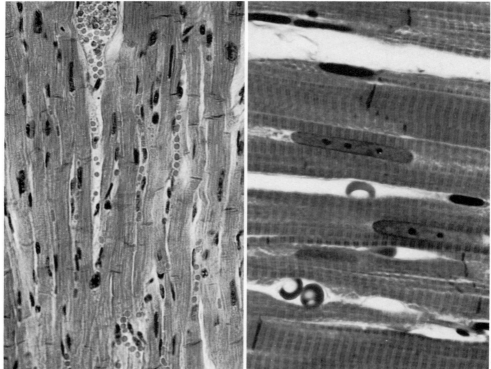

Figure 6–17. Photomicrographs of human cardiac muscle in longitudinal section. Note the branching muscle fibers, central nuclei with perinuclear (nonfibrillar) sarcoplasm, cross bands as in striated muscle, and intercalated discs crossing the muscle fibers transversely, and often in a stepwise fashion (top, *right*), but always at the site of a Z band. Note also the large number of blood vessels between muscle fibers. Left, × 250; right, plastic section, × 750.

contain nuclei in a row. Afferent nerve fibers terminate on nuclear bag fibers in a spiral form (the annulospiral endings) and on nuclear chain fibers as clusters (flower spray endings); the fibers also have a motor supply. The sensory endings are proprioceptive and respond to stretch, being involved in stretch reflexes. *Neurotendinous endings* (organs) are found in tendons near muscle-tendon junctions and show sensory nerve fibers terminating between bundles of tendon (collagen) fibers. These fibers are stimulated by tension or stretching of the tendon during muscle contraction.

Regeneration

After damage, degenerated muscle fibers have a limited capacity for regeneration, but gross damage is repaired by fibrous connective tissue, thus leaving a scar. Similarly, if the nerve or blood supply is interrupted, the muscle fibers degenerate and are replaced by fibrous tissue. However, in adult muscle there are *satellite* cells. These small cells with single nuclei lie between the sarcolemma and endomysium and probably represent a reservoir of embryonic myoblasts. During life, they can divide and play a role in the repair and regeneration that can occur in mature muscle.

CARDIAC MUSCLE

Cardiac muscle, which is involuntary but striated, contracts rhythmically and automatically. It is found only in the myocardium (muscle layer of the heart) and in the walls of the large vessels joining the heart. A cardiac muscle fiber is shown by light microscopy to be a linear unit composed of several cardiac muscle cells joined end to end at specialized junctional zones called *intercalated discs.* Each cell is about 100 microns (μm)

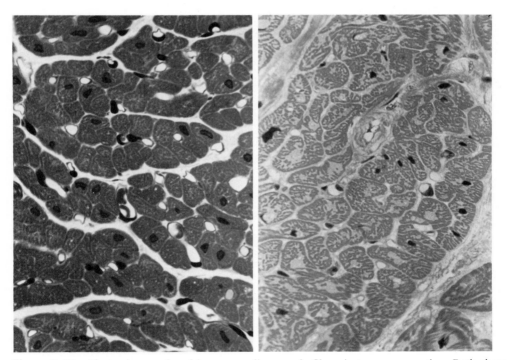

Figure 6–18. Photomicrographs of human cardiac muscle fibers in transverse section. Both show nuclei centrally located in fibers and, in the right figure, myofibrils are seen. Note the numerous capillary blood vessels between fibers. Left, × 400; right, plastic section, × 450.

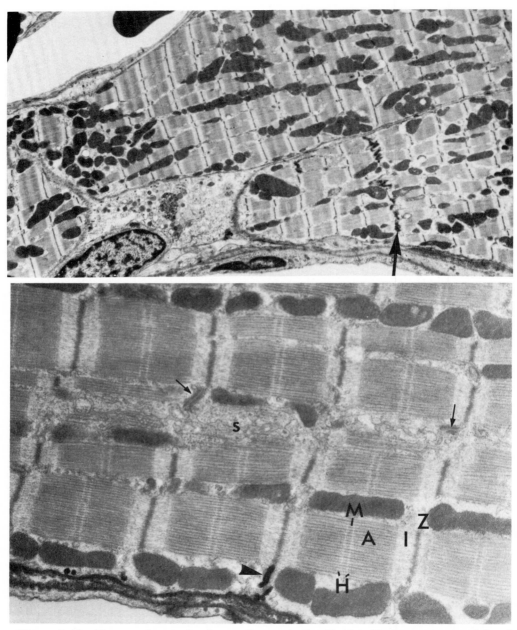

Figure 6–19. Electron micrographs of rat cardiac muscle. *Top:* Blood capillaries are seen at top left and bottom with muscle cells between. Note in the muscle cells numerous mitochondria between myofibrils, banding of myofibrils as in striated muscle, and an intercalated disc (arrow) crossing a muscle fiber at the site of a Z band. × 4,000. *Bottom:* A, I, Z, H., and M bands are seen in myofibrils with sarcoplasmic reticulum (s), triads located at Z lines (arrows), and a darkly staining T tubule (arrowhead) adjacent to (and would be continuous with) the sarcolemma. × 22,000.

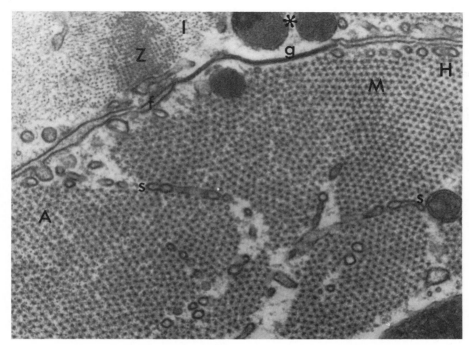

Figure 6–20. Electron micrograph of rat cardiac muscle in transverse section. The myofilaments are grouped into irregular myofibrils separated by sarcoplasm containing elements of sarcoplasmic reticulum (s) and mitochondria. They are sectioned at different levels of the sarcomere through A, I, Z, M, and H bands. Parts of two cells are seen with a gap junction (g) and a small intermediate junction or fascia adherens (f). This is atrial muscle and the upper cell shows two "atrial specific granules" (asterisk). × 48,000.

long and 15 microns (μm) in diameter, often partially divided into two or more branches at its ends, these branches meeting adjacent cells, or parts of them, at intercalated discs. The overall appearance thus is one of mainly parallel fibers with numerous cross beams, giving the false impression of a syncytial network. Between the fibers, but not extending into the intercalated discs, is fine connective tissue, the endomysium, containing small blood vessels and lymphatics.

The cardiac muscle fiber is enveloped by a thin sarcolemma similar to that of skeletal muscle, and sarcoplasm is abundant with numerous mitochondria. Myofibrils are separated by mitochondria arranged in rows between them, with consequent obvious longitudinal striation. A pattern of cross striations of the myofibrils, with A, I, Z, M, and H bands identical to those of skeletal muscle, also is obvious, but the bands are less conspicuous than those

of skeletal muscle. Nuclei are elongated and situated centrally in the fiber between diverging myofibrils. Around the nuclei are fusiform areas of sarcoplasm containing many mitochondria, a small Golgi apparatus at one pole of the nucleus, a few lipid droplets, and, with increasing age, some deposits of lipofuchsin pigment (secondary lysosomes). This pigment may be so extensive as to give a brownish tinge to the fresh myocardium, a condition known as "brown atrophy of the heart." The sarcoplasm also contains larger deposits of glycogen than are found in skeletal muscle. By light microscopy, intercalated discs appear as dark lines which may cross the fiber transversely but which usually pass in an irregular, zigzag, or steplike manner across the fibers at irregular intervals. They always cross fibers at the level of the Z lines and are more obvious in adult tissue, first appearing in late fetal life. Intercalated discs are areas of cell adhesion between

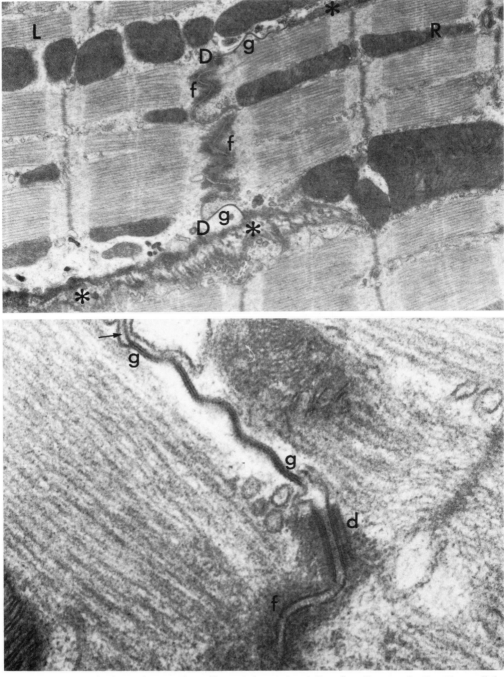

Figure 6–21.   Electron micrographs to illustrate intercalated disc of cardiac muscle. *Top:* Extracellular (intercellular) space is indicated by an asterisk and parts of two cells (left and right, L and R) meet at an intercalated disc (D) located at a Z line. The disc shows fasciae adherentes (f) and gap junctions (g). × 24,000. *Bottom:* A higher magnification showing an extensive gap junction (g), a spot desmosome (d), and intermediate junction or fascia adherens (f). The intercellular space appears above (arrow). × 84,000.

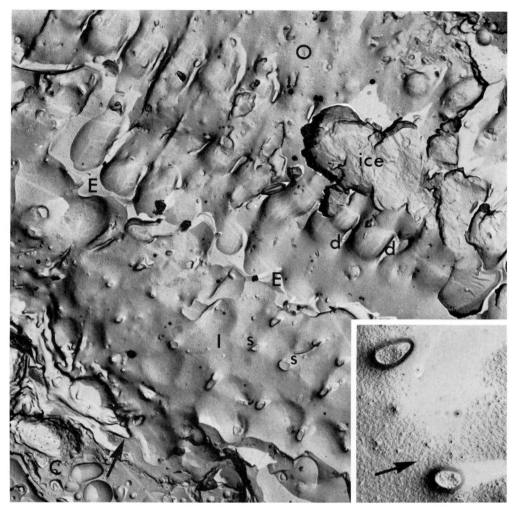

Figure 6–22. Electron micrograph of a freeze-etch preparation of cardiac muscle. Portions of two muscle cells are shown running obliquely from upper left to lower right. The upper cell (O) has fractured to show the outer surface of the plasma membrane with depressions or pits (d) as apertures of transverse tubules. In this cell also is an ice crystal as an artifact. In the lower cell (I) the fracture has exposed the inner, cytoplasmic surface of the plasma membrane with stumps (s) of transverse tubules. A capillary (C) is present at lower left. × 8300. Insert (lower right) shows the stumps of two transverse tubules at higher magnification. × 55,400. The broad arrows indicate the direction of metal shadowing. (Courtesy of Dr. D. G. Rayns.)

adjacent cardiac muscle cells, specialized to transmit tension of the myofibrils along the axis of an entire fiber.

Fine Structure

Myofilaments containing actin and myosin are identical to those of skeletal muscle and show a similar arrangement although they are less numerous. They are limited to individual muscle cells and do not cross cell junctions. However, grouping of myofilaments into myofibrils is not complete as it is in skeletal muscle, and cross sections show that myofibrils are incompletely surrounded and delineated by sarcoplasmic reticulum and sarcoplasm. Mitochondria characteristically are large, about 2.5 microns (μm) long (the length of a sarcomere), and show closely packed cristae.

The *T tubules* of cardiac muscle resemble those of skeletal muscle in that they are invaginations of the sarcolemma but differ in that they are of greater diameter and lie at the Z lines and not at

A-I junctions. The tubules are an extension of the extracellular space and contain extracellular basal lamina material continuous with that of the sarcolemma. The *sarcoplasmic reticulum* consists of longitudinal, interconnected tubules that couple with a T tubule at the Z line, but no large terminal cisternae are present. Thus, the total area of contact between the sarcoplasmic reticulum and the T tubules is less than in skeletal muscle. However, also present are cisterns of sarcoplasmic reticulum located subjacent to the sarcolemma (subsarcolemmal cisterns). These often make couplings with the sarcolemma and function like triads in the release of calcium necessary for contraction.

The *intercalated discs* are specialized cell junctions located at Z lines. If two cells could be separated at a disc, the opposing surfaces would show a complex pattern of blunt papillae and ridges with reciprocal pits and grooves. As indicated, they usually cross a fiber in a stepwise pattern and thus have transverse and longitudinal parts, the latter parallel to the axis of the fiber and therefore the axis of contraction. In the transverse regions are scattered spot desmosomes or maculae adherentes, presumably for firm cell adhesion, and extensive intermediate junctions or fasciae adherentes. Here, the intercellular space is about 20 nm wide, with some dense material on the cytoplasmic surfaces of each plasmalemma, to which are anchored the thin myofilaments. These regions also function in firm cell adhesion. In longitudinal regions particularly are extensive gap junctions or nexuses with some less extensive gap junctions in transverse regions. These permit rapid impulse conduction between cells.

Contraction

From early embryonic life, spontaneous myogenic contractions occur in cardiac muscle cells. The mechanism of contraction is identical to that of skeletal muscle, i.e., a sliding filament. In the adult, in various regions of the heart, cardiac muscle cells are modified to form the impulse conducting system (see Chapter 8), which regulates the beat of the heart. Transmission of impulses occurs from cardiac muscle cell to cell via the nexuses.

Purkinje fibers are specialized cardiac muscle cells and part of the impulse conducting system. They are located just beneath the endocardium on the internal surface of the heart, particularly in relation to the interventricular septum. As with cardiac muscle, the Purkinje fibers form a network composed of separate cellular units. By light microscopy, in comparison to cardiac muscle fibers, Purkinje fibers are larger, thicker (about 50 microns or μm in diameter), and more palely staining, with abundant central sarcoplasm and relatively few myofibrils, which usually are found in a peripheral position. Purkinje fibers contain large quantities of glycogen. Intercalated discs are present but not seen commonly. Regions exist where there is a gradual transition between Purkinje and ordinary cardiac muscle fibers.

Connective Tissue

Connective tissue is not prominent in cardiac muscle but extends between fibers as a delicate endomysium containing a very rich capillary network, more extensive than that of skeletal muscle. Lymphatic capillaries also are numerous, and fine autonomic nerves may be seen occasionally.

Regeneration

Cardiac muscle is more resistant to injuries than are the other types of muscle but shows very little evidence of regeneration after injury. Damaged cardiac muscle is repaired by fibroconnective scar tissue.

SMOOTH MUSCLE

This type is also called unstriped, nonstriated, or involuntary muscle. Individual cells are fusiform, elongated, and closely associated with connective tissue. Smooth muscle mainly is visceral in distribution, forming the contractile portion of the wall of the digestive tract from the midpoint of the esophagus to the anus, including the ducts of glands associated with the system. It is found in the respiratory, urinary, and genital systems and in arteries, veins, and larger lymphatic vessels. In addition it is present in the dermis and in the iris and ciliary body of the eye.

Shape and Size

Smooth muscle fibers are elongated, spindle-shaped cells with fine tapering ends and a wider central region in which the nucleus is situated. In size, they vary with location, being only 20 microns (μm) or less in length around small ducts and blood vessels, but reaching 0.5 mm in the pregnant uterus. Generally throughout the intestinal tract and in association with larger blood vessels, they are about 0.2 mm long and about 6 microns (μm) in diameter at the midpoint of the cell. The

sarcoplasm of a smooth muscle cell in a stained preparation is acidophil and usually appears homogeneous but may show small, clear areas which probably indicate the location of glycogen. In special preparations—for example, after gentle maceration in acid—fine longitudinal striations can be demonstrated. These are the myofibrils or contractile elements. In thin, plastic sections, small darkly staining patches are visible both along the surface plasmalemma and in the sarcoplasm; these have been called attachment plaques and dense bodies. Cytoplasmic organelles are few and are grouped near the nucleus. The nucleus in cross section of the fiber is central or slightly eccentric in position. Owing to the length of the fibers, nuclei are seen in only a few cells in cross section. The nucleus is elongated, ovoid, or cylindrical, has a fine chromatin network, and thus does not stain darkly. It contains one or more nucleoli. In cells fixed during contraction, nuclei characteristically show a folded or twisted shape.

Organization

In many regions of the body, particularly in the dermis, smooth muscle cells are scattered singly or in small groups and are associated intimately with connective tissue. Individual cells are embedded in bundles of reticular or thin elastic fibers, and small groups of cells, e.g., in association with hairs, often are held in a small cylindrical mass or fascicle, covered by a fine envelope or sheath of fibroelastic tissue. The other common arrangement is in sheets, the fibers all being oriented in the same direction in each sheet. Often two such sheets form the contractile wall of a duct with the fibers of the two sheets lying at right angles to each other. For example, in the intestine the inner layer of muscle is circular around the tube, the outer layer longitudinal along the length of the tube. Probably these orientations really are spiral in type, the "circular" being a closed and the "longitudinal" an open helix. In these sheets, muscle cells are arranged so that the nuclear (broad) region of one is adjacent to the thin tapering end of its neighbors. The space

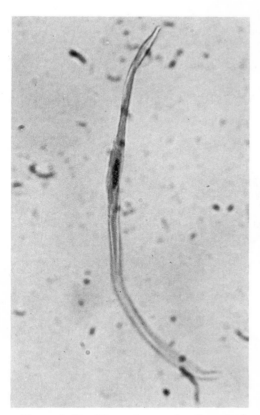

Figure 6–23. Photomicrograph of a single teased smooth muscle cell from the tunica muscularis of the human duodenum. × 660.

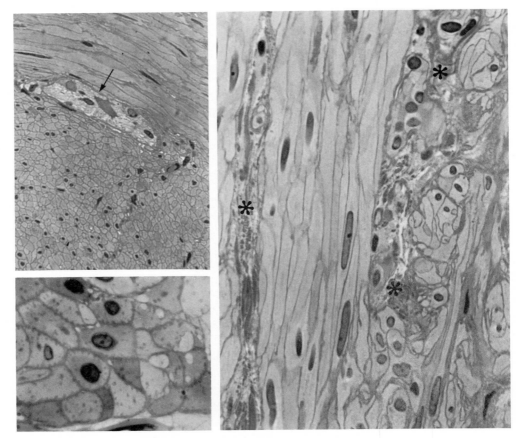

Figure 6–24. Photomicrographs of smooth muscle, all plastic sections. *Top left:* From the small intestine, cut in longitudinal (above) and transverse (below) section. Between the layers, the arrow points to a small collection of ganglion cells (Auerbach's plexus). × 160. *Right:* From the wall of a gallbladder, longitudinal (left) and transverse (right) sections, the muscle cells in bundles with strands of connective tissue (asterisks) between the bundles. × 400. *Bottom left:* From the bladder wall, transverse section with darker staining attachment plaques at the surface and dense bodies (small dark dots) within the sarcoplasm. × 1000.

between adjacent muscle fibers is narrow and in the order of 500 to 800 Å (50 to 80 nm). Fine reticular and elastic fibers extend between individual fibers, but fibroblasts are few, and the extracellular fibers between the muscle cells probably are formed by the muscle cells themselves. A large bundle or sheet of muscle is surrounded by more dense fibroconnective tissue with fibroblasts and other connective tissue cells, blood vessels, and nerves. In such a sheet, the pull of a contracting fiber first is transmitted to the fine reticular-elastic network surrounding it and then to the stronger connective tissue of the muscle bundle, thus giving a steady, general force to the enclosed or surrounded tissue, e.g., in constriction of a blood vessel.

Fine Structure

In electron micrographs, the noncontracted smooth muscle cell is elongated, has a regular outline, and shows a nucleus also of smooth, ovoid shape. When contracted, the cell surface usually is irregular, as is the nucleus. In the sarcoplasm around the nucleus, and particularly at its poles, are mitochondria, a

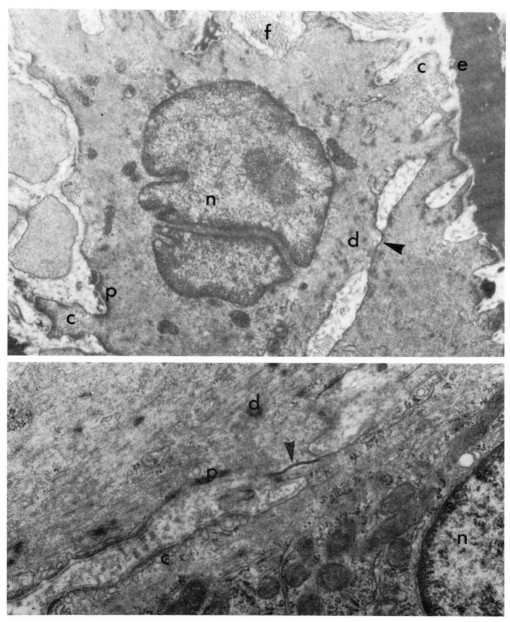

Figure 6–25. Electron micrographs of smooth muscle of musculus trachealis. *Top:* Transverse section, one cell cut through the nuclear area (n) and making a nexus (arrowhead) with an adjacent cell. Note the subsarcolemmal caveolae (c), attachment plaques (p) at the surface and dense bodies (d) in the sarcoplasm, and elastin (e) and collagen microfibrils (f) in the interstitium. × 12,000. *Bottom:* Longitudinal section with myofilaments running longitudinally, a nexus, and most organelles in a paranuclear position. × 36,000.

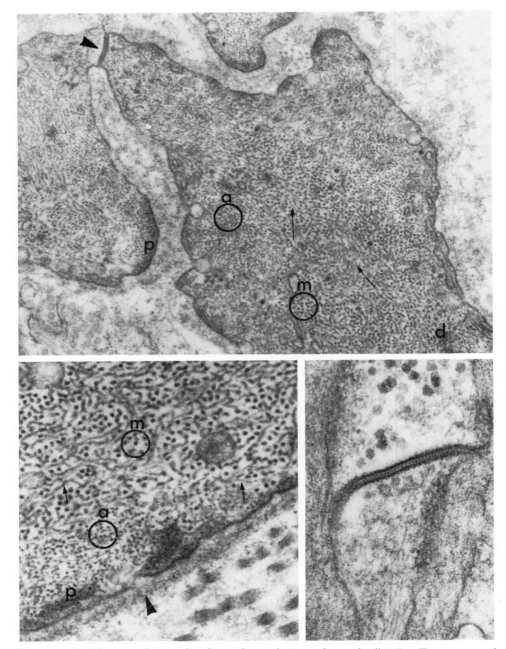

Figure 6–26. Electron micrographs of smooth muscle (musculus trachealis). *Top:* Transverse section showing a nexus (arrowhead) and cytoplasmic filaments of three sizes: thick (myosin — m) myofilaments, thin (actin — a) myofilaments, and intermediate 10-nm filaments (arrows). Attachment plaques (p) and dense bodies (d) also are seen. × 44,000. *Bottom left:* A higher magnification to show filament types. Also seen is the basal lamina (arrowhead) and collagen microfibrils (below). × 180,000. *Bottom right:* A nexus or gap junction between two smooth muscle cell processes, above and below. × 68,000.

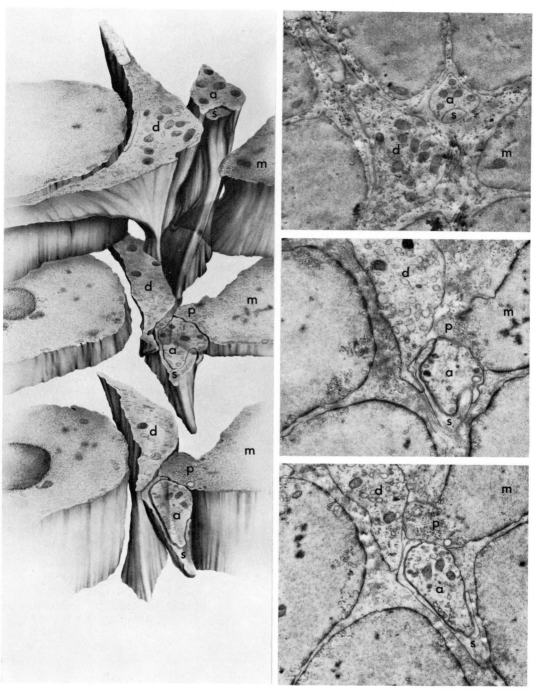

Figure 6–27. Three-dimensional illustration and electron micrographs of a neuromuscular junction in smooth muscle tissue. The illustration was drawn in perspective from serial sections of the inner layer of the muscularis externa of the duodenum of a frog. The electron micrographs on the right represent the visible surfaces in the illustration on the left. The total depth of the three slices in the illustration is 6.1 microns, which represents approximately 60 sections of 1000 angstroms thickness. A vesiculated nerve process (a), which is invested partially by a portion of a Schwann cell (s), is making intimate contact with a protrusion (p) of a smooth muscle cell (m). The expanded process (d), which actually emanates from the cell body of a neuron within the myenteric plexus, is presumably a dendrite. The semitransparency of the nerve process and the Schwann cell investment in the illustration permits the visualization of the edges of the smooth muscle cells. × 20,000, (Courtesy of Dr. J. C. Thaemert.)

few elements of granular endoplasmic reticulum, free ribosomes, a small Golgi apparatus, glycogen, and a few lipid droplets. In the remainder of the sarcoplasm are mostly myofilaments, both thick and thin, arranged in irregular bundles, a few mitochondria, and glycogen particles. Also present at the periphery, adjacent to the sarcolemma, are a few elements of agranular sarcoplasmic reticulum and numerous caveolae, some of which open to the surface. These subsarcolemmal caveolae probably function like T tubules in conducting contraction impulses and may function like sarcoplasmic reticulum in regulating calcium flow.

The sarcolemma is a typical unit membrane of about 7 nm width, covered externally by a basal lamina. While usually of smooth outline, it may show blunt, finger-like processes abutting against adjacent cells or contacting similar processes from adjacent cells. Fine reticular and elastic fibers occupy narrow spaces between adjacent cells, but there are regions where sarcolemmae of adjacent cells form *nexuses* or *gap junctions* that permit rapid passage of an electrical impulse from one cell to another (see page 91).

Myofilaments and Contraction. Both thin (5 to 8 nm) and thick (14 to 15 nm) myofilaments are present, but they do not show the regular arrangement seen in striated and cardiac muscle. In a sense, the contractile unit is the cell, not the sarcomere, which is not present in smooth muscle. Involved in the process also are the densities of the sarcolemma (attachment plaques), those lying in sarcoplasm (dense bodies), and a third, intermediate type of filament of 10 nm diameter. Bundles of thin filaments attach to the cell surface at the attachment plaques and extend into the interior of the cell, probably to attach also to dense bodies. As in other types of muscle, these filaments contain F actin, tropomyosin, and the troponin complex. The thick filaments are 2000 nm long and about 15 nm in diameter and occur as discrete elements between thin filaments. While both types of myofilament are mainly parallel and longitudinally oriented in the relaxed smooth muscle cell, in the contracted fiber the orientation is less regular. Thin filaments are more numerous than in striated muscle, with a ratio of about 15 thin to 1 thick myofilament.

The intermediate, 10-nm filaments contain the protein desmin and attach to the attachment plaques and dense bodies, forming a framework or skeleton in the cell. The dense bodies contain α-actinin, a protein found in Z lines of striated muscle, and thus the dense bodies may function like Z lines for the attachment of thin myofilaments. It is believed that the contractile force is generated by a sliding filament mechanism between actin and myosin and transmitted by the dense bodies and cytoskeleton of 10 nm filaments to decrease cell length. This actin-myosin interaction requires calcium ions for activation, and, while the reservoir for calcium is not known for certain in smooth muscle, it is believed to be the subsarcolemmal caveolae.

Nerve Supply. Smooth muscle is supplied by both sympathetic and parasympathetic divisions of the autonomic nervous system, all nerve fibers being postganglionic and unmyelinated. On the basis of innervation and function, two types of smooth muscle are recognized. The *multiunit* type has a rich nerve supply with all, or nearly all, muscle cells receiving nerve terminals. Such an arrangement is found in the muscle of the iris, larger arteries, and ductus deferens, the muscle fibers contracting together and relatively fast. The second type shows much fewer terminal nerve endings, the stimulus passing from cell to cell via nexuses. This *unitary* type gives a relatively slow contraction and is found in the viscera and smaller blood vessels. Intermediate types also are found.

Origin, Growth, and Regeneration

The great majority of smooth muscle develops by the differentiation of mesenchymal cells, although that of the iris is derived from ectoderm. In association with some glands and their ducts, e.g., salivary, sweat, and lacrimal glands, cells with many of the characteristics of smooth muscle differentiate from ectoderm and are called myo-epithelial cells (see Chapter 2). Smooth muscle cells can increase in size in response to physiological stimuli (e.g., in the uterus in pregnancy) and pathological stimuli (e.g., in arterioles in hypertension). There also is evidence that although the increase in bulk (for example, of the uterus in pregnancy) is due mainly to an increased size of individual muscle cells, there also may be an increase in the number of cells following differentiation of mesenchymal cells present in the uterus. There is some evidence that smooth muscle cells themselves can divide by mitosis.

Differentiation Between Smooth Muscle and Collagen Fibers

One of the most common difficulties in identification of tissues is that of distinguishing between smooth muscle and connective tissue. Muscle fibers are cellular and usually stain more intensely with eosin than do collagen fibers. Nuclei are situated within the fibers, may be wrinkled, and are larger than the nuclei of fibroblasts, which are situated between collagen fibers. Certain staining techniques, e.g., Mallory and van Gieson, readily distinguish between the two.

REFERENCES

Ashton, F. T., Somlyo, A. V., and Somlyo, A. P.: The contractile apparatus of vascular smooth muscle: intermediate high voltage stereo electron microscopy. J. Mol. Biol., *98*:17, 1975.

Bois, R. M.: The organization of the contractile apparatus of vertebrate smooth muscle. Anat. Rec., *177*:61, 1973.

Butler, R.: A new grouping of intrafusal muscle fibers based on developmental studies of muscle spindles in the cat. Am. J. Anat., *156*:115, 1979.

Ellisman, M. H., Rash, J. E., Staehelin, A., and Porter, K. R.: Studies of excitable membranes. II. A comparison of specializations at neuromuscular junctions and nonjunctional sarcolemmas of mammalian fast and slow twitch muscle fibers. J. Cell Biol., *68*:752, 1976.

Forssmann, W. G., and Girardier, L.: A study of the T system in rat heart. J. Cell Biol., *44*:1, 1970.

Franzini-Armstrong, C.: The structure of a simple Z line. J. Cell Biol., *58*:630, 1973.

Gabella, G.: I. Cellular structures and electrophysiological behaviour. Fine structure of smooth muscle. Phil. Trans. R. Soc. Lond. B., *265*:7, 1973.

Goldstein, M. A., Schroeter, J. P., and Sass, R. L.: The Z-lattice in canine cardiac muscle. J. Cell Biol., *83*:187, 1979.

Hanson, J., and Huxley, H. E.: The structural basis of contraction in striated muscle. Symp. Soc. Exp. Biol., *9*:228, 1955.

Huxley, H. E.: The contractile structure of cardiac and skeletal muscle. Circulation, *24*:328, 1961.

Huxley, H. E.: The mechanism of muscular contraction. Sci. Am., *213*:18, 1965.

Kelly, D. E.: Models of muscle Z-band fine structure based on a looping filament configuration. J. Cell Biol., *34*:827, 1967.

Kelly, R. E., and Rice, R. V.: Ultrastructural studies on the contractile mechanism of smooth muscle. J. Cell Biol., *42*:683, 1959.

Knappeis, G. G., and Carlsen, F.: The ultrastructure of the Z disc in skeletal muscle. J. Cell Biol., *13*:323, 1962.

Leeson, C. R.: The electron microscopy of the myoepithelium in the rat exorbital lacrimal gland. Anat. Rec., *137*:45, 1960.

Leeson, T. S.: Sarcotubules and subsarcolemmal caveolae and their continuity with the sarcolemma in frog striated muscle. Am. J. Anat., *150*:185, 1977.

Leeson, T. S.: The transverse tubular (T) system of rat cardiac muscle fibers as demonstrated by tannic acid mordanting. Can. J. Zoo., *56*:1906, 1978.

Ovalle, W. K., Jr.: Fine structure of rat intrafusal muscle fibers. The equatorial region. J. Cell Biol., *52*:382, 1972.

Philpott, C. W., and Goldstein, M. A.: Sarcoplasmic reticulum of striated muscle: localization of potential calcium binding sites. Science, *155*:1019, 1967.

Porter, K. R., and Franzini-Armstrong, C.: The sarcoplasmic reticulum. Sci. Am., *212*:72, 1965.

Rayns, D. G.: Myofilaments and cross bridges as demonstrated by freeze-fracturing and etching. J. Ultrastruct. Res., *40*:103, 1972.

Schultz, E.: Fine structure of satellite cells in growing skeletal muscle. Am. J. Anat., *147*:49, 1976.

Shoenberg, C. F., and Needham, D. M.: A study of the mechanism of contraction in vertebrate smooth muscle. Biol. Rev., *51*:53, 1976.

Simpson, F. O., and Rayns, D. G.: The relationship between the transverse tubular system and other tubules at the Z disc levels of myocardial cells in the ferret. Am. J. Anat., *122*:193, 1968.

Sommer, J. R., and Johnson, E. A.: Cardiac muscle: a comparative study of Purkinje fibers and ventricular fibers. J. Cell Biol., *36*:497, 1968.

Stromer, M. H., Hartshorne, D. J., and Rice, R. V.: Removal and reconstitution of Z-line materia in a striated muscle. J. Cell Biol., *65*:C23, 1967.

Thaemert, J. C.: Intercellular bridges as protoplasmic anastomoses between smooth muscle cells. J. Biophys. Biochem. Cytol., *6*:67, 1959.

Thaemert, J. C.: Ultrastructural interrelationships of nerve processes and smooth muscle cells in three dimensions. J. Cell Biol., *28*:37, 1966.

Zubrzycka, E., and MacLennan, D. H.: Assembly of the sarcoplasmic reticulum. J. Biol. Chem., *251*:7733, 1977.

NERVOUS TISSUE

The nervous system includes the total mass of nervous tissue in the body. Nervous tissue is widely distributed and with a few minor exceptions all organs of the body include a nervous element. Basically, the nervous system consists of tissue which collects stimuli from the environment, transforms such stimuli into nervous impulses, and passes them to a large, highly organized reception and correlation area. Here the impulses are received and interpreted and, in turn, are issued to effector organs to institute appropriate responses. The nervous system also includes structural areas for all conscious experience. All these functions are performed by a highly specialized collection of cells called *neurons* which, together with their supporting cells and associated extracellular material, form the nervous system.

Anatomically, the nervous system can be divided into the *central nervous system* and the *peripheral nervous system.* The central nervous system is composed of the brain and spinal cord located in the cranium and vertebral canal, i.e., it is protected by bone; the peripheral nervous system includes all other nervous structures. The central nervous system receives all nervous impulses from the body (interoceptive) and all impulses following stimuli originating outside the body (exteroceptive). The peripheral nervous system serves to interconnect all other tissues and organs with the central nervous system. Functionally, the nervous system is divided into *somatic* and *autonomic* parts, each with central and peripheral divisions.* The

somatic portion is concerned with structures derived from the embryological somites, i.e., muscles, bones, and skin. Muscles derived from branchial arches are included in this part because, histologically, the muscles of the two groups are identical. The autonomic nervous system is concerned with the innervation of smooth and cardiac muscle and the glands of the body. To a great extent its functions are independent of the rest of the nervous system.

In the neuron, two properties of protoplasm are developed to a great degree. These are *irritability,* which is the capacity for response to physical and chemical agents with the initiation of an impulse, and *conductivity,* the ability to transmit such an impulse from one locality to another. The extreme degree to which these two properties of protoplasm are developed in neurons, together with the great diversity of shape and size of the cell bodies and the length of their processes, distinguishes neurons from all other cell types. Most of the nerve cell bodies are collected in or near the central nervous system. Their processes, which are capable of transmitting impulses, may lie totally within the central nervous system, may extend from the central nervous system for great distances, or may lie entirely outside the central nervous system. All neurons are capable of exciting other neurons in contact with them. Such specialized contacts between neurons are called *synapses.* The term neuron, then, refers to a complete nerve cell, including the nucleus and its surrounding cytoplasm (the perikaryon) and one or more protoplasmic extensions or processes. The latter

---

*Note on terminology: *soma* = body; *autos* = self, *nomos* = control, i.e., automatic.

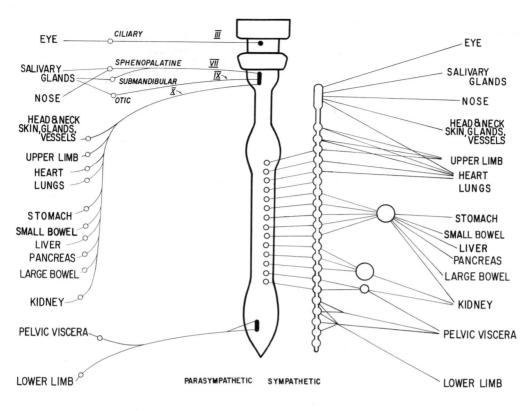

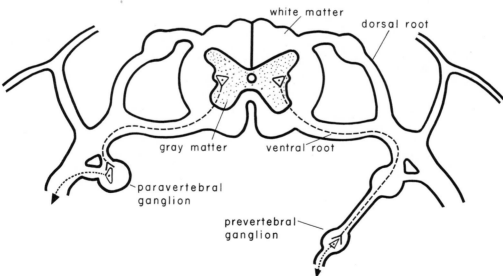

Figure 7–1. *Top:* Diagram of the peripheral distribution of components of the autonomic system; parasympathetic division on the left, symphathetic division on the right. The three peripheral or prevertebral ganglia represented by circles on the right are the celiac, superior mesenteric, and inferior mesenteric. *Bottom:* Diagram of a cross section of the spinal cord to show two possible courses taken by preganglionic (----) and postganglionic (....) fibers of the sympathetic nervous system.

usually comprise several *dendrites* and one *axon* or *axis cylinder*. Connections with other neurons at synapses are by contact only. Thus, the neuron is the structural and functional unit of the nervous system.

(The student may experience some confusion in terminology. The nerve cell body of a neuron often is called the nerve cell and its threadlike processes the nerve fibers, both being constituent parts of the neuron.)

THE REFLEX ARC

The basic unit of the nervous system is the neuron, but the integrative unit is the reflex arc. Any nervous activity involves the activity of many neurons with numerous potential interconnections by their synapses. However, the basic pattern is best exemplified by the simple reflex arc. Most of the actions in man involve such reflex arcs. The simplest reflex arc involves only two

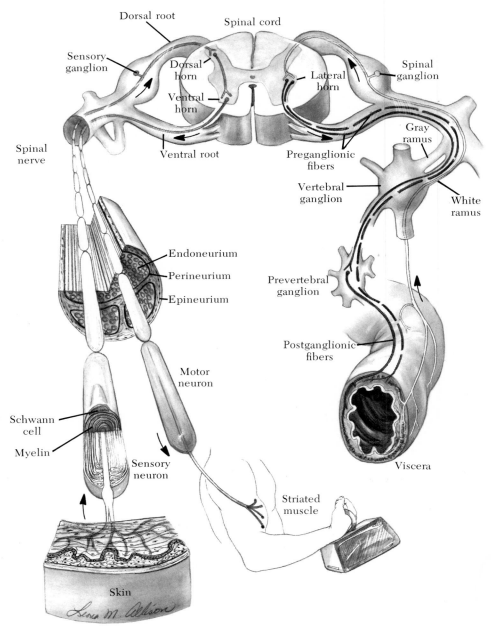

Figure 7–2.   Diagram to illustrate somatic (left) and sympathetic (right) reflex arcs.

neurons. These are illustrated in Figure 7–2 (top). One example of this is the *knee jerk*, commonly used clinically in the examination of patients. With the knees crossed in a sitting, relaxed patient, the patellar tendon of the uppermost leg is tapped sharply but gently. Normally the quadriceps muscle contracts to kick forward the foot. This reflex response involves one afferent or sensory neuron and an efferent, motor neuron. A peripheral process (a dendrite) of the afferent neuron lies in the **substance of the quadriceps muscle** tendon and passes centrally to the cell body lying in a posterior root ganglion near the spinal cord. From the cell body, a second nerve process (an axon) passes into the substance of the spinal cord. Here it synapses with an efferent (motor) neuron cell body from which a nerve fiber (an axon) passes in a peripheral nerve to terminate by supplying muscle fibers in the quadriceps muscle. This is a very simple mechanism and, of course, most reflex arcs in the body are more complex. By inserting a third neuron (a connector, association, or internuncial neuron) between the afferent and efferent neurons, potentially numerous connections within the central nervous system are established

(Figure 7–2, left). Thus more complex reflex arcs can be built. It must be emphasized that once a nervous impulse reaches the central nervous system in an intact animal, there is widespread activity within the central nervous system and that, in fact, the simple reflex arc as just described does not exist. It is a simplification of a basic principle that such activity involves inflow to the central nervous system (by the afferent neuron), modification and integration (by the internuncial neuron), and outflow to an effector organ (by the efferent neuron).

STRUCTURE OF THE NEURON

Neurons vary greatly in size and shape, but each consists of a cell body, or *perikaryon*, and one or more processes. These processes are of two types, the *axon*, always a single process, and the *dendrites*. A neuron with just one process, which branches beyond the cell body into an axon and a dendrite, is termed *unipolar*. A neuron with two processes is *bipolar;* with more than two it is *multipolar*. For convenience, the cell body, or perikaryon,

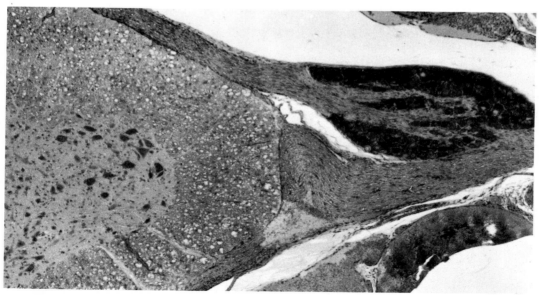

Figure 7–3. Photomicrograph of a transverse section of the spinal cord in the spinal canal, only the left half being seen. The posterior surface is above. In the spinal cord (left), the central gray matter, with large motor neurons (dark) in the anterior horn, and peripheral white matter are seen. Anterior (motor) and posterior (sensory) roots of a spinal nerve join at the right edge, and the dorsal (sensory) root ganglion with nerve cell bodies is well seen. × 50.

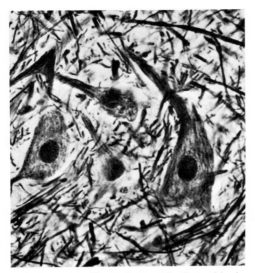

Figure 7–4. Photomicrograph of a multipolar ganglion cell from the spinal cord. Neurofibrils are seen. Cajal silver method. × 500.

and the processes will be described separately.

Perikaryon

The cell body usually is large in comparison to other cells and varies from 4 to 135 microns (μm) in diameter. The shape is variable in the extreme and is dependent upon the number and orientation of cell processes. Unipolar cells are globular in shape and have a single process which bifurcates. They are found in the cranial and spinal ganglia (a ganglion being a collection of nerve cell bodies situated outside the central nervous system). A bipolar cell is elongated, spindle-shaped, and with a process at each end or pole of the cell. Examples are found in organs of special sense, e.g., in the retina of the eye, in the olfactory epithelium, and in the acoustic ganglion. Multipolar cells, by far the most common, have numerous processes and vary from stellate to pyramidal to pear-shaped. They are found throughout the central nervous system and in autonomic ganglia. The total number of nerve cells in the body never has been estimated accurately, but there are probably 14 billion in the cerebral cortex alone.

Nucleus

The nucleus usually is large (up to 20 microns or μm in diameter), spherical, and centrally situated in the cell body. The nuclear envelope is distinct and shows numerous pores. Heterochromatin is small in amount and usually marginated at the inner aspect of the nuclear envelope. In general, the nucleus is pale-staining and contains one or more large nucleoli. A Barr body (sex chromatin) may be present as a nucleolar satellite. The large, pale, vesicular nucleus with a prominent, dark-staining nucleolus is often referred to as having the "owl's-eye" appearance.

Cytoplasmic Organelles

The plasma membrane is 70 to 80 Å (7 to 8 nm) thick and shows specializations in regions of intercellular adhesion and at synapses where there are accumulations of dense material in the adjacent cytoplasm. Mitochondria are usually small, ovoid or spherical, with cristae of both tubular and lamellar types. The Golgi apparatus may be quite large, and while often perinuclear in position, it may be multiple with several dictyosomes scattered throughout the perikaryon. One characteristic feature of the perikaryon is the presence

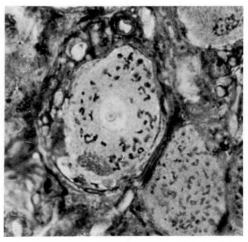

Figure 7–5. Photomicrograph of a nerve cell body from a spinal ganglion stained to demonstrate the Golgi apparatus. Note the pale-staining nucleus with darker nucleolus. × 550.

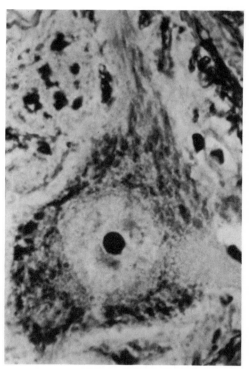

Figure 7–6. Photomicrograph of a nerve cell body of the spinal cord (anterior horn cell) stained to demonstrate the granular chromophil substance or Nissl bodies. Note that Nissl substance not only is found in the perikaryon but extends into the dendrite (top). It is not present in the axon or axon hillock (lower right). The large vesicular nucleus and prominent nucleolus are well seen. × 950.

drites. Agranular endoplasmic reticulum usually is not found in the perikaryon, although a few slender, tubular elements may be found in some dendrites.

A second prominent feature of neurons is the presence of neurofibrils, present throughout the cytoplasm and extending into dendrites and axon. A bundle of neurofibrils may branch, although the individual elements do not, the bundles extending from the perikaryon to the tips of nerve cell processes. Electron microscopy demonstrates in these bundles both microtubules (neurotubules) and microfilaments (neurofilaments). Microtubules resemble those found in other cells, are 25 nm in diameter, but may contain a thin central filament within the hollow core. Microfilaments are 70 to 100 Å (7 to 10 nm) in diameter. Both elements are believed to be involved in intracellular transport of ions and metabolites and in cell support and maintenance of cell shape.

Centrioles are not prominent in nerve cells, which are incapable of cell division, but when present are usually found at the cell periphery adjacent to a single cilium. A single cilium, protruding from a basal body, is often present and in neurons of the CNS is believed to be vestigial and without any apparent function. In other specialized cells, e.g., bipolar neurons of rods and cones, a modified cilium performs a sensory function. Primary lysosomes are common, usually located near the Golgi apparatus, and are associated with hydrolysis of end products of cellular metabolism and, perhaps, with degradation of lipids. With increasing age, secondary lysosomes increase in numbers, some of these being lipofuchsin granules.

The reaction of the Nissl bodies to injury of the neuron is characteristic, the Nissl bodies apparently breaking up and diffusing generally throughout the neuroplasm. This results in a general, dark staining of the entire neuroplasm. If such an effect follows injury of the axon, it is termed the Nissl reaction or primary irritation of the nerve cell. The dissolution of the Nissl bodies after damage to the nerve cell itself is termed *chromatolysis.*

of clumps of *Nissl substance* or *Nissl bodies,* representing the basophilic component of the cytoplasm, stainable by toluidine blue, thionin, and other basic aniline dyes. Nissl bodies are widely distributed in the cytoplasm, more numerous in large motor neurons and in lesser amounts in sensory neurons. Nissl bodies are formed by short, flat cisternae of granular endoplasmic reticulum with ribosomes and polysomes in the adjacent cytoplasm. They also are present in dendrites but are absent in the axon and the *axon hillock,* which is a clear conical area at the origin of the axon from the perikaryon. It is accepted generally that this extensive development of granular reticulum, associated with prominent nucleoli and numerous mitochondria, is concerned with the formation of new cytoplasmic protein, this material passing to all regions of the neuron, including its axon and den-

Cytoplasmic Inclusions

Fat droplets commonly are seen in the perikaryon and either represent reserve material or are a product of normal or pathological metabolism. Glycogen, although present in embryonic nerve cells, is not present in adult neurons. Pigment granules of various types are widespread. Lipofuscin granules, which probably are secondary lysosomes, are found in large neurons, the quantity increasing with age. The granules are yellow-brown in color. Melanin, as brownish-black granules, is present particularly in cells of certain regions, for example, in the substantia nigra of the midbrain, in spinal and sympathetic ganglia, and in the locus ceruleus in the floor of the fourth ventricle. Its significance is unknown. Iron-containing granules, demonstrable by the Prussian blue technique, are found in nerve cells in various regions, for example, the globus pallidus. Like granules of lipochrome, such iron-containing granules tend to increase in number with age.

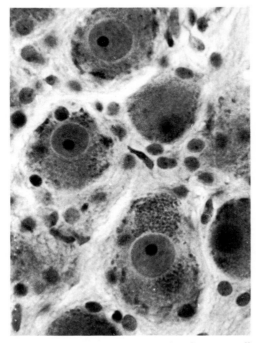

Figure 7–7. Photomicrograph of nerve cell bodies of a sympathetic ganglion to demonstrate lipochrome pigment. Note vesicular nuclei with prominent nucleoli. × 500.

Nerve Cell Processes

The processes, or nerve fibers, of neurons are a remarkable feature developed to provide conduction pathways and to provide greater surface areas for contact. These processes, as explained previously, are cytoplasmic extensions of the nerve cell body, there being one axon and one or more dendrites to each cell. The dendrites conduct impulses toward the cell, and the single axon or axis cylinder conducts impulses away from the cell.

Dendrites.   The single dendrite or peripheral process of a sensory ganglion cell resembles an axon of the peripheral nervous system. Such dendrites are associated with unipolar and bipolar ganglion cells. In multipolar cells, dendrites are short and numerous, branch widely, and lack myelin sheaths. They are thicker at their bases or origins from the cell body, and, while they vary greatly in size and shape, most do not have a regular surface but are covered by numerous, small spine-like processes, the "gemmules" or *dendritic spines.* The main branches of a dendrite contain microtubules and some microfilaments, elongated mitochondria, a few tubular profiles of agranular endoplasmic reticulum, and Nissl bodies. Nissl bodies do not extend into the terminal branches. The dendritic spines, usually about 0.2 micron (μm) long, show a narrow stalk with an ovoid terminal expansion. They contain only some fine filamentous material and the so-called "spine apparatus," composed of flat membranous cisternae with thin laminae of dense material between the cisternae. The spines are the sites of the majority of synapses between axons and the dendrite whereby the parent neuron makes contact with, and receives impulses from, many functionally related neurons. The number, extent of branching, and length of dendrites vary from neuron to neuron and are not dependent upon the size of the perikaryon. It is the dendrites which constitute much of the feltlike "neuropil" of the central nervous system (see page 242).

Axon.   The axon, or axis cylinder, is single and arises usually from the pe-

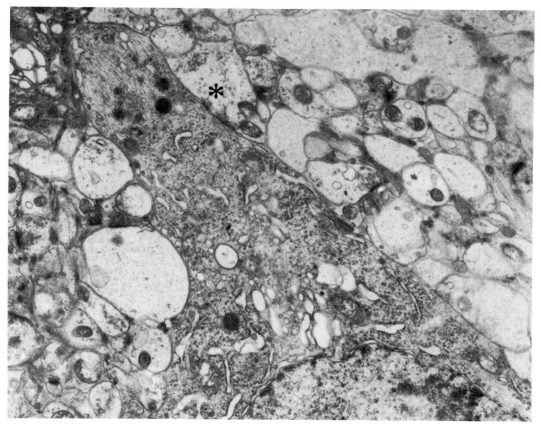

Figure 7–8. Electron micrograph of part of a small pyramidal cell from the rat cerebral cortex showing part of the nucleus (bottom right) and perikaryon with a dendritic process extending to the top left corner. The cell is surrounded mainly by small axons, one of which (asterisk) forms a synapse with the root of the dendrite. × 11,500.

riphery of the nerve cell body at a region termed the axon hillock. This area contains no chromophil substance, but passing through it is a concentration of neurofibrils which then enters the axon. There is no chromophil substance in the axon. An axon is more slender and usually much longer and straighter than the dendrites of the same neuron. Axons vary from less than a micron to several microns (μm) in diameter and from a fraction of a millimeter to a meter or more in length. Along the course of an axon, there may or may not be a series of side branches, called collaterals, which usually leave the axon at right angles near the axon hillock. The surface of the axon is smooth and its diameter constant, unlike a dendrite. Terminally, an axon ends in twiglike branchings, the *telodendria*, which touch the cell body,

dendrites or axons of one or more neurons at synapses. In some cases, the telodendria are so numerous as to surround the neuron on which they terminate in a basket-like arrangement. As will be described later in more detail, axons are covered with accessory sheaths. The plasma membrane or axolemma covering an axon is continuous with that of the nerve cell body. Within it are elongated mitochondria, a few tubular elements of agranular endoplasmic reticulum, and numerous microtubules and microfilaments, the last being more numerous in larger axons (which conduct impulses faster than small axons).

It now is accepted generally that the nerve cell body, with its extensive ergastoplasm, continuously synthesizes new protoplasm which flows down the nerve cell processes to

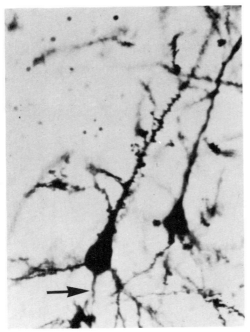

Figure 7–9. Photomicrograph of pyramidal cells from the cerebral cortex showing cell bodies and branching dendrites with dendritic spines or gemmules. The cell on the left also shows the origin of the axon (arrow). × 250.

replace protoplasm used in metabolism, protoplasm which cannot be synthesized in the cell processes themselves. This newly synthesized protein probably is distributed via the neurotubules. The rate of flow has been estimated at about 1 mm per day.

TYPES OF NEURONS

As indicated earlier, neurons can be uni- or multipolar depending on the number of dendrites. They also vary considerably in size and shape. Some of these neuron types are described here in more detail.

Golgi Type I. The majority of these neurons have many dendrites and very long axons, which leave the cell body in the gray matter of the central nervous system, and pass in white matter, some of them leaving the central nervous system to become peripheral nerve fibers. This type includes neurons whose axons contribute to peripheral nerves and those whose axons form the main fiber tracts of the brain and spinal cord.

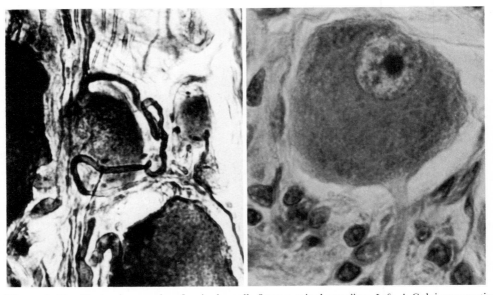

Figure 7–10. Photomicrographs of unipolar cells from a spinal ganglion. *Left:* A Golgi preparation showing the glomerulus formed by the coiled cell process. *Right:* The single process is seen leaving the nerve cell body. Left, × 550. (Courtesy of W. R. Ingram.) Right, × 1100.

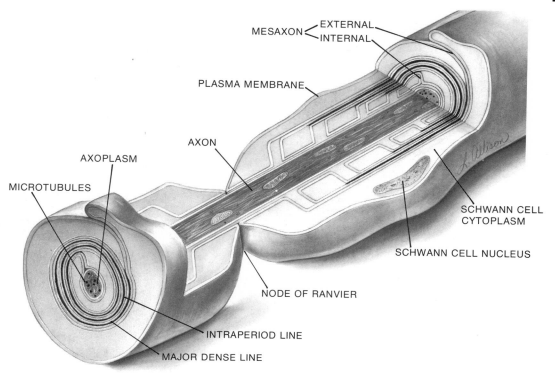

Figure 7–25. Diagram to show a myelinated nerve fiber and a node of Ranvier in longitudinal and transverse section as seen with the electron microscope.

gin and are essential to the vitality and function of peripheral nerve fibers. They form myelin but also are necessary for regeneration of axons. After division, an axon is regenerated from the central stump, i.e., from the end continuous with the nerve cell body, and grows peripherally to its termination along a channel formed by Schwann cells. Schwann cells also can become phagocytic after nerve injury, removing cellular debris.

Nerve Fibers in the CNS. Schwann cells are not present in the CNS, and their function is performed by oligodendrocytes, one type of neuroglia (discussed later). In myelinated fibers in the CNS, a single oligodendrocyte can form myelin sheaths around several separate axons, each axon being wrapped in a cytoplasmic process of the oligodendrocyte. The cell body of the oligodendrocyte thus is not directly opposed to the myelin sheath, as is the case with Schwann cells in the PNS, but lies between myelinated fibers, these fibers being myelinated by processes of the oligodendrocyte. Further, adjacent oligodendrocytes are not always in close contact, as are Schwann cells, thus leaving a short segment of the axon without a sheath.

Staining of Nerve Fibers. Myelinated fibers are highly refractile in fresh preparations. In fixed preparations, myelin is darkened by osmium tetroxide or Weigert's method. The axon remains unstained. Myelin, being a lipoprotein complex, is dissolved by fat solvents. Silver impregnation and methylene blue vital staining methods are used to demonstrate axons and are of particular value for unmyelinated fibers which are not easily seen in routine histological preparations.

PERIPHERAL NERVES

Peripheral nerves are composed of bundles of nerve fibers held together by connective tissue and include spinal

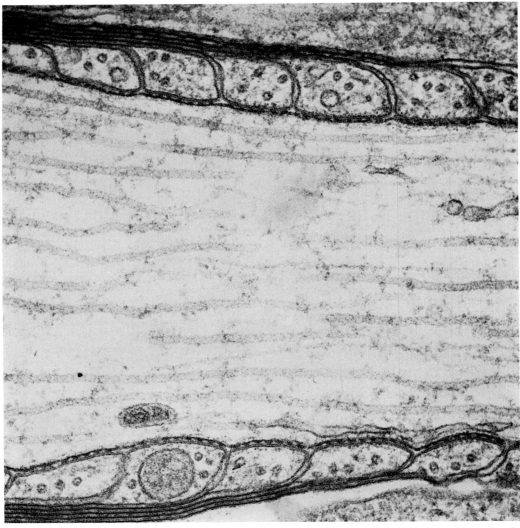

Figure 7–26.   Electron micrograph of a longitudinal section of a myelinated axon near a node of Ranvier from a rat brain. × 100,000. (Courtesy of Dr. A. Hirano. Reproduced by permission from the Editors, The Journal of Cell Biology, *34*:561, 1967.)

nerves connected to the spinal cord and cranial nerves connected with the brain. Most peripheral nerves appear white due to their content of myelinated fibers, although most contain also unmyelinated fibers. Most nerves are mixed, containing both sensory (afferent) and motor (efferent) fibers, although they are indistinguishable structurally; a few are sensory only, a few motor.

Surrounding the entire nerve is a sheath of relatively strong connective tissue termed the *epineurium.* It is composed of fibroblasts and collagenous fibers, mainly longitudinal in orientation, and a few elastic fibers, and contains the major blood vessels to the nerve. Within the epineurium, nerve fibers are grouped into bundles or fascicles, each fascicle being surrounded by a connective tissue sheath called the *perineurium.* This perineural sheath is formed by concentric layers or sleeves of flattened, fibroblast-like cells, each sleeve being one cell thick. Between adjacent cells in a sleeve are occluding junctions so that each sleeve is a complete cylinder around the nerve fascicle, with basal laminae between the cel-

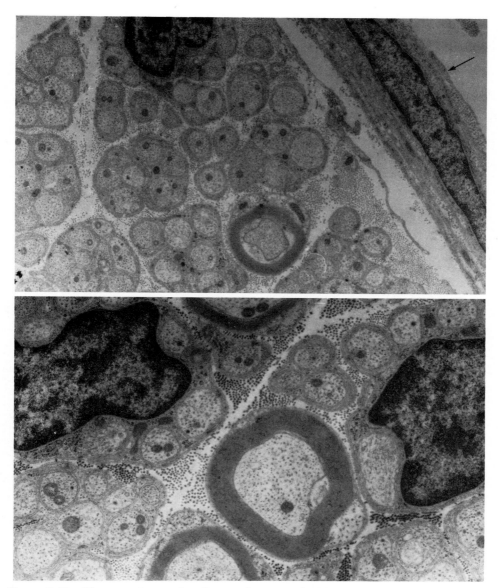

Figure 7–27. Electron micrographs of part of a nerve fascicle. *Top:* At the upper right is the perineurium (arrow) consisting of concentric layers or sleeves of flattened cells with basal laminae and collagen fibrils. Within the fascicle, part of a nucleus of a Schwann cell is seen (top center) with one myelinated and many unmyelinated nerve fibers. × 5000. *Bottom:* The nuclei of two Schwann cells are seen, each cell enclosing several unmyelinated fibers. Part of three myelinated fibers are seen with collagen fibrils of the endoneurium between the nerve fibers. × 9500.

lular sleeves. The number of sleeves decreases as the nerve branches and becomes smaller, the last sleeve terminating just before the nerve ending. Traced centrally, the perineurium is continuous with the pia arachnoid membrane of the central nervous system (see page 246). The perineurium provides a barrier to the passage of material into or out of the nerve fascicle. Within the perineurium are strands of delicate connective tissue extending around and between individual nerve fibers. This is the *endoneurium,* composed of delicate collagenous and reticular fibers and flattened, elongat-

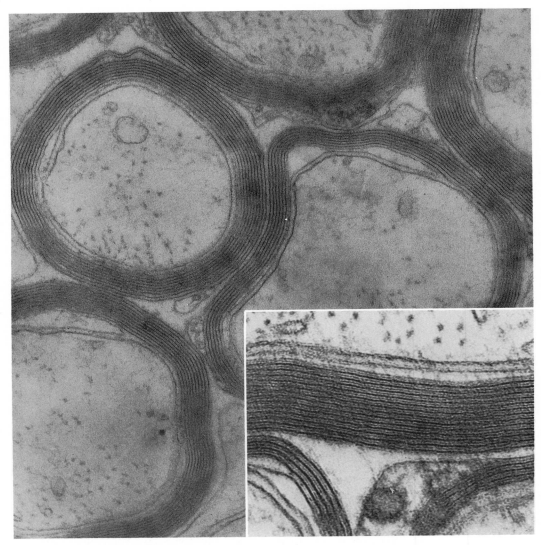

Figure 7–28.   Electron micrograph of myelinated nerve fibers in a cross section of the rat optic nerve. ×
70,000. *Inset,* bottom right: Higher magnification to show major dense and intraperiod lines. × 125,000.
(Preparation by A. Peters.)

ed fibroblasts. It is closely adherent to
the neurilemma, although separated
from it by the basal lamina that surrounds the neurilemma cells.

The blood supply to a peripheral
nerve is rich with branches from adjacent arteries entering the epineurium,
anastomosing, and coursing mainly in
a longitudinal manner. From these,
smaller vessels pass into the perineurium with an extensive capillary network located in the endoneurium,
where lymphatic vessels also are present.

THE SYNAPSE

A synapse is a specialized membranous contact between nerve cells or between nerve cells and effector organs,
e.g., muscle and gland cells. Physiologically, a synapse is the site of transneuron-
al transmission of an impulse. In a few
instances, the electrical signal may be
passed directly to the adjacent cell by a
gap junction or nexus, structurally similar to junctions described already in
various epithelia, smooth muscle, and
intercalated discs of heart muscle. Such

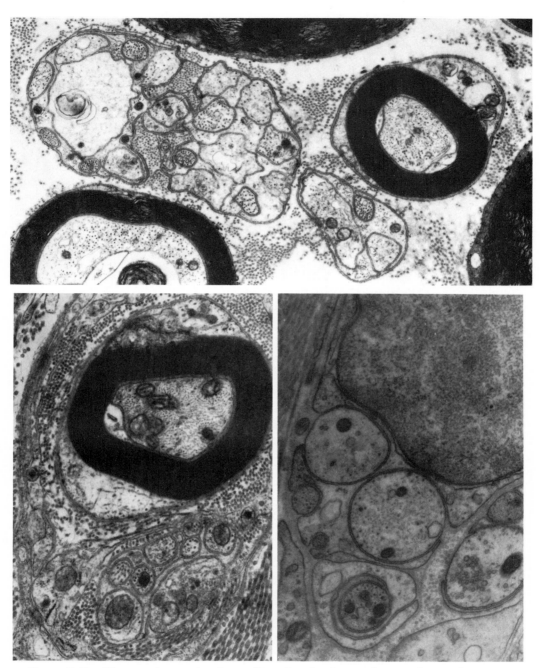

Figure 7–29. Electron micrographs of nerve fibers. *Top:* One large and one small unmyelinated fibers are seen between myelinated nerve fibers. × 18,000. *Bottom left:* A small nerve bundle with one myelinated and several unmyelinated fibers, still with a thin perineural sheath (left). × 18,000. *Bottom right:* A small, unmyelinated nerve with well-defined mesaxons around axons in Schwann cell cytoplasm. × 28,000.

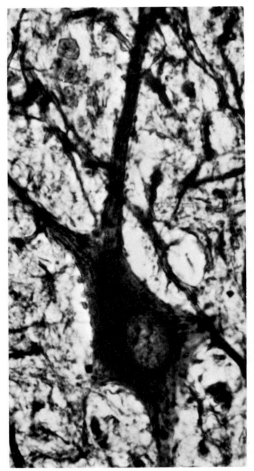

Figure 7–30. Photomicrograph of an anterior horn cell to show boutons terminal on the cell body and its dendrites. × 1100. (Preparation by E. G. Bertram.)

Basically, a synapse is formed by the expanded termination of an axon called the *presynaptic terminal* or *element*, the *postsynaptic element* or area of the cell contacted, and the intervening extracellular space of 20 to 30 nm width called the *synaptic cleft*. The preterminal part of the axon is expanded into a small bulb or *bouton terminal* (end foot), but similar expansions occur along the course of an axon *(boutons en passage)*, so that a single axon may make synapses with many different neurons. Presynaptic terminals contain numerous mitochondria and abundant small vesicles of 40 to 60 nm diameter called *synaptic vesicles*. The presynaptic membrane, i.e., the plasmalemma of the axon terminal, is thickened by the presence on its cytoplasmic face of electron-dense particles projecting into the presynaptic terminal and connected by fine filaments with an associated network of actin-like filaments in the adjacent cytoplasm. In the synaptic cleft there is some electron-dense filamentous material that appears to be associated with the outer (extracellular) surfaces of both pre- and postsynaptic membranes, probably related to cell coat material (glycocalyx), and that appears to hold the two membranes firmly together. At neuronal synapses,

junctions are termed *electrical synapses.* More commonly, the impulse is transmitted from cell to cell by a chemical mediator or neurotransmitter substance. Usually, the contact is between the axon of one neuron and a dendrite (axodendritic) or perikaryon (axosomatic) of another neuron, but occasionally contact occurs between one axon and another axon (axoaxonic). Functionally, both excitatory and inhibitory synapses occur, and there are morphological differences seen in the various types. All, however, have some common features. Synapses are numerous, and nearly all the surface of its dendrites and approximately half the surface of the perikaryon of a neuron may be involved in synaptic contacts with other neurons.

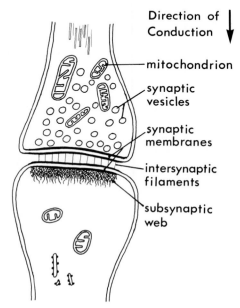

Direction of Conduction ↓

mitochondrion

synaptic vesicles

synaptic membranes

intersynaptic filaments

subsynaptic web

Figure 7–31. Diagram of a typical synaptic region as seen with the electron microscope.

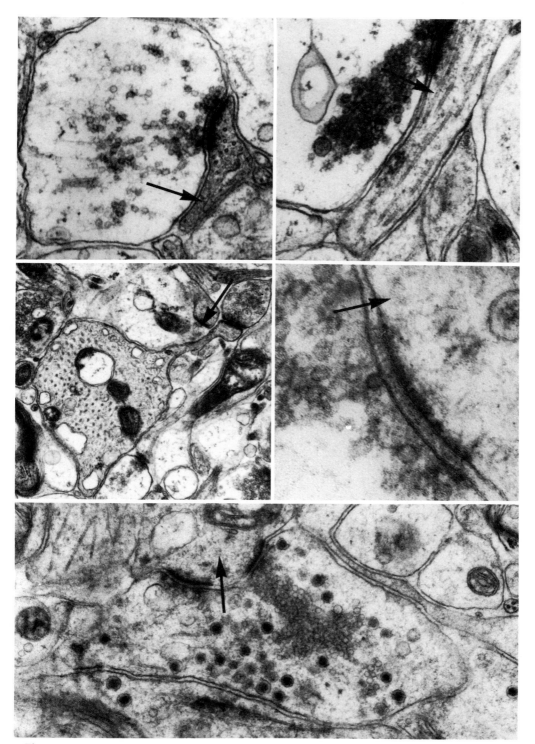

Figure 7–32. Electron micrographs of synapses. In all figures, the arrow indicates the direction of conduction. *Top left:* Axodendritic, the dendrite in cross section at right. Presynaptic vesicles are seen at left. × 45,000. *Top right:* Axodendritic, the dendritic process containing neurotubules in longitudinal section. × 52,000. *Center left:* A dendrite in cross section shows a dendritic spine extending up and to the right to a synapse. × 22,500. *Center right:* Axodendritic at higher magnification. One presynaptic vesicle appears to be fusing with the axolemma at the synapse. Unit membrane structure is seen both in synaptic membranes and in presynaptic vesicles. × 98,000. *Bottom:* The axon terminal here contains small, spherical, clear synaptic vesicles and dense-cored vesicles of the neurosecretory type. × 37,000.

no basal lamina is present between the two membranes, although a basal lamina does occur at motor nerve endings. The postsynaptic membrane often is more dense than the presynaptic membrane due to the presence on its cytoplasmic side of dense granular material in the form of perforated plates or networks, or as patches of material. This has been called the subsynaptic or postsynaptic web.

While synaptic vesicles vary in both size and shape, they also vary in content, some containing clear material, others containing a dense core. Synapses known to release the neurotransmitter acetylcholine (cholinergic synapses) contain clear vesicles, while terminals that release noradrenalin (adrenergic synapses) contain dense-core vesicles. Physiologically, it appears that the transmitter substances are released in "packets," probably by exocytosis of synaptic vesicles and discharge of their contents into the synaptic cleft, where the neurotransmitter in turn affects the postsynaptic neuron. It is known also that the synaptic complex contains mechanisms for the breakdown or uptake of released neurotransmitter. In cholinergic synapses, acetylcholinesterase is present and hydrolyzes acetylcholine, while in adrenergic endings the neurotransmitter is not broken down but is removed from the extracellular space and recycled. In addition to acetylcholine and noradrenalin, other neurotransmitters such as γ-aminobutyric acid and serotonin have been identified. After release, all combine with receptor sites on the postsynaptic membrane and affect membrane permeability to certain ions, either to generate an action potential (excitatory) or to inhibit one (inhibitory synapses).

Unlike a nerve fiber, which is capable of conduction in either direction, a synapse is dynamically polarized and can conduct only from the axon to the dendrites or perikaryon of the receiving neuron.

AUXILIARY TISSUES OF THE NERVOUS SYSTEM

As stated at the beginning of the chapter, the nervous system includes all nervous tissue of the body, the basic functional unit of which is the neuron. However, like other tissues in the body, nervous tissue includes associated connective and supporting elements. Some of these, e.g., the neurolemma of the peripheral nervous system and the capsule cells of peripheral ganglia, have been described already. Others will be described in this section.

NEUROGLIA

As the name suggests (neuron, nerve, and glia, "glue"), this tissue functions to bind together the nervous tissue proper. The neurolemma, capsule, and satellite cells of the peripheral nervous system probably subserve functions in the peripheral nervous system similar to those of neuroglia in the central nervous system. The term neuroglia includes the *macroglia* (astrocytes and oligodendrocytes), the *ependyma*, and *microglia*, the last being of mesodermal origin, the others of ectodermal origin. These cells form myelin, are phagocytic under normal and pathological conditions, and provide a supporting framework for the neurons. Together, they should be regarded as a dynamic system of functional significance in fluid and respiratory interchange between the neurons of the central nervous system and their environment. In addition, some of the glial cells are mobile.

Neuroglial cells are not seen well in ordinary preparations, for their processes are not visible. In an H and E preparation, for example, only the nuclei are visible, and identification of neuroglial cells is dependent upon the size and shape of nuclei and the arrangement of chromatin granules within them.

Astrocytes

As the name suggests, astrocytes are star-shaped cells with many branching, cytoplasmic processes. Nuclei are large, ovoid or spherical, and pale-staining with fine, sparse chromatin granules, most lying adjacent to the nuclear envelope. Nucleoli are not obvious. The cytoplasm is characterized by the pres-

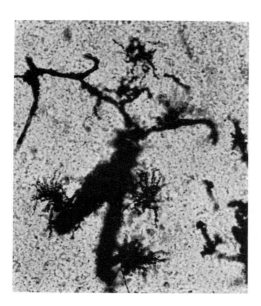

Figure 7–33. Photomicrograph of protoplasmic astrocytes. Note the end-feet attached to the wall of a capillary (solid black). Golgi method. × 300.

ence of glycogen, dense bodies or lysosomes, and cytoplasmic filaments. These filaments lie in bundles, extending from one cytoplasmic process through perinuclear cytoplasm and into another process, and are 8 to 9 nm in diameter. They provide rigidity for astrocytic processes. Cytoplasmic processes extend to blood vessels (perivascular feet), to the surfaces of neurons, and to the basement membrane at the surface of the CNS. Two types of astrocytes are distinguished.

Protoplasmic astrocytes have many branching processes and are found mainly within the gray matter of the brain and spinal cord. In addition to perivascular feet, their processes contact neuronal surfaces between synapses and, in some regions, protoplasmic astrocytes connect one to another by gap junctions. *Fibrous astrocytes* have fewer processes than the protoplasmic type and these are usually long and straight

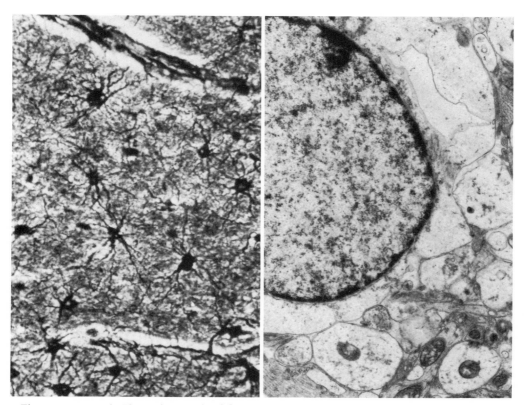

Figure 7–34. *Left:* Photomicrograph of fibrous astrocytes in the white matter of the brain. Golgi method. × 300. *Right:* Electron micrograph of an astrocyte. Note the vesicular nucleus and pale-staining, "watery" cytoplasm. × 11,500.

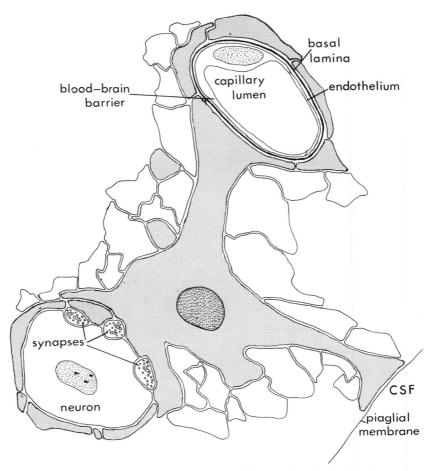

Figure 7–35. Diagram of a protoplasmic astrocyte to illustrate the relationships between it and other components of the gray matter. Note that by its cytoplasmic processes it contacts a capillary (top), a nerve cell (bottom left), and the piaglial membrane (bottom right).

and branch infrequently. Cytoplasmic filament bundles are very prominent. These cells lie mainly in white matter, frequently show gap and desmosomal type junctions, and are particularly numerous at the surface of brain and spinal cord, with numerous end feet abutting against the surface basement membrane. In brain damage with loss of neurons, it is the fibrous astrocyte that proliferates to result in "scarring" or "sclerosis." The processes of astrocytes and other glial elements lying between nerve cell bodies and their axons and dendrites constitute the neuropil.

Oligodendrocytes

Oligodendrocytes (oligodendroglia) have few cell processes, are smaller than astrocytes (only 6 to 8 μm), and contain heterochromatic ovoid or spherical nuclei. Cytoplasm is scanty and appears as a perinuclear rim with mitochondria, microtubules, some free ribosomes and a few profiles of granular endoplasmic reticulum, and a small Golgi apparatus. Oligodendrocytes occur in three general locations. They occur in groups around blood vessels (perivascular), directly adjacent to nerve cell bodies in gray matter (perineuronal or satellite cells), and in white matter where they lie in rows between myelinated fibers (interfascicular). In this last situation, leaflike cytoplasmic processes extend from the oligodendrocyte cell body to wrap around nerve fibers forming the myelin sheath, thus serving the same function as Schwann cells in the PNS. However, each oligodendrocyte has

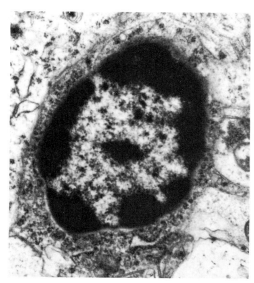

Figure 7–36. Electron micrograph of an oligodendrocyte showing heterochromatic, ovoid nucleus and free cytoplasmic ribosomes. × 7500.

several processes and thus forms myelin sheaths around several adjacent nerve fibers.

Three types of oligodendrocyte have been described. One, probably immature and actively involved in myelin formation, is large and light staining, while, in the adult, most are small and darkly staining. Cells intermediate between these two constitute the third type.

Astrocytes and oligodendroglia are derived from *spongioblasts,* a primitive ectodermal cell. Spongioblasts may be present in adult nervous tissue as a fourth type of neuroglial cell. Such cells have spherical nuclei, smaller than those of astrocytes and oligodendroglia, which contain much chromatin and thus are darkly staining. Cytoplasm is extremely scanty.

Microglia

Microglia, unlike the other two types, are of mesodermal origin and comprise fibroblast-like cells, presumably derived from the pia mater or from connective tissue which penetrated nervous tissue with ingrowing blood vessels. Nuclei are small and elongated with chromatin granules distributed throughout the karyoplasm. Cytoplasm is scanty and often appears as a slender thread at each pole of the elongated or kidney-shaped nucleus, but frequently shows numerous, small "spiny" processes. Characteristically, the cytoplasm contains lysosomes, and these cells are capable of phagocytic activity. Microglial cells are distributed throughout gray and white matter, usually near blood vessels or as nerve satellites.

Ependyma

The entire central nervous system develops as a hollow cylinder—the neural tube—and cavities remain in the adult as the ventricles of the brain and the central canal of the spinal cord. The lining of these cavities is the ependyma, which retains the epithelial character present in the early embryo. In the embryo, the cells of the ependyma are ciliated, but in the adult the cells appear to be of the cuboidal epithelial type with few cilia. By electron microscopy, it can be shown that on the luminal aspect ependymal cells have numerous microvilli and the cytoplasm contains fibrils which may extend into basal cytoplasmic processes. Desmosomes and junctional complexes between cells are present.

Blood-Brain Barrier

Many substances are exchanged rapidly between the blood and brain tissue;

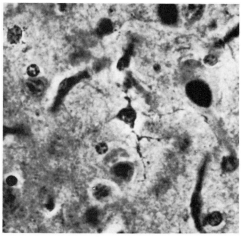

Figure 7–37. Photomicrograph of a microglial cell from the cerebral cortex. Golgi method. × 750.

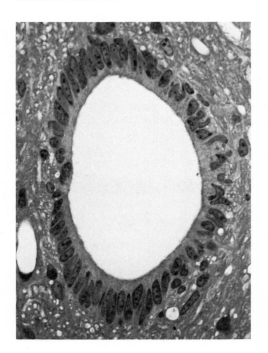

others are not. In the adult human brain, nervous elements do not abut directly upon capillaries except in certain special situations, e.g., parts of the hypothalamus. Usually they are separated from capillaries by intervening neuroglial cells or their processes; the majority of these cells are astrocytes. The apposed plasma membranes of adjacent end bulbs of the neuroglial cells fit closely together by specialized "closed contacts" so that diffusion from capillaries may be regulated by neuroglial cells. However, a diffusion barrier also exists at the capillary itself in that endothelium of capillaries in the CNS is markedly impermeable to macromolecules.

Figure 7–38. Photomicrograph of the central canal of the spinal cord to show its lining ependyma. Note its epithelium-like arrangement. × 400.

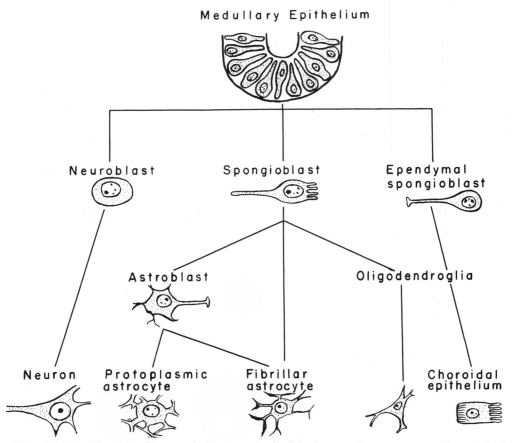

Figure 7–39. Diagram to illustrate the histogenesis of cells in the central nevous system. All are derived from the medullary epithelium of the neural tube. Microglial cells (not illustrated) are derived from mesenchymal cells which invade the developing nervous system.

MEMBRANES AND VESSELS OF THE CENTRAL NERVOUS SYSTEM

Living nervous tissue of the central nervous system is soft and delicate and requires both adequate protection and nourishment. Protection is provided in the first place by a complete bony case covering brain and spinal cord in the form of the cranium (skull vault) and the vertebral column. Within the bony case are three membranous investments called the meninges. The outermost, the *dura mater* or *pachymeninx*, is fibrous, tough, and relatively inelastic and lines the cranium, being attached firmly to bone. At the foramen magnum, it continues as a tubular invest-ment surrounding the spinal cord within the vertebral canal but is sepa-rated from bone by an *epidural* or ex-tradural space. The middle membrane is the *arachnoid*, composed of fine, cobweb-like strands of interlacing retic-ular fibers. The most internal layer, which closely invests the brain and spi-nal cord, is the *pia mater*. In this layer are found the blood vessels supplying the central nervous system. Pia and arachnoid have a similar structure and sometimes are regarded as a single layer called the *leptomeninx* or *leptomen-inges*.

Dura Mater

The cranial dura mater usually is described as consisting of two layers.

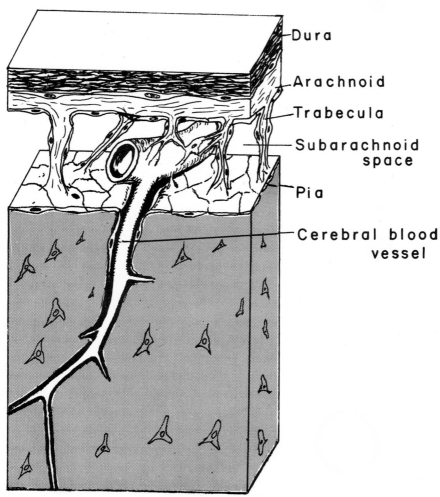

Figure 7–40. Diagram to illustrate the relationship of the meninges to the brain.

The first is an outer layer of dense connective tissue, containing numerous blood vessels and nerves. This layer is in direct contact with the inner surface of bone. It is, quite simply, the periosteum on the inner surface of the cranial bones and is termed the *endosteal layer*. The second is an inner layer of dense fibrous tissue with a single layer of flat, mesothelial cells on its inner surface. This, the *fibrous layer*, is separated from the outer layer in regions to form the large venous sinuses of the brain and also is reflected inward to extend into large fissures of the brain as partitions. Such partitions occur in the midsagittal plane (the falx cerebri) between the two cerebral hemispheres, horizontally between the occipital lobes of the cerebrum and the upper surface of the cerebellum (the tentorium cerebelli), and between the two cerebellar hemispheres as the small falx cerebelli. In addition, there is an extension of dura forming the roof of the pituitary fossa (the diaphragma sellae). The spinal dura corresponds to the inner fibrous layer of the cranial dura, with which it is continuous at the foramen magnum. The vertebrae have their own periosteum. Both inner and outer surfaces of the spinal dura are covered by a single layer of flat cells, and dura is separated from periosteum by a slender *epidural space* in which are anastomosing venous channels lying in fatty, areolar tissue.

Between dura and arachnoid is a narrow capillary interval, the subdural space, containing lymphlike fluid.

Arachnoid

The arachnoid is a delicate nonvascular membrane lining the dura and covering the brain surface without passing into the sulci. It is separated from the pia by an interval of varying extent which is crossed by numerous trabeculae passing between arachnoid and pia, thus subdividing this space into numerous interconnected *subarachnoid spaces*. Over the spinal cord the trabeculae are few and thus the subarachnoid space is continuous.

The membrane lining the dura and the trabeculae is composed of fine collagenous fibers with some elastic fibers. Surfaces of the membrane lining the dura and trabeculae and the surface overlying the pia are covered with a continuous, single layer of flat cells with large, pale, oval nuclei. These cells can become phagocytic.

The subarachnoid spaces are filled with cerebrospinal fluid. In certain regions, arachnoid is separated from pia by a considerable distance, the spaces so formed containing large quantities of cerebrospinal fluid. Such spaces are termed *cisternae*.

Pia Mater

The pia matter is a delicate membrane closely investing the surface of the brain, and unlike the arachnoid, it extends into the depths of the cerebral sulci. It often is described in two layers. The inner, membranous layer (intima pia) is composed of a close network of fine reticular and elastic fibers. This layer is adherent to underlying nervous tissue and sends a fibrous, posterior median septum into the substance of the spinal cord. As blood vessels enter nervous tissue, they take with them a covering of the intima pia, with an intervening perivascular space containing cerebrospinal fluid in the case of the larger vessels. The more superficial layer of the pia, the epipial tissue, is composed of a network of collagenous fibers with, of course, a few fibroblasts. This layer is continuous with the tissue of the arachnoid. The external surface of the epipial layer is covered with a single layer of flattened mesothelial cells continuous with those covering arachnoid tissue. The epipial layer is more obvious over the spinal cord and contains the spinal blood vessels. That over the brain is less obvious, and vessels here appear to lie upon the intima pia within the subarachnoid space.

Branches of the internal carotid and vertebral arteries pass from the pia mater into the substance of the central nervous system. Capillary networks are richer in the gray matter than in the white. Venous return is to veins in the pia mater and thence to the dural venous sinuses. No lymphatics have been described in the central nervous system. Dura and pia contain a rich plexus of nerve fibers, mainly of the autonomic system to the blood vessels, but

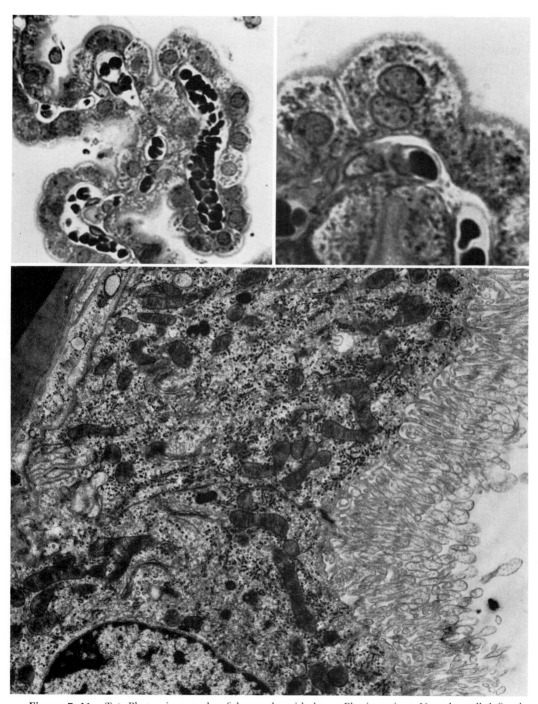

Figure 7–41. *Top:* Photomicrographs of the rat choroid plexus. Plastic sections. Note the well-defined brush border. Left, × 250; right, ×1250. *Bottom:* Electron micrograph of the choroid plexus. Note the bulbous microvilli on the apical surface (right) and some basal infoldings of the basal plasma membrane (left center). There is a portion of a capillary containing a red blood corpuscle at top left. × 8500.

some sensory fibers are present also, these traveling from sensory receptors in the meninges.

CHOROID PLEXUS AND CEREBROSPINAL FLUID

The central nervous system is made up of delicate tissue and, as stated previously, is protected by the bones of the cranium and spinal column, within which is the pia arachnoid containing fluid to function as a water cushion. This fluid is the cerebrospinal fluid, which also fills the ventricles of the brain and the central canal of the spinal cord. Fluid within the ventricular system of the brain freely communicates with fluid in the subarachnoid space and constantly is being replenished, for not only does it subserve a protective function but it also plays an important role in the metabolism of nervous tissue.

Cerebrospinal fluid is secreted by the *choroid plexuses,* which are areas where brain tissue retains its embryonic character as a thin, non-nervous epithelium and is closely associated with pia mater which is extremely vascular. The plexuses are located in the roof of the third and fourth ventricles and in the medial walls of part of the lateral ventricles. In these sites the ventricular lining (ependyma) is composed of a regular layer of cuboidal cells with large, central, spherical nuclei and a free, brushlike border. By electron microscopy, this surface shows many bulbous microvilli, and at both lateral and basal borders the plasma membrane is infolded into the cytoplasm. Both microvilli and membrane infoldings presumably are structures for increasing surface area. This epithelium rests upon a delicate connective tissue derived from pia-arachnoid and in which are numerous thin-walled blood vessels lined by fenestrated (type II) endothelium. The entire tissue of the choroid protrudes into the ventricular cavities, and this is the site of secretion of the cerebrospinal fluid. In the roof of the fourth ventricle are three foramina—one central (the foramen of Magendie) and one lateral on each side (the foramina of Luschka)—and through these foramina

cerebrospinal fluid can pass from the ventricles into the subarachnoid space. All the ventricles and the central canal of the spinal cord are continuous. Flow of cerebrospinal fluid usually is from the ventricles into the subarachnoid space.

Absorption of cerebrospinal fluid occurs mainly into the large venous sinuses inside the cranium. These are enclosed by the fibrous tissue of the dura, but in certain sites arachnoid protrudes into the lumina of the sinuses as finger-like projections termed the *arachnoid villi.* In these villi, cerebrospinal fluid is separated from blood within the sinuses only by arachnoid mesothelium and can diffuse back into the blood. Small amounts of cerebrospinal fluid return to the circulation via extracranial lymphatics which are in continuity with perineural spaces of the cranial nerves.

Thus, there is a constant secretion of cerebrospinal fluid by the choroid plexuses and a consequent absorption back into the venous system.

Cerebrospinal fluid, a clear, colorless liquid similar to if not identical with the aqueous humor of the eye and tissue fluid, contains small amounts of protein and glucose, and some inorganic salts. It has a specific gravity of only 1.004 to 1.007. A few lymphocytes usually are present also.

CYTOARCHITECTURE OF THE CENTRAL NERVOUS SYSTEM

Although this subject is described fully in textbooks of neuroanatomy, a brief outline of the arrangement of nerve cells and their processes in the more important parts of the brain and spinal cord follows.

Spinal Cord

As shown in Figure 7–42, in cross section the spinal cord is oval in shape. Posteriorly, the cord is divided partially into right and left halves by the dorsal median septum while anteriorly there is a deep longitudinal cleft called the anterior (ventral) median fissure. The entire cord is surrounded by pia mater

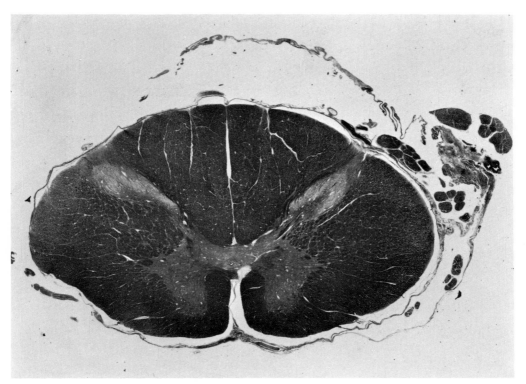

Figure 7–42. Photomicrograph of a transverse section of the spinal cord. Weil method. × 3.

which extends into the anterior median fissure.

Although there are variations in shape and structure at different levels—cervical, thoracic, lumbar, and sacral—the basic pattern of the cord is similar at all levels. Centrally in the cord in cross section is an H-shaped area of gray matter composed of nerve cells. On each side, the limbs of the H are called the anterior and posterior horns. In addition, extending throughout the thoracic and upper one or two lumbar segments, there is a lateral horn of gray matter. The central canal, lined by ependyma, is situated in the horizontal bar of the H. Nerve cell bodies lie in groups in the gray matter, the large motor neurons lying in the anterior horn.

The white matter, formed by nerve fibers, surrounds the gray matter and is divided into longitudinal columns or *funiculi.* Between the posterior horn of gray matter and the dorsal median septum is the posterior or dorsal funiculus. The remainder of the white matter is divided by the ventral horn and nerve roots and the anterior median fissure into lateral and ventral columns respec-

tively. Between the tip of the posterior horn and the surface of the cord is a small area of white matter containing fine nerve fibers, called the *zone of Lissauer.*

Nerve cells in the gray matter are multipolar. The axons of some leave the cord as ventral root fibers, others send axons into the white matter of ipsilateral and contralateral sides, and still others have short axons which terminate on neurons near their origin, confined to the gray matter (Golgi type II). Generally the white matter contains no nerve cell bodies or dendrites and is formed by myelinated and nonmyelinated fibers. At the surface of the cord there is a narrow marginal area composed only of neuroglia.

Cerebellum

The cerebellum consists of right and left *hemispheres* and a central *vermis,* divided into lobules by transverse fissures. Each lobule comprises a part of the vermis with two lateral, winglike extensions into the hemispheres. The sur-

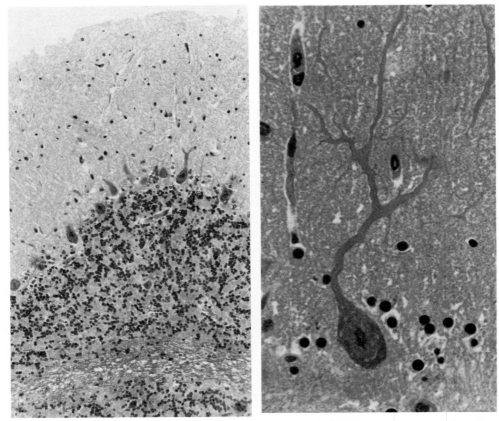

Figure 7–43.   Photomicrographs of cerebellar cortex. *Left:* Total thickness of cortex, surface above, white matter below. *Right:* A Purkinje cell of the cerebellar cortex. Plastic section. × 400.

face of the hemispheres shows numerous folds, or folia, arranged parallel to the main fissures so that in sagittal section there is the appearance of a central stem with numerous branches (the arbor vitae). Gray matter of the cerebellum is located on the surface as a thin cortex overlying the centrally placed white matter, but there are also small collections of nerve cells (nuclei) in the central parts of the cerebellum.

The cerebellar cortex on section shows three layers: an outer molecular layer of a few small nerve cells and many nonmyelinated fibers, a central layer of a single row of large cells, called Purkinje cells, and an innermost granular layer of numerous small nerve cell bodies. Cells of the granular layer are small, with three to six short dendrites, and a nonmyelinated axon which ascends to the molecular layer where it divides into two lateral

branches running along the length of a folium. The Purkinje cells are large and flask-shaped with several main dendrites which enter the molecular layer as a fan-shaped network of branching processes at right angles to the folium, and thus at right angles to the parallel terminal axonal branches of the granular cells. Axons from Purkinje cells arise from part of the cell opposite to the dendrites, acquire myelin sheaths, and give off collaterals, and the main, myelinated axonal stem then traverses the granular layer to terminate in one of the deep cerebellar nuclei or to go to another part of the cortex. Cells of the molecular layer are small and stellate in form. Dendrites and axons of those situated near the surface are short, but those of the deeper layer, i.e., near Purkinje cells, have longer axons with collaterals in relation to several Purkinje cells.

In the cortex also are terminations of

the *mossy* and *climbing* fibers, these passing into the cerebellar cortex from the white matter of the brain stem and spinal cord. The mossy fibers are thick and synapse on cells of the granular layer. Climbing fibers pass through the granular layer to terminate on Purkinje cells.

The cerebellum functionally is related to movements of striated muscle, being concerned with coordination, posture, and equilibrium.

Cerebrum

In the cerebral hemispheres, gray matter is located on the surface as *cere-* *bral cortex* and centrally, surrounded by white matter, as ganglia or nuclei.

The surface of the hemispheres is convoluted, by which means the surface area is increased, the projecting folds being called the *gyri* with intervening depressions or *sulci*. The surface area of the cortex is about 200,000 sq mm and it varies from 1.5 to 4 mm in thickness, containing nerve cells, fibers, neuroglia, and blood vessels. Most of the cells are pyramidal, stellate (granule), and fusiform or spindle in type, and they are arranged in a laminated manner so that six layers are recognizable in a section. These are, from superficial to deep: the molecular layer, composed mainly of fibers from cells in the

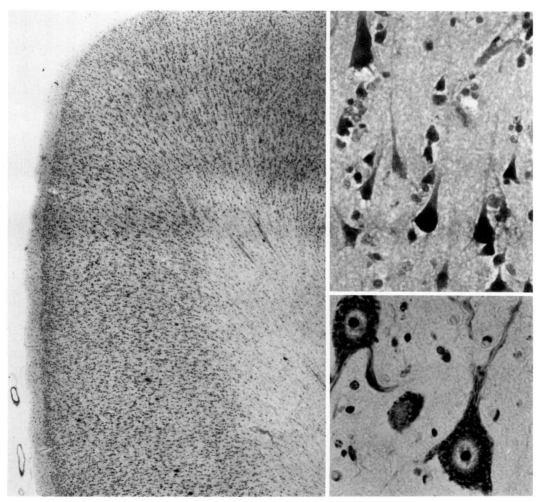

Figure 7–44. Photomicrographs of cerebral cortex. *Left:* All layers. Methylene blue, × 10. *Top right:* Layer five showing pyramidal cells. H and E, × 250. *Bottom right:* Large pyramidal cells to show Nissl substance. Cresyl violet, plastic section, × 550.

deeper layers, these running parallel to the surface, and a few small nerve cell bodies; the external granular layer of small, triangular nerve cell bodies; the pyramidal cell layer of large, pyramidal cells and many small granule cells; the internal granular layer of small stellate granule cells; the internal pyramidal or ganglionic layer of large and medium-sized pyramidal cells; and the multiform or polymorphic cell layer of cells of varying shape.

It should be emphasized that the layers blend with each other and that all layers contain neuroglia. Cells thus lie in the *neuropil*, a feltwork of naked nerve fibers and processes of neuroglia cells. The thickness of the different layers varies in different regions of the cerebral cortex, this being related to the particular functions of different regions.

The white matter underlying the gray cortex is composed of bundles of myelinated fibers passing in all directions. These fibers, of course, are supported by neuroglia and, functionally, are of three main groups. Some fibers connect different parts of the cortex of one hemisphere and are called *association fibers*. Others connect areas of the cortex of one hemisphere with other areas of the opposite hemisphere and are termed *commissural fibers*. *Projection fibers* connect the cortex with lower centers.

DIFFERENTIATION AND PROLIFERATION

The details of development of the nervous system are given in textbooks of embryology and neurology. The *neural tube* is developed from an infolding of the ectoderm along the dorsum of the embryo, from which cells detach to form the *neural crests* on each side. From neural crests are developed the craniospinal ganglia and perhaps also the autonomic ganglia. The cells of the neural tube, the wall of which at first is composed of a single layer of epithelium, undergo rapid division and differentiate into neuroblasts, later forming neurons, and spongioblasts, which later form neuroglia. Ependyma develops from the primitive lining of the neural tube. In the neural crests, differentiation occurs and neurons, satellite cells, and neurolemma are formed. Microglia probably are formed by mesenchymal cells which enter the central nervous system with the blood vessels. A simplified scheme of development in the central nervous system is illustrated in Figure 7–39.

Throughout life, neuroglia, neurolemma, and capsule cells are capable of proliferation, but neurons become incapable of reproduction at about the time of birth. After destruction, they cannot be replaced.

DEGENERATION AND REGENERATION

Although after birth neurons cannot reproduce, they are capable of withstanding and recovering from a certain degree of injury. If a nerve fiber is crushed or severed, changes occur in both the central and peripheral portions of the neuron. As explained previously, the cell body undergoes chromatolysis, whereby the Nissl substance breaks down to a powder-like mass and becomes spread diffusely throughout the cell body. Reconstitution of Nissl substance after such an injury may occur rapidly in a few days or, depending on the nature of the injury, may take months. Peripherally, the axis cylinder swells and fragments within a period of days, and, in myelinated fibers, the myelin also is broken up. The degenerated and fragmented material of axis cylinder and myelin is removed by phagocytosis of macrophages which enter the neurolemmal tubes. These degenerative changes are accompanied by proliferation of neurolemma to form a band or cord of cells.

After an interval of about a week, the divided axon from its central end starts to grow peripherally at a rate of 1 to 2 mm per day. It shows numerous fine branches or sprouts, and these grow across the scar tissue at the site of the injury and enter the cords of neurolemma, and thence follow them to reach the original site of termination. However, in such injuries usually many axons are divided and obviously may reach a termination which is functionally inappropriate. Others are lost in scar tissue. Myelin is re-formed but the process is slow. Unmyelinated fibers undergo a similar process but, of course, without a myelin sheath. In the central nervous system where a neurolemma sheath is lacking, regeneration is not possible.

SPECIAL STAINS

Ordinary staining methods show few details of nervous tissue, and it is necessary to employ special staining methods. However, no single stain shows more than a few features. Of the basic dyes, cresyl violet is useful as a stain for nuclei and Nissl substance and can be used to demonstrate chromatolysis. After mordanting in potassium bichromate, hematoxylin stains myelin, and methylene blue used supravitally is useful for demonstrating axons and nerve endings.

Various silver reduction methods, e.g., Golgi and Cajal, impregnate entire neurons (cell body and processes) with a silver deposit, but the results often are difficult to reproduce. Silver carbonate with gold toning is a good method for neuroglia. Osmium tetroxide blackens myelin and, when used with potassium bichromate (Marchi stain), demonstrates degenerating fibers.

REFERENCES

Adrian, E. D.: The Mechanism of Nervous Action. London, Oxford University Press, 1932.

Akert, K., Sandri, C., Weibel, E. R., Peper, K., and Moor, H.: The fine structure of the perineural epithelium. Cell Tissue Res., 165:281, 1976.

Bischoff, A., and Moor, H.: Myelin ultrastructure revealed by freeze etching. Med. Biol. Illustration, 19:89, 1969.

Bondareff, W., and McLone, D. G.: The external glial limiting membrane in Macaca: ultrastructure of a laminated glioepithelium. Am. J. Anat., 136:277, 1973.

Carlsen, F., Knappeis, G. G., and Behse, F.: Schwann cell length in unmyelinated fibres of human sural nerve. J. Anat., 117:463, 1974.

DeRobertis, E. D. P.: Histophysiology of Synapses and Neurosecretion. Oxford, Pergamon Press Ltd., 1964.

DeRobertis, E. D. P.: Ultrastructure and cytochemistry of the synaptic region. Science, 156:907, 1967.

Geren, B. B.: The formation from the Schwann cell surface of myelin in peripheral nerves of chick embryos. Exp. Cell Res., 7:558, 1954.

Glees, P.: Neuroglia: Morphology and Function. Springfield, Ill., Charles C Thomas, 1955.

Hirano, A., and Dembitzer, H. M.: A structural analysis of the myelin sheath in the central nervous system. J. Cell Biol., 34:555, 1967.

Jones, D. G.: Some current concepts of synaptic organization. Advances in Anatomy, Embryology and Cell Biology, Vol. 55, Part 4. Berlin, Springer-Verlag, 1978.

Landen, D. N. (editor): The Peripheral Nerve. London, Chapman and Hall, 1976.

Morales, R., and Duncan, D.: Specialized contacts of astrocytes with astrocytes and other cell types in the spinal cord of the cat. Anat. Rec., 182:255, 1975.

Morse, D. E., and Low, F. N.: The fine structure of the pia mater of the rat. Am. J. Anat., 133:349, 1972.

Palay, S. L., and Palade, G. E.: The fine structure of neurons. J. Biophys. Biochem. Cytol., 1:69, 1955.

Peters, A.: Observations on the connections between myelin sheaths and glial cells in the optic nerves of young rats. J. Anat., 98:125, 1964.

Peters, A., Palay, S., and Webster, H. deF.: The Fine Structure of the Nervous System. The Neurons and Supporting Cells. Philadelphia, W. B. Saunders Co., 1976.

Ranson, S. W., and Clark, S. L.: The Anatomy of the Nervous System, ed. 10. Philadelphia, W. B. Saunders Co., 1959.

Robertson, J. D.: The ultrastructure of adult vertebrate peripheral myelinated nerve fibers in relation to myelinogenesis. J. Biophys. Biochem. Cytol., 1:271, 1955.

Robertson, J. D.: The ultrastructure of Schmidt-Lanterman clefts and related shearing defects of the myelin sheath. J. Biophys. Biochem. Cytol., 4:39, 1958.

Ross, M. H., and Reith, E. J.: Perineurium: evidence for contractile elements. Science, 165:604, 1969.

Santini, M. (editor): Golgi Centennial Symposium: Perspectives in Neurobiology. New York, Raven Press, 1975.

Shanthaveerappa, T. R., and Bourne, G. H.: Perineural epithelium: a new concept of its role in the integrity of the peripheral nervous system. Science, 154:1464, 1966.

Uzman, B. G., and Nogueira-Graf, G.: Electron microscope studies of the formation of nodes of Ranvier in mouse sciatic nerves. J. Biophys. Biochem. Cytol., 3:589, 1957.

Van Deurs, B., and Koehler, J. K.: Tight junctions in the choroid plexus epithelium. A freeze-fracture study including complementary replicas. J. Cell Biol., 80:662, 1979.

Van Harreveld, A., and Steiner, J.: The magnitude of the extracellular space in electron micrographs of superficial and deep regions of the cerebral cortex. J. Cell Sci., 6:793, 1970.

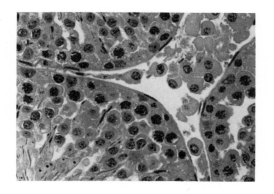

THE CIRCULATORY SYSTEM

The circulatory system comprises the blood vascular system and the lymph vascular system. The blood vascular system, which distributes nutritive materials, oxygen, and hormones to all parts of the body and removes the cellular products of metabolism, includes the heart and a series of tubular vessels, the *arteries, capillaries,* and *veins.* The heart is a modified blood vessel, specialized as an organ of propulsion. The arteries, which by branching constantly increase in number and decrease in caliber, conduct blood from the heart to the capillary bed. The capillaries, where most of the interchange of elements between the blood and the other tissues takes place, form a meshwork of anastomosing tubules. Veins return blood from the capillaries to the heart.

The lymph vascular system (commencing in the tissues as blind tubules) consists of lymphatic capillaries and various-sized lymphatic vessels which return fluid (lymph) from tissue spaces to the blood stream via the large veins in the neck.

Frequently nerve fascicles lie in company with arteries and veins as they course through the various tissues. These are the so-called *neurovascular bundles.*

THE BLOOD VASCULAR SYSTEM

The blood vascular system has a continuous lining which consists of a single layer of endothelial cells. In the capillaries this single layer of cells forms the major component of the wall. Thereafter the addition of accessory coats can be traced progressively in larger vessels. Since the structure of the capillary is simpler than that of any of the other components of the vascular system, we shall describe the capillary first instead of following the system in its functional order of heart, arteries, capillaries, and veins.

Capillaries

The capillaries are simple, endothelial tubes that connect the arterial and venous sides of the circulation. They have an average diameter of about 7 to 9 microns or μm (i.e., approximately the diameter of a single red blood corpuscle) and form a network of narrow canals. The meshes of the network vary in size and in shape in the different tissues and organs. The intensity of metabolism in a region determines the closeness of the mesh. There is a close network in the lungs, liver, kidneys, mucous membranes, glands, and skeletal muscle and in the gray matter of the brain. The network has a large mesh and is sparse in tendon, nerve, smooth muscle, and serous membranes. The network is best visualized in thick, cleared sections of material in which the capillaries have been injected with a colored gelatin or in living preparations such as the web of a frog's foot. Since capillaries pursue irregular courses, it is seldom that they are cut longitudinally in thin sections.

The wall of a capillary consists of a

257

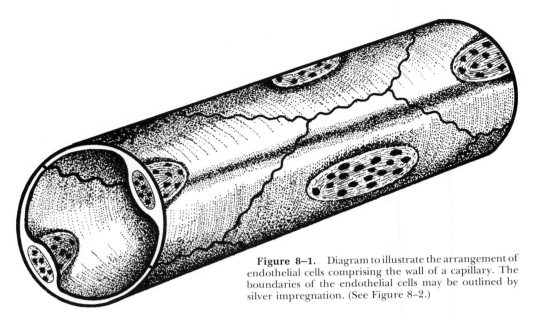

Figure 8–1. Diagram to illustrate the arrangement of endothelial cells comprising the wall of a capillary. The boundaries of the endothelial cells may be outlined by silver impregnation. (See Figure 8–2.)

single layer of flat endothelial cells which is separated from a supporting bed of connective tissue by a basal lamina. Each endothelial cell is a curving, thin plate, with an ovoid or elongated nucleus. Usually the cells are stretched along the axis of the capillary and have tapering ends. The cell borders, which can be made visible readily by the injection of silver nitrate, are serrated or wavy. The cytoplasm is clear or finely granular. Two or three cells, occasionally only one, line the circumference of a capillary at any level of section. Capillaries are surrounded by a thin sheath of delicate collagenous and reticular fibers and are accompanied by occasional perivascular cells or *pericytes.* These slender, elongated cells often show a highly branched cytoplasm. Generally they appear similar to fibroblasts, and their cytoplasm is characterized by the presence of numerous filaments and some dense bodies. Each pericyte is invested by a basal lamina that occasionally is deficient where the cell membrane of the pericyte is in close proximity to that of the endothelial cells. In the past, it was suggested that pericytes may be contractile and thus exert some influence upon the luminal diameter of the capillary network. However, recent evidence indicates that endothelial cells themselves are capable of contraction and are able to change their shape and reduce the diameter of the capillary lumen. The pericytes probably are relatively undifferentiated cells that can differentiate into other cell types, including smooth muscle.

Recent electron microscopic studies have added considerably to our knowl-

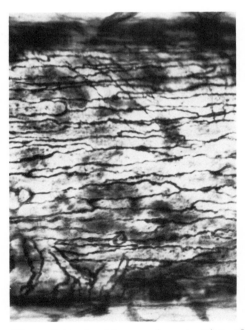

Figure 8–2. In this spread preparation of mesentery, a portion of a small vein is shown. The lining endothelial cells have been outlined with silver. They are elongated in the long axis of the vessel and show simple intercellular boundaries. × 450.

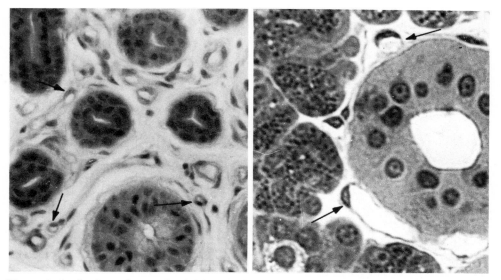

Figure 8–3. Sections of sweat gland *(left)* and of submandibular gland *(right)*. Capillaries, which form close networks around the glandular elements, generally are sectioned transversely or obliquely (arrows). The wall consists of a single layer of endothelial cells, the nuclei of which project slightly into the lumen. Left, × 275; right, Plastic section, × 650.

edge of capillary structure. Described variations in the structure of the capillary wall now form the basis of a classification of capillaries into two major types, *continuous* and *fenestrated*.

Continuous (type 1) capillaries are found in many tissues, including muscle, lung, the central nervous system, and skin. The cytoplasm of each endothelial cell is relatively thick opposite

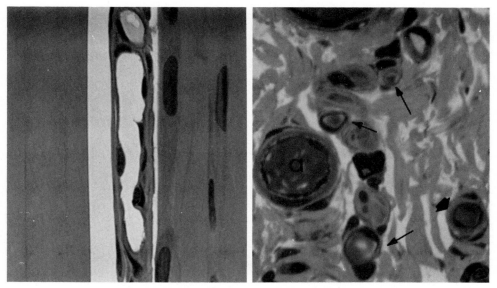

Figure 8–4. *Left:* Section of tendon showing a capillary, sectioned both transversely (above) and longitudinally (below). Endothelial nuclei project into the lumen and the cytoplasm of these cells is attenuated. The capillary lies within delicate connective tissue of the peritendineum. Plastic section. × 550. *Right:* Capillaries (arrows) lie within loose connective tissue of the submucosa of the stomach. Also present are an arterial capillary (arrowhead) and an arteriole (a). Plastic section. × 500.

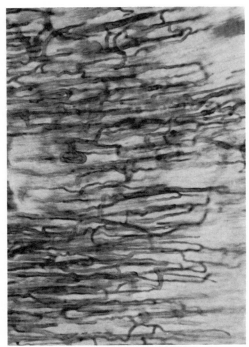

Figure 8–5. Unstained section of cardiac muscle in which the capillary network had been made visible by the injection of colored gelatin into the main arteries of supply. Note the close meshwork of capillaries between the individual cardiac muscle fibers. × 120.

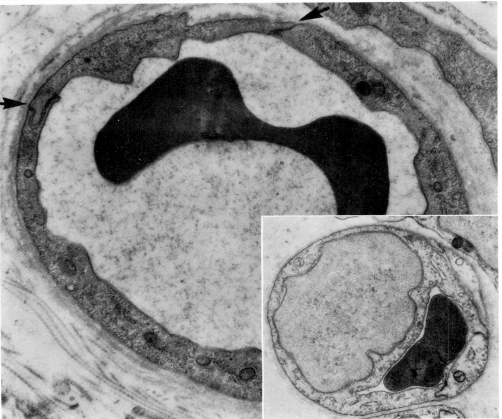

Figure 8–6. Electron micrograph of a continuous capillary in loose areolar connective tissue. The lumen contains a portion of a red blood corpuscle. Note the numerous pinocytotic vesicles in relation to the cell membrane of the endothelium and the two interphases between endothelial cells (arrows). × 18,500. *Inset:* A capillary, the wall of which is composed of two endothelial cells, one showing a prominent nuclear area. Present in the lumen is a red blood corpuscle. × 7500.

the nucleus, but it becomes attenuated elsewhere. Characteristically, it contains fine filaments and numerous small vesicles (*pinocytotic vesicles* or *caveolae intracellulares*) along both the luminal and basal surfaces. The vesicles or caveolae, which have a diameter of 50 to 70 mμ (or nm), are thought to form on one surface by invagination of the cell membrane, to detach, to cross the cytoplasm and fuse with the opposite surface, thus discharging their contents. Functionally, it appears that they are involved in the transport of fluid across the capillary wall and that they represent the sites of a so-called "large-pore" system of capillary permeability. The endothelial cells are held together by simple or interdigitated junctions. In most regions there is a narrow gap between opposed cell membranes, which contains some electron-dense material, but in certain regions, the opposed cell membranes fuse to form tight junctions (e.g., CNS). True desmosomes (maculae adherentes) are infrequent.

Fenestrated (type II) capillaries are found in the intestinal mucosa, many endocrine glands, the renal glomerulus, and the pancreas. Within the endothelium, the cytoplasm on each side of the nucleus is extremely thin and is perforated at intervals by "pores" ranging in diameter from 30 to 50 mμ (nm). The pores, or circular fenestrations, may be closed by a thin diaphragm. The diaphragm, which is thinner than the cell membrane, has a complex structure, and its chemical composition is unknown. The endothelial cells in these capillaries are separated by gap junctions.

In some organs, the capillaries have a luminal diameter much greater than that of normal capillaries. These large capillaries are termed *sinusoids* or *sinusoidal capillaries*, and they possess features not characteristic of ordinary capillaries. They may be 30 microns (μm) or more in diameter and have irregular, tortuous walls. The walls are not formed by a continuous layer of endothelial cells, as in true capillaries, and wide gaps exist between cells. Macrophages are closely associated with the endothelial cells, both within and around the sinusoidal wall. The basal lamina is incomplete and the lining of the sinusoids is separated from the parenchyma of the organs only by a fine network of reticular fibers.

The ability to transfer substances

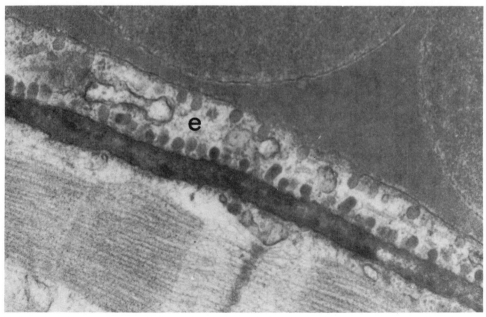

Figure 8–7. Electron micrograph of endothelial lining (e) of a capillary within cardiac muscle. Numerous pinocytotic vesicles occur along both the luminal and basal surfaces. Portions of two erythrocytes are present within the lumen. Tannic acid mordanted. × 25,000.

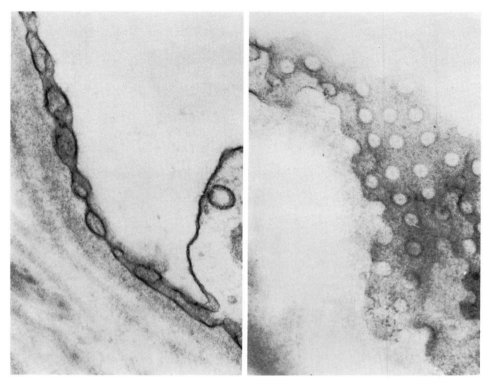

Figure 8–8.   Electron micrographs of segments of two fenestrated capillaries from the choroid plexus. In the left figure, the circular fenestrations (pores), each covered by a thin diaphragm, are cut transversely; in the right figure, the endothelium has been sectioned obliquely and the fenestrations are seen in surface view. Left, × 50,000; right, × 40,000.

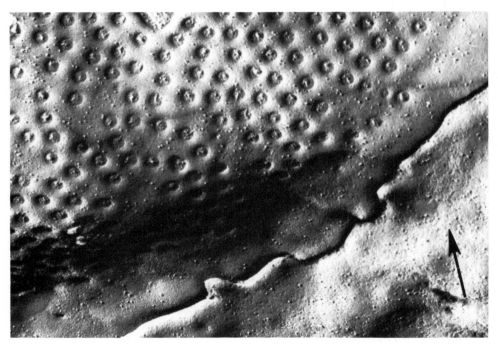

Figure 8–9.   Freeze-etch preparation of a fenestrated capillary, showing a surface view of portions of two endothelial cells. The interface between the two cells runs obliquely across the figure, and in the upper cell, circular fenestrations, each closed by a diaphragm, are frequent. The arrow indicates the direction of shadowing during preparation. Compare with Figure 8–8 (right). × 38,000.

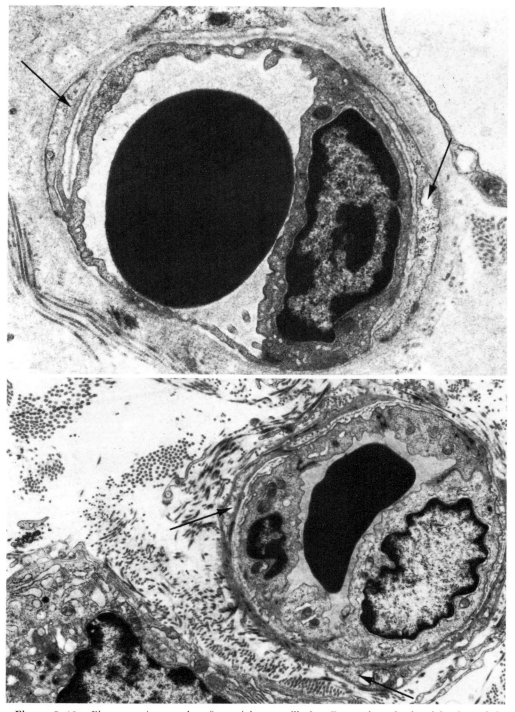

Figure 8–10. Electron micrographs of arterial precapillaries. External to the basal lamina of the continuous endothelium, there are scattered smooth muscle cells (arrows). The surrounding perivascular connective tissue merges with the neighboring connective tissue of the organ. In the lower figure, a plasma cell also is present (lower left). Top, × 15,000; bottom, × 7000.

through the wall of capillaries is referred to as permeability. Permeability varies regionally and, under changed conditions, locally. Whether the interchange occurs through the endothelial protoplasm or between adjacent endothelial cells is not known, and at present it is the subject of considerable investigation. Many physiologists are of the opinion that most changes in permeability can be accounted for by changes in the nonliving component of the capillary wall (i.e., changes at the interphase between adjacent cells). In continuous capillaries it is generally accepted that the vesicles or caveolae participate in carrying metabolites and perhaps fluid across the capillary wall. The pores of fenestrated capillaries are considered by many authorities to be devices that allow interchange of much more fluid and other substances, principally proteins, between the capillaries and the tissues than is possible with continuous capillaries. Thus, both pino-

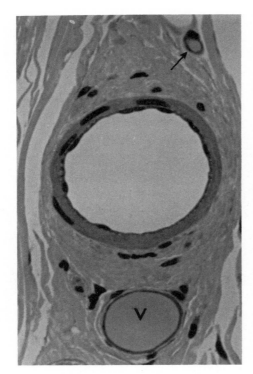

Figure 8–11. Section of loose areolar connective tissue containing a small arteriole. Note the single layer of smooth muscle surrounding the endothelial lining. Also present are a capillary (arrow) and a postcapillary venule (v). Plastic section. ×400.

cytotic vesicles and fenestrae may represent the morphological counterparts of the large pore system of physiologists. The basal lamina, present around both continuous and fenestrated capillaries, does not represent a major barrier to the passage of most substances or to the formed elements of blood.

Arterial (pre-) and *venous (post-)* capillaries are vessels intermediate between arteries and capillaries and capillaries and veins, respectively. Arterial capillaries (or *metarterioles*) have a wider lumen than that of the capillary network and contain scattered smooth muscle cells in their walls. The smooth muscle cells have branching processes and generally are oriented longitudinally, unlike the transversely oriented muscle cells of the smaller arteries (arterioles). The vessels are surrounded by a sparse perivascular connective tissue that merges with the surrounding connective tissue of the organ. They are of variable length, and most of them are joined directly to capillary networks. *Precapillary sphincters* are said to exist at the sites where capillaries arise from metarterioles or arterioles proper and to control the amount of blood flowing through the capillary bed. Venous capillaries, or *postcapillary venules,* not infrequently have a considerable diameter (up to 30 microns or μm or more) and may be 500 microns (μm) in length. The wall consists of an endothelial lining, a basal lamina, and a thin connective tissue coat containing pericytes. The latter occur in greater numbers than in the capillary network. Functionally, postcapillary venules are related closely to true capillaries in that these segments aid in the exchange of metabolites and fluid between the blood and the intercellular spaces. The concept of arterial and venous capillaries, although somewhat indefinite, has received wide acceptance and is helpful in understanding the transitions between capillaries and vessels with clearly defined coats.

Arteries

All arteries show a common pattern of organization. The wall of a typical artery is composed of three tunics or coats. The innermost coat, the *tunica intima* (or *interna*), consists of an inner en-

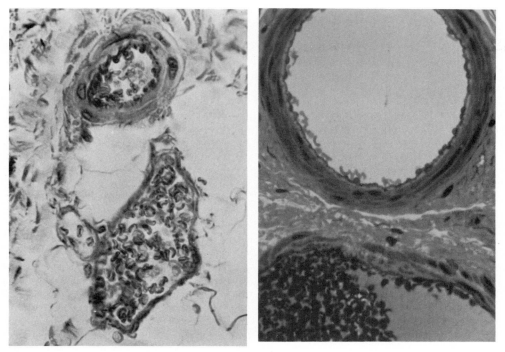

Figure 8–12. Section of loose areolar connective tissue containing an arteriole and a venule. The prominent muscular wall and the internal elastic lamina of the arteriole distinguish it readily from the venule. Left: Paraffin section, × 300. Right: Plastic section. × 450.

dothelial lining, a *subendothelial layer* of delicate fibroelastic connective tissue, and an external band of elastic fibers, the *internal elastic membrane*, which may be absent in many vessels. The middle coat, the *tunica media*, consists chiefly of smooth muscle cells, circularly arranged. Interspersed between the smooth muscle cells are varying amounts of elastic and collagenous fi-

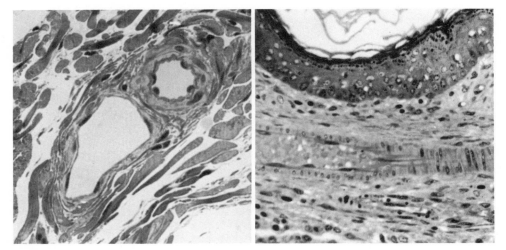

Figure 8–13. Sections of small arterioles in the dermis of the skin. In the left figure, the arteriole (above) is sectioned transversely and is accompanied by a venule. In the right figure, the arteriole is sectioned longitudinally: to the left, the section passes through the lumen, which contains red blood cells; to the right, it passes through the wall and shows the circular arrangement of smooth muscle cells. Plastic sections, both × 300.

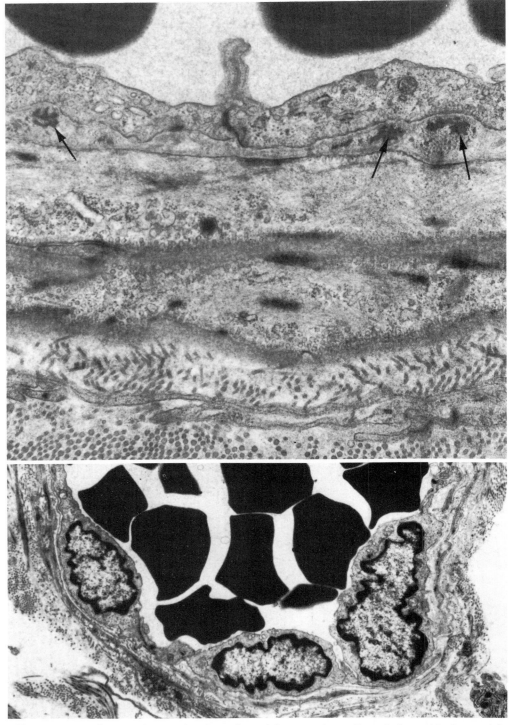

Figure 8–14. Electron micrographs of a small arteriole *(top)* and a small venule *(bottom.)* In the arteriole, the internal elastic membrane is represented by a network of fibers, here sectioned transversely (arrows). In the venule, the endothelium is bounded externally by a sheath of collagenous fibrils. Top, × 22,000; bottom, × 8000.

bers. The outer coat, the *tunica adventitia*, is composed principally of connective tissue, most of the elements of which run parallel to the long axis of the vessel. Closest to the media there may be a definite *external elastic membrane.* The structure and relative thickness of each of the tunics vary according to the type and size of the vessel.

Arterial blood vessels can be classified in three groups: *large arteries,* which contain a preponderance of elastic fibers; *small* to *medium-sized arteries,* containing numerous muscular elements; and *arterioles,* the smallest arterial vessels.

Arterioles. These vessels, with a diameter of 100 microns (μm) or less, have a tunica intima which consists only of endothelium and an internal elastic membrane. No subendothelial tissue is recognizable. The internal elastic membrane is really a network of fibers which by light microscopy appears as a thin, bright line just beneath the endothelium. The media is muscular and is composed of one to five complete layers of muscle cells, among which are some scattered elastic fibrils. The number of layers of muscle cells decreases as the caliber of

the vessel decreases, and at about a diameter of 20 microns (μm), the muscle coat becomes a single layer. The adventitia, which usually is thinner than the media, is a layer of loose connective tissue with longitudinally oriented collagenous and elastic fibers. It merges into the surrounding connective tissue. No definite external elastic membrane is present.

The arterioles have relatively thick walls and narrow lumina. They are able to control the distribution of blood to different capillary beds by vasodilation and vasoconstriction in localized regions. They are the prime controllers of systemic blood pressure. Most of the fall in blood pressure occurs within the arterioles so that only a gentle stream passes into the delicate capillary beds. Arterioles, in comparison with capillaries, have relatively impermeable walls and are not involved in interchange between blood and tissue fluid.

Small and Medium-sized Arteries. This group comprises all arteries belonging to the *muscular type* and includes most of the arteries that bear names and all small unnamed ones. There is a gradual transition between

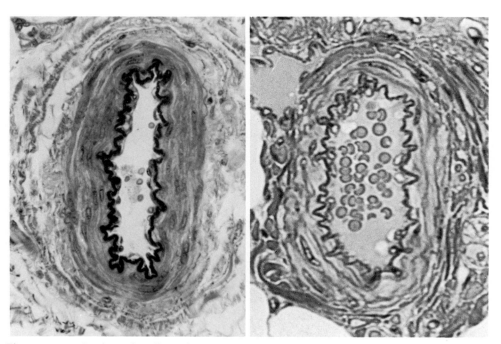

Figure 8–15. Sections of small arteries. Note the prominent internal elastic lamina and the thickness of the tunica media. Left, aldehyde fuchsin stain, × 250. Right, Plastic section, × 400.

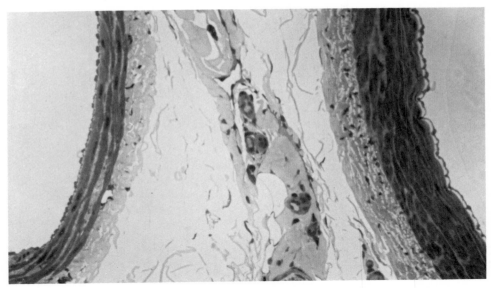

Figure 8–16.   Comparison of vein (left) and artery (right) within loose areolar connective tissue. The artery is identified by the overall thickness of its wall, the thick tunica media, and the prominent internal elastic lamina (unstained.) See also Figure 8–17. Plastic section. × 125.

these vessels and the arterioles described above. The walls of the muscular arteries are relatively thick, owing principally to the large amount of muscle in the media. They also have been called *distributing arteries* because they distribute blood to different organs and regulate the supply of blood in response to different functional demands.

The tunica intima exhibits three definite layers. Beneath the endothelium, which lies upon a thin basal lamina,

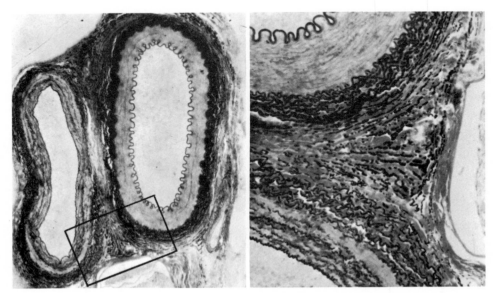

Figure 8–17.   Comparison of small artery and small vein. The artery is identified by the thickness of the tunica media. Elastic fibers are stained specifically by resorcin fuchsin. Left, × 40; right, (enlargement of blocked area of left figure), × 120.

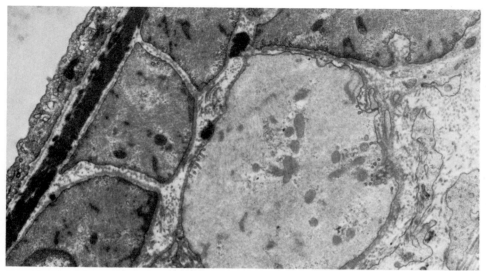

Figure 8–18. Electron micrograph of the tunica intima and a portion of the tunica media of an artery. A complete internal elastic lamina (darkly stained) is interposed between the endothelium and transversely sectioned smooth muscle cells of the tunica media. Compare with Figure 8–14. × 20,000.

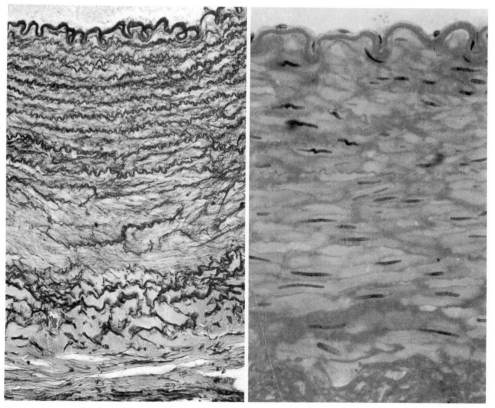

Figure 8–19. Sections through the walls of medium-sized arteries. *Left:* The tunica media, in which numerous elastic fibers may be seen, lies between the prominent internal and external elastic laminae. Resorcin fuchsin stain. × 120. *Right:* Individual smooth muscle cells may be identified clearly in the tunica media. Plastic section. × 350.

there is the subendothelial layer comprising delicate elastic and collagenous fibers, occasional fibroblasts, and, in some of the larger muscular arteries, a few bundles of longitudinally oriented smooth muscle fibers. The internal elastic membrane, or lamina, is prominent and forms a thick fenestrated band composed of closely interwoven elastic fibers. In histological sections, it typically is thrown into folds because of postmortem contraction of the muscular elements of the media. In many arteries the membrane is split into two or more layers.

The media consists almost exclusively of circularly disposed smooth muscle cells. Between the layers of muscle (up to 40 in number) there are small amounts of connective tissue, the constituents of which are elastic, collagenous, and reticular fibers, and a few fibroblasts. In the larger muscular arteries, elastic fibers are prominent between the layers of smooth muscle, where they form close networks, circularly oriented.

The adventitia often is as thick as the media. It is composed of loose connective tissue containing collagenous and elastic fibers, most of which course helically or longitudinally. The elastic fibers are concentrated in the inner layer of the coat, where they commonly form a definite external elastic membrane. The outer layer of the adventitia blends into the surrounding connective tissue without a sharp boundary between the two.

Large Arteries. The large arteries belong to the elastic type. The wall is relatively thin for the size of the vessel. The amount of elastic tissue present is sufficient to impart a yellow color to the freshly cut wall. This group includes the aorta and its largest main branches, the brachiocephalic, the common carotid, the subclavian, and common iliac.

The endothelial cells of the intima are polygonal in shape, not elongate as in the smaller vessels. The subendothelial layer consists of collagenous and elastic fibers and scattered fibroblasts, and in the deeper portion of the intima small bundles of smooth muscle cells are present. A distinct internal elastic membrane is difficult to discern. Numerous elastic fibers, arranged mainly longitudinally, course in the deeper zone of the subendothelial layer and pass to the innermost elastic membrane of the media. This zone, by its location, corresponds with the internal elastic membrane.

The media is characterized by numerous distinct elastic membranes, 40 to 60 in number, which are arranged concentrically. They anastomose to form complex elastic nets. Interspaces between the concentric membranes contain fibroblasts, an amorphous ground substance, a fine elastic network, and smooth muscle cells which pursue a spiral course. The smooth muscle cells have numerous short processes that are attached to the meshes of the elastic membranes.

The adventitia is a thin coat and is not highly organized. It cannot be distinguished sharply from the surrounding connective tissue. There is no dis-

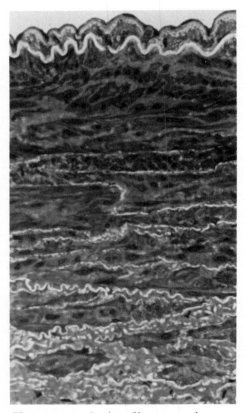

Figure 8–20. Section of large muscular artery, showing a prominent subendothelial layer and internal elastic lamina and numerous elastic fibers (unstained) between the muscle layers of the tunica media. Plastic section. × 250.

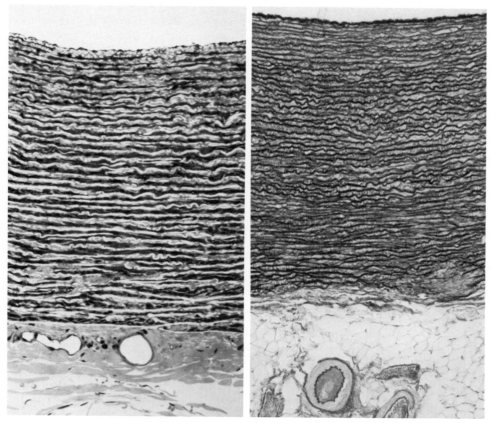

Figure 8–21. Sections of the aorta (large elastic artery). *Left:* Plastic section. × 125. *Right:* Resorcin fuchsin. × 100. In both, note the distinct elastic membranes, concentrically arranged (unstained in left figure) and the small blood vessels (vasa vasorum) in the tunica adventitia (below).

tinctive external elastic layer or membrane. The collagenous fibers present within the adventitia are oriented in an open spiral.

The elastic arteries absorb some of the pulse beat by the expansion of the elastic tissue within their walls and make the blood flow less intermittent than it would be if the vessels were rigid tubes. Often they are termed *conducting arteries*, emphasizing their function of conducting blood to the smaller ramifications of the vascular system.

Specialized Arteries. Certain arteries exhibit pronounced structural deviations from the generalized plan. These variations reflect adaptations to special locations and functional demands. Arteries protected within the skull have a thin wall and a well-developed internal elastic membrane. Arteries of the lung have thin walls owing to a reduction of both muscle and elastic tissue. This is correlated with a lower blood pressure in the pulmonary circulation. The umbilical arteries possess a media composed of two thick, muscular layers: an inner longitudinal layer and an outer circular layer. These arteries either lack an internal elastic membrane or exhibit an incomplete one. In the penile arteries the intima is greatly thickened and contains many longitudinal muscle fibers. These groups of smooth muscle cells form the cores of *intimal cushions* that serve functionally as valves. Cardiac muscle extends into the roots of the aorta and pulmonary artery.

Age Changes in Arteries. Arteries do not complete their differentiation until adult life. It is difficult to separate some of the final stages of differentiation from the retrogressive changes which develop gradually with age. Arteries of the elastic type show greater changes with age than do arteries of the muscular type. In the aging process the principal changes occur in the intima and media. The elastic tissue shows irregular thickenings, individual elastic fibers tend to fragment, fat infiltrates the interstitial substance, and in the medium-sized arteries, calcification occurs within the media.

Veins

Blood in the venous system is under a pressure one-tenth of that in the arteries and hence must accommodate a volume of blood greater than that within the arterial system. The caliber of veins in general is larger than that of arteries, but their walls are much thinner, chiefly owing to a reduction of muscular and elastic components. Venous blood vessels are classified into three groups: venules, small to medium-sized veins, and large veins. This classification is somewhat unsatisfactory since the divisions are not rigid categories and there is greater individual variation within a group than occurs in arteries. The structure may be quite different in veins of the same caliber, and even the same vein may show great structural differences along its course. Thus a description of the venous wall is not so practical as that of arteries and can concern only the most general features.

Venules. The transition from capillary or venous capillary to venule is a very gradual one and involves the acquisition of connective tissue elements first and smooth muscle fibers later. The smallest venules possess an intima consisting of endothelium only and an outer sheath of collagenous fibers. These venules participate in the interchange of metabolites between blood and tissues. When the vessel attains a diameter of about 50 microns (μm), smooth muscle fibers appear between the endothelium and the connective tissue. In venules of 200 microns (μm) or more, the circular muscle fibers form a continuous layer (media), one to three cells thick, external to the endothelium. The muscle cells are more

widely spaced than in an arteriole of corresponding size and are separated by bundles of collagenous and elastic fibers. The adventitia is thick in comparison to the overall thinness of the wall and consists of longitudinally oriented collagenous fibers and scattered elastic fibers and fibroblasts. The latter often are irregular in shape, with attenuated processes.

Small and Medium-sized Veins. These include practically all the named veins and their principal branches, excepting the main trunks. The diameter ranges from 1 to 9 mm. The tunica intima is thin. Endothelial cells are short and polygonal in shape. The subendothelial layer of connective tissue is inconspicuous. Sometimes it may be bounded externally by a network of fine elastic fibers, but they do not form a distinct internal elastic membrane.

The media is thin compared with that of arteries of the same size. It is composed of small bundles of circularly arranged muscle fibers separated by collagenous fibers and delicate net-

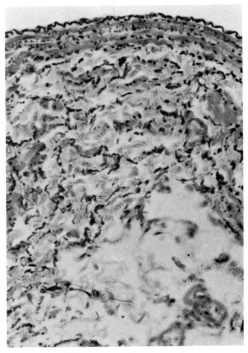

Figure 8–22. A segment of a medium-sized vein, lumen above. The tunica media is thin and the tunica adventitia, composed principally of collagenous fibers, comprises the bulk of the wall of the vein. Aldehyde fuchsin stain. × 135.

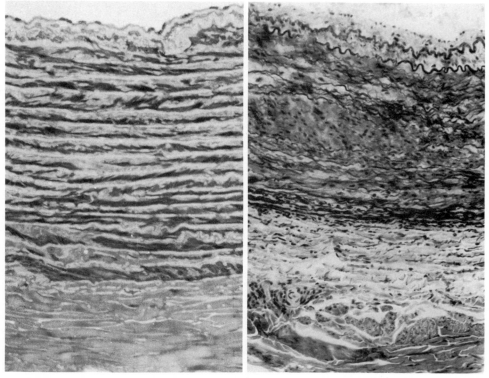

Figure 8–23. Sections of the inferior vena cava, a large vein, with the lumina above. *Left:* Plastic section, × 250. *Right:* Aldehyde fuchsin stain, × 120. In the latter note the bundles of longitudinally arranged smooth muscle fibers, here sectioned transversely, in the tunica adventitia.

works of elastic fibers. The media is best developed in the veins of the lower limbs.

The adventitia is well developed and forms the bulk of the wall. It is composed of loose connective tissue with thick longitudinal collagenous bundles and frequently a few smooth muscle fibers. These are arranged in small fascicles and are oriented longitudinally along the vessel.

Large Veins. This group includes the superior and inferior venae cavae, the portal vein, and the main tributaries of these trunks. The intima has the same structure as that of the

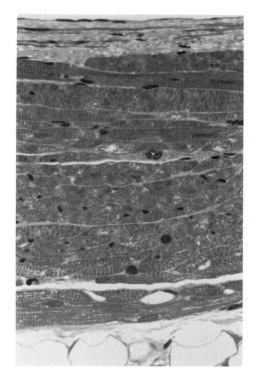

Figure 8–24. Section of the inferior vena cava immediately prior to its entry into the right atrium. Note the thin tunica media composed principally of connective tissue elements, and the thick tunica adventitia containing principally cardiac muscle. Plastic section. × 250.

smaller veins but may be a little thicker. The media is poorly developed and smooth muscle elements within it are much reduced or absent. The adventitia is the thickest of the three coats and shows three zones. Immediately external to the tunica media is a zone of dense fibroelastic connective tissue with coarse collagenous fibers, frequently arranged in open spirals. The middle zone contains many longitudinal muscle fibers, and the outermost zone consists only of a coarse network of collagenous and elastic fibers.

Special Features of Certain Veins. Some veins lack smooth muscle and thus are without a media. In this group belong cerebral and meningeal veins, dural sinuses, and veins of the retina, bones, penile erectile tissue, and the maternal component of the placenta. Veins which are rich in smooth muscle include those of the gravid uterus and of the limbs, the umbilical vein, some

mesenteric veins, and certain other veins. Cardiac muscle extends for a distance into the adventitia of the venae cavae and pulmonary veins near their entrance into the heart.

Valves. Many small and medium-sized veins, particularly those of the lower limbs, are provided with valves which prevent the flow of blood away from the heart. The valves are semilunar folds or pockets produced by local folding of the intima. They usually are arranged in pairs and project into the lumen with their free margins directed toward the heart. Both surfaces of the valve are covered with endothelium, and on the side facing the current the subendothelial connective tissue contains a network of elastic fibers. Generally the valves lie against the wall of the vein, but when regurgitation of blood occurs, the valves become distended, their free margins come into contact, and backflow of blood is prevented. Since the venous wall is dilated on the cardiac side of attachment of the valves, the vein appears knotted when distended with blood.

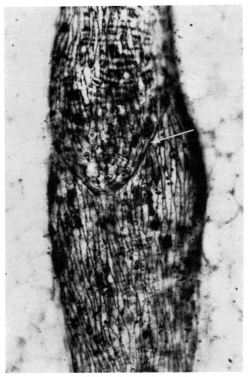

Figure 8–25. A spread preparation of mesentery, stained with silver nitrate. Shown is a segment of a small vein. The cell borders of endothelial cells and a valve (arrow) may be identified readily. × 120.

Arteriovenous Anastomoses

In addition to capillary and sinusoidal connections between arteries and veins, in certain regions arteries are connected directly to veins by *arteriovenous anastomoses*. In the anastomoses endothelium lies directly upon a specialized tunica media comprising a sphincter. These vascular shunts are especially numerous in the skin of exposed parts of the body, such as the palm, sole, lips, and nose, and in tissues where metabolic activity is intermittent, such as the thyroid gland and the digestive system. When the shunt is closed, arterial blood passes into the regular capillary bed. When the shunt is open, much of the blood is passed directly into the veins and thus bypasses the capillary bed.

In many regions the anastomosis is convoluted in outline and is surrounded by a definite connective tissue sheath, forming a *glomus*. Smooth muscle cells in the anastomosis are modified in shape and may be epithelioid in appearance. They are richly innervated by fibers of the autonomic nervous system.

Blood Vessels of Blood Vessels (Vasa Vasorum)

Arteries and veins with a diameter over 1 mm are supplied with small, nutrient blood vessels, the *vasa vasorum*. These vessels enter the adventitia and terminate in a dense capillary network which penetrates as far as the deepest layers of the media. Generally, no capillaries are found in the intima; however, in some of the large veins, probably due to the low venous pressure and oxygen tension, capillaries do penetrate as far as the intima.

Networks of lymph vessels are found in the adventitia of many of the larger arteries and veins.

Nerves

The walls of blood vessels, particularly the arteries, have a rich nerve supply. Unmyelinated axons, which are vasomotor, arise from sympathetic ganglia, penetrate the adventitia, and end in relation to smooth muscle cells of the media. Myelinated nerve fibers, receptor or sensory in function, terminate in free sensory endings within the walls of the vessels.

The Heart

The heart, a highly specialized portion of the vascular system, propels blood through the blood vessels. It consists of four main chambers: a right and left *atrium* and a right and left *ventricle*. The superior and inferior venae cavae bring venous blood from the body to the right atrium, through which blood passes to the right ventricle. Blood is forced from the right ventricle through the pulmonary arteries to the lungs, where gaseous exchange occurs, and is returned by the pulmonary veins to the left atrium. Blood passes from the left atrium to the left ventricle and then is circulated to the body by the aorta and its branches.

The wall of the heart consists of three layers: the inner layer, or *endocardium;* the middle layer, the *myocardium*, which forms the main mass of the heart; and the outer layer, or *epicardium*.

Endocardium. The endocardium is homologous to the tunica intima of blood vessels and covers all internal surfaces of the heart. It is lined by endothelium continuous with that of the blood vessels entering and leaving the heart. Beneath the endothelium there is a narrow zone of fine collagenous fibers forming a *subendothelial layer*. Still deeper there is a stouter layer containing numerous elastic fibers and some smooth muscle fibers. A *subendocardial layer* of loose connective tissue, which binds the endocardium proper to the underlying myocardium, lies farthest from the lumen. This layer contains numerous blood vessels and nerves and branches of the conduction system of the heart.

Myocardium. The myocardium, or middle coat, which corresponds to the tunica media, is composed of cardiac muscle, already described in Chapter 6. Its thickness varies in different parts of the heart, being thinnest in the atria and thickest in the left ventricle. In the atria the muscle fibers tend to be arranged in bundles which form a latticework. Internally, the muscle bundles project as irregular ridges, the pectinate muscles, in the auricular portions of the atria. In the ventricles, the muscle sheet is arranged in two layers, superficial and deep. The superficial fibers run a spiral course from the base of the ventricles to the apex, where they pass deeply to terminate in the papillary muscles. Fibers of the deep layer follow a circular course around each ventricle, with some fibers describing an S-shaped pattern as they pass from one ventricle to the other through the interventricular septum. Deeply, some bundles are present in a more or less isolated fashion on the internal surface, covered by endocardium. These bundles are called *trabeculae carnae*. The spaces between muscle fibers and bundles contain reticular, collagenous, and elastic fibers.

The muscle sheets of the atria and ventricles are attached by way of their interstitial connective tissue (endomysium) to the central supporting structure of the heart, the *cardiac skeleton.*

Cardiac Skeleton. The central support of the heart is dense fibrous connective tissue on which cardiac muscle inserts and valves attach. Its main components are the *septum membranaceum,* the *trigona fibrosa,* and the *anuli fibrosi.* The anuli fibrosi, or fibrous rings, surround the origins of the aorta and pulmonary artery and the atrioventricular canals. These rings form the principal site of attachment of the muscular fibers of the atria and the ventricles, and they also serve for the attachment of the atrioventricular valves. The trigona fibrosa are masses of fibrous tissue between the arterial foramina and the atrioventricular canals. The septum membranaceum, the fibrous portion of the interventricular septum,

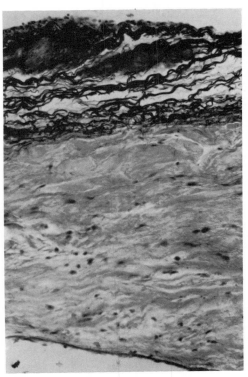

Figure 8–27. A portion of an atrioventricular valve, atrial surface above. Note the concentration of elastic fibers beneath the atrial surface. Resorcin fuchsin stain. × 120.

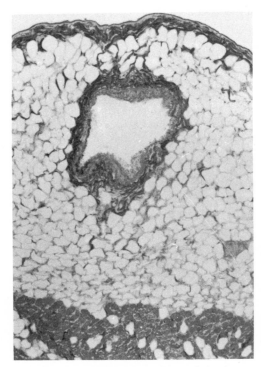

Figure 8–26. The epicardium of the heart. Above is the visceral pericardium (a mesothelium). The subepicardial layer, containing numerous fat cells and a coronary artery, is prominent, and beneath it a portion of the myocardium is shown. × 75.

also provides attachment for the free ends of some fibers of cardiac musculature. In certain large mammals, the dense connective tissue of the anuli and trigona may become chondroid in nature and give rise to either cartilage or bone.

Epicardium. The external coat (also called the *visceral pericardium*) is a serous membrane. It is covered externally by a single layer of mesothelial cells. Beneath the mesothelium is a thin layer of connective tissue containing numerous elastic fibers. At the arterial and venous openings, the connective tissue fibers continue into the adventitia of the major blood vessels. A *subepicardial layer,* composed of areolar tissue containing blood vessels, many nervous elements, and fat, attaches the epicardium to the myocardium.

Cardiac Valves. The atrioventricular valves (*tricuspid* and *mitral*) are reduplications of endocardium containing a core of dense connective tissue continuous with that of the anuli fibrosi. The endocardium is thicker on the atrial than on the ventricular surface and contains more elastic tissue. The valves are connected to papillary muscles of the ventricles by fibrous cords, the *chordae tendineae*, which serve to restrain the valves and prevent eversion of the valves when the ventricles contract.

The *semilunar valves* of the aorta and pulmonary artery are similar in structure to the atrioventricular valves. Each valve has three cusps. The central, fibrous plate of each cusp forms a thickening (the *nodule of Arantius*) at the free border.

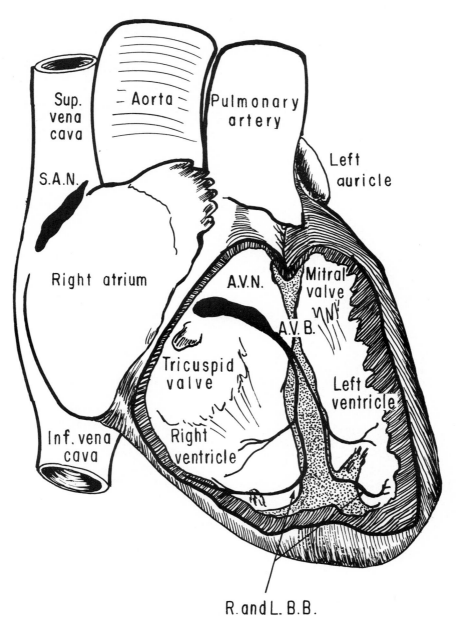

Figure 8–28. Drawing of the heart, with the interior of the ventricles exposed, to show the main components of the conducting system. S.A.N., sinoatrial node; A.V.N., atrioventricular node; A.V.B., atrioventricular bundle (of His); R. and L.B.B., right and left branches of the bundle.

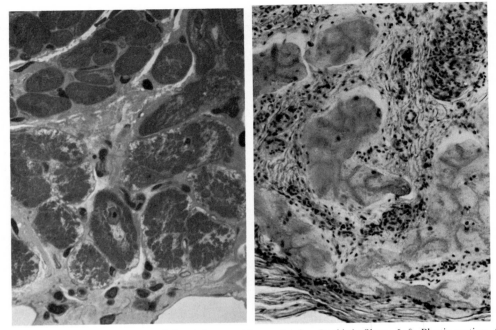

Figure 8–29. Endocardium of the right ventricle, containing Purkinje fibers. *Left:* Plastic section. × 400. *Right:* Hematoxylin and eosin, × 60. In the left figure, the larger Purkinje fibers, with distinct peripheral myofibrils, may be identified readily from the ordinary cardiac musculature above. In the right figure, groups of Purkinje fibers are separated by connective tissue containing numerous nerve fibers.

Impulse-conducting System. The heart possesses a system of specialized cardiac muscle fibers whose function is to coordinate the heart beat by regulating the contractions of the atria and ventricles. The modified fibers of this system (*Purkinje fibers*), which have a faster rate of conduction than ordinary cardiac muscle fibers, lie in the subendocardium. Purkinje fibers generally have a larger diameter than ordinary cardiac muscle fibers and contain relatively more sarcoplasm. The sarcoplasm often has a large amount of glycogen. Myofibrils are reduced in number and usually are limited to the periphery of the fibers. Purkinje fibers ultimately lose their specific characteristics and pass by a gradual transition into ordinary cardiac fibers.

An impulse begins at the *sinoatrial node*, which lies at the junction of the superior vena cava with the right atrium. This node consists of a dense network of small conduction fibers. From here, since the modified fibers are in close association with typical cardiac muscle fibers, the impulse spreads to the *atrioventricular node*, which lies in the median wall of the right atrium. The atrioventricular node also consists of conduction fibers which form a dense tangled network whose meshes are filled with connective tissue. The fibers of the node are continuous with the cardiac muscle fibers of the atrial system on the one hand and on the other with Purkinje fibers of the *atrioventricular bundle (bundle of His)*. The bundle passes through the cardiac skeleton in the region of the right fibrous trigone to reach the posterior margin of the membranous portion of the interventricular septum. The bundle then divides into two trunks, one to each ventricle. Each trunk, composed of Purkinje fibers, ultimately breaks up into a large number of branches which pass to all parts of the ventricle and terminate in the myocardium, where they connect with ordinary cardiac muscle fibers.

Blood Vessels of the Heart. Two *coronary arteries* supply blood to the heart, and the *cardiac veins* drain it. The arteries break up in the myocardium into a rich capillary plexus. The capillary plexus drains into cardiac veins, which empty into the right atrium via the *coronary sinus.* A small number of veins empty directly into the lumen of the heart.

The conducting system is abundantly supplied with special fine branches of the coronary arteries. The capillary network here is less dense than in the ordinary cardiac musculature.

Lymphatics of the Heart. Lymph channels are abundant within the heart and are intimately associated with muscle fibers. In addition to the network within the myocardium, there are lymphatic networks in the subendocardial and subepicardial connective tissue.

Nerves of the Heart. The nerve supply is from the vagus and the sympathetic division of the autonomic system. The vagus and sympathetic fibers are antagonistic, the vagus fibers inhibiting and the sympathetic fibers accelerating the heart action. These fibers form extensive plexuses, often asso-

ciated with small autonomic ganglia, and terminate principally in relation to the sinoatrial and atrioventricular nodes and along the atrioventricular bundle and the coronary vessels. Both sensory and motor endings are represented.

THE LYMPH VASCULAR SYSTEM

The lymphatic system is composed of lymphatic vessels and organs. The lymphatic vessels are tubes which collect tissue fluid and return it by a roundabout route to the blood stream. Lymph drainage is a one-way flow, not a circulation. The smallest lymphatic vessels, *lymph capillaries,* end blindly. Centrally the converging lymphatic vessels run into one of two main trunks, the large *thoracic duct* or the smaller *right lymphatic duct,* which empty into the great veins. Lymphatic nodes are located along the course of lymphatic

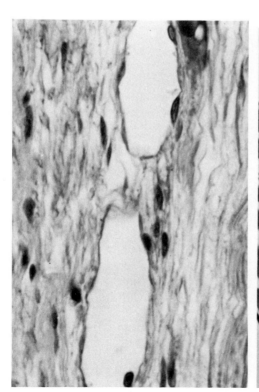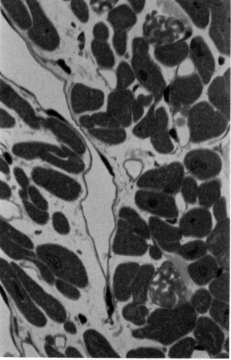

Figure 8–30. Lymph capillaries in the epicardium *(left)* and in the myocardium *(right).* Note the large lumen and the distinct endothelial wall. Left, × 550; right, plastic section, × 400.

vessels, where lymph is filtered and lymphocytes added to it before it reaches the main lymphatic trunks.

Lymph capillaries and vessels are found in most tissues and organs. They are not found in the central nervous system, the bone marrow, the internal ear, and the coats of the eyeball.

Lymph Capillaries

Lymph capillaries, like blood capillaries, are delicate tubes but are somewhat broader and are not uniform in caliber. The wall is composed only of a continuous endothelium which exhibits numerous small pinocytotic vesicles. Junctional complexes between endothelial cells are rare, and gaps readily appear between the cells in active regions. The capillaries lack a complete

basal lamina and are surrounded by a thin layer of collagenous and reticular fibers. They form dense networks which often run in company with blood capillaries. Near surfaces they frequently end in loops or in blind, swollen projections.

Lymphatic Vessels (Collecting Vessels)

Lymph passes from capillaries into larger vessels which have thicker walls and valves. The endothelium is surrounded by collagenous and elastic fibers and a few smooth muscle cells. In the larger vessels three coats — intima, media, and adventitia — may be distinguished, but usually they are poorly demarcated. These vessels resemble the veins in structure, but their walls

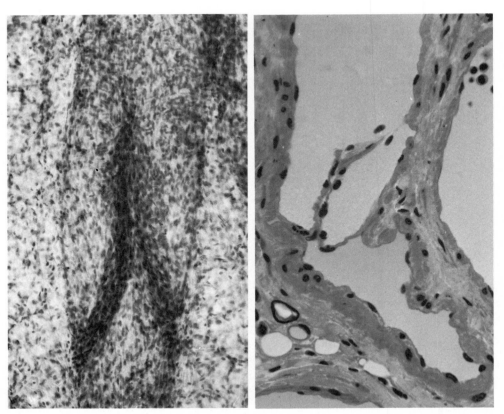

Figure 8–31. *Left:* Whole mount preparation of the mesentery, showing a lymphatic vessel. × 120. *Right:* Section of lymphatic vessel in the hilum of a lymph node. Plastic section. × 250. Note the pair of valves and the dilated lumen above the attachment of the valves.

tend to be thinner than those of veins of equal caliber.

The tunica intima consists of endothelium and a thin layer of delicate elastic and collagenous fibers. The media is composed of helically arranged smooth muscle fibers, between which are a few elastic fibers. The adventitia is the thickest layer and consists of interlacing collagenous and elastic fibers and a few smooth muscle fibers.

Lymphatic vessels contain numerous valves which are more closely spaced than those found in veins. The valves occur in opposed pairs, and their free margins are directed centrally. Each valve is a fold of the intima. Between valves the vessels are swollen; thus they have a beaded appearance.

Main Lymphatic Trunks

These are the thoracic and the right lymphatic ducts. In structure they are much like a vein of equal size except for the greater development of smooth muscle in the media. The intima consists of an endothelial lining, a subendothelial layer containing some longitudinal muscle, and a thin, inconstant, elastic membrane. The media is the thickest coat and consists of longitudinal and circular muscle bundles, separated by abundant connective tissue. The adventitia, which consists of coarse collagenous fibers and a few longitudinal muscle fibers, is poorly defined and blends into the surrounding connective tissue.

Blood vessels supply the wall of the main lymphatic trunks in much the same way as do the vasa vasorum of the larger blood vessels. Nerve fibers, both motor and sensory, are found in the walls of the larger vessels.

DEVELOPMENT OF THE CIRCULATORY SYSTEM

The blood vessels and heart first appear as a collection of endothelial cells which differentiate from mesenchymal cells. The heart, main blood vessels, and peripheral vessels develop independently and later unite to establish a blood circulation.

Arteries and veins of all types first appear as ordinary capillaries, which later increase in size and acquire smooth muscle and connective tissue by differentiation from the surrounding mesenchyme. After the establishment of the circulation, new vessels arise by budding from pre-existing vessels.

The heart in the earliest human embryos is a tube with a double wall: the internal endothelium, from which the endocardium develops, and the external *myoepicardial* layer. From the myoepicardial layer are formed both myocardium and epicardium. The endocardium has important roles in the formation of partitions to separate the primary single cavity of the heart into chambers, and in the formation of the valves.

There are two opinions concerning the mode of development of the lymphatic vessels. According to one view the lymphatic vessels arise as evaginations or buds from veins. Most observers, however, believe that the lymphatics first arise independently of the veins as isolated intercellular clefts in

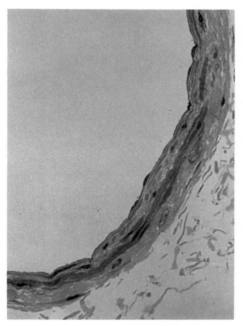

Figure 8–32. Section of the thoracic duct. Note the smooth muscle fibers within the tunica media. Plastic section. × 250.

the mesenchyme. The mesenchymal cells lining the clefts differentiate into endothelial cells, and the clefts enlarge and fuse to form the primary lymphatic vessels. These later establish communication with the veins. Later development of the lymphatic system occurs mainly by budding from the walls of pre-existing lymphatics in much the same way as in the blood vessels.

REFERENCES

Bennett, H. S., Luft, J. H., and Hampton, J. C.: Morphological classification of vertebrate blood capillaries. Am. J. Physiol., *196*:381, 1959.

Boggon, R. P., and Palfrey, A. J.: The microscopic anatomy of human lymphatic trunks. J. Anat., *114*:389, 1973.

Bojsen-Møller, F., and Tranum-Jensen, J.: Rabbit heart nodal tissue, sinuatrial ring bundle and the atrioventricular connexions identified as a neuromuscular system. J. Anat., *112*:367, 1972.

Bruns, R. R., and Palade, G. E.: Studies on blood capillaries. I. General organization of blood capillaries in muscle. II. Transport of ferritin molecules across the wall of muscle capillaries. J. Cell Biol., *37*:244, 277, 1968.

Casley-Smith, J. R.: The functioning and interrelationships of blood capillaries and lymphatics. Experientia, *32*:1, 1976.

Chambers, R., and Zweifach, B. W.: Topography and function of the mesentine capillary circulation. Am. J. Anat., *75*:173, 1944.

Clark, E. R.: Arterio-venous anastomoses. Physiol. Rev., *18*:229, 1938.

Clementi, F., and Palade, G. E.: Intestinal capillaries. I. Permeability to peroxidase and ferritin. J. Cell Biol., *41*:33, 1969.

Fawcett, D. W.: The fine structure of capillaries, arterioles and small arteries. *In* The Microcirculation: A Symposium on Factors Influencing Exchange of Substances across Capillary Wall, edited by S. R. M. Reynolds and B. W. Zweifach. Urbana, University of Illinois Press, 1959, p. 1.

Florey, H.: The endothelial cell. Biol. Med. J., *2*:487, 1966.

Karnovsky, M. J.: The ultrastructural basis of capillary permeability studied with peroxidase as a tracer. J. Cell Biol., *35*:213, 1967.

Leak, L. V.: Studies on the permeability of lymphatic capillaries. J. Cell Biol., *50*:300, 1971.

Majno, G., Shea, S. M., and Leventhal, M.: Endothelial contraction induced by histamine-type mediators. An electron microscopic study. J. Cell Biol., *42*:647, 1969.

Muir, A. R.: Observations on the fine structure of the Purkinje fibers in the ventricles of the sheep's heart. J. Anat., *91*:251, 1957.

Palade, G. E., and Bruns, R. R.: Structural modulations of plasmalemmal vesicles. J. Cell Biol., *37*:633, 1968.

Rhodin, J. A. G.: The ultrastructure of mammalian arterioles and precapillary sphincters. J. Ultrastruct. Res., *18*:181, 1967.

Rhodin, J. A. G.: Ultrastructure of mammalian venous capillaries, venules and small collecting veins. J. Ultrastruct Res., *25*:452, 1968.

Simionescu, M., Simionescu, N., and Palade, G. E.: Morphometric data on the endothelium of blood capillaries. J. Cell Biol., *60*:128, 1974.

Simionescu, N., Simionescu, M., and Palade, G. E.: Recent studies on vascular endothelium. Ann. N.Y. Acad. Sci., *275*:64, 1976.

Thaemert, J. C.: Fine structure of the atrioventricular node as viewed in serial sections. Am. J. Anat., *136*:43, 1973.

Williams, M. C., and Wissig, S. L.: The permeability of muscle capillaries to horseradish peroxidase. J. Cell Biol., *66*:531, 1975.

LYMPHOID ORGANS

Several organs and structures within the body consist largely of *lymphoid (lymphatic) tissue*, which is not one of the primary tissue types but is merely a variety of connective tissue. It has two principal components: reticular tissue, comprising a framework of reticular cells and reticular fibers, and free cells, chiefly lymphocytes, which lie within the interstices of the reticular tissue. In many regions of the body the lymphoid tissue is not sharply delineated from the surrounding connective tissue and is known as *diffuse lymphoid tissue* in contrast to the more dense form (*lymph nodules*) in which the component cells are densely aggregated. Numerous gradations between the two varieties of lymphoid tissue are found.

Diffuse lymphoid tissue occurs principally as an infiltration of the lamina propria of mucous membranes, particularly those of the digestive and respiratory systems. It shows no special organization. The reticular cells are arranged in an apparent syncytium in close relation to the reticular (argyrophil) fibers. Some cells have little cytoplasm and are relatively undifferentiated. Others possess more cytoplasm and have acquired phagocytic properties. These are fixed macrophages which, on detachment from the reticular network, become free macrophages. Small lymphocytes are the commonest of the free cells present. In addition, hemocytoblasts (lymphoblasts), monocytes, and plasma cells are found within the meshes of the stroma.

Lymph, or *primary*, *nodules* are dense aggregations of lymphoid tissue arranged in spherical masses. They have been called the structural units of lymphoid tissue. Nodules vary in diameter from a few hundred microns (μm) to a millimeter or more, and the periphery of each nodule is poorly defined. It is represented by a diffuse border of small lymphocytes separating the nodule from the surrounding connective tissue. Each nodule may be homogeneous or may consist of a darker *cortex*, containing closely packed small lymphocytes, and a lighter central area, the *germinal center* (or *secondary nodule*). The central area develops in response to an

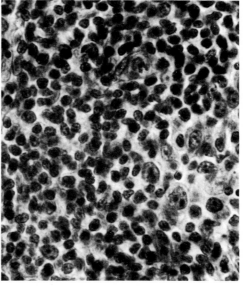

Figure 9–1. Section through a portion of the wall of the small intestine. There is an accumulation of lymphocytes (diffuse lymphatic tissue) in the connective tissue of the lamina propria. Most cells are small, with dense nuclei. A few cells, principally large lymphocytes, contain large, pale nuclei with distinct nucleoli (right center). × 400.

283

antigenic stimulation and contains lymphoblasts and large and medium-sized lymphocytes in addition to small lymphocytes. It is a zone of rapid proliferation, and the size of the center is an indication of the level of the immunological response. Generally, many more lymphocytes are produced in the center than are released, and these are phagocytosed by the macrophages present within the supporting reticular tissue. It should be emphasized that lymph nodules are not constant features, either in structure or in position. They appear, remain for a time, and then disappear. Nodules are rare in the newborn and in animals maintained in an aseptic environment, since their formation is dependent upon antigenic stimuli. Similarly, new nodules may arise in diffuse lymphatic tissue at any time as an expression of the cytogenetic and defense functions of the lymphatic tissue.

Lymph nodules may be isolated or may occur in aggregations in specific lymphoid organs such as lymph nodes, tonsils and spleen. The *solitary nodules*

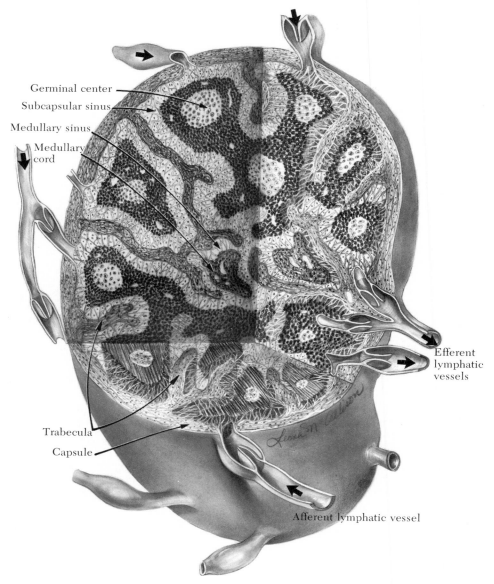

Figure 9-2. Diagram to illustrate the general structure of a lymph node. The arrows indicate the direction of lymph flow.

or *follicles* of the digestive system are examples of isolated nodules. Nodules also may be aggregated into less highly organized structures than lymph nodes, forming the unencapsulated *Peyer's patches* of the intestine.

The lymph nodes are the only lymphoid organs which are interposed in the course of lymph vessels. Thus they possess both afferent and efferent lymphatic vessels. The tonsils, spleen, and thymus have efferent vessels draining from them, but they are not associated with afferent lymphatic vessels.

THE LYMPH NODES

Lymph nodes are variable in number but are found more or less constantly in certain definite regions of the body such as the prevertebral region, the mesentery, and the loose connective tissue of the axilla and groin. Frequently they occur in chains or groups. Each node is an oval or bean-shaped body, ranging from 1 to 25 mm in diameter. It has a convex contour except at an indented region, the *hilum* (or *hilus*) on one side, where the blood vessels enter and leave the node. Afferent lymphatic vessels enter at multiple points on the convex surface of the node. Efferent vessels leave only at the hilum.

Lymph nodes are covered by a definite *capsule* of connective tissue which is continuous with a number of *septa* or *trabeculae* extending into the substance of the organ. The latter, in turn, connect with a fine meshwork of reticular tissue. The parenchyma of each node is specialized into two regions, an outer *cortex*, characterized by the presence of lymph nodules, and an inner *medulla*, in which the lymphoid tissue is arranged chiefly in the form of irregular, anastomosing cords.

Framework

The capsule is a firm covering composed mostly of densely packed collagenous fibers. A loose network of elastic fibers, particularly on its inner surface, is found also in the capsule. At the hilum the capsule is greatly thickened. Trabeculae of dense collagenous

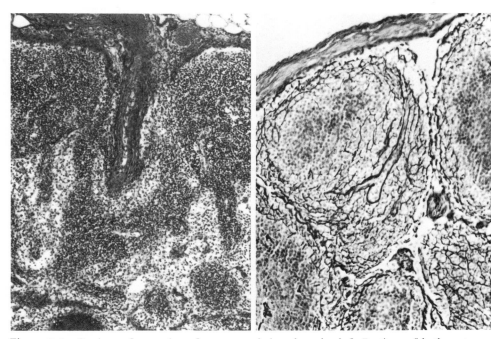

Figure 9–3. Sections of a portion of a mesenteric lymph node. *Left:* Portions of both cortex and medulla are visible. × 60. *Right:* Section stained to visualize the reticular framework. Silver stain. × 75. In both sections, a portion of the capsule is present above.

fibers arise from the inner aspect of the capsule and project into the interior of each node, dividing the cortex into a number of incomplete compartments. In the medulla the trabeculae become highly branched and finally fuse with the connective tissue of the hilum. A few smooth muscle fibers occur in the capsule, particularly at sites where lymphatic vessels enter the node, and in the trabeculae. The functional significance of their presence is unknown. The capsule, the hilum, and the trabeculae constitute the collagenous framework. Within the framework there is a delicate meshwork of reticular connective tissue, comprising reticular fibers, reticular cells, and fixed macrophages. The spaces within this reticulum form the *lymph sinuses,* through which lymph percolates, and these sinuses contain the free cells.

Cortex

The degree of development of the trabeculae and the separation of the cortex into compartments vary in nodes of different animals and in nodes taken from different regions of the body. In man the compartments are not so definite as in many lower mammals. Within the cortical compartments the lymphocytes are closely packed into nodules which are attached indirectly by reticulum to the nearby capsule and trabeculae. The nodules are separated from the capsule and trabeculae by spaces, the lymph sinuses, through which the lymph circulates. Although the cortex usually is found surrounding the medulla except at the hilum, it shows considerable variation in thickness.

The cortical nodules often contain germinal centers but, as in solitary nodules, these are inconstant features. Component cells of each germinal center are larger and possess more cytoplasm and paler nuclei than do the small lymphocytes. Hence the whole central area appears lighter in stained sections. Most of the cells are medium-sized lymphocytes. A few are large, undifferentiated lymphocytes (lympho-

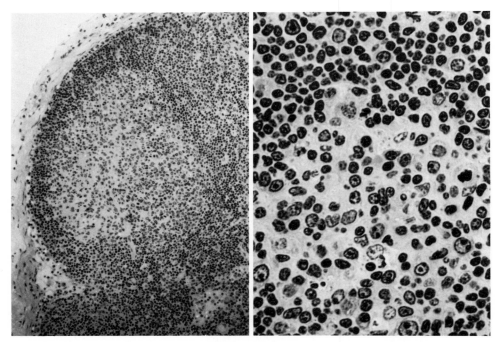

Figure 9-4. Sections of the cortex of a mesenteric lymph node. *Left:* A cortical nodule with a large germinal center. A portion of the capsule is present above and to the left. Plastic section. × 100. *Right:* A portion of a cortical nodule. Component cells of the germinal center are large with pale nuclei. Above is a portion of the cortex containing closely packed small lymphocytes. Plastic section. × 350.

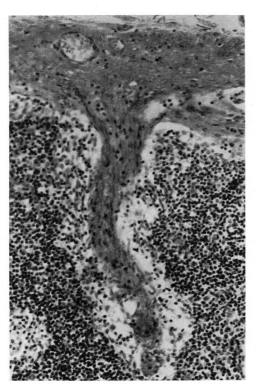

Figure 9–5. Section of a portion of a lymph node, showing the capsule, a trabecula, cortical sinuses, and portions of two cortical nodules. × 100.

blasts) and plasma cells. During an active phase small lymphocytes are produced by the cells of the germinal center and are pushed outward into a peripheral zone, which becomes the *cortex of the nodule.* After a time mitotic activity diminishes, the former growth pressure subsides, and the sharp boundary between the germinal center and the cortex disappears. The center becomes inactive and the nodule returns to its homogeneous, resting appearance. Under certain pathological conditions some of the pale centers contain numerous free macrophages. These areas have been called *reaction centers.*

Internal to the major cortical zone, which contains the nodules, there is a zone composed principally of small lymphocytes, the *paracortex.* This zone characteristically contains numerous postcapillary venules, recognized by their relatively thick endothelium and many lymphocytes within their walls. Recent experimental studies have shown that the lymphocytes of this zone, unlike those of the cortex proper, are of thymic origin (T lymphocytes) and are concerned with cell-mediated immune responses. On the other hand, the cortex itself, and particularly its nodules, is a region where B lymphocytes are concentrated and where stimulation by an antigen leads to the proliferation of small lymphocytes and plasma cells concerned with the production of specific humoral antibody.

Medulla

The cellular components of the medulla and cortex are similar but there is a difference in arrangement. In the medulla the lymphoid tissue takes the form of dense lymphoid strands, or *lymph cords,* containing B lymphocytes and numerous plasma cells, which run between the irregular branching and anastomosing trabeculae. Some lymph *(medullary)* cords are continuous with the deep surface of the cortical tissue and appear as extensions of it into the underlying medulla. They are surrounded by medullary lymph sinuses. Reticulum, which bridges the sinuses, attaches the cords to adjacent trabeculae. This arrangement of dense lymph tissue, sinuses, and trabeculae is similar to that found in the cortex.

Lymphatic Vessels and Sinuses

The circulation of lymph through a lymph node involves afferent lymphatic vessels, a system of lymph sinuses within the node, and efferent lymphatic vessels. Several afferent vessels pierce the capsule on the convex side of the node and open into the system of lymph sinuses. The afferent vessels are provided with valves which open toward the node. Each node contains a tortuous system of irregular channels, the *sinuses,* within the lymphoid tissue. Unlike the endothelium-lined blood vascular and lymphatic vessels, the sinuses generally have walls which are not continuous. They are incompletely lined by reticular cells and fixed macrophages *(littoral cells),* supported by reticular fibers. The sinuses are bridged by further reticular cells that are inter-

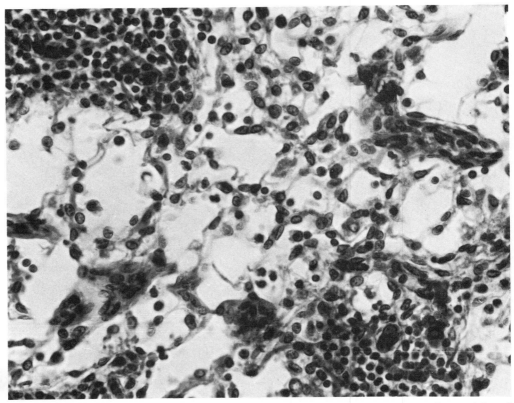

Figure 9–6. Portion of the medulla of a lymph node, showing two medullary cords (top left and bottom right), delicate trabeculae, and medullary sinuses. The latter are irregular spaces delineated by the network of reticular cells. × 325.

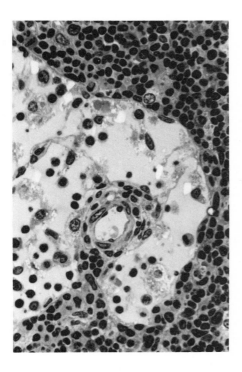

connected by delicate cytoplasmic processes to form a network that is three-dimensional. The walls allow the free movement of lymphocytes from the nodules and medullary cords into the sinuses and thus into the efferent lymphatic vessels. The sinus system comprises three parts. Afferent vessels enter the *marginal* or *subcapsular* sinus, which separates the capsule from the cortical parenchyma. From the marginal sinus lymph flows into the *cortical sinuses,* which lie between the cortical nodules and the trabeculae. Recent electron microscopic studies indicate that the outer

Figure 9–7. Portion of a medulla of a lymph node. The irregular medullary sinuses are bounded by reticular cells. Also shown are a medullary cord containing closely packed small lymphocytes and a small arteriole. Plastic section. × 350.

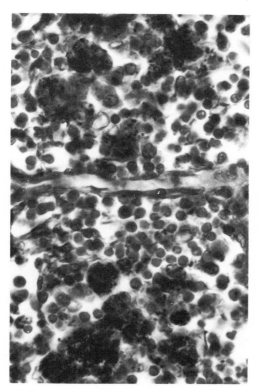

Figure 9–8. Portion of the cortex of a bronchial lymph node. Notice the accumulation of carbon particles in macrophages. × 400.

wall of the marginal sinus and the trabecular side of cortical sinuses possess an intact, continuous endothelium with a basal lamina. Thus, sinus walls adjacent to connective tissue limit movement of lymphocytes, whereas those adjacent to lymphoid tissue have gaps that permit free movement of cells. Cortical sinuses are continous with *medullary sinuses,* which are interposed between medullary trabeculae and medullary cords. The medullary sinuses pierce the thickened portion of the capsule at the hilum and continue into the efferent lymphatic vessels. The efferent vessels are fewer in number and wider than the afferent vessels and contain valves which open away from the nodes. The arrangement of valves in the afferent and efferent vessels allows a flow of lymph only in one direction through the node.

Blood Vessels and Nerves

Arteries enter the lymph node at the hilum and give branches to the medul-

lary cords and to the trabeculae. The branches to the cords continue into the cortex to supply the cortical nodules. Branches to the trabeculae supply the connective tissue of the trabeculae and ultimately reach the capsule. Dense capillary plexuses are present within the medullary cords and the cortical nodules. From the capillaries, blood is collected into postcapillary venules which, in the deep (paracortical) cortex, are lined by cuboidal endothelial cells. Lymphocytes of the recirculating type, principally T lymphocytes, apparently recognize the cuboidal endothelium as a site for migration. The migration may occur either by an intercellular or intracellular (transcellular) route, but recent evidence favors the latter. Lymphocytes that leave the venules penetrate the paracortical zone and medullary sinuses and leave the node by the efferent vessels to return via the thoracic duct to the blood vascular system. By this route, most T lymphocytes recirculate many times. The postcapillary venules then drain into veins which follow the same general route taken by the arteries and leave the node at the hilum.

Nerves, which are mostly vasomotor, enter the hilum with the blood vessels and follow them into the interior of the node.

Functions of Lymph Nodes

One of the primary functions of lymph nodes is the production of lymphocytes, which enter the sinuses partly by ameboid activity and partly by crowding pressure. Lymph is not markedly cellular until it has passed through a lymph node. The development of new lymphocytes from undifferentiated cells has been described previously (see Chapter 5). The actual stimuli for lymphopoiesis both in physiological and in pathological conditions are unknown. In certain pathological conditions extramedullary hemopoiesis occurs and the lymph nodes produce myeloid elements. The fact that lymph in efferent vessels is more cellular than that in afferent vessels is not due principally to production of lymphocytes in lymph nodes, however. Studies using transfused labeled cells have shown that the majority of lymphocytes leaving a

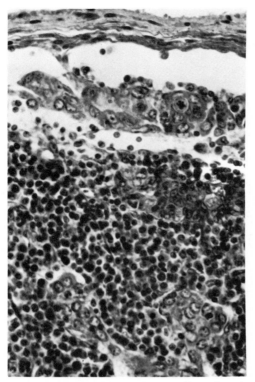

Figure 9–9. Portion of an axillary lymph node from a patient with carcinoma of the breast. Groups of cancer cells (metastatic growths) are present within the subcapsular sinus and the cortex. Notice that one cancer cell in the subcapsular sinus is in the process of dividing. × 250.

lymph node are of the recirculating type.

Lymph nodes filter lymph by means of the phagocytic activity of the fixed and detached reticular cells. They remove degenerating cells, including erythrocytes, and particulate matter from the lymph. A good example of the latter is provided by the bronchial lymph nodes. Inhaled carbon particles eventually reach the bronchial lymph nodes where they are taken up by the macrophages, often in such quantity that the entire nodes appear black.

The lymph nodes also play a role in the elaboration of antibodies and in the production of immunity. They provide a pool of stem cells capable of transforming into antibody-producing cells and of mounting an immune response that is both humoral and cellular. Additionally, lymph nodes constitute a portal of entry of lymphocytes from the blood stream back into the lymphatic channels.

Development of Lymph Nodes

Lymph nodes develop after the formation of the primary lymphatic vascular system. In connective tissue associated with plexuses of lymph vessels, condensations of mesenchymal cells occur which later infiltrate the vessels. Lymphocytes form *in situ* from the mesenchymal cells. Lymph sinuses develop as isolated lymph spaces within the mesenchyme. The spaces fuse to form a system of anastomosing sinuses throughout the developing node. Later this system comes into contact with the afferent and efferent lymphatic vessels. The connective tissue outside the marginal sinus becomes thickened to form the capsule and extends into the node as the trabeculae, which always remain separated from concentrations of lymphoid tissue by the sinuses. The medullary region differentiates in advance of the cortex, and germinal centers within the latter usually do not appear until after birth.

Hemal (Hemolymph) Nodes

In certain animals, structures exist which are very similar to lymph nodes except that they contain large numbers of erythrocytes. These structures, the *hemal nodes*, are common in ruminants such as the sheep but probably do not occur in man. The general organization is similar to that of a lymph node in that the hemal node consists of a mass of lymphatic tissue covered by a connective tissue capsule. The sinuses, however, are purely blood sinuses. In the hog there are structures which are intermediate between a lymph node and a hemal node. Both blood vessels and lymphatics connect with the sinuses. In this instance the term *hemolymph node* is most appropriate.

Hemal nodes are lymphopoietic and also function to filter blood.

THE TONSILS

Three tonsillar groups, the *palatine tonsils*, the *lingual tonsil*, and the *pharyngeal tonsil*, form a ring of lym-

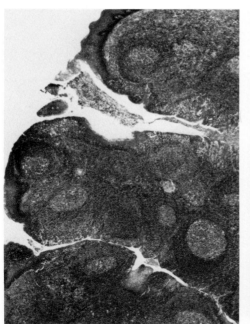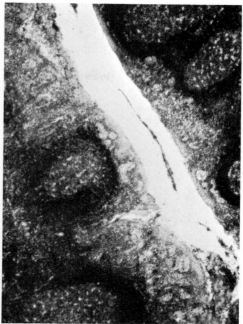

Figure 9–10. Sections of the palatine tonsil, showing the accumulation of lymph nodules, many with germinal centers, covered by epithelium lining the tonsillar crypts. Left, × 15; right, × 30.

phoid tissue surrounding the pharynx, where nasal and oral passages unite. The tonsils are characterized by depressions of the surface epithelium around which aggregations of lymph nodules are grouped.

The palatine, or *faucial*, tonsils are paired, ovoid masses of lymphoid tissue which occupy the intervals between the glossopalatine and pharyngopalatine arches. They lie in the connective tissue of the mucosa and are covered on their free surface by a stratified squamous epithelium which is continuous with the lining of the mouth and pharynx. The epithelium rests upon a basal lamina, under which there is a thin layer of fibrous connective tissue. At various places on the surface of the tonsil, deep indentations, ten to twenty in number, occur. These indentations, or *tonsillar crypts*, penetrate into the interior of the tonsil and are lined by a continuation of the surface epithelium. Frequently, secondary crypts, also lined by epithelium, extend from the bases and sides of the main, or primary, crypts. Lymphoid tissue surrounds the crypts as a diffuse mass in which are embedded lymph nodules. The nodules, like those of

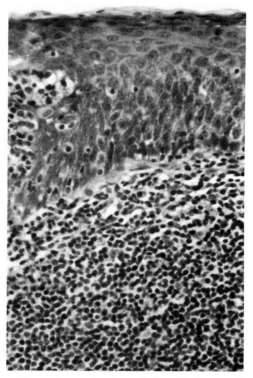

Figure 9–11. Portion of the palatine tonsil. Notice the invasion by lymphocytes of the stratified squamous epithelium. × 250.

lymph nodes, may contain germinal centers. In the deeper parts of the crypts there is no clear delineation between epithelium and lymphoid tissue because of an intense infiltration of the epithelium with lymphocytes. Adjacent to the deepest portions of the tonsil the fibrous tissue is condensed to form a thin capsule which covers the base and sides of the tonsil. Connective tissue septa extend into the interior of the tonsil and separate the various crypts, with their surrounding zones of lymphatic tissue, from one another. Small mucous glands lie in the connective tissue beneath the tonsil and its capsule. Their ducts open for the most part on the free surface; occasionally they may open into the tonsillar crypts.

The *lingual tonsil* is located in the root of the tongue, behind the circumvallate papillae. It consists of an aggregation of wide-mouthed epithelial pits, each surrounded by lymphoid tissue. Each simple pit or crypt is lined by a continuation of the surface stratified squamous epithelium. The lymphoid tissue comprises a layer of lymph nodules, often with germinal centers. In most crypts there is marked infiltration of the epithelium with lymphocytes. Ducts of underlying mucous glands open onto the surface or into the crypts.

The *pharyngeal tonsil* is an accumulation of lymphoid tissue in the median posterior wall of the nasopharynx. The lymphatic tissue is similar to that of the palatine tonsils. The epithelium over the free surface is folded but no true crypts occur. In general the epithelium is pseudostratified, with cilia and goblet cells, but in the adult there may be islands of stratified squamous epithelium. The epithelium is extensively infiltrated with lymphocytes. A thin capsule surrounds the pharyngeal tonsil and sends septa into the cores of epithelial folds. Mixed seromucous glands occur in the connective tissue beneath the capsule, and their ducts open onto the free surface or into the furrows between the folds. Hypertrophy of the pharyngeal tonsil, with consequent obstruction to the nasal openings, is common and is known clinically as *adenoids*.

The *tubal tonsils* sometimes are considered as a separate tonsillar group. Each tubal tonsil lies around the pharyngeal orifice of the pharyngotympanic (auditory) tube and constitutes a lateral extension of the pharyngeal tonsil. The tubal tonsil is covered with ciliated columnar epithelium.

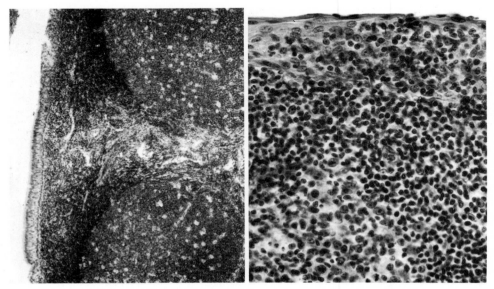

Figure 9–12. Sections of a portion of the pharyngeal tonsil. *Left:* Pseudostratified columnar epithelium covers the masses of tonsillar tissue. × 40. *Right:* A region where the epithelium is stratified squamous and shows extensive infiltration with lymphocytes. × 200.

Blood vessels course in the capsule and septa of the tonsils and supply the lymphoid tissue. The tonsils possess no afferent lymphatic vessels. Plexuses of lymph capillaries occur around the lymphoid tissue and drain into efferent lymphatic vessels. The tonsils, which reach their maximum development in childhood and thereafter decline, constitute a discontinuous ring of lymphoid tissue around the pharynx. They participate in lymphocyte production and aid in the protection of the body against invading bacteria, viruses, and other foreign proteins. As in other lymphoid tissue, the foreign proteins (antigens) stimulate the production of antibodies in plasma cells, which themselves are derived from lymphocytes. On the other hand, epithelial erosion would seem to enhance an invasion by microorganisms, and the tonsils are known to be frequent portals of infection.

THE THYMUS

The thymus varies in size and development with the age of the individual.

It attains its maximum development about puberty, after which it becomes inconspicuous.

It consists of two *lobes* closely applied and united by connective tissue, and it is situated in the anterior mediastinum behind the upper portion of the sternum. A lobe is composed of thousands of *lobules*, each containing *cortical* and *medullary* components. The lobules are not completely separate units since the medulla constitutes a central core to each lobe and sends prolongations into each lobule. A capsule encloses each lobe and extensions from it *(septa)* delineate the lobules. The capsule consists of collagenous fibers together with a few elastic fibers, and interlobular septa extend from it as far as the medulla and partially separate the lobules from each other. In addition intralobular *trabeculae* arise from the capsule and pass into the cortex of the lobules. The reticular connective tissue of the thymus differs in some respects from that of other lymphoid organs. The reticular cells, which support the parenchyma, arise from entoderm rather than from mesenchyme and in tissue

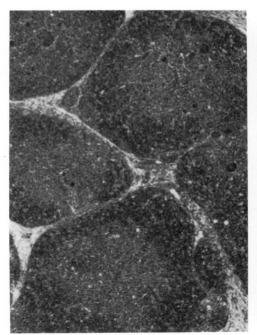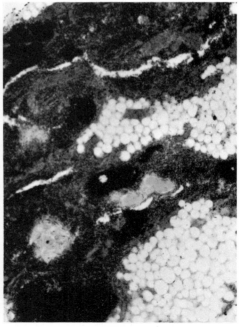

Figure 9–13. *Left:* Section through the thymus of a seven-year-old child. The cortex of the lobules is dark, the medulla light. The dark-staining bodies in the medulla of the lobule at the top are thymic corpuscles. Plastic section. × 40. *Right:* Portion of the thymus from an adult. Notice the involution of the organ and the replacement with fat. × 40.

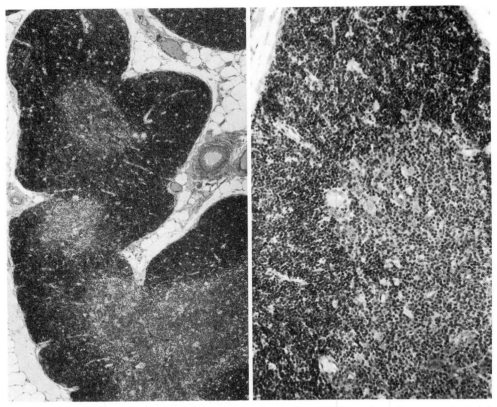

Figure 9–14.   Sections of a portion of the thymus of an infant. *Left:* Note the delicate capsule and the irregular lobulation. × 40. *Right:* Thymocytes are densely packed within the cortex. Thymic corpuscles are not apparent within the medulla. × 120.

culture have been shown to possess epithelioid characteristics. These *epithelial reticular cells* are stellate and possess ovoid, pale-staining nuclei with distinct nucleoli. The cells form an interconnecting meshwork by opposition of their branching cytoplasmic processes. The junctions between processes of neighboring cells show typical desmosomes with associated tonofibrillae. The cytoplasm is characterized by the presence of lysosomes, vacuoles, and electron-dense granules, possibly secretory in nature. The arrangement of the meshwork varies with location: in the cortex, it is open and has large interstices, and in the medulla it forms a system of incomplete anastomosing sheets. Additionally, the meshwork occurs as incomplete sheets over the connective tissue of the capsule and the trabeculae and ensheaths the major blood vessels of the cortex and the medulla. Many investigators believe that the latter ar-

rangement constitutes a *blood-thymic barrier,* similar to the blood-brain barrier in the central nervous system formed by the glial cells, and that it limits access of certain circulating materials, particularly proteins, into the thymic parenchyma. The epithelial reticular cells, unlike true reticular cells of mesenchymal origin, do not phagocytose colloidal dyes and generally are not associated with reticular fibers.

Cortex and Medulla

The cortex contains small lymphocytes, sometimes called *thymocytes,* that are densely and uniformly packed. The thymocytes appear similar in structure to lymphocytes elsewhere, although their origin differs. They arise by division of stem cells that originally migrated to the thymus from the bone marrow. The thymocytes occupy the in-

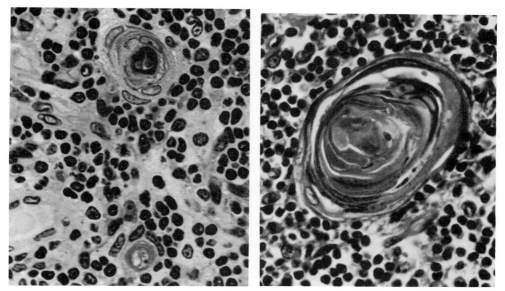

Figure 9–15. Portions of the thymic medulla containing thymic corpuscles. The concentric arrangement of epithelial cells is most apparent in the left hand figure. Left, Plastic section. Both × 400.

terstices of the sparse reticular meshwork and obscure the epithelial reticular cells. The lymphatic tissue, unlike that of lymph nodes, is not arranged in nodules. The medulla stains more lightly and is less compact than the cortex. The thymocytes are less numerous in the medulla, and consequently the epithelial reticular cells are prominent. In addition to thymocytes, lymphocytes of medium and large size are present, particularly in the medulla. Myoid cells also have been described in the medulla of some species.

True macrophages vary in number but are most common in the cortex in perivascular regions and in relation to the capsule and to the trabeculae. They are similar in structure to macrophages elsewhere and are concerned with the phagocytosis of thymocytes. It has been estimated that the majority of thymocytes produced in the cortex are destroyed and that only a small minority of cells is released.

A further feature of the thymus is the presence of *thymic corpuscles* (of Hassall). They are spherical or ovoid bodies composed of concentrically arranged epithelial cells and are localized principally in the medulla. They are acido-phil and vary in diameter from 20 to more than 100 microns (μm). The central cells are large and often show evidence of hyalinization and degeneration. The surrounding cells are flattened and may retain connections with nearby reticular cells. The corpuscles become increasingly prominent during periods of intense destruction of thymocytes and during involution. Their significance is as yet unknown.

Blood Vessels

The arteries supplying the thymus are derived from the internal thoracic and the inferior thyroid arteries. They branch and pass along the trabeculae before giving off arterioles, ensheathed by epithelial reticular cells, that enter the lobules at the junction between cortex and medulla. Numerous capillary branches pass from the arterioles into the cortex and less regular branches into the medulla. Epithelial reticular cells surround all smaller vessels in the thymus and, although incomplete, they constitute a layer that separates blood from the thymocytes, particularly in the cortex. From the capillary bed, blood passes through postcapillary venules which, unlike those of lymph nodes, do not show a thickened endothelium. Thymocytes (lymphocytes) that proliferate in the cortex enter the blood vascular system through the walls of these vessels. Returning venules pass mainly into the medulla and from there to veins in the interlobular trabeculae. The latter drain into the left brachiocephalic and thyroid veins.

Lymphatics

There are no afferent vessels and no lymph sinuses in the thymus. Efferent lymphatics run mainly in the interlobular connective tissue.

Nerves

A few branches of the vagus and cervical sympathetic nerves reach the thymus. They are distributed mainly to the walls of the blood vessels.

Involution

The thymus reaches its maximum size at puberty, and then begins to involute, a process which continues into old age. Involution first involves a gradual loss of lymphocytes from the cortex with the result that the boundary between cortex and medulla becomes indistinct. The medulla also begins to atrophy at puberty. Adipose tissue replaces the thymocytes and epithelial reticular cells. The last elements to be replaced are the thymic corpuscles which may be recognizable even in old age.

Functions

Lymphopoiesis is a known thymic activity and occurs principally during fetal and early postnatal life. Plasma cells and myelocytes also are formed in small numbers. In mice, removal of the thymus shortly after birth results in lymphocyte deficiency and in some form of immunity lack. The mice grow for several months and then die, pre-

sumably owing to an inability to produce antibodies. In the meantime the mice do not resist bacterial infections and will not reject skin grafts from other strains of mice. These phenomena do not occur if thymectomy is delayed until a few days after birth. Thus it is postulated that the thymus is responsible for the production of a pool of circulating lymphocytes (T cells), which then migrate to the other lymphoid organs, principally lymph nodes and spleen. Here they settle down in so-called *thymus-dependent* zones, including the paracortical zones of lymph nodes, the periarterial sheaths in the white pulp of the spleen, and the lymphoid tissue of Peyer's patches in the small intestine. They give rise to immunologically competent cells. In the adult the thymus continues to be an important source of small lymphocytes, particularly if the individual has suffered depletion of his lymphoid organs by irradiation. There is evidence that, in addition, the thymus exerts a humoral effect upon other lymphoid tissues, particularly with regard to the stimulation of lymphocyte production and the development of immunological competence. The nature and origin of the humoral factor, called *thymosin* by some authors, are unknown, but it is believed that it may be synthesized by the epithelial reticular cells.

The thymus has some relations with the gonads, adrenals, and thyroid gland. Gonadal hormones induce involution, and thyroidectomy hastens it.

There appears to be some relation between the thymus and *myasthenia gravis*, a clinical condition characterized by muscle weakness. Many individuals suffering from this disease have either a thymic tumor or an enlarged thymus, but the significance of the relationship remains obscure.

Development

In man the thymus arises as a paired ventral outgrowth from the third branchial pouch. Each outgrowth has a narrow lumen at first, but this quickly is obliterated by proliferation of the lining epithelial cells. The epithelial cells differentiate, and some transform into epithelial reticular cells at about the end of the second month of pregnancy. Thymocytes (or lymphocytes) appear at this time also. It is thought that they arise from mesenchymal cells which invade the developing thymus. The lymphocytes proliferate rapidly and the epithelium is converted into a reticular cell mass. Lobules form at this time and connective tissue invades the lobes to form septa and trabeculae. Hassall's corpuscles first appear during fetal life and continue to form until involution is initiated. They are thought to arise from hypertrophied and degenerating epithelial cells.

THE SPLEEN

The spleen is the largest of the lymphoid organs, and with the possible exception of the hemal nodes, it is the only organ specialized for filtering blood. It has no afferent lymphatic vessels and its sinuses, as in the hemal nodes, are filled with blood instead of lymph.

The spleen, like the lymph nodes, has a collagenous framework within which is suspended a reticular network. It is surrounded by a capsule which itself is covered by a serous membrane, the peritoneum. Many trabeculae pass

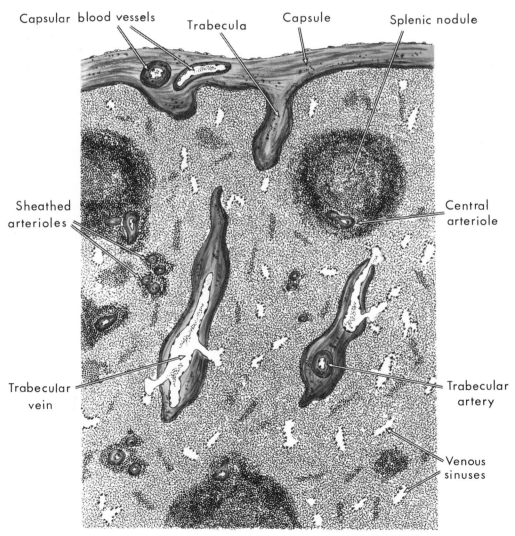

Figure 9–16. Diagram of a section of spleen. The white pulp consists of nodules and aggregations of lymphocytes, and the red pulp is an open mesh with sinusoids.

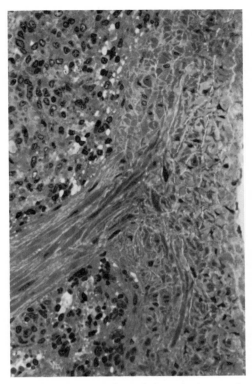

Figure 9–17. Section of the splenic capsule. Smooth muscle cells with densely staining cytoplasm are prominent in the dense connective tissue of the capsule and of a trabecula (left center). The external surface of the capsule is covered by flattened mesothelial cells of the peritoneum. Plastic section. × 225.

from the capsule into the interior of the organ. At one point on the surface of the spleen there is a deep indentation, the *hilum*, where blood vessels enter and leave. The parenchyma (*splenic pulp*) is of two distinct types. *White pulp* is typical lymphatic tissue which surrounds and follows the arteries. At intervals it is thickened into ovoid masses, the *splenic nodules* (or *malpighian bodies*). The *red pulp* is more abundant, often forms plates, the *pulp cords*, and is associated with numerous erythrocytes. The structure of the spleen and the relations between the red and white pulp depend upon the arrangement and distribution of blood vessels. Arteries are connected closely with the white pulp, and the terminal blood vessels (sinuses and veins) with the red pulp.

The trabeculae delineate many compartments, or *lobules*, within the spleen. A lobule is about 1 mm in diameter and is bounded by several trabeculae. Each lobule is supplied by a central artery

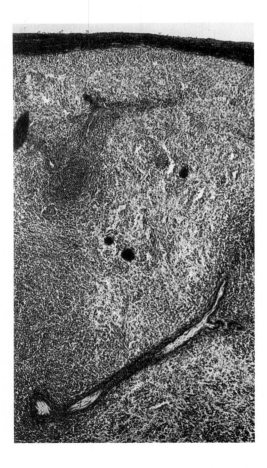

Figure 9–18. Section through a portion of spleen showing capsule (top), densely staining segments of trabeculae, and white pulp in association with splenic arterial branches. × 40.

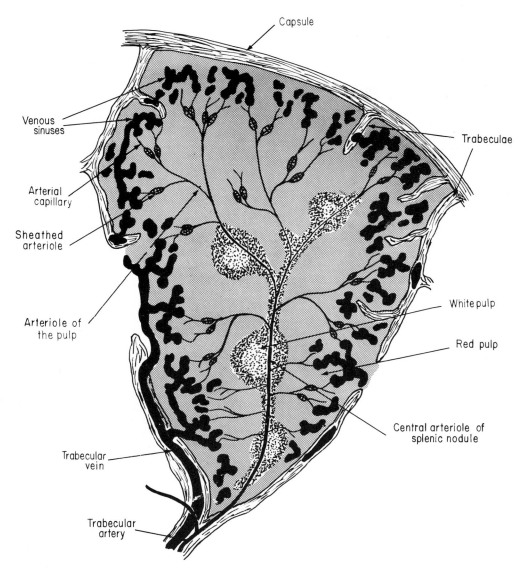

Capsule

Venous
sinuses

Trabeculae

Arterial
capillary

Sheathed
arteriole

White pulp

Red pulp

Arteriole of
the pulp

Central arteriole of
splenic nodule

Trabecular
vein

Trabecular
artery

Figure 9–19. Diagram of a splenic lobule. The principal vascular relations within a lobule are depicted diagrammatically.

and is drained by veins which run in trabeculae to leave the lobule. The lobules are not distinct since they are not outlined completely by trabeculae.

Framework

The capsule and trabeculae of the spleen consist of dense collagenous connective tissue with some elastic fibers and some smooth muscle fibers. The capsule is thickest at the hilum where it surrounds the major blood vessels. The external surface of the capsule is covered by a layer of flattened mesothelial cells, a component of the peritoneum. Trabeculae radiate inward from the hilum and from the internal surface of the capsule. They branch and anastomose repeatedly to form a fairly complex framework throughout the interior. Smooth muscle elements within the capsule and trabeculae are responsible for the slow, rhythmical changes in volume of the spleen. The splenic pulp is supported by a fine meshwork of reticular fibers

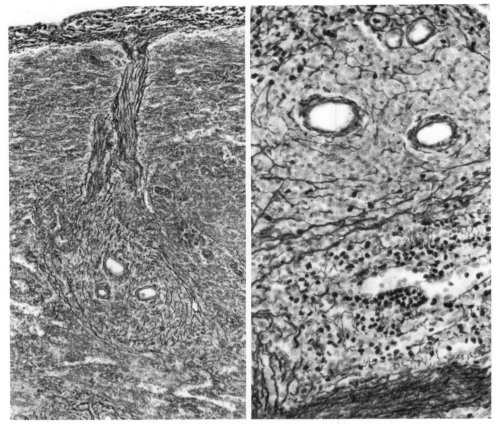

Figure 9–20. Sections of spleen stained to visualize reticular fibers. *Left:* Fibers are concentrated within the capsule and a trabecula. They also occur in relation to a splenic nodule (below). Silver stain. × 100. *Right:* Between a splenic nodule (above) and a trabecula (below), there is red pulp. Within the latter, note an irregular-shaped venous sinus, bounded by delicate reticular fibers. × 250.

which blends with the capsule, trabeculae, and walls of the blood vessels. The cells in relation to the reticulum are, as in other lymphoid organs, primitive reticular cells and fixed macrophages.

White Pulp

White pulp appears on a cut surface as scattered gray areas of compact pulpal tissue. It forms a *periarterial sheath* of lymphocytes about the arteries, the adventitia of which is largely replaced by reticular tissue. The reticular tissue is infiltrated with lymphocytes, which form areas of diffuse and nodular lymphatic tissue. The cells present within this tissue are predominantly small lymphocytes, but in addition there are medium-sized and large lymphocytes, monocytes, and plasma cells. The

amount of lymphoid tissue is not constant but varies as it does in all lymphatic tissue in response to certain stimuli. *Splenic nodules* are denser accumulations of lymphocytes along the strands of white pulp. They are typical lymph nodules which may show germinal centers. In the spleen the nodules are arranged around a blood vessel, the so-called *central artery,* which in most instances is an arteriole, and is eccentric in position since it avoids the germinal center.

Between the white and red pulp are poorly delineated *marginal zones* of diffuse lymphatic tissue containing few lymphocytes and numerous macrophages. These zones trap circulating antigens and are important in the immunological activity of the spleen. In the white pulp, T and B lymphocytes generally are segregated in two different sites. T lymphocytes populate the

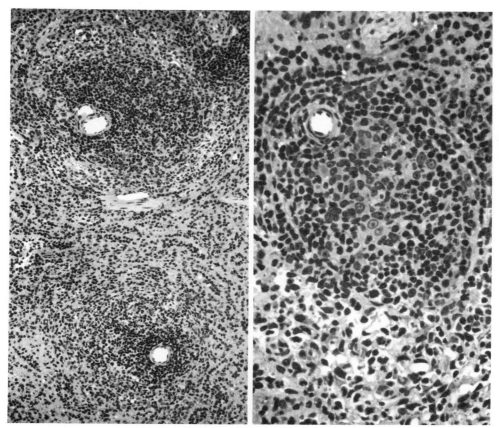

Figure 9–21. Plastic sections of a portion of the spleen. *Left:* Between a splenic nodule (above) and a splenic arteriole, surrounded by a cuff of lymphocytes (below), there is a small trabecular vein. × 100. *Right:* A splenic nodule, with the arteriole in an eccentric position, shows a small, ill-defined germinal center. × 275.

periarterial sheath, and B lymphocytes are concentrated in the marginal zones and in the nodules. From birth to early adulthood, the white pulp forms the greater volume of the spleen, but with increasing age it regresses, the number of splenic nodules decreases, and the red pulp becomes increasingly prominent.

Red Pulp

The red pulp is a pastelike, red mass which can be scraped from a freshly cut surface. It is looser in texture than white pulp and is infiltrated with all elements of circulating blood. It occupies all space not utilized by trabeculae and white pulp. It contains numerous ve-

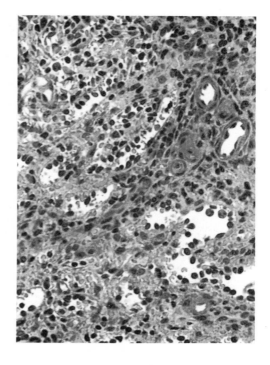

Figure 9–22. Portion of the red pulp of spleen, showing pulp arterioles (top right), venous sinuses, and splenic cords. Plastic section. × 250.

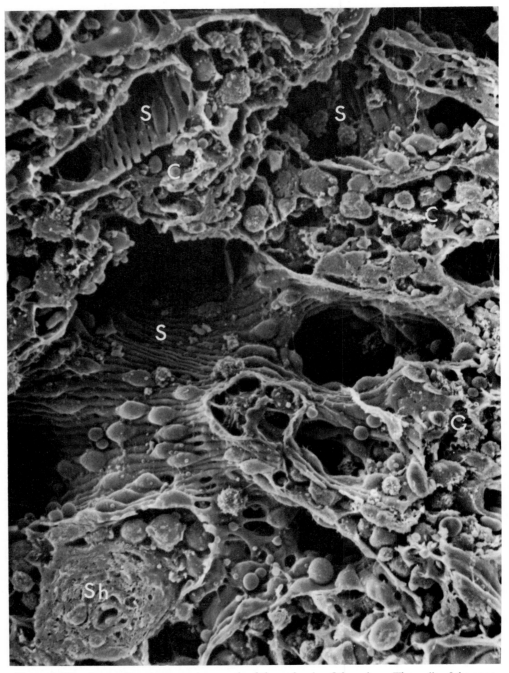

Figure 9–23.   A scanning electron micrograph of the red pulp of the spleen. The walls of the venous sinuses (S) are seen mainly in surface view. Also shown are splenic cords (C) and a sheathed arteriole (Sh). × 700. (Courtesy of Dr. T. Fujita.)

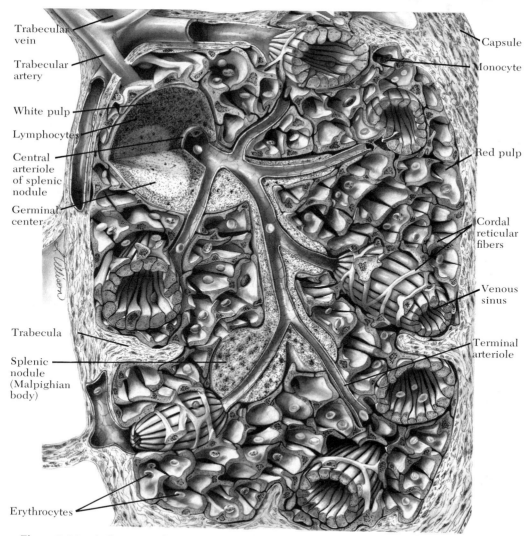

Trabecular vein

Trabecular artery

White pulp

Lymphocytes

Central arteriole of splenic nodule

Germinal center

Trabecula

Splenic nodule (Malpighian body)

Erythrocytes

Capsule

Monocyte

Red pulp

Cordal reticular fibers

Venous sinus

Terminal arteriole

Figure 9–24. A diagrammatic representation of a splenic lobule. The white pulp consists of nodules and aggregations of lymphocytes that surround and follow the arterial blood vessels, and the red pulp is an open mesh with sinusoids.

nous sinuses. Between the sinuses the pulp appears as cellular cords (*splenic* or *Billroth cords*). which form a spongy network of modified lymphatic tissue that merges gradually into the white pulp.

The support of the pulp is a typical reticulum with its associated reticular cells, both primitive and phagocytic. Within the meshes of this framework are lymphocytes, free macrophages, and all the elements of circulating blood. Lymphocytes of large, medium,

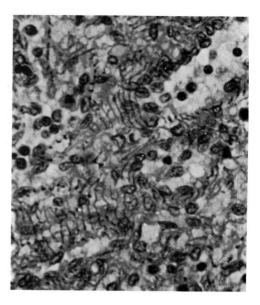

Figure 9–25. Section of red pulp of spleen stained by the periodic acid–Schiff (PAS) reaction to show reticular fibers in relation to splenic sinuses. × 425.

and small sizes are numerous in the white pulp but are less numerous and more loosely arranged in the red pulp. The various types of lymphocytes arise in the white pulp and spread to the red pulp by amebism. Monocytes also are fairly numerous. Some are brought by the blood stream; others arise within the spleen by proliferation of existing cells or by differentiation from hemocytoblasts. The red pulp also contains numerous plasma cells, granular leukocytes, and erythrocytes.

In many mammals and in mammalian embryos the red pulp of the spleen contains megakaryocytes, myelocytes, and erythroblasts. These myeloid elements are absent from the spleen in adult man except in certain pathological conditions when the spleen undergoes *myeloid metaplasia*.

Blood Vessels

The distribution and organization of the red and white pulp depend upon the vascular arrangement. An appreciation of this arrangement is necessary also to an understanding of the structure of the spleen as a whole.

The arteries enter the spleen at the hilum and divide into branches that are typical muscular arteries which pass along the trabeculae as *trabecular* or *interlobular arteries*. As the trabeculae branch, the arteries subdivide also. When reduced to a diameter of approximately 0.2 mm, they leave the trabeculae to enter the splenic parenchyma. As they do so, the tunica adventitia of the arteries loosens, takes on the character of reticular tissue, and becomes infiltrated with lymphocytes. At various points along the course of the vessels the lymphatic sheath is increased in amount to form the splenic nodules. These vessels, which are called "central arteries or arterioles" although they are eccentric with reference to the corpuscles, give off capillaries that supply the white pulp and continue into the red pulp. After numerous divisions, the arterioles become reduced in size, lose their investment of white pulp, and enter the red pulp. Here each arteriole subdivides into several small branches that lie close together like a brush or *penicillus*. The

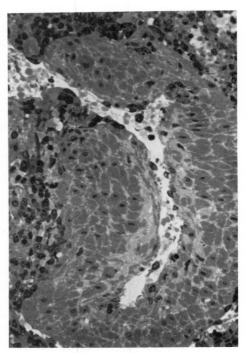

Figure 9–26.   Section of the spleen to show a trabecular vein, the wall of which contains large numbers of smooth muscle cells, here sectioned transversely. A pulp vein enters the trabecular vein at top left. Plastic section. × 250.

penicilli vessels show three successive segments. The first portion, the longest segment, is the *pulp arteriole (artery of the pulp),* which possesses a thin tunica of smooth muscle. This vessel becomes narrow and divides into the *sheathed arterioles,* or *ellipsoids,* which have markedly thickened walls, the *Schweigger-Seidel sheath.* The thickened sheath, which is not so well developed in man as in many lower mammals, is spindle-shaped and is composed of a mass of concentrically arranged cells and fibers continuous peripherally with the reticulum of the red pulp. Each sheathed arteriole divides into two or more *terminal arterial capillaries,* lined by a continuous endothelium. The terminations of the arterial capillaries are the subject of considerable controversy. Some authors claim that the arterial capillaries open directly into the pulp reticulum and that the blood gradually filters back into the venous sinuses (the "open" or slow circulation theory). Other authors consider that the arterial capillaries empty directly into the venous sinuses (the "closed" or rapid circulation theo-

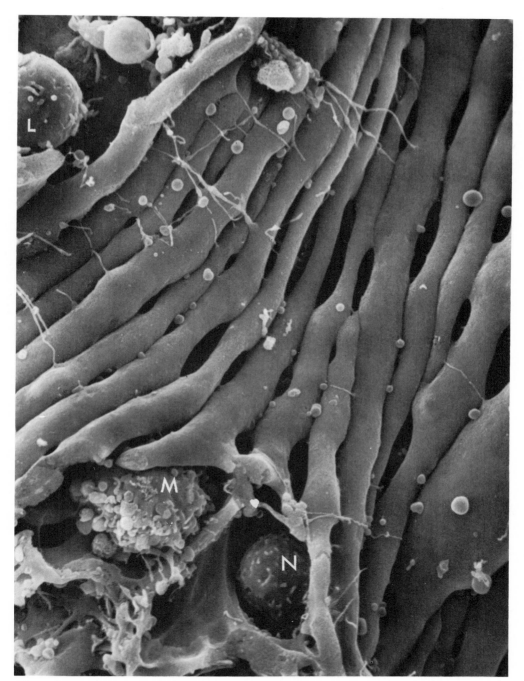

Figure 9–27. A scanning electron micrograph of a venous sinus. The littoral (rod) cells show deficiencies between them. Also present are a lymphocyte (L), a macrophage (M), and a neutrophil leukocyte (N). × 3700. (Courtesy of Dr. T. Fujita.)

ry). There is considerable evidence for both theories, and it is possible that structurally and functionally both systems exist in the spleen. The exact routing of the blood is, in a sense, a detail of academic interest only, since there is an interchange of cells between the red pulp and the sinuses.

The venous sinuses constitute a system of irregular, anastomosing tunnels throughout the red pulp. They occupy more space than that occupied by the splenic cords which lie between them. These vessels are called *sinuses* since they have an irregular lumen and are highly distensible. The sinus wall is composed of specialized endothelial cells which are rod-shaped and run longitudinally in the vessel wall. The cell bodies bulge into the lumen of the sinus. This bulging is most pronounced in the region of the nucleus. The lining cells, termed *littoral, rod,* or *stave cells,* are connected by short transverse processes, and large gaps, or oval clefts, are present between them. These deficiencies are large enough to allow formed elements of blood to cross the sinusoidal wall. The cells rest upon an incomplete basal lamina and the wall of the sinus is supported by thick, anastomosing reticular fibers circularly arranged.

The venous sinuses empty into the *pulp veins,* large thin-walled vessels lined by endothelium. These veins leave the pulp and unite to form larger veins which pass into the trabeculae as *trabecular* or *interlobular* veins. The trabecular veins, which consist only of endothelium supported by the fibromuscular tissue of the trabeculae, travel to the hilum, where they drain into the splenic vein.

Lymphatics

Efferent vessels are present in the capsule and in the larger trabeculae. A few deep efferent lymphatic vessels, which follow the arteries, may be present also in the white pulp.

Nerves

Unmyelinated nerve fibers follow the arteries and terminate in the smooth muscle of their walls. Nerves also terminate in the capsule and in the trabeculae in species which possess smooth muscle cells in these sites. A few branches enter both the red and white pulp but their endings here are unknown. Occasional myelinated fibers, which probably are sensory in function, are seen also.

Functions of the Spleen

Splenic functions are not understood completely. The spleen is said to be not essential for life. However, although in some cases it can be removed without harm to the individual, in others morbidity may follow the operation. Often the morbidity is related to an increase in the number of lymphocytes in the blood due to excessive compensation by the lymph nodes. After extirpation the spleen's functions are taken over by various organs, principally other lymphoid organs and the bone marrow.

The spleen is an important hemopoietic organ, producing principally lymphocytes which are formed chiefly in the white pulp, in particular in its nodules. From the white pulp they pass to the red pulp, and so into the sinuses and splenic vein. In the embryo the spleen also produces myeloid elements. In certain pathological conditions it may undergo myeloid metaplasia, as mentioned previously, and produce all types of blood cells.

The spleen also acts as a store for red blood cells. It is an elastic, controllable reservoir that is important in adjusting the volume of the circulating blood. From time to time large numbers of red blood cells are retained in the spleen, principally within the venous sinuses, and then expelled when needed into the general circulation by contraction of the smooth muscle fibers and the stretched elastic fibers in the trabeculae and capsule.

The spleen filters the blood in much the same way as the lymph nodes filter lymph. The phagocytic cells of the spleen, both free and attached, remove foreign particles, bacteria, degenerating leukocytes, and erythrocytes. In the latter instance the spleen functions as an organ of blood destruction. Erythrocytes are engulfed by the phagocytic cells, and iron recovered from the hemoglobin is stored in the cells. The iron is given up as needed and is utilized in the formation of new hemoglobin.

The production of antibodies is another important function of the spleen. Under antigenic stimulation, B lymphocytes proliferate and give rise to antibody-producing plasma cells, and lymphoblasts proliferate and produce additional plasma cells and lymphocytes.

Development

The primordium of the spleen in human embryos appears as a thickening of the mesenchyme in the dorsal mesentery of the stomach during the fifth week of embryonic development. At this time it consists of a mass of mesenchymal cells which later divide actively. The mass of the primordium is added to by apposition of cells from the covering mesothelium of the body cavity. The mesenchymal cells differentiate into cells of the reticulum and into primitive free cells resembling lymphocytes. Later the tissue becomes myeloid in type, containing all stages in the development of megakaryocytes, granulocytes, and erythrocytes. The development of lymphocytes and monocytes continues throughout life, but myeloid elements disappear shortly after birth.

In the early stages of development the spleen is supplied by a rich capillary plexus, but as a characteristic distribution of vessels is established, lymphocytes become compactly arranged around the arteries to form the white pulp. Definite nodules do not appear until later in fetal life, and germinal centers are not present until after birth. The venous sinuses develop as irregular spaces which later become connected with the established blood vessels.

REFERENCES

Ackerman, G. A., and Hostetler, J. R.: Morphological studies of the embryonic rabbit thymus: the *in situ* epithelial versus the extrathymic derivation of the initial population of lymphocytes in the embryonic thymus. Anat. Rec., *166*:27, 1970.

Bellanti, J. A.: Immunology II. Philadelphia, W. B. Saunders Co., 1979.

Bearman, R. M., Bensch, K. G., and Levine, G. D.: The normal human thymic vasculature: an ultrastructural study. Anat. Rec., *183*:485, 1975.

Caso, L. V.: Some endocrine aspects of the thymus gland. Japan J. Med. Sci. Biol., *28*:289, 1976.

Chapman, W. L., and Allen, J. R.: The fine structure of the thymus of the fetal and neonatal monkey (*Macaca mulatta*). Z. Zellforsch., *114*:220, 1971.

Chen, L.-T.: Microcirculation of the spleen: an open or closed circulation. Science, *201*:157, 1978.

Chen, L.-T., and Weiss, L.: Electron microscopy of the red pulp of human spleen. Am. J. Anat., *134*:425, 1972.

Cho, Y., and De Bruyn, P. P. H.: Passage of red blood cells through the sinusoidal wall of the spleen. Am. J. Anat., *142*:91, 1975.

Cho, Y., and De Bruyn, P. P. H.: The endothelial structure of the postcapillary venules of the lymph node and the passage of lymphocytes across the venule wall. J. Ultrastruct. Res., *69*:13, 1979.

Clark, S. L., Jr.: The reticulum of lymph nodes in mice studied with the electron microscope. Am. J. Anat., *110*:217, 1962.

Daniels, J. C., Ritzmann, S. E., and Levin, W. C.: Lymphocytes: morphological, developmental, and functional characteristics in health, disease, and experimental study — an analytical review. Texas Rep. Biol. Med., *26*:5, 1968.

Folse, D. S., Beathard, G. A., and Granholm, N. A.: Smooth muscle in lymph node capsule and trabeculae. Anat. Rec., *183*:517, 1975.

Forkert, P.-G., Thliveris, J. A., and Bertalanffy, F. D.: Structure of sinuses in the human lymph node. Cell Tiss. Res., *183*:115, 1977.

Fujita, T.: A scanning electron microscope study of the human spleen. Arch. Histol. Jap., *37*:187, 1974.

Kohnen, P., and Weiss, L.: An electron microscopic study of thymic corpuscles in the guinea pig and the mouse. Anat. Rec., *148*:29, 1964.

Lewis, O. J.: The blood vessels of the adult mammalian spleen. J. Anat., *91*:245, 1957.

Maximow, A. A.: The lymphocytes and plasma cells. *In* Special Cytology, ed. 2, edited by E. V. Cowdry. New York, Paul B. Hoeber, 1932, vol. 2, p. 601.

Miyoshi, M., and Fujita, T.: Stereo-fine structure of the splenic red pulp. A combined scanning and transmission electron microscope study on dog and rat spleen. Arch. Histol. Jap., *33*:225, 1971.

Moe, R. E.: Electron microscopic appearance of the parenchyma of lymph nodes. Am. J. Anat., *114*:341, 1964.

Nopanjaroonsri, C., Luk, S. C., and Simon, G. T.: Ultrastructure of the normal lymph node. Am. J. Pathol., *65*:1, 1971.

Peck, H. M., and Hoerr, N. L.: The intermediary circulation in the red pulp of the mouse spleen. Anat. Rec., *109*:447, 1951.

Raviola, E., and Karnowsky, M. J.: Evidence for a blood-thymus barrier using electron opaque tracers. J. Exp. Med., *136*:466, 1972.

Roberts, D. K., and Latta, J. S.: Electron microscopic studies on the red pulp of the rabbit spleen. Anat. Rec., *148*:81, 1964.

Sasou, S., Satodate, R., and Katsura, S.: The marginal sinus in the perifollicular region of the rat spleen. Cell Tiss. Res., *172*:195, 1976.

Suzuki, T., Furusato, M., Takasaki, S., Shimizu, S., and Hataba, Y.: Stereoscopic scanning electron microscopy of the red pulp of dog spleen with special reference to the terminal structure of the cordal capillaries. Cell Tiss. Res., *182*:441, 1977.

Weiss, L.: A study of the structure of the splenic sinuses in man and in the albino rat, with the light microscope and the electron microscope. J. Biophys. Biochem. Cytol., *3*:599, 1957.

Weiss, L.: The structure of fine splenic arterial vessels in relation to hemoconcentration and red cell destruction. Am. J. Anat., *111*:131, 1962.

Weiss, L.: An electron microscopic study of splenic white pulp. J. Cell Biol., *19*:74A, 1963.

THE SKIN AND ITS APPENDAGES (THE INTEGUMENT)

The integument comprises the skin that covers the surface of the body together with certain specialized derivatives of the skin. These include nails, hair, and several kinds of glands.

The skin protects the organism from injurious substances and influences; it provides a barrier to invasion by microorganisms; it helps to regulate the temperature of the body; by sweating it excretes water and various waste products of catabolism; it is the most extensive sense organ of the body for the reception of tactile, thermal, and painful stimuli.

THE SKIN

The skin is composed of two layers: the *epidermis*, a specialized epithelium derived from the ectoderm, and beneath this, the *dermis* (or *corium*), of vascular dense connective tissue, a derivative of mesoderm; the dermis corresponds to the lamina propria of a mucous membrane. These two layers are firmly adherent to each other and form a membrane that varies in thickness from about 0.5 to 4 mm or more in different parts of the body. Beneath the dermis is a layer of loose connective tissue which varies from areolar to adipose in character. This is the superficial fascia of gross anatomy, sometimes referred to as the *hypodermis*, but it is not considered to be part of the skin. The dermis is connected to the underlying hypodermis by connective tissue fibers which pass from one layer to the other. The superficial fascia permits great mobility of skin over most regions of the body. It is only in local areas such as the palm and the sole, where there is considerable interlocking of fibers between dermis and hypodermis, that mobility is limited.

The free surface of the skin exhibits numerous ridges which can be seen with the naked eye. They run in various directions and are most apparent on the palms of the hands and the soles of the feet. The patterns, which consist of loops, whorls, and arches, are determined in the main by hereditary factors and correspond to similar patterns on the surface of the dermis, the *dermal ridges*. Thus, in sections, the boundary between epidermis and dermis appears uneven. However, variations in the degree of development of ridges do occur, and ridges are absent on the forehead, external ear, perineum, and scrotum. The ridges seen on the skin of the palmar surface of the fingers constitute the basis for the prints used in personal identification, since they are subject to marked individual variation and never change (apart from enlargement) after they are formed during the third and fourth months of fetal life.

Skin is classified commonly as thick or thin, thick skin being found on the palms of the hands and soles of the feet, thin skin covering the remainder of the body. It should be emphasized that these terms, thick and thin, do not refer to the thickness of the skin as a whole, only to the epidermis. Thin skin itself varies greatly in thickness in different parts of the body and these variations are due, in actual fact, almost entirely to variations in the thickness of the dermis. The dermis of extensor surfaces is usually thicker than that of flexor surfaces. Both regions, however, have an epidermal component which is classified as thin.

The Epidermis

The epidermis, a stratified squamous epithelium, is composed of cells of two separate origins. The bulk of the epithelium, of ectodermal origin, undergoes a process of *keratinization* resulting in the formation of the dead superficial layers of skin. The second component comprises the melanocytes which produce melanin. The latter cells do not undergo keratinization. The superficial keratinized cells are continuously lost from the surface and must be replaced by cells that arise as a result of mitotic activity of cells of the basal layers of the epidermis. Cells which result from this proliferation are displaced to higher levels, and as they move upward they elaborate keratin. Keratin eventually replaces the majority of the cytoplasm, the cell dies and finally is shed. Thus it should be appreciated that the structural organization of the epidermis into layers reflects stages in the dynamic processes of cellular proliferation and differentiation.

Epidermis of the Palms and Soles. The epidermis here is particularly thick and exhibits maximal layering and cellular differentiation. It consists of five layers or strata: stratum germinativum or stratum basale, resting upon the dermis; stratum spinosum or prickle cell layer; stratum granulosum; stratum lucidum; and stratum corneum, the outermost horny layer.

The *stratum germinativum* consists of a single layer of columnar cells, each cell of which has short, thin, cytoplasmic processes on its basal surface. These toothlike processes fit into pockets of

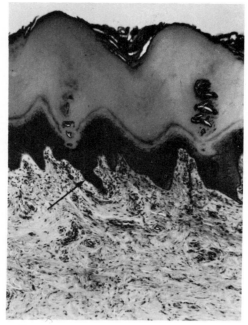

Figure 10–1. Low-power photomicrograph of a section of thick skin of sole of foot. Note that the epidermis consists chiefly of keratin (stratum corneum), in which portions of two ducts of sweat glands can be seen as they pass through to the surface. The junction between the epidermis and the dermis (arrow) is irregular. × 100.

the basal lamina and appear to anchor the epithelium to the underlying dermis. The plasma membrane in relation to the basal lamina exhibits numerous hemidesmosomes. Desmosomes occur frequently at the lateral and upper surfaces of the cells and serve to bind the cells together. Electron microscopy shows that the cells contain bundles of fine filaments randomly distributed throughout the cytoplasm. Aggregates of these filaments are visible on light microscopy as *tonofibrils*. Mitotic figures occur frequently in this layer, thus producing new cells which are displaced into the layer above.

The *stratum spinosum* is several layers thick and is composed of irregular, polyhedral cells, slightly separated from each other. Toward the surface the cells become flattened. The surface of the cells (*prickle cells* or *keratocytes*) is covered with short cytoplasmic spines or projections which meet with similar projections of adjacent cells to form "intercellular bridges." It should be emphasized that these do not indicate cy-

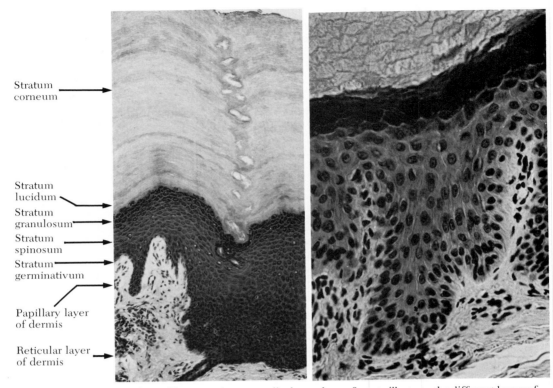

Stratum
corneum

Stratum
lucidum
Stratum
granulosum
Stratum
spinosum
Stratum
germinativum

Papillary layer
of dermis

Reticular layer
of dermis

Figure 10–2. Sections of human sole, perpendicular to the surface, to illustrate the different layers of the skin. Left, ×175; right, ×300.

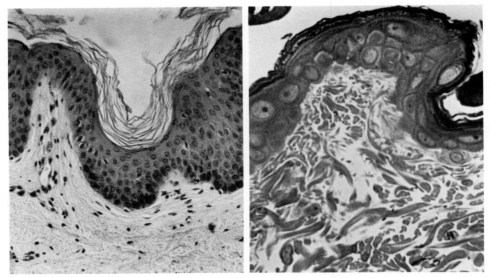

Figure 10–3. *Left:* Section of thin skin of a Negro. Compare with Figure 10–2 (thick skin). Note the scattered cells representative of the stratum granulosum and the thinness of the stratum corneum. There is marked deposition of pigment (melanin) in the lower layers of the epidermis, particularly in the stratum germinativum. × 180. *Right:* Section of thin skin of Caucasian. Plastic section. × 550.

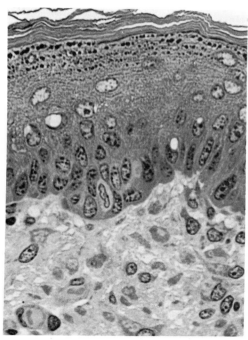

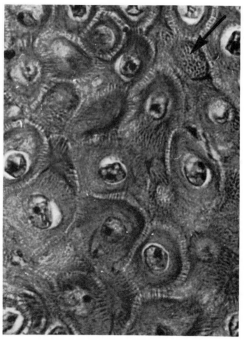

Figure 10–4. Section through the skin of the palm of the hand in a human fetus. At this stage, dermal ridges are low and cells of the stratum spinosum appear immature. Note the accumulation of keratohyalin granules within the stratum granulosum and the thin stratum corneum. Plastic section. × 450.

Figure 10–5. Oil immersion photomicrograph of a section of human palm, stained with iron hematoxylin, showing junctions between cells of the stratum spinosum. In one region (arrow), the contacts are seen in cross section. × 1200.

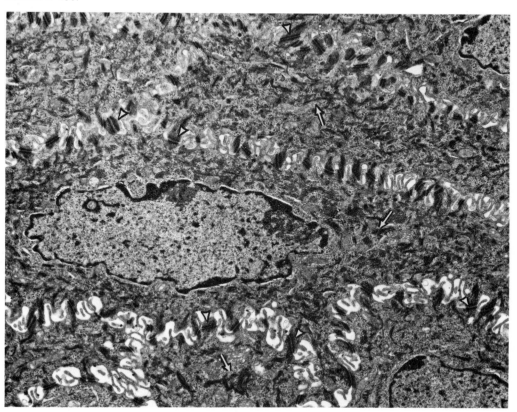

Figure 10–6. Electron micrograph of cells of the stratum spinosum. Note the presence of tonofibrils (arrows) and the wide intercellular spaces crossed by cytoplasmic processes. The areas of contact between the latter are marked by desmosomes (arrowheads). × 7500.

toplasmic continuity between cells. Electron micrographs demonstrate that the short processes constituting a "bridge" make intimate contact at a desmosome. Hence the cells are independent entities. The cytoplasm of these cells is basophil, indicating a considerable content of RNA, in this case associated with protein synthesis for growth and division of cells. The cytoplasm also contains numerous bundles of filaments which form the *tonofibrils.* Many of these pass into cytoplasmic processes and terminate in the desmosome. They do not extend across cell membranes. It is thought that the tonofibrils are the principal precursor of keratin. Additionally, the cytoplasm contains a number of membrane-bound granules, the significance of which is uncertain. It has been suggested that they may contribute to the intercellular material or that they may deposit dense material on the inner aspect of the cell membrane.

It should be mentioned at this point that the two layers just described, the stratum germinativum and stratum spinosum, are grouped together as the Malpighian layer (stratum [or rete] Malpighii) by many authors. This layer

is responsible for proliferation and for initiation of the keratinization process. The Malpighian layer also contains *melanocytes,* which produce the pigment, melanin, described below under "Pigmentation." Additionally, scattered in this layer are Langerhan's and Merkel cells whose functional significance is unknown.

The next layer, the *stratum granulosum,* consists of three to five layers of flattened cells whose long axis is parallel to the skin surface. The cytoplasm of these cells contains granules of *keratohyalin,* which stain with some acid dyes and with certain basic dyes. On electron microscopy, the granules appear as irregularly shaped masses of electron-dense material in association with bundles of filaments. The origin of these granules is obscure, but they appear to be involved in the process of formation of soft keratin. With increase in size and number of these granules, the nuclei become pale and indistinct, and show degenerative changes. The granules later become intimately associated with tonofibrils, and cell contacts become indistinct. It is in this layer that the cells of the epidermis die.

The *stratum lucidum* is a clear translu-

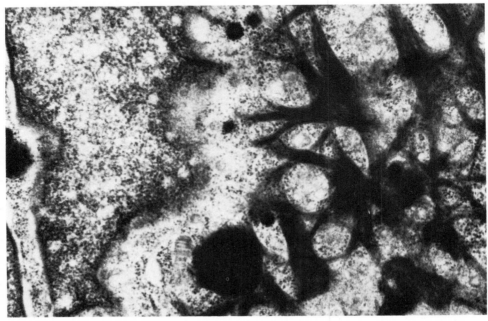

Figure 10–7.   Electron micrograph of a cell of the stratum granulosum, with a portion of the nucleus (left). Note the irregular granules of keratohyalin. × 35,000.

cent layer, three to five cells deep. Cells are not distinguishable clearly as separate entities. They are flattened and closely packed. Nuclei are indistinct or absent. The cytoplasm contains a semifluid substance, *keratohyalin*, which is presumed to be a product of the granules noted in subjacent layers. The keratohyalin is distributed among the tonofibrils, which generally now are arranged parallel to the surface of the skin.

The fifth and outermost layer, the *stratum corneum*, is composed of clear, dead, scalelike cells which become progressively flattened and fused. The nucleus is absent and the cytoplasm is replaced with keratin, thought to be derived principally from the tonofibrils of the deeper layers of the epidermis.

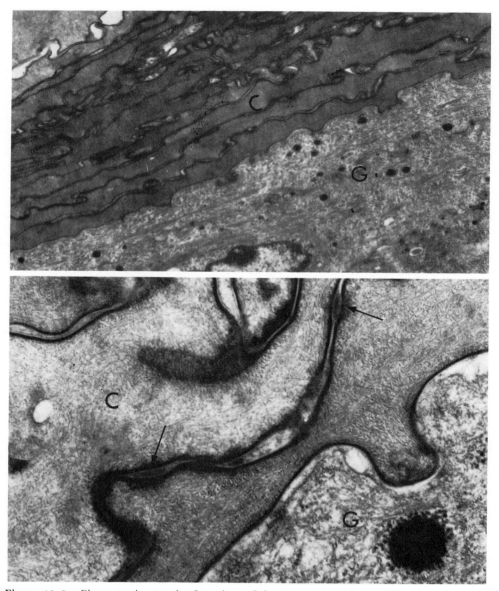

Figure 10–8. Electron micrograph of portions of the stratum granulosum (G) and of the stratum corneum (C). Cells of the latter are filled with keratin which, at low magnification, appears amorphous. Desmosomes (arrows) between the cells are relatively well preserved. Top: ×20,000. Bottom: ×70,000.

This is "soft keratin," low in sulfur content, as distinct from "hard keratin" found in nails and the cortex of hairs. The most superficial layers of the stratum corneum (sometimes called *stratum disjunctum*) are flat horny plates which are desquamated constantly. The stratum corneum stains pink with eosin and often is shredded during specimen preparation. Thus, from the surface of the epidermis, there is a constant loss of dead cells which are replaced by new cells formed as a result of mitoses in the deeper layers, principally in the stratum germinativum and the stratum spinosum, and pushed toward the surface during the process of keratinization.

Epidermis of the General Body Surface. The epidermis of the rest of the body is both thinner and simpler than that of the palms and soles. All layers of the epidermis are reduced and the stratum lucidum is usually absent. The stratum germinativum is similar to that of thick skin but the stratum spinosum is not so extensive. The granular layer may be present as one or two rows of cells or may be represented by scattered cells along the line where this layer might be expected. The reduction in thickness of the epidermis of thin skin is due probably to the fact that keratinization here is less marked and is not a continuous process.

Pigmentation. The color of the skin is dependent upon three factors. The color of skin itself is yellow, owing to the presence of carotene. Blood, showing through from the underlying vascular dermis, imparts a reddish hue. Finally, the presence of varying amounts of melanin pigment is responsible for shades of brown. Melanin is present mainly in the stratum germinativum and in the deeper layers of the stratum spinosum.

As cells move toward the surface, the granules of melanin (*melanosomes*) become dustlike and cannot be identified as definite entities in the stratum corneum. In colored races, pigment is present in greater amounts in all layers of the epidermis. The pigment is not elaborated in the general cell population of the epidermis but in specialized cells derived from the neural crest, the *melanocytes*, which then distribute it to the epidermal cells. Melanocytes are scattered within the basal layer of the epidermis and send numerous cytoplasmic processes between the cells of the stratum spinosum. These cells contain an enzyme, *tyrosinase*, which is involved in synthesis of the pigment. Exposure to x-rays and to ultraviolet light increases the enzymic activity of these cells and thus leads to increased melanin production and deposition in the epidermis and to tanning. Melanocytes cannot be identified in normal preparations but can be made visible with a special reagent, "dopa," which they oxidize, coloring them black. The fate of the pigment in the epidermis is not clearly understood, but it is thought that it is probably broken down and eliminated with the epidermal scales. Characteristically, melanin granules in cells of the stratum germinativum are found related to the superficial aspect of the nucleus.

Dermis

It is difficult to define the exact limits to the dermis since it merges into the underlying subcutaneous layer (hypodermis). However, the average thickness varies from 0.5 mm to 3 mm or more. It is composed of dense irregularly arranged connective tissue and is subdivided into two strata, the *papillary layer* superficially and the *reticular layer* beneath. The papillary layer includes the ridges and papillae that protrude into the epidermis. Papillae tend to occur in double rows and often are branched. Some papillae contain special nerve terminations (nervous papillae); others possess loops of capillary blood vessels (vascular papillae). The papillary layer is composed of thin collagenous, reticular, and elastic fibers arranged in an extensive network. Just beneath the epidermis, reticular fibers of the dermis form a close feltwork of fibrils which insert into the basal lamina beneath the epidermis and extend perpendicularly into the dermis as anchoring fibrils.

The reticular layer is the main fibrous bed of the dermis. It consists of coarse, dense, and interlacing collagenous fibers, in which are intermingled a few reticular fibers and .numerous elastic fibers. The predominant direction of all fibers is parallel to the surface. Owing to the direction of the fibers, lines of skin tension, *Langer's lines,* are formed. The direction of these lines is of surgical importance since incisions made parallel with the lines gape less and heal with less scar tissue than incisions made at right angles to or obliquely across the lines.

The predominant cellular elements of the dermis are fibroblasts and macrophages. In addition, fat cells may be present, either singly or, more commonly, in groups. Apart from the usual types of connective tissue cells, pigmented, branched, connective tissue cells, *chromatophores,* may be present. They are numerous only in areas where the overlying epidermis is heavily pigmented, for example, in the areola of the nipple and the circumanal region. They do not elaborate their pigment but obtain it apparently from melanocytes. True *dermal* melanocytes are rare. These, like the melanocytes of the epidermis, are dopa-positive. They may accumulate in the sacral region, where they form the "mongolian spot," or in certain tumors of the dermis (blue nevi). Generally, the papillary layer contains more cells and smaller and finer connective tissue fibers than the reticular layer.

Smooth muscle fibers may be found in the dermis. They are arranged in small bundles in connection with hair follicles (*arrectores pilorum* muscles) and are scattered throughout the dermis in considerable numbers in the skin of the nipple, penis, scrotum, and parts of the perineum. Contraction of the fibers gives the skin of these regions a wrinkled appearance. In the face and neck, fibers of some skeletal muscles terminate in delicate elastic fiber networks of the dermis.

Hypodermis. The subcutaneous layer (superficial fascia) is not part of the skin, but appears as a deep extension of the dermis. The density and arrangement of the subcutaneous layer determine the mobility of the skin. Depending upon the region of the body and the general state of nutrition of the organism, varying numbers of fat cells occur in the hypodermis. When continuous lobules of fat are present, the hypodermis forms a fat pad, the *panniculus adiposus.* On the abdomen this layer may reach a thickness of 3 cm or more. In the eyelids, penis, and scrotum the subcutaneous layer is devoid of fat. The superfical zone of the hypodermis contains parts of the hair follicles and sweat glands.

THE NAILS

The nails are horny plates that form a protective covering on the dorsal surface of the terminal phalanges of the fingers and toes. Their structure and relationship to the epidermis and

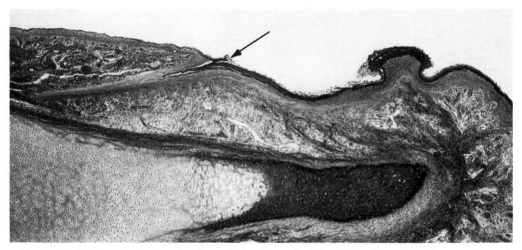

Figure 10–9. Longitudinal section through the finger of a human fetus. Note the nail groove (arrow), the developing nail bed, and the cartilaginous model of the terminal phalanx (below). ×50.

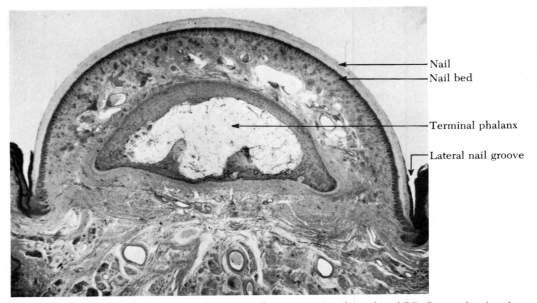

Figure 10–10. Low-power photomicrograph of a cross section through a child's finger, showing the nail and nail bed. × 30.

dermis are understood best if consideration is given to their early development. Toward the end of the third month of intrauterine life, the epidermis over the dorsal surface of the terminal phalanx of each finger and toe invades the underlying dermis. Unlike the early development of a gland, which is a tubular ingrowth of epithelial cells into the underlying connective tissue, in the case of the nail the invasion occurs along a transverse curved line and slants proximally with relation to the surface. The invading plate of epidermis later splits to form a *nail groove*, and the epidermal cells of the deep (distal) wall of the groove proliferate to form the matrix of the nail. With continuing proliferation and differentiation of cells in the lower part of the matrix, the forming *nail plate* is pushed out of the groove and slowly advances over the dorsal surface of the digit toward the distal end. The epidermis immediately beneath the nail plate constitutes the *nail bed.* The nail

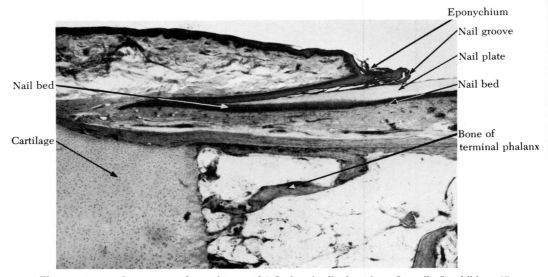

Figure 10–11. Low-power photomicrograph of a longitudinal section of a nail of a child. × 45.

plate itself is contained within the nail groove, which becomes U-shaped as seen from the dorsum, flanked by a skin fold, the *nail wall*. The nail bed, which underlies both the exposed and concealed portions of the nail, consists of only the deeper layers of the epidermis and the underlying dermis, which is ridged longitudinally. It lacks sweat glands and hair follicles. The epidermis of the nail bed, the matrix, is thickest proximally, and it is here that nail growth chiefly occurs and the rate of cell division is rapid. Component cells contain numerous cytoplasmic fibrils which are lost at a later stage as the cells become homogeneous, cornify, and join the nail plate. At no time can keratohyalin granules be recognized in cells of the matrix, and the keratin of the nail is termed hard.

Epidermis of the nail bed is continuous distally with epidermis of the finger tip under the free edge of the nail. At the junction, the stratum corneum of the epidermis is thickened. This thickened epidermis is known as the *hyponychium*. The nail plate itself consists of intimately fused epidermal scales that do not desquamate. The body of the plate is translucent and transmits the pink color of blood vessels in the nail bed. The root is more opaque than the body since cornification and drying are incomplete. The root becomes continuous with the body of the nail over a crescentic margin, a portion of which junction is visible distal to the nail groove. This is the *lunule*. The nail groove is lined by modified epidermis of the nail wall. Cells of the stratum corneum extend from the nail wall onto the free surface of the nail plate as the *eponychium*, or cuticle.

The addition of newly keratinized cells to the nail root results in a slow movement of the nail plate over the nail bed. On the average, nails grow at the rate of about 0.5 mm a week; growth is quicker in the finger nails than in toe nails. If a nail is removed forcibly, a new nail will grow if the matrix is not destroyed.

THE HAIR

Hairs are elastic keratinized threads that develop from the epidermis. They vary from 1 mm or less to 1.5 meters in length and from 0.05 to 0.5 mm in thickness. They are distributed over the entire skin except for the palms, soles, dorsal surfaces of the distal phalanges, and region of the anal and urogenital apertures. Each hair has a free *shaft* and a *root* embedded in the skin. Enclosing the hair root is a tubular *hair follicle*, which consists of epidermal (epithelial) and dermal (connective tissue) portions. At its lower end the follicle expands into a *hair bulb*, which is indented at the basal end by a connective tissue *papilla*. Associated with the hair follicle are one or more sebaceous glands and a bundle of smooth muscle. The muscle, the *arrector pili*, is attached at one end to the connective tissue sheath of the follicle and at the other to the papillary layer of the dermis. By its contraction it causes erection of the hair since the hair is not set perpendicularly to the skin surface but slopes at an obtuse angle.

Structure of the Hair

The hair consists of epidermal cells arranged in three concentric layers: the medulla, cortex, and cuticle. The medulla forms the loose central axis and consists of two or three layers of shrunken, cornified, cuboidal cells which are separated partially by air spaces. The medulla is absent in fine short hairs of the downy type and is missing also from some of the hairs of the scalp and from "blonde" hair. The cells often contain pigment. The keratin of medullary cells is of the "soft" type.

The cortex makes up the main bulk of the hair and is composed of several layers of long, flattened, spindle-shaped cornified cells in which the keratin is of the "hard" type. The keratin fibrils are oriented parallel to the long axis of the hair, and pigment granules are found in and between cells. Black hair contains pigment that is oxidized. Air also accumulates in the intercellular spaces of cortical cells and modifies the hair color. Superficially there is a single layer of thin clear cells, the cuticle. These are cornified cells which, except for those in the base of the root, have lost their nuclei. The cells overlap, like shingles on a roof,

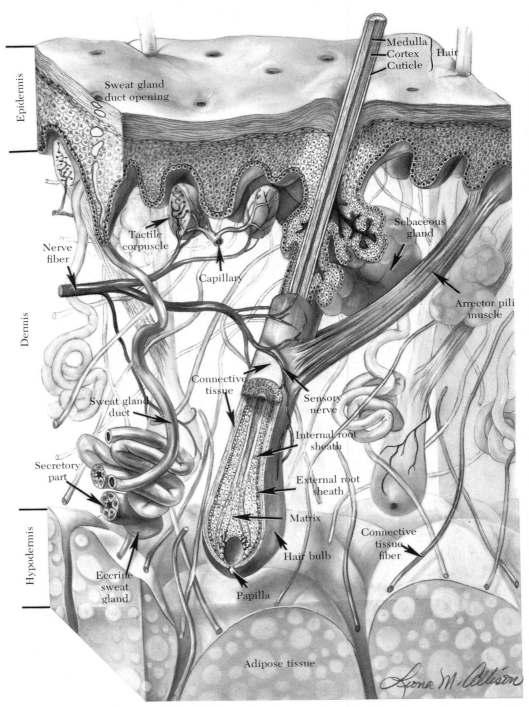

Figure 10–12.   Diagram of hair follicle to show the general relationships between it, arrector pili muscle, and sebaceous and sweat glands.

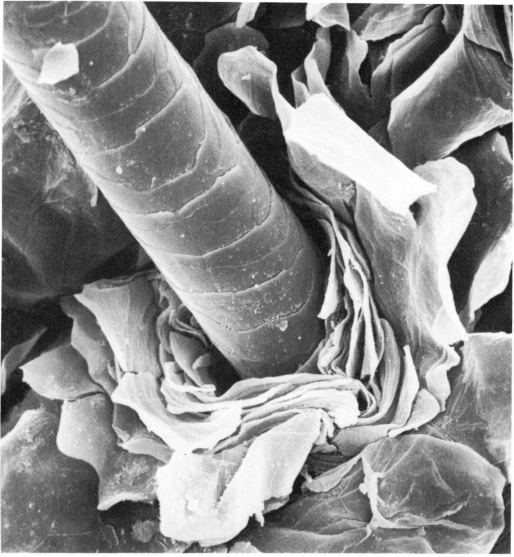

Figure 10–13. Scanning electron micrograph of a hair. Note the way in which cells of the cuticle overlap. Monkey scalp. × 1400 (Courtesy of Dr. P. M. Andrews.)

with their free edges directed upward. The appearance of hair in cross section varies from race to race. The straight hair of the Mongol races (Chinese, Eskimos, and American Indians) is round whereas the wavy hair of many people, including Caucasians, is oval in cross section. The cross section of the wooly hair of Negroes is elliptical or reniform.

The Hair Follicle

The hair follicle is a compound sheath which consists of an external connective tissue sheath (the *dermal root sheath*) derived from the dermis and an internal *epithelial root sheath* from the epidermis. The epithelial root sheath is subdivided into inner and outer components. Toward its deep end, the follicle is expanded into a hair bulb where the hair root and its sheath blend in a mass of primitive cells, the matrix. The base of the bulb is invaginated by a connective tissue papilla, and it is in relation to the papilla that the hair root and its sheaths merge. The hair papilla, although much larger, is similar in structure to other dermal papillae and

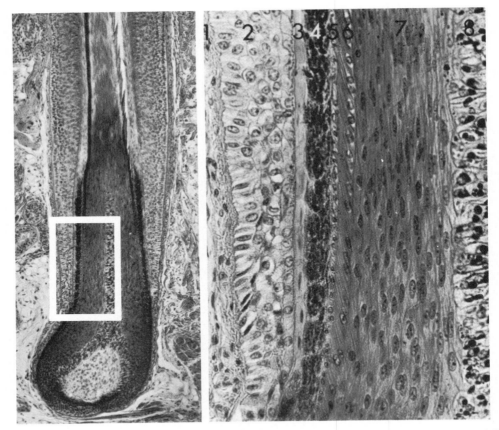

Figure 10–14.   Longitudinal section of human hair follicle. Note that the section passes tangentially through the connective tissue papilla. (1) Glassy membrane. (2) External root sheath. (3) Henle's layer. (4) Huxley's layer. (5) Cuticle of the root sheath. (6, 7, 8) Cuticle, cortex and medulla of the hair respectively. Left, × 50; right, × 275.

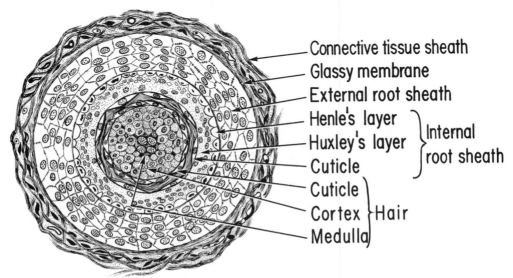

Connective tissue sheath
Glassy membrane
External root sheath
Henle's layer   ⎫ Internal
Huxley's layer   ⎬ root sheath
Cuticle   ⎭
Cuticle   ⎫
Cortex   ⎬ Hair
Medulla   ⎭

Figure 10–15.   Diagram of a hair follicle in cross section beneath the level of entry of a sebaceous gland.

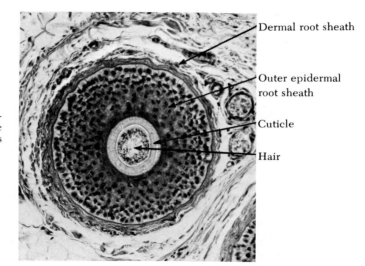

Figure 10–16. Cross section of human hair follicle above the level of entry of a sebaceous gland. ×180.

Dermal root sheath

Outer epidermal root sheath

Cuticle

Hair

contains delicate connective tissue fibers, cellular elements, and a rich plexus of blood vessels and nerves. All layers of the follicle are not found at all levels but are represented best in the portion of the follicle between the bulb and the entry of a sebaceous gland.

The dermal root sheath is composed of three layers, corresponding to similar strata of the dermis. The outer layer is poorly defined and consists of coarse bundles of collagen fibers running in a longitudinal direction. It corresponds to the reticular layer of the dermis. The middle layer is thicker and corresponds to the papillary layer of the dermis. It is cellular and contains fine connective tissue fibers, circularly arranged. The inner layer is a homogeneous narrow band, the *glassy membrane*, corresponding to the basal lamina beneath the epidermis. It consists of reticular fibers and amorphous ground substance.

The epidermal root sheath has an outer component, continuous with the deeper layers of the epidermis, and an inner component, which corresponds to the more specialized, superficial layers. The outer epithelial root sheath possesses a single row of tall cells directly in relation to the glassy membrane and an inner stratum of polygonal cells (with cell contacts) which resemble cells of the stratum spinosum of the epidermis. The inner epithelial root sheath is a keratinized sheath enveloping the growing hair root and,

like the hair, it is pushed up by addition of cells from the bulb. It elaborates "soft keratin" with a keratohyalin stage that is similar to that found in epidermis. The inner sheath does not extend above the point of entry of the duct of the sebaceous gland into the follicle. It has three distinct strata: *Henle's layer, Huxley's layer,* and the *cuticle of the root sheath.* Henle's layer, directly in relation to the outer epithelial root sheath, is a single layer of flattened, clear cells which contain hyaline fibrils. Immediately internal to this is Huxley's layer, which consists of several rows of elongated cells whose cytoplasm contains *trichohyalin* granules, much like keratohyalin, and bundles of tonofibrils. In the deeper portion of the hair follicle the cells contain nuclei, but superficially nuclei are pyknotic or absent. The cuticle of the root sheath lies against the cuticle of the hair and is similar to the latter in structure. It is a single layer of transparent, horny scales, the free edges of which project downward and interdigitate with the upward projecting scales of the hair cuticle. This interlocking explains why the inner root sheath is also removed when a hair is extracted.

Growth of the hair occurs following mitosis in cells of the undifferentiated matrix of epidermal cells above and around the dermal papilla of the follicle. Cells immediately above the apex of the papilla form the medulla; those above the slope and sides form the cortex and cuticle of the hair respectively. Cells immediately lateral to the papilla transform into the inner root sheath which, like the hair root, grows upward. Cells at the bottom of the follicle continue into the outer root sheath. The cells of the hair matrix are analogous to the Malpighian layer of the epidermis in that the life cycle of each terminates with the formation of cornified cells. In the case of the epidermis the product is soft keratinous material and the process is continuous. The product of matrix cells is a hard keratinous material and the process is intermittent and is dependent upon an inductive influence of

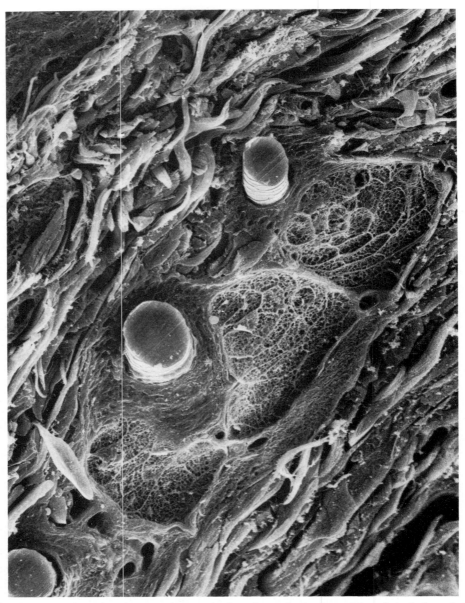

Figure 10–17.   Scanning electron micrograph of monkey scalp. Portions of three hair shafts and of the sebaceous glands associated with them are shown. They lie embedded within the coarse connective tissue of the dermis. × 300. (Courtesy of Dr. P. M. Andrews.)

a particular portion of the dermis. Pigment is acquired from melanocytes present within the matrix in a manner similar to that occurring in the epidermis.

Hair has a definite period of growth. For the head it is about two to four years, for eyelashes only three to four months. Upon cessation of growth, multiplication of the undifferentiated cells at the base of the follicle ceases. The root of the hair then becomes detached from the matrix and the hair either falls out or is pulled out. After a resting phase, the remaining cord of epithelial cells of the follicle undergoes a period of growth and contacts either the old papilla or a new one. A new germinal matrix develops and a new hair begins to grow up the re-forming follicle.

GLANDS OF THE SKIN

Glands of the skin include sebaceous, sweat, and mammary glands. Mammary glands, which are specialized sweat glands, are described with the female genital system (p. 508).

Sebaceous Glands

The sebaceous glands are, with a few exceptions, connected with hair follicles. Usually several drain into a single hair follicle but where they are independent of hairs, their ducts open directly upon the free surface of the skin, for example, in glans penis, labia minora, and tarsal (meibomian) glands of the eyelids. They are lacking entirely in the palms and the soles. Sebaceous glands are located in the dermis, where each gland is encapsulated by a thin layer of connective tissue. They are alveolar (saccular) glands which synthesize lipid. In most glands several alveoli open into a short wide duct, which itself empties into the neck of a hair follicle. The alveoli themselves are filled completely with a stratified epithelium. The epithelium of the secretory portion lies upon a delicate basal lamina, on the internal surface of which is a single row of small cuboidal cells, continuous with the basal cells of the epidermis at the neck of the hair follicle. These cells acquire increased amounts of agranular endoplasmic reticulum before they become active in lipogenesis. Toward the center of the

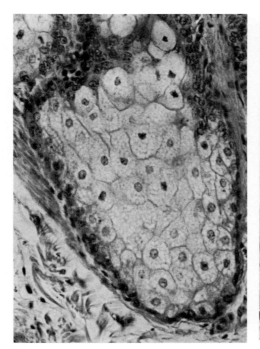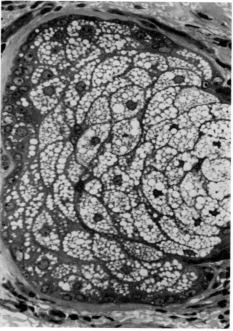

Figure 10–18. High-power photomicrographs of human sebaceous glands. *Left:* Paraffin section. ×275. *Right:* Plastic section. ×400.

alveolus, cells become progressively larger and the cytoplasm is distended with fat droplets. The droplets contain cholesterol, phospholipids, and triglycerides. Nuclei gradually shrink and then disappear and the cells break down into a fatty mass and cellular debris. This is the oily secretion (*sebum*) of the gland, which is of the holocrine type since it results from total destruction of epithelial cells. Cells lost in the secretory process are replaced by proliferation from the basal cells and from cells close to the wall of the excretory duct. The short, wide duct of sebaceous glands is lined by stratified squamous epithelium continuous with the external root sheath of the hair and with the Malpighian layer of the epidermis. Toward the alveolus, the layering decreases progressively until finally it merges with the row of low basal cells of the alveolus. Discharge of secretion is aided by contraction of the arrector pili muscle and by general pressure owing to an increase in the size of cells centrally within the alveolus.

Sweat Glands

The ordinary sweat glands (*eccrine* type) are unbranched, coiled, tubular glands distributed throughout the skin, except upon the nail bed, margins of the lips, glans penis, and eardrum. They are most numerous in the palms and soles. The secretory portion is situated deeply in the dermis, or in the hypodermis, and is coiled into a discrete mass. The excretory portion, or duct, rises to the epidermis by a slightly tortuous course, joins the epidermis, and spirals through it to reach the free surface where it opens by a minute pit, the *sweat pore*.

The coiled secretory portion of the gland is lined by a simple columnar or cuboidal epithelium supported by a distinct basal lamina. Three distinct cell types are present in the epithelium. The principal (clear) cells are serous and vary in height, depending upon the activity of the gland. The nucleus is spherical and occupies a midposition within the cell. The cytoplasm is vacuolated and contains fat droplets and, occasionally, pigment granules. Secretory capillaries (intercellular canaliculi) can be demonstrated between the cells. Scattered between serous cells are mucigenous (dark) cells, which contain small basophilic secretory granules. Between the bases of the cells and the bounding basal lamina, there is a zone occupied by spindle-shaped myoepithelial cells, which wind in longitudinal

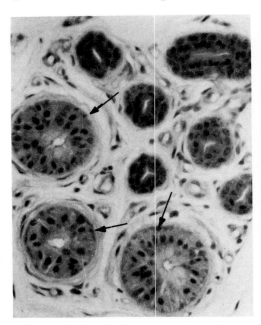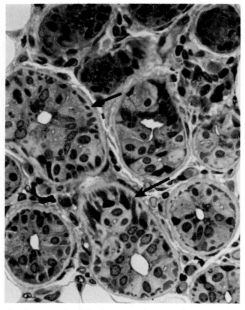

Figure 10–19.   Medium power photomicrographs of a human (eccrine) sweat gland — duct portion top right, secretory portion bottom left. Processes of myoepithelial cells are present in relation to the secretory portion (arrows). *Left*, Paraffin section, ×225; *right*, Plastic section. ×250.

spirals around the tubule. The nucleus of such cells is elongated and the cytoplasm deeply acidophil. They are thought to be specialized smooth muscle cells which are contractile and aid in emptying the gland of secretion.

The secretory tubule narrows into a slender excretory duct which is lined with a double layer of darkly staining cuboidal cells. The cells which form the inner layer of the duct wall bear a specialized fibrous border along their free surface, where the cytoplasm appears homogeneous and stains intensely because of the concentration of tonofilaments. The duct is surrounded by a basal lamina, but no myoepithelial elements are interposed between it and the lining epithelium. Where the duct joins the epidermis, it loses its own wall, becoming a specialized channel through the epithelium.

The ordinary sweat glands (eccrine type) are merocrine in their secretion, but certain large sweat glands found in the axilla, areola of the nipple, labia majora, and circumanal region produce a thicker secretion than the sweat formed by the smaller glands. In these large glands, the apices of the gland cells frequently are broken off in the process of preparation, but this is an artifact and secretion is merocrine in type, although the glands traditionally still are called apocrine glands. No clear cells are present; the mucigenous (dark) cells are similar to those of eccrine sweat glands and contain secretory granules and numerous secondary lysosomes. These large sweat glands show less coiling than do ordinary sweat glands and the lumen of the secretory portion is much wider. Myoepithelial cells are larger and form a more complete layer between the epithelial cells and the basal lamina. The wax-secreting *ceruminous* glands of the external auditory canal and the *glands of Moll* in the margin of the eyelid also belong to this group of larger sweat glands.

BLOOD VESSELS, LYMPHATICS, AND NERVES OF THE SKIN
Blood Vessels

The blood supply to the skin is from large arteries in the subcutaneous layer.

These vessels send branches superficially to form a horizontally oriented network (*rete cutaneum*) at the junctional zone between dermis and hypodermis. From this network, branches pass on one side to supply the subcutaneous tissue including sweat glands and the deeper portions of hair follicles, and on the other side to the dermis where they form a further network between the papillary and reticular layers (the *rete subpapillare*). From the latter plexus, small arteries are given off to the papillae, where they break up into capillary networks to supply the papillae, sebaceous glands, and the intermediate portion of the hair follicle.

Veins collecting blood from the area supplied by the rete subpapillare form a network immediately beneath the papillae. This network communicates with a second plexus just deeper than the first and via this with a third plexus at the junction of the dermis with the hypodermis. Into the latter plexus pass most of the veins from the fat lobules and sweat glands. From the third plexus, veins pass to a deeper network of large veins in the subcutaneous tissue which is drained by large veins accompanying the arteries. Arteriovenous anastomoses are common within the deeper layers of the dermis.

Lymphatics

The lymphatics begin in the papillae as endothelium-lined clefts, which pass to a horizontal network of lymph capillaries in the papillary layer. This network communicates with a network of larger lymph capillaries in the subcutaneous tissue, which also receives lymph from delicate plexuses surrounding sebaceous and sweat glands and hair follicles.

Nerves

The skin, together with its accessory organs, receives stimuli from the external environment and thus is abundantly supplied with sensory nerves. In the subcutaneous tissue, there are bundles of large nerves which send branches to several plexuses in the reticular, papillary, and subepithelial zones. In all layers of the skin and hypodermis there

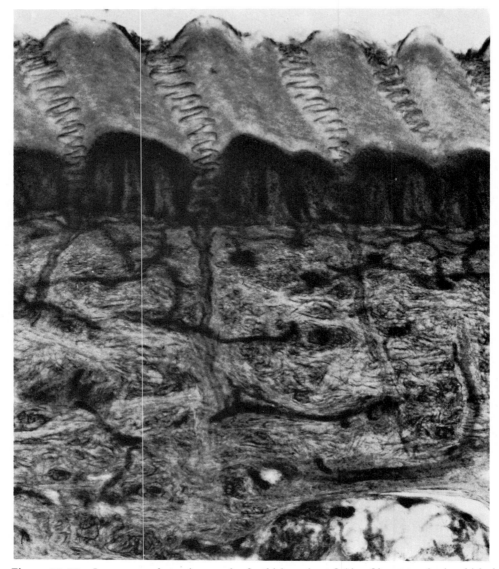

Figure 10–20. Low-power photomicrograph of a thick section of skin of human palm in which the blood vessels were injected with red gelatin. In this thick section, one also has a good demonstration of the spiral course taken through the epidermis by ducts of sweat glands. ×80.

are numerous nerve endings of various kinds (see Chapter 17). Apart from free endings of unmyelinated sensory fibers in or close to the epidermis, there are numerous fibers supplying hair follicles. In addition to sensory nerves, there are efferent sympathetic fibers supplying the blood vessels, the arrectores pilorum, and the secretory cells of the sweat glands.

REFERENCES

Bell, M. A.: A comparative study of sebaceous gland ultrastructure in subhuman primates. I. Anat. Rec., *166*:213, 1970.

Bertalanffy, F. D.: Mitotic and renewal rate of sebaceous gland cells in the rat. Anat. Rec., *129*:231, 1957.

Birbeck, M. S. C., and Mercer, E. H.: Electron microscopy of the human hair follicle. J. Biophys. Biochem. Cytol., *3*:203, 1957.

Braverman, I. N., and Yen, A.: Ultrastructure of the human dermal microcirculation. II. The capillary loops of the dermal papillae. Invest. Dermatol., *68*:53, 1977.

Breathnach, A. S.: An Atlas of the Ultrastructure of Human Skin. London, J. & A. Churchill, 1971.

Brody, I.: Variations in the differentiation of the fibrils in the normal human stratum corneum as revealed by electron microscopy. J. Ultrastruct. Res., *30*:601, 1970.

Brody, I.: Ultrastructure of the stratum corneum. Dermatology, *16*:245, 1977.

Bunting, H., Wislocki, G. B., and Dempsey, E. W.: The chemical histology of human eccrine and apocrine sweat glands. Anat. Rec., *100*:61, 1948.

Chase, H. B.: Growth of the hair. Physiol. Rev., *34*:113, 1954.

Ellis, R. A.: Fine structure of the myoepithelium of the eccrine sweat glands of man. J. Cell Biol., *27*:551, 1965.

Fukuyama, K., Weir, K. A., and Epstein, W. L.: Dense homogeneous deposits of keratohyalin granules in newborn rat epidermis. J. Ultrastruct. Res., *38*:16, 1972.

Hashiomoto, K.: Ultrastructure of the human toenail. J. Ultrastruct. Res., *36*:391, 1971.

Hibbs, R. G., and Clark, W. H., Jr.: Electron microscope studies of the human epidermis. J. Biophys. Biochem. Cytol., *6*:71, 1959.

Laidlaw, G. F.: The dopa reaction in normal histology. Anat. Rec., *53*:339, 1932.

Montagna, W.: The Structure and Function of Skin, ed. 3. New York, Academic Press, 1974.

Montagna, W., and Lobitz, W. C. (editors): The Epidermis. New York, Academic Press, 1964.

Odland, G. F.: The fine structure of the interrelationship of cells in the human epidermis. J. Biophys. Biochem. Cytol., *4*:529, 1958.

Rogers, G. E.: Some aspects of the structure of the inner root sheath of hair follicles revealed by light and electron microscopy. Exp. Cell Res., *14*:378, 1958.

Spearman, R. I. C.: The Integument. London, Cambridge University Press, 1973.

Squier, C. A., and Rooney, L.: The permeability of keratinized and nonkeratinized oral epithelium to lanthanum in vivo. J. Ultrastruct. Res., *54*:286, 1976.

Zelickson, A. (editor): The Ultrastructure of Normal and Abnormal Skin. Philadelphia, Lea & Febiger, 1967.

THE DIGESTIVE TRACT

GENERAL ORGANIZATION

The digestive tract is a long tube extending from the mouth to the anus, and basically each part of the tube has a similar structure. In addition to the digestive tube, there are associated glands situated outside the tube but delivering their secretions into it by duct systems. The process of digestion involves first the breaking down of food material to a small particulate size, accomplished primarily by the cutting and grinding action of the teeth and also by the action of hydrochloric acid and digestive enzymes. Digestive enzymes help to split or hydrolyze complex food materials (proteins, carbohydrates, and fat) into smaller residues and thus are to be classed as hydrolytic enzymes or hydrolases. Secondly, digestion involves the absorption of such food materials into the circulation. It should be appreciated that any material within the lumen of the digestive tract virtually is outside the body and thus has to pass through the lining of the tract to enter the circulation. *Digestion, then, is the process whereby food material is converted into substances which can be absorbed into the circulation.* Materials which are useless, and some which even are toxic, are eliminated by fecal excretion.

The digestive tract will be described in three major sections: the oral cavity (including salivary glands and oropharynx), the tubular digestive tract (esophagus, stomach, small intestine, large intestine, rectum, and anal canal), and the major digestive glands (pancreas, liver, and biliary passages).

SECTION I. THE ORAL CAVITY

THE LIP

The oral cavity is closed anteriorly by apposition of upper and lower lips. The substance of each lip is composed of striated muscle fibers of the orbicularis oris muscle embedded in elastic fibroconnective tissue. Externally, the lip is covered by skin containing hair follicles, sebaceous glands, and sweat glands. At the free margin of the lip, the epithelium is modified by a high content of keratohyalin and a thick stratum lucidum, which renders it more transparent, and the underlying dermis shows high papillae with a very rich plexus of blood capillaries. It is blood in this plexus which is responsible for the red color of the free margin of the lip. In this region, there are no hairs, sweat glands, or sebaceous glands, and the surface epithelium can be kept moist only by licking with the tongue. On the internal aspect, the lip is covered by a mucous membrane consisting of a stratified squamous nonkeratinizing epithelium lying upon a connective tissue lamina propria with high papillae. Within the connective tissue are numerous small mucous glands (the la-

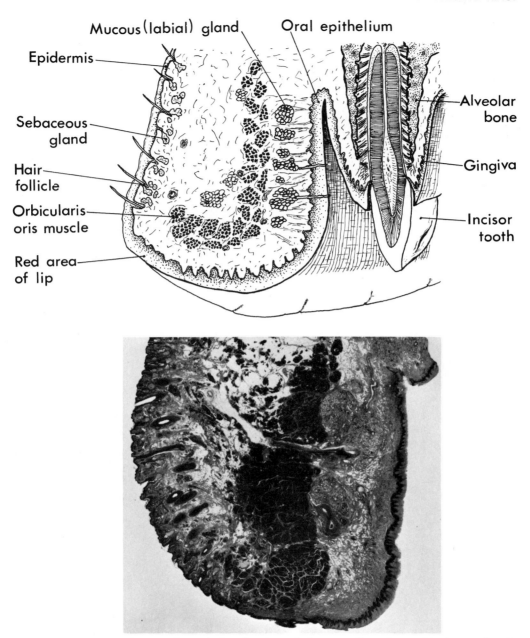

Epidermis

Mucous (labial) gland

Oral epithelium

Sebaceous gland

Hair follicle

Orbicularis oris muscle

Red area of lip

Alveolar bone

Gingiva

Incisor tooth

Figure 11–1. *Top:* Diagram of a vertical section through the upper lip and central incisor tooth. ×6. *Bottom:* Photomicrograph of a section through the upper lip, outer (skin) surface on the left. ×6.

bial glands), the secretion of which passes to the surface via short ducts. In the epithelium, some keratohyalin granules can be found in the more superficial layers and the surface cells constantly are worn off and appear in the saliva. Numerous sensory nerve endings are found both in the dermis of the red lip margin and in the lamina propria of the oral mucous membrane.

THE CHEEK

The cheek has a structure similar to the lip, with a core of striated muscle and elastic fibroconnective tissue lined internally by a mucous membrane covered by stratified squamous nonkeratinizing epithelium. A submucosa is present also, consisting of elastic connective tissue containing a rich vascular

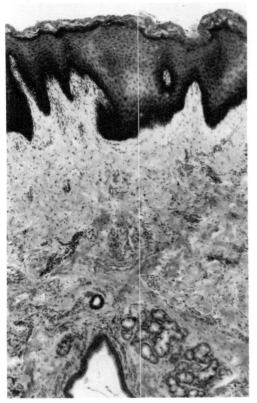

Figure 11–2. Photomicrograph of a section of the oral mucous membrane. Note the mucous glands in the submucosa. × 40.

plexus. The elastic fibers are continuous externally with those around the striated muscle and internally with those of the lamina propria. They serve to bind the mucous membrane (mucosa) quite firmly to the muscle and prevent folds of the mucous membrane from being formed and bitten between the teeth when the jaws are closed. Mucous (labial) salivary glands are present in the lamina propria of the cheek.

THE TONGUE

The tongue consists of a freely movable portion (the body) located in the oral cavity and a base or root attached to the floor and forming part of the anterior wall of the pharynx. On the upper or dorsal surface of the tongue is a V-shaped groove, the *sulcus terminalis*, with the apex of the V directed pos-

teriorly. This sulcus divides the tongue into anterior and posterior regions. The tongue is covered by a mucous membrane, and its bulk consists of striated muscle fibers and glands. The muscle fibers are both intrinsic and extrinsic; i.e., some are confined to the tongue, whereas others originate outside, principally on the mandible and hyoid bone, and pass into it. Between muscle fibers are glands. These glands are mainly mucous in the base of the tongue with their ducts opening behind the sulcus terminalis, serous in the body of the tongue with their ducts opening anterior to the sulcus (near circumvallate papillae), and mixed acini near the tip, their ducts opening on the inferior surface of the tongue.

The posterior third of the tongue has a nodular, irregular surface owing to the presence of lymphatic nodules (the lingual tonsil) (see p. 292). Between the protrusions are cleftlike depressions of the surface epithelium termed *crypts*. Here the epithelium is infiltrated with numerous lymphocytes.

The mucous membrane on the under-

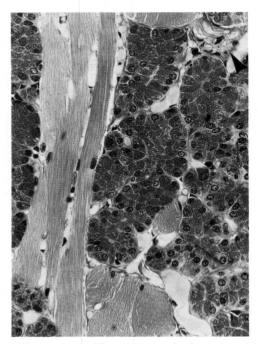

Figure 11–3. Photomicrograph of a section of the body of the tongue showing striated muscle fibers, serous acini, fat cells, and a small peripheral nerve (arrowhead, top right). × 250.

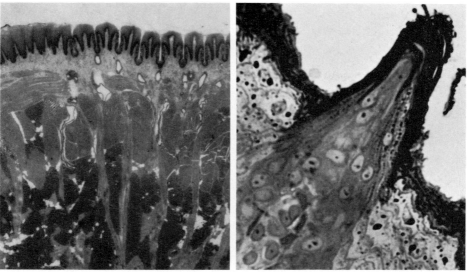

Figure 11–4. *Left:* Photomicrograph of a vertical section through the tongue. The surface mucosa shows filiform (left) and foliate (right) papillae, and deep to it are bundles of striated muscle, glands, and adipose tissue. *Right:* One filiform papilla from rabbit tongue, Plastic section. Left, × 15; right, × 450.

surface of the tongue is smooth and underlain by a submucosa, but on the upper surface the mucosa shows numerous small protuberances called *papillae*, which give the tongue a "furred" or roughened appearance. The papillae are of three main types in man: filiform, fungiform, and circumvallate. The *filiform papillae* are located mainly in rows parallel to the V-shaped sulcus and are 2 to 3 mm in height; each has a primary, pointed, conical core of the connective tissue of the lamina propria with secondary papillae. The covering epithelium, although not fully keratinized, is quite hard. *Fungiform papillae* are disposed singly among the rows of filiform papillae and are more numerous toward the tip of the tongue. They are shaped like a mushroom (fungus) with a short stalk and a broader cap. The connective tis-

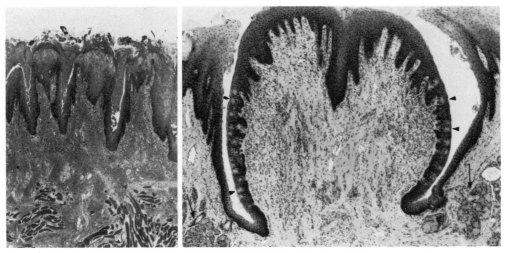

Figure 11–5. Photomicrographs of, *left,* fungiform papillae and, *right,* a circumvallate papilla of human tongue. Note taste buds in the walls of the latter (arrowheads) and parts of serous (Ebner's) glands and ducts below (arrows). Both × 40.

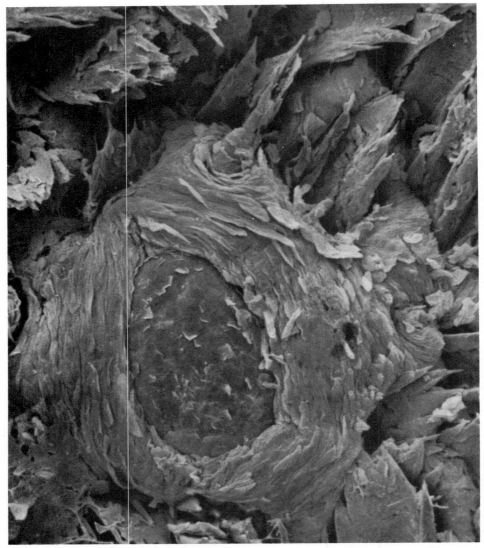

Figure 11–6. Scanning electron micrograph of monkey tongue to show a fungiform papilla surrounded by filiform papillae. × 80. (Courtesy of Dr. P. M. Andrews.)

sue core shows secondary papillae, over which the epithelium may be quite thin, so that the rich vascular plexus within the lamina propria imparts a pinkish or reddish tinge to the papillae. Taste buds may be present in the epithelium.

Circumvallate papillae (vallum, a wall), numbering only 10 to 14 in man, are located along the V-shaped sulcus. Each protrudes slightly from the surface and is surrounded by a moatlike, circular furrow. Secondary papillae are present but the surface epithelium is smooth. Taste buds are located on the lateral walls, viz., in the side of the circular furrow. Opening into the depths of the circular furrow are the ducts of specialized serous or albuminous glands (Ebner's glands), the glands themselves being located more deeply in the muscle tissue of the tongue.

At lateral borders of the tongue and toward its posterior part may be found leaflike folds of the mucosa, sometimes called foliate papillae, with taste buds in the grooves between the folds. These are poorly developed in man but fully formed and important areas of taste sensation in animals such as the rabbit.

All papillae contain numerous sensory nerve endings for touch, and in addition, taste buds are located on vallate, fungiform, and foliate papillae.

TASTE BUDS

The taste buds, containing gustatory (taste) receptor cells, lie in oral epithelium of the tongue mainly in relation to circumvallate and fungiform papillae, but also are found elsewhere in the oral cavity and in the palate and epiglottis. In sections at low power, they are recognizable as pale, barrel-shaped bodies in the darkly staining epithelium and have a laminated or layered appearance. They extend through the full thickness of the epithelium with a small external opening, the outer taste pore, and a small basal pit, the inner taste pore.

By light microscopy, three cell types are distinguished. At the periphery of the taste bud and arranged like staves of a barrel around the outer taste pore are *supporting* or *sustentacular cells,* generally darkly staining with spheroidal or ovoid pale-staining nuclei. Between them, and toward the center of the bud, are lighter staining *neuroepithelial taste cells,* usually only 10 to 14 in each taste bud, often

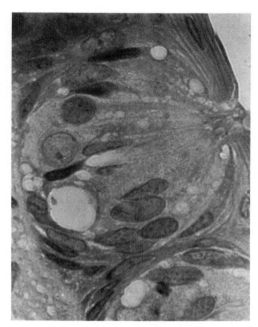

Figure 11–7. Photomicrograph of taste bud with outer taste pore at the surface (right). Plastic section. × 1000.

with slender, ovoid dark nuclei. Both types show apical microvilli protruding through the outer taste pore. The third cell type is the basal cell lying peripherally toward the base and believed to be the stem cell for the other cell types. Within a taste bud, there is a quite rapid cell turnover, the life span being of the order of only 10 days, with movement of cells from the periphery to the center of the bud. Electron microscopy confirms the presence of these cell types but, at least in some animals, shows the presence of an additional cell type with, in its basal region, presynaptic densities of the plasmalemma and synaptic vesicles. This cell type may be the true gustatory cell in that it shows synapses with nerve terminals. The sustentacular cell contains quite extensive granular endoplasmic reticulum and some apical secretory droplets that probably are released to provide polysaccharide material found in the outer taste pore. The cell types in fact may represent different developmental (and functional) stages of a single cell.

Gustatory cells are stimulated by substances in solution which enter the outer taste pore and which must pass through the polysaccharide material to reach the sensory surface. Only four fundamental taste sensations can be detected, and there is a regional sensitivity on the tongue. Sensations of sweet and salt are appreciated at the tip, acid (sour) at the sides, and bitter in the region of the circumvallate papillae. The nerves from taste buds in the anterior two-thirds of the tongue pass by way of the chorda tympani branch of the facial (seventh) cranial nerve, those from the posterior third by the glossopharyngeal (ninth) nerve, and taste buds in the epiglottis and lower pharynx by the vagus (tenth) nerve. All nerves lose their myelin before reaching the taste buds and terminate as club-shaped endings. They pass between all cell types but make synaptic endings only with the gustatory cells.

TEETH

Basically, teeth are derivatives of ectoderm and mesoderm. Each consists of a specially developed dermal papilla covered by calcified material originat-

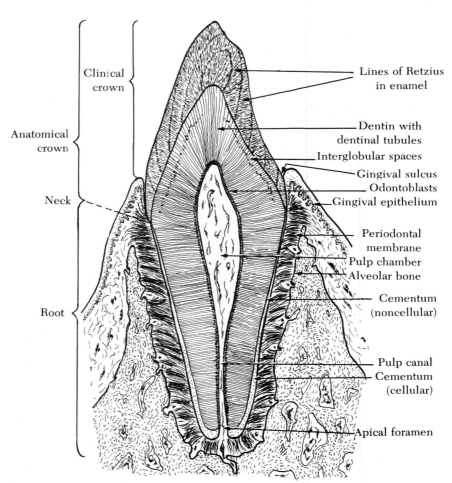

Figure 11–8. Diagram of a longitudinal section through a lower lateral incisor tooth. × 6.

ing chiefly in connective tissue but also in epithelium. Teeth, embedded in the bone of upper and lower jaws, are arranged in two arcs, the upper arc being larger than the lower with the result that the lower teeth are overlapped slightly by the upper. In man, two sets of teeth are distinguished. The *primary, milk,* or *deciduous* teeth of childhood number five in each half jaw (total 20), first erupt six to seven months after birth, and are a complete set by two years of age. They are shed between six and 12 to 13 years of age, being replaced gradually by the *permanent* set of adulthood. Permanent teeth number eight in each half jaw (total 32), the anterior five replacing milk teeth, the posterior three not being represented in the primary dentition.

Although individual teeth are modified for specific functions, e.g., incisors

for biting, molars for grinding, all show a similar histological structure. Each tooth has a *crown* projecting above the gum or gingiva, which thus is visible, and a *root* (or roots), which is buried in the alveolus of the maxilla or mandible. Crown and root meet at a region termed the *neck*. Each tooth is hollow, containing a *pulp cavity* filled in life with connective tissue, and at the apex of the root this cavity communicates via one or more small pores or *apical foramina* with the connective tissue or *periodontal membrane* which holds the tooth in its socket or alveolus. This arrangement of a calcified tooth held in a bony socket by fibroconnective tissue is classified as a *gomphosis* or peg-and-socket type of fibrous joint.

The hard tissues of the tooth consist of *dentin*, which forms the bulk of the tooth and which surrounds the pulp

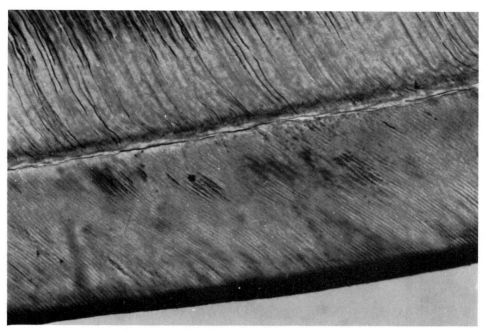

Figure 11–9. Photomicrograph of a ground section of a tooth, showing from above down, dentin with dentinal tubules, dentinoenamel junction, and enamel with enamel rods. × 100. (Courtesy of K. J. Paynter.)

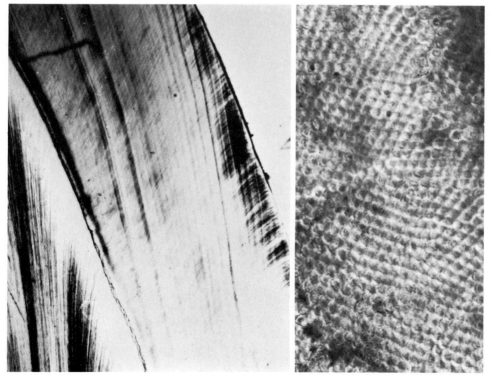

Figure 11–10. Ground sections, *left,* in a longitudinal plane, of enamel to show the striae of Retzius (dentinal tubules also seen at lower left) and, *right,* in a transverse plane, to show enamel rods. Notice the scalelike appearance. Left, × 100; right, × 550. (Courtesy of K. J. Paynter.)

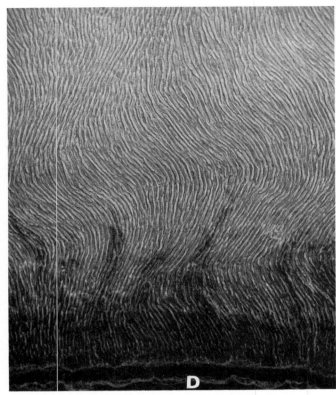

Figure 11–11.   Scanning electron micrograph of transversely sectioned human tooth, acid-etched. The enamel prisms follow a wavy course toward the enamel surface (above), with dentin (D) below. The cleft between dentin and enamel is artefactual. × 200. (Courtesy of Dr. S. Risnes.)

cavity; *enamel,* which covers the dentin of the crown; and *cementum,* covering dentin of the root. The edge of the enamel thus contacts cementum at the neck of the tooth. The soft tissues include the pulp filling the pulp cavity, the periodontal membrane between bone of the alveolus and cementum covering the root, and the gingiva or gum. The last is continuous with the periodontal membrane and is that portion of the oral mucous membrane which surrounds a tooth at the neck and lower part of its crown. In a young person, gingiva is attached to enamel but gradually recedes from it in the adult so that the entire crown is exposed.

Dentin.   Dentin, or dentine, is a substance harder than compact bone, but is of a similar chemical composition, being 72 per cent inorganic salts and 28 per cent organic material. In sections, dentin has a radially striated appearance owing to a multitude of fine canals

or tubules termed the *dentinal tubules.* These run from the pulp cavity to the periphery of the dentin and are 3 to 4 microns (μm) in diameter at the bases and somewhat narrower near the periphery. Each pursues a wavy course through the dentin in the form of an open S. In the outer layers of dentin, the tubules may branch and anastomose, and some show slender, lateral branches communicating with adjacent tubules. The dentinal tubules are occupied by processes of odontoblasts termed *Tomes' dentinal fibers.* The material between the dentinal fibers consists of a meshwork of collagenous fibers embedded in calcified ground substance. Immediately surrounding each dentinal tubule is a thin layer or peritubular sheath (of Neumann), which appears more dense and more highly refractile than the remainder of the intercellular substance between dentinal tubules. This sheath contains less collagen and is more highly calcified than

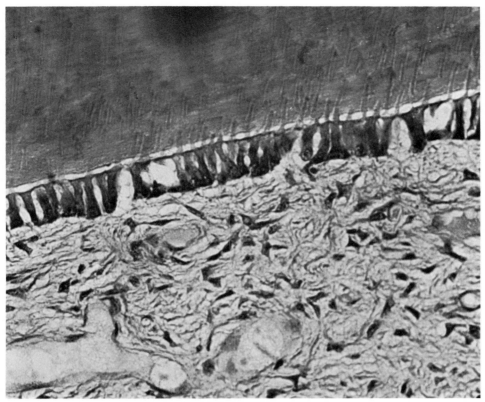

Figure 11–12. Photomicrograph of a demineralized section of tooth, showing odontoblasts with their processes entering dentinal tubules. The pulp chamber filled with mesenchyma-like tissue is below and contains a branching blood vessel (lower left). × 900. (Courtesy of K. J. Paynter.)

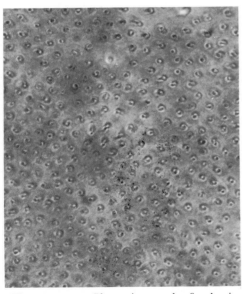

Figure 11–13. Photomicrograph of a demineralized section of tooth, showing dentinal tubules in cross section. The black central dot in each hole is an odontoblast process; the dark area of modified matrix around the hole is the sheath of Neumann. × 900. (Courtesy of K. J. Paynter.)

the remainder of the dentin matrix. With age, the peritubular sheath thickens, particularly in the root, with consequent narrowing and eventual obliteration of dentinal tubules. In addition, small areas of matrix remain incompletely calcified. These are termed the *interglobular spaces.*

The bundles of collagenous fibers of the dentin are 2 to 4 microns (μm) thick. In general they are oriented at right angles to the dentinal tubules and parallel to the long axis of the tooth, but in the crown of the tooth they run tangentially to the surface. The ground substance between the collagenous bundles is a mucopolysaccharide and is similar to that of bone but with a lower organic content. Dentin formation is cyclic and not regular, and in the fully developed tooth there are growth or incremental lines (of Owen) which appear as growth rings in transverse section.

Dentin is sensitive to touch, cold, and

hydrogen ion concentration, sensation being received by the Tomes' fibers and not directly by nerve fibers.

Odontoblasts covering the pulp cavity remain viable throughout life and if stimulated, e.g., by excessive wear of the crown or irritation originating in the region of the periodontal membrane, new and excessive dentin or "reparative dentin" will be laid down at the periphery of the pulp cavity. This is irregular in structure and may be so excessive as to obliterate the pulp cavity.

Enamel. Enamel covers only the crown of the tooth. As mentioned previously, it is of epithelial origin and is the hardest substance in the body. It contains about 97 per cent inorganic material, mainly calcium phosphate in the form of apatite crystals about 200 nm long and 50 nm wide.

The structural unit of enamel is the *enamel prism,* and between the prisms is *interprismatic* substance. Both the prisms and interprismatic substance are composed of apatite crystals in an organic matrix. Each prism, formed by a single ameloblast, is about 4 μm in diameter, being somewhat thicker at the tooth surface, and in cross section appears scalelike and basically hexagonal. Each prism traverses the entire thickness of the enamel but does not run a straight course. Near the dentin and at the surface, the orientation is perpendicular to the surface, but in the central region prisms bend spirally and also show small curvatures. The protein matrix of enamel has a cross-β configuration with a high content of proline and is neither keratin nor collagen.

Like dentin, enamel is laid down rhythmically, and cross sections of the tooth crown show concentric, parallel, incremental lines (of Retzius). When the enamel is fully formed, the ameloblasts on its surface form a membrane about 1 micron (μm) thick and then disappear. Covering this membrane is a second membrane composed of a glycoprotein and derived from the enamel organ. Both membranes are worn off gradually after eruption. Unlike dentin, new enamel obviously cannot be added in the adult after the degeneration and disappearance of ameloblasts.

Cementum. Cementum covers dentin of the root of the tooth from the neck to the apex and serves to attach the tooth to the periodontal membrane. Histologically, it is similar to bone with coarse bundles of collagen fibrils in a calcified matrix. In general, it is thin

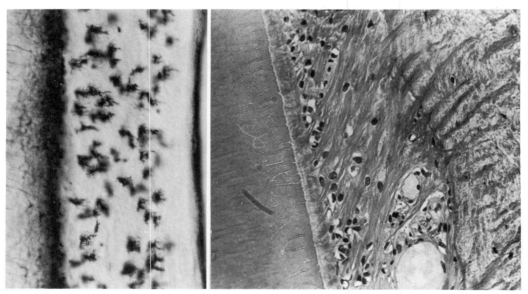

Figure 11–14. *Left:* Ground section showing cementocytes in cellular cementum; a little dentin with dentinal tubules is seen at left. × 350. (Courtesy of K. J. Paynter.) *Right:* Plastic section, just below the neck of the tooth, showing, from left to right, dentin with dentinal tubules, a thin layer of noncellular cementum, periodontal membrane, and alveolar bone. Note strands of collagen crossing the periodontal space and anchored in cementum and bone by Sharpey's fibers. × 250.

and acellular in the upper third, but bone cells (*cementocytes*) are present in the lower part, the cells lying in lacunae interconnected by canaliculi. The coarse bundles of collagen are continuous with fibers from the periodontal membrane which penetrate the cementum as Sharpey's fibers. These do not calcify, and thus they appear as clear canals in ground sections.

Cementum, like bone, is a labile tissue that reacts to stresses and under certain circumstances can undergo resorption or hyperplasia. Increase in thickness, which may develop near the apex in old age, occurs by appositional growth, i.e., by addition of new layers to its surface. Occasionally, the thickness is such that Haversian systems with blood vessels will form. Destruction of cementum occurs rarely, e.g., in periodontal membrane disease.

Pulp.   The pulp of the tooth fills the main pulp chamber and the root canals and is derived from mesenchyme of the embryonic dental papilla. Pulp consists of both cells and intercellular material, the majority of the cells resembling mesenchymal cells in shape (stellate with long cytoplasmic processes) but not in potentiality. Also present are lymphocytes, macrophages, and plasma cells in limited numbers. In the gelatinous, metachromatic ground substance are reticular and thin collagen fibrils. Peripherally, bounding the pulp cavity and underlying dentin is a single layer of epithelium-like, columnar cells, the *odontoblasts,* also of mesenchymal origin. Each odontoblast has a long, cytoplasmic process (a dentinal fiber of Tomes) extending into a dentinal tubule, the cell body showing a basally located nucleus, prominent mitochondria, and a Golgi apparatus. The odontoblasts are responsible for dentin formation. Immediately subjacent to the layer of odontoblasts is a cell-poor zone (of Weil) containing slender bundles of reticular fibers passing from the pulp, between odontoblasts, into dentinal matrix.

Usually, a single arteriole and two venules enter the pulp cavity through the root canal(s) to supply an extensive capillary bed in the pulp chamber, with capillaries underlying, and even extending between, odontoblasts. All pulpal blood vessels are thin-walled and thus are pressure-sensitive, lying as they do in an unexpandable chamber. Thus, a relatively mild inflammation of the pulp with associated edema can cause occlusion of the blood vessels and consequent death of the pulp. The pulp also has a rich nerve supply with small nerve endings passing between odontoblasts and, perhaps, for a short distance into dentinal tubules. With age, the pulp becomes more fibrous with coarser collagen fibrils and fewer cells and the pulp cavity usually becomes smaller by the formation of dentin peripherally. Local, irregular dentin (secondary dentin) may form, for example, in relation to a cavity.

Periodontal Membrane.   The periodontal membrane is a modified periosteum of alveolar bone and is a dense fibrous connective tissue. At the neck of the tooth it supports the gingiva. Strong, thick bundles of collagenous fibers run between alveolar bone and cementum. At the extremities of a bundle, collagen fibers extend into bone and cementum respectively as Sharpey's fibers. However, the fibers of each bundle are not taut and run a slightly wavy course, being attached somewhat deeper to the root of a tooth than to the alveolar bone. Thus, the tooth is "slung" in its socket and can move slightly in each direction, the periodontal membrane functioning as the suspensory ligament of the tooth. Between the fiber bundles are a few fibroblasts and some osteoblasts. The turnover rate in collagen of the periodontal membrane is high, permitting remodelling (and orthodontic procedures). Blood vessels and nerves pass through the membrane to reach the pulp cavity of a tooth but are not prominent in the membrane itself. However, the periodontal membrane has a relatively rich vascular supply, although the vessels are not seen readily in histological preparations. It also is highly sensitive to pressure changes and has a good nerve supply. There are lymph vessels and nerves in the membrane and small, scattered islands of epithelial cells derived from the embryonic root sheath. These may form dental cysts or calcify to form small bodies termed cementicles.

Gingiva.   The gingiva or gum surrounds each tooth like a collar and is the oral mucous membrane extending between and connected to the periosteum of alveolar bone at its crest and the tooth above its neck. Near the tooth, the gingiva extends around the tooth as the gingival crest, between the summit of which and the tooth is a narrow gingival crevice. More deeply at the bottom of the gingival crevice, the gingiva is attached around the circumference of the tooth crown. This attachment is to enamel cuticle and it extends deeply to the upper part of the cementum. The attachment to the enamel is not firm and with age the gingival sulcus deepens until the gingiva is attached only to cementum, thus exposing the entire crown.

The connective tissue papillae underlying the stratified squamous epithelium of the gingiva are high. The connective tissue itself consists of interlacing bundles of collagenous fibers with relatively few fibroblasts and numerous blood capillaries which form a rich vascular network immediately below the epithelium. It is blood in this network which is responsible for the pink color of the gums.

Development of the Teeth

Each tooth has a mesodermal and an ectodermal component, the latter forming only the enamel. During the fifth week, ectoderm of the oral cavity develops horseshoe-shaped linear thickenings in the developing upper and lower jaws. Each thickening, a *labiodental lamina*, is at first solid and bifid, extending deeply into underlying mesenchyme. The outer labial limb later splits to form the groove between the lip and the alveolar process of the jaw (i.e., the vestibule). The inner limb, the *dental lamina*, develops a series of bud-like thickenings, or *tooth germs*, there being five in each half jaw or one for each deciduous tooth. Later, at 10 to 12 weeks, a second series of tooth germs develops on the lingual side of each developing deciduous tooth (five) plus three more posteriorly for each adult molar (the molar is not preceded by a deciduous tooth). The tooth germs for the adult teeth do not appear until later (fourth month of intrauterine life for the first permanent molar, and first and fourth years after birth for the second and third molars). Each tooth germ, both deciduous and adult, develops further in identical fashion.

The epithelial tooth germ is invaginated from below by a papilla of mesenchymal connective tissue and thus becomes bell-shaped, still attached above by a cord of epithelial cells to the dental lamina. The bell-shaped epithelial bud, now termed the *enamel organ*, sits like a cap on the dental papilla. The whole is embedded in a layer of connective tissue, the dental sac, which soon completely invests the developing tooth when the connecting strand between the dental lamina and the enamel organ breaks down and disappears. The central cells of the enamel organ become separated by intercellular

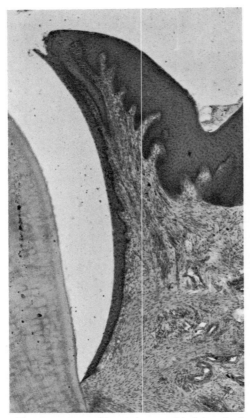

Figure 11–15. Photomicrograph of the gingiva and gingival sulcus. The sulcus is excessively wide owing to the loss of the enamel. × 150. (Courtesy of K. J. Paynter.)

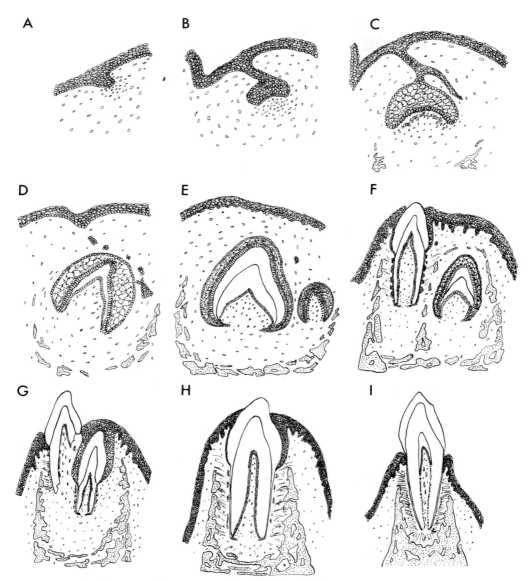

Figure 11–16. Diagram to illustrate stages in development of the lower central incisor. The approximate time is indicated in parentheses. *A,* Dental lamina formation from oral epithelium. (Six weeks intrauterine.) *B,* Early formation ("cap" stage) of the enamel organ of the deciduous tooth with condensation of underlying mesenchyme. (Seven to eight weeks intrauterine.) *C,* Early "bell" stage of the enamel organ with extension (to the right) of the dental lamina indicating formation of the permanent tooth. Alveolar bone is forming. (Ten weeks intrauterine.) *D,* Advanced "bell" stage with a cap of dentin now formed at the tip of the dental papilla. Connection between the tooth bud and the oral epithelium now is discontinuous. (Sixteen weeks intrauterine.) *E,* The crown of the deciduous tooth is complete with enamel formation, and the permanent tooth is in the bell stage. (Birth.) *F,* Early eruption of the deciduous tooth, the root of which now is formed, with the crown of the permanent tooth nearly completed, showing enamel and dentin. (Six months postnatal.) *G,* The deciduous tooth shows resorption of the root and the process of shedding is commencing. In the permanent tooth, root formation is complete (Six to seven years.) *H,* The permanent tooth now is erupting. (Seven to eight years.) *I,* In the permanent tooth, early attrition is shown with some recession in the neck and formation of secondary dentin. (After 20 years.) Stages A to E drawn at higher magnification than stages F to I. (Based on diagrams supplied by J. G. Dale and K. J. Paynter.)

spaces, the cells remaining in contact only by long cytoplasmic processes to become reticulum-like in appearance. This is the stellate reticulum. Peripherally around the stellate reticulum, the epithelial cells are arranged in a regular sheet, one cell thick. The cells of the outer enamel epithelium remain small, but those of the inner enamel epithelium adjacent to the dental papilla become tall and columnar. These are the *ameloblasts*, responsible for enamel formation. Cells of the stellate reticulum which lie adjacent to the inner enamel epithelium (ameloblasts) form a single layer of cuboidal cells. This is termed the stratum intermedium and it plays an important role in attaching the epithelial tissues around the crown of the tooth to the oral mucous membrane during eruption of the tooth. By the time that ameloblasts have differentiated, the peripheral cells of the dental papilla in contact with ameloblasts become arranged in a regular manner, one cell thick. These are the *odontoblasts*

(dentinoblasts); they are separated from the ameloblasts only by basal lamina material.

By about 20 weeks of gestation, the hard tissues of the tooth begin to form. Dentin appears first between the two layers of cells (ameloblasts and odontoblasts) and at first is uncalcified and thus usually is called *predentin*. It gradually extends down toward the neck and increases in thickness by apposition on the internal surface. As it increases in thickness, cytoplasmic processes of the odontoblasts remain within the dentin as the dentinal fibers. Predentin thus is composed of odontoblast processes, collagen fibers, and ground substance. The collagen fibers originate in the pulp, and as mineralization occurs the fibers condense and thicken around odontoblast processes. Electron microscopy shows that odontoblasts form an acid mucopolysaccharide which is concentrated in granules. These granules, situated mainly at the bases of odontoblast processes, are extruded later

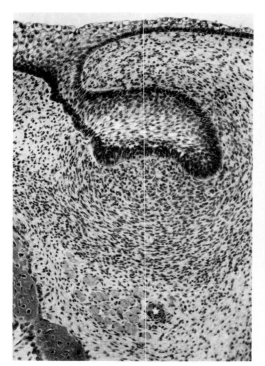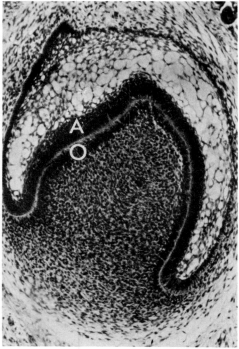

Figure 11–17. Photomicrographs of developing teeth. *Left:* In the early "bell" stage with enamel organ attached to oral mucosa by the dental lamina. (Compare with Figure 11–16C.) × 100. *Right:* In late "bell" stage with ameloblasts (inner enamel epithelium, A) differentiated and in contact with odontoblasts (O). (Compare with Figure 11–16D.) × 45.

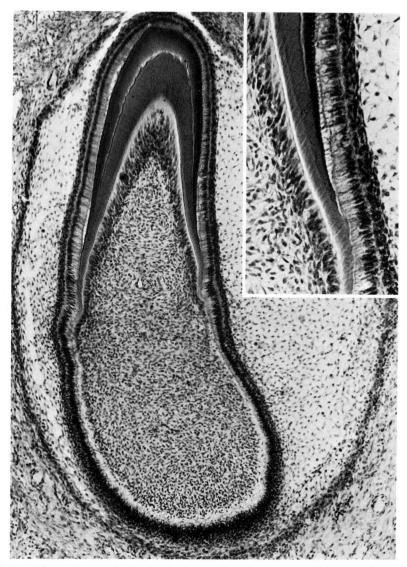

Figure 11–18. Photomicrograph of a developing tooth at the stage in which crown formation is well advanced. (Compare with Figure 11–16*E*.) Enamel and dentin are present with a thin layer of predentin in relation to odontoblasts. Note the connective tissue dental sac enveloping the entire developing tooth. ×75. *Top right, inset:* A higher magnification of part of the tooth showing, from left to right, pulp, odontoblasts, predentin, dentin, enamel (black), ameloblasts, stratum intermedium, and stellate reticulum. ×175.

into the surrounding matrix where the polysaccharide lies on the surface of collagen fibers and in the interfibrillar spaces. Mineralization occurs in the patches of mucopolysaccharide and, later, upon the surface of fibers. Throughout dentin formation, collagen fibers invade the developing matrix and appear to be derived from fibroblasts within the pulp. Because mineralization occurs after the presence of fibers and ground substance, there is always a thin layer of predentin adjacent to the odontoblasts. As soon as dentin formation has been initiated, the ameloblasts commence to form enamel, layer by layer on the surface of the dentin. Ameloblasts, as seen by electron microscopy, contain abundant ergastoplasm, presumably associated with protein synthesis. Ameloblasts form enamel matrix which later is mineral-

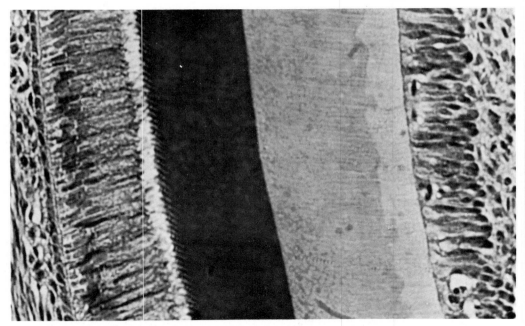

Figure 11–19. Photomicrograph of a developing monkey tooth, showing from left to right, stratum intermedium, ameloblasts, enamel (black), dentin, predentin, odontoblasts, and pulp. × 900. (Courtesy of K. J. Paynter.)

ized extracellularly. With the increase in thickness of the enamel, the ameloblasts recede from the dentin. It must be emphasized that enamel does not develop as a homogeneous mass but as enamel rods, each rod corresponding to a single ameloblast. Complete calcification in the enamel does not occur until late. Before the ameloblasts disappear, they elaborate the inner enamel cuticle which covers the bases of the enamel rods.

The development of the tooth as described above accounts only for the formation of the crown. At the periphery of the enamel organ in the future neck region, i.e., at the edge of the bell, where inner and outer enamel epithelia come together, a fold of epithelial cells develops and grows downward toward the root. This is the *epithelial root sheath* (of Hertwig). Root development occurs shortly before tooth eruption and gradually progresses as the crown emerges through the gingiva. Odontoblasts develop in relation to the epithelial sheath of Hertwig and form dentin. Cementum develops from mesenchyme of the periodontal membrane. The epithelial sheath of Hertwig disappears only when the root is formed completely.

During eruption of a permanent tooth, the deciduous tooth superficial to it gradually is resorbed by growth pressure, osteoclasts being prominent during the process. The deciduous tooth when finally shed consists only of the upper portion of the crown, the remainder having been resorbed.

THE MAJOR SALIVARY GLANDS

There are numerous small, intrinsic glands associated with the oral cavity which continuously secrete a liquid, *saliva*. This secretion moistens the mucous membrane of the oral cavity proper, the vestibule of the mouth, and the lips. In addition to these glands, there are three pairs of large, extrinsic glands, the ducts of which open into the oral cavity. These major salivary glands are the *parotid*, the *submandibular* or *submaxillary* and the *sublingual*, and they secrete copious amounts of saliva intermittently on nervous stimulation. Secretions occur following mechanical, thermal, chemical, psychic, or olfactory stimuli owing to the presence or anticipated presence of food in the mouth cavity.

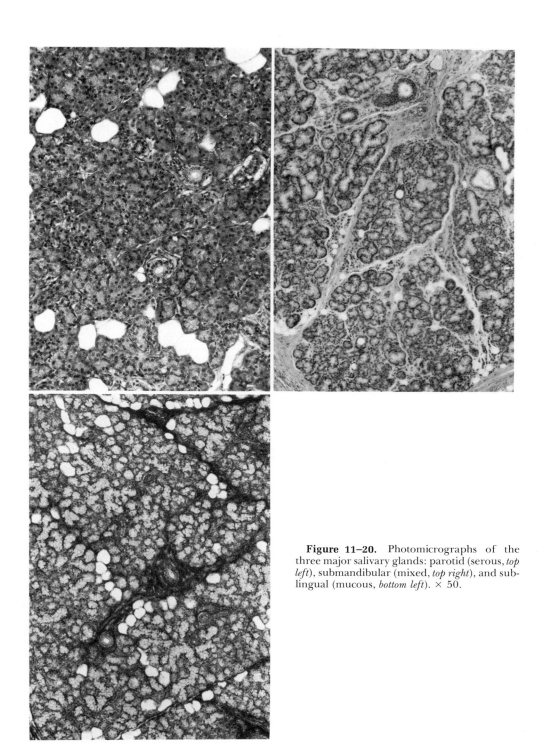

Figure 11–20. Photomicrographs of the three major salivary glands: parotid (serous, *top left*), submandibular (mixed, *top right*), and sublingual (mucous, *bottom left*). × 50.

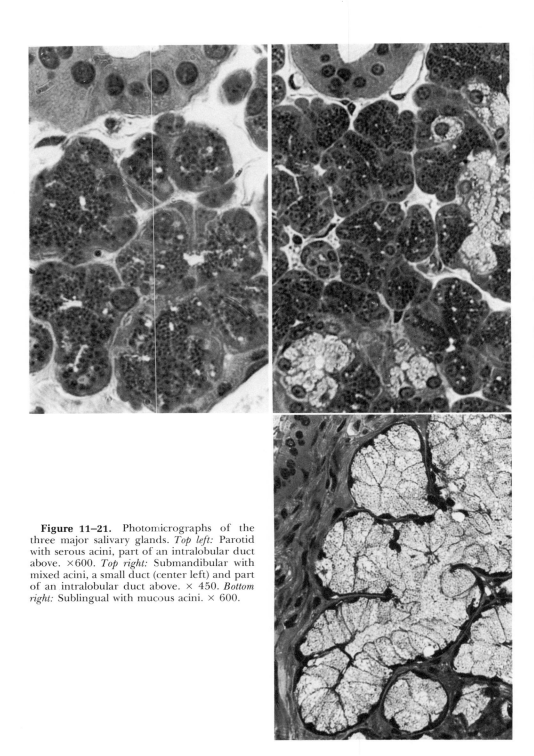

Figure 11–21. Photomicrographs of the three major salivary glands. *Top left:* Parotid with serous acini, part of an intralobular duct above. ×600. *Top right:* Submandibular with mixed acini, a small duct (center left) and part of an intralobular duct above. × 450. *Bottom right:* Sublingual with mucous acini. × 600.

Saliva

Saliva, the mixed secretions of *all* the salivary glands, may amount to 1000 to 1500 ml in 24 hours. Saliva is a viscid liquid containing water, mucin, proteins, salts, and two enzymes, *ptyalin* and *maltase*. Ptyalin splits starch, which is relatively insoluble in water, into less complex, soluble carbohydrates. Maltase splits the disaccharide maltose. Saliva also contains desquamated, degenerated, squamous epithelial cells from the oral epithelium and degenerated lymphocytes and granulocytes called "salivary corpuscles." These arise mainly from the tonsils. It should be noted that the quality as well as the quantity of saliva varies with different stimuli. The quality is affected by the varying contributions made by the different major salivary glands in response to different food materials.

The secretion of saliva subserves several functions. It constantly moistens the oral cavity and aids in cleaning the mouth of food debris which otherwise would provide a culture medium for bacterial growth, bacteria always being present in the oral cavity. Obviously, it moistens food and this permits both ease of swallowing and the appreciation of taste, for the chemical substances responsible for taste must be in solution to cause stimulation of the taste buds. Enzymatic digestion of carbohydrates by ptyalin and amylase commences in the mouth but ceases in the stomach where both enzymes are inactivated in an acid medium. The secretion of saliva is one important factor in the maintenance of fluid balance, a decreased secretion occurring when the body is dehydrated, giving rise to a sensation of thirst. Much of the fluid in saliva, of course, is returned to the circulation by absorption in the digestive tract. Finally, some heavy metals are secreted in the saliva.

The salivary glands are classified as merocrine and tubuloacinar in type. The student is referred to Chapter 2 for a general description of exocrine glands.

Parotid Gland

This, the largest of the major salivary glands, is situated below and anterior to the ear, being related to the mastoid process behind and the mandibular ramus in front. There is an anterior extension onto the face beneath the zygomatic arch and from this border the main duct (Stensen's duct) passes forward, through the cheek, and opens into the vestibule of the mouth opposite the second upper molar tooth. The gland is enclosed in a fascial sheet and contains serous acini composed of pyramid-shaped cells, and intercalated and striated ducts.

From the fibrous capsule, relatively dense septa pass into the gland to divide it into lobes and lobules. The connective tissue of the septa often contains fat cells. Slips of fine connective tissue surround acini and ducts, and contained in this tissue are numerous blood capillaries.

Acini are elongated and enclosed in a basal lamina with some myoepithelial cells. All acinar cells have spherical nuclei situated toward the base and show infranuclear cytoplasmic basophilia and apical secretion granules. By electron microscopy, serous cells contain extensive granular endoplasmic reticulum and free ribosomes and mitochondria below and around the nucleus with a supranuclear Golgi apparatus and apical secretory and presecretory droplets. Cell interfaces characteristically are complex and apical microvilli are present. By electron microscopy, two regions of the *intercalated duct* are identified. Cells in the proximal part are small, arranged in a tubular fashion from the lumen of an acinus, and show the presence of secretory granules. In the distal part, the cells contain no secretion granules, the lumen usually is of greater diameter, and myoepithelial cells may be present between the duct cells and the surrounding basal lamina. The intercalated duct continues into the *striated duct*. Cells here are tall and polygonal or columnar in shape and show basal striation, which by electron microscopy is resolved as basal invaginations of the plasma membrane with numerous elongated mitochondria in the pockets of cytoplasm so formed. The apical cytoplasm contains vesicles. The morphology of these cells is similar to that of cells in the distal convoluted tubules of the kidney, and it is

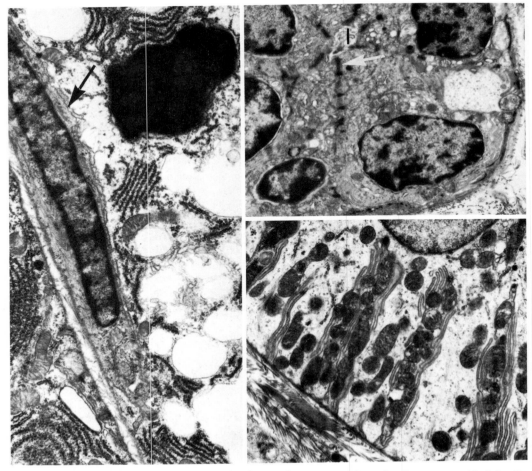

Figure 11–22. *Left:* Electron micrograph of part of a mucous acinus showing a myoepithelial cell (arrow). × 9000. *Top right:* A small intralobular duct showing small lumen (1) and junctional complexes (arrow) with desmosomes. × 7200. *Bottom right:* Part of a cell of a striated duct showing basal infoldings of the plasmalemma. × 7200.

suggested that they subserve a similar function of fluid resorption from the lumen to the interstitium. *Excretory ducts* commence with simple columnar epithelium which then becomes pseudostratified and finally stratified. Intralobular ducts particularly are prominent in this gland. (They are less so, for example, in the pancreas.)

Submandibular (Submaxillary) Gland

This gland is located in the floor of the mouth underlying the body of the mandible and extending beneath its lower border into the side of the neck. Its duct (Wharton's) opens into the floor of the mouth just behind the lower incisor teeth and beneath the tip of the tongue. It also is a tubuloacinar or compound acinar gland, the majority of the acini being serous. The remainder are mucous but usually with serous crescents, i.e., mixed acini. Like the parotid, the submandibular gland has a capsule, septa, and a prominent duct system. Intercalated ducts are similar to those of the parotid, but with fewer secretion granules in the proximal part. By electron microscopy, striated ducts contain, in addition to the cell type described previously, a cell with masses of endoplasmic reticulum and some secretion granules. Striated ducts tend to be longer than those in the parotid and thus are more conspicuous in sections of this gland.

Sublingual Gland

The sublingual gland really is not a single gland but a collection of glands lying beneath the mucous membrane of the floor of the mouth in close relation to the duct of the submandibular gland, and each part has a duct opening separately. It is a mixed gland, the majority of the acini being mucous, but with some mixed units. Pure serous units are rare. There is no definite capsule but septa are present. Myoepithelial cells usually are found in relation to acini. Intercalated ducts are short and not prominent, and the cells contain no secretory granules. The striated ducts are similar in appearance to those of the parotid and submandibular but are short and thus less commonly seen.

Each of the major salivary glands is provided with sensory nerve endings and motor nerves from both the sympathetic and parasympathetic nervous systems. The latter supplies both secretory acini and blood vessels of the glands, the sympathetic being derived from the superior cervical ganglion and the parasympathetic from salivary nuclei located in the brain stem and associated with the seventh and ninth cranial nerves. There is some experimental evidence that stimulation of the glands by the sympathetic system causes secretion of a thick, mucous saliva and by the parasympathetic causes a profuse watery secretion. The actual mechanism by which nervous stimulation causes acinar cell secretion is not well understood.

Palate

The roof of the mouth or palate is also the floor of the nasal cavity. The anterior part, termed the *hard palate,* contains bone (palatine processes of maxillae and palatine bones) and thus is rigid. The posterior portion, called the *soft palate,* has a core of strong fibroconnective tissue and thus is movable. The hard palate provides a rigid surface against which the tongue, a powerful muscular organ, can bring force to mix food material and expedite the swallowing mechanism. The oral surface of the hard palate correspondingly is covered by stratified squamous keratinizing epithelium, the lamina propria of which blends with the periosteum. Within the lamina propria are numerous small glands and some fatty tissue. In the midline, the lamina propria is thin and attached to a median ridge of bone. This linear region is called the *raphe.*

The soft palate functions to close off the nasopharynx from the oropharynx during swallowing, thus preventing aliment from entering the nasal cavity. It is covered inferiorly by stratified squamous nonkeratinizing epithelium, the lamina propria of which contains numerous glands. A layer of striated muscle (the musculus uvulus) lies between the lamina propria and the palatine aponeurosis, a sheet of fibroconnective tissue. On the nasal side, the soft palate is covered by the pseudostratified ciliated columnar epithelium of the nasal cavity, although posteriorly the oral type of epithelium extends around the posterior border of the soft palate and onto its superior, nasal surface. The lamina propria of this epithelium also contains a few glands.

Tonsils

The oral cavity is continuous with the oropharynx (see page 405) through a region termed the *fauces.* There are two mucosal folds, each containing a muscle, on each side between the palate and the side of the tongue and pharynx respectively. These are called the palatoglossal and palatopharyngeal folds and between them is a depression in which is located a mass of lymphoid tissue. This is the *palatine tonsil* (see page 291). Lymphoid tissue also is present in the nasopharynx (adenoids), around the openings of the pharyngotympanic (eustachian) tubes ("tubal tonsil"), and in the posterior part of the tongue ("lingual tonsil"). The parts of the pharynx are discussed on page 405.

SECTION II.   THE TUBULAR DIGESTIVE TRACT

LAYERS OF DIGESTIVE TRACT

Each part of the digestive tube has four coats or layers, their nature and thickness varying with functional requirements in the different regions. These layers are the tunicae mucosa, submucosa, muscularis, and serosa (adventitia).

Mucous Membrane (Tunica Mucosa)

This is a wet, surface epithelial membrane, lubricated by mucus, resting upon a basal lamina, in turn supported by a layer of connective tissue termed the lamina propria, and, in many regions, with a thin, outer layer of smooth muscle, the muscularis mucosae. The last usually is arranged in two layers oriented as an inner circular layer and an outer longitudinal layer. In most regions, the mucous membrane is irregular and shows finger-like projections, the *villi*, which greatly increase surface area, and deep epithelial-lined invaginations, the *intestinal glands* or *crypts*. These glands extend deeply within the lamina propria to the muscularis mucosae in many regions and thus make the lamina propria difficult to identify as a separate entity. The lamina propria is classified as a loose, areolar, connective tissue but with lymphatic tendencies, the lymphoid material presumably functioning as a defense barrier against bacterial infection. Contained within the lamina propria are numerous blood and lymph capillaries into which absorbed food materials pass.

Submucosa (Tunica Submucosa)

This extends from the mucosa to the muscularis externa and comprises

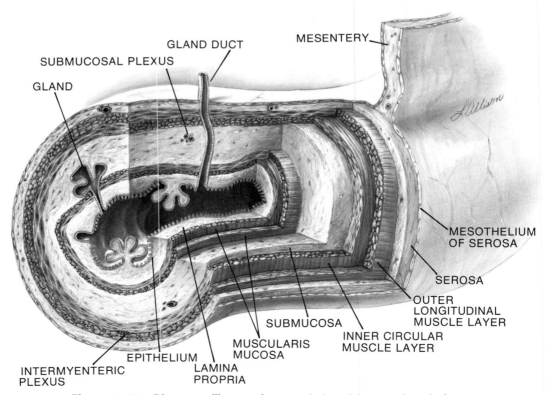

Figure 11–23.   Diagram to illustrate the general plan of the gastrointestinal tract.

coarse areolar connective tissue with some elastic fibers. It permits mobility of the mucosa. Contained in it are plexuses of larger blood vessels and nerves with some ganglion cells which are part of the autonomic nervous system, some being postganglionic fibers of the sympathetic system and others preganglionic fibers of the parasympathetic system. The ganglion cells are all parasympathetic. This is termed *Meissner's* or the *submucous plexus*. In some regions, e.g., the duodenum, there are submucosal glands.

Muscularis Externa (Tunica Muscularis)

This characteristically consists of an inner layer of circularly oriented and an outer layer of longitudinally oriented smooth muscle fibers, although there is striated muscle in the upper esophagus. Both layers actually are arranged in a spiral fashion, the inner following a tight helix and the outer a very open helix. Between the two layers is a vascular plexus and a nerve plexus associated with numerous small ganglia. This is *Auerbach's myenteric plexus* and is mainly parasympathetic with some postganglionic sympathetic fibers. The muscularis functions to propel onward food material in the lumen of the digestive tube, a process termed peristalsis, and by churning movements aids in mixing the food material with the digestive enzymes. It varies in thickness with the region of the tube; for example, a third layer is identified in the wall of the stomach.

Serosa or Adventitia (Tunica Serosa or Adventitia)

The outermost layer comprises a relatively dense areolar connective tissue, often blending with the connective tissue of surrounding structures. This is termed an adventitia. In many regions it is covered with peritoneum, i.e., by a single layer of mesothelial cells, and in these sites is termed a serosa rather than an adventitia. Blood vessels, lymphatics, and nerves are present and pass through it to the other layers.

Developmentally, the epithelial lining of the digestive tube is derived from endoderm with the exception of the external parts of the oral cavity and anal canal. These are ectodermal in origin. The connective and muscular tissues are derived from splanchnic or visceral mesoderm.

THE ESOPHAGUS

The esophagus, about 20 cm long, is a relatively straight muscular tube, continuous with the lower extremity of the pharynx at the inferior border of the cricoid cartilage (see Figure 12–7) and extending through the lower neck and the mediastinum of the thorax to perforate the diaphragm and terminate by opening into the stomach. Its wall shows the four layers as described previously.

The mucous membrane consists of a stratified squamous nonkeratinizing epithelium continuous with that lining the pharynx, a lamina propria, and a muscularis mucosae. The epithelium is thick and shows mitotic figures in its basal layer of cells, indicating a constant shedding and renewal of cells. Cells of the superficial layer contain keratohyalin granules, although they do not undergo true cornification. Characteristically, this epithelium is indented by peglike protrusions of the underlying lamina propria. At the lower end, the epithelium undergoes an abrupt transition to the epithelium lining the stomach. The lamina propria is relatively acellular with scattered lymphocytes and a few lymphatic nodules. At the level of the cricoid cartilage, the muscularis mucosae is continuous with the elastic layer of the pharynx.

The submucosa shows relatively coarse collagenous and elastic fibers and, in the empty esophagus, is thrown into several longitudinal folds. This gives the lumen a characteristic irregular outline. During passage of a food bolus the esophagus dilates and these longitudinal folds are "ironed out." The muscularis shows inner circular and outer longitudinal layers of muscle, although many bundles are spiral or oblique in orientation. In the upper third of the esophagus, muscle fibers are en-

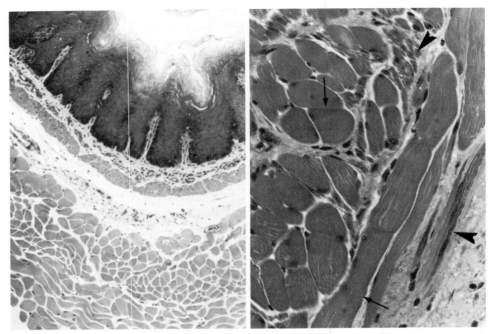

Figure 11–24. *Left:* Transverse section of the upper third of the esophagus showing mucosa with its stratified squamous epithelium, lamina propria and muscularis mucosae of smooth muscle, submucosa, and muscularis of striated muscle. × 40. *Right:* The muscularis of the middle third showing striated (arrows) and smooth (arrowheads) muscle fibers in transverse and longitudinal section. × 400.

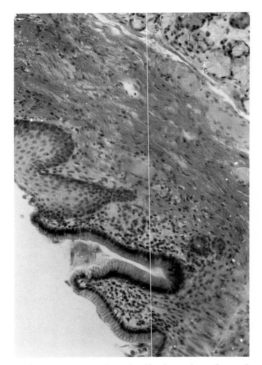

Figure 11–25. Longitudinal section through esophagogastric junction, showing abrupt change in epithelium from stratified squamous to simple columnar. Note the mucous glands in the submucosa. × 275.

tirely skeletal, striated muscle, often variable in orientation. In the middle third, smooth muscle bundles are mixed with striated fibers, and the proportion gradually increases until only smooth muscle is present in the lower third, where the arrangement into inner circular and outer longitudinal layers is more regular. While there is no local thickening of muscle, at upper and lower ends of the esophagus there appear to be regions of higher muscular tone. The lower or gastroesophageal sphincter functions to prevent reflux of gastric contents into the esophagus. External to the muscularis is an adventitia that blends with surrounding structures.

Food material in the esophagus passes rapidly downward and has been mixed previously with saliva, so little additional lubrication is needed. However, some glands are present, not only scattered throughout the length of the esophagus as small, submucosal, tubuloalveolar mucous glands but as the so-called esophageal cardiac glands at upper and lower ends. These are confined to the lamina propria, are mucous-secreting, and resemble cardiac glands of the stomach.

Functionally, the esophageal epithelium is of a type to resist abrasion from rough food material; some mucous glands aid its lubrication; the thick, loose submucosa permits great dilation during swallowing; and the thick muscularis, particularly in the upper portion where it is composed of striated muscle, provides the motive power for rapid propulsion of food material from the pharynx to the stomach. Indeed, swallowing is possible in the inverted position when the muscularis must work against gravity. Little or no absorption of aliment occurs in the esophagus.

THE STOMACH

The stomach when empty is of only slightly larger caliber than the large gut but is capable of considerable distention and can accommodate two to three liters of material when distended. As indicated, there is a *gastroesophageal or cardiac sphincter* at the entrance of the stomach

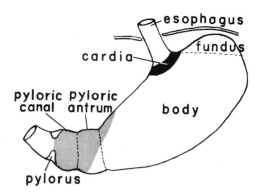

Figure 11–26. Diagram showing the anatomical and histological (shaded) areas of the stomach.

and a more powerful *pyloric sphincter* at its junction with the small intestine, where there is marked thickening of the muscularis. To the left of and above the cardiac orifice (esophageal opening) is a dilatation or bulge termed the *fundus*. The main *body* of the stomach passes into a region called the *pyloric antrum*, in turn narrowing to the *pyloric canal* that narrows to the *pylorus*, the opening into the duodenum. The stomach is flat-

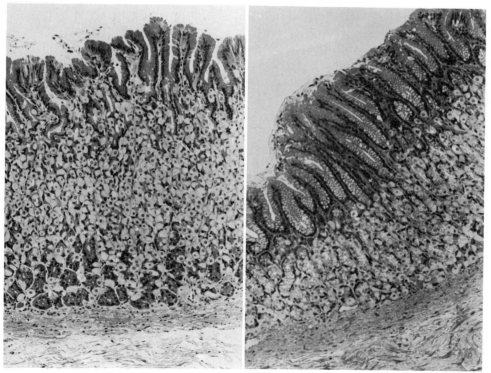

Figure 11–27. Photomicrographs of the mucosa of the body of the stomach *(left)* and the pyloric part of the stomach *(right)* showing gastric pits and glands, the muscularis mucosae below. × 50.

tened anteroposteriorly with upper concave and lower convex borders called the *lesser* and *greater curvatures.* In the empty, contracted stomach, the lining is thrown into longitudinal folds or *rugae* formed by the lining mucosa with a core of submucosa, these rugae disappearing with distention.

Food enters the stomach as boli (bolus, a ball) of semisolid, masticated material, partially moistened by saliva, but leaves it intermittently after a period of three to four hours as a semifluid, pulplike mass termed *chyme.* The thick muscularis of the stomach functions to churn the contained material, mixing it thoroughly with the digestive juices secreted by the stomach. The *gastric juice* contains hydrochloric acid, enzymes, and mucus. One of the enzymes, *pepsin,* in an acid medium commences the digestion of proteins; *rennin* functions to curdle milk; and *lipase* starts fat digestion. In addition, the gastric mucosa secretes a factor necessary for the absorption of vitamin B_{12} (essential for hemopoiesis), and some absorption occurs, although this is limited to salts, water, glucose, alcohol, and some drugs.

The stomach wall is composed of four layers.

Mucosa

The mucous membrane of the living stomach is pale, grayish-pink, paler at the cardia and pylorus, and its entire thickness is occupied by a mass of *gastric glands* which open on the surface by *gastric pits* or *foveolae.* These pits usually are interpreted as tubular, but they also probably take the form of linear crevices that outline irregular areas of 1 to 5 mm diameter at the surface, these areas further subdivided by slender grooves. The gastric glands are simple tubular or branched tubular and extend deeply to reach the muscularis mucosae. Between them is the lamina propria, split up to such a degree to occupy the spaces between glands and pits that it is difficult to recognize it as a separate entity. On the basis of differences in the glands and pits, three zones are recognized: a narrow, ring-shaped area around the cardia containing *cardiac glands,* a main

area comprising the fundus and body (the proximal two-thirds or more of the stomach) containing the *fundic* or *main glands,* and a distal area, the pyloric region, containing *pyloric glands,* this extending more proximally on the lesser than the greater curvature. The surface epithelium of the mucosa, however, is similar in form from cardia to pylorus.

Surface Epithelium

This is a tall, columnar epithelium (only one cell type being present) which distinguishes the stomach from all other regions of the digestive tract. At the cardia, it commences abruptly, adjoining the stratified squamous epithelium of the esophagus, and it is continuous at the pylorus with the intestinal epithelium. The columnar cells are mucin-secreting, the secreted neutral mucopolysaccharide material providing a protective coat for the epithelium. These mucin granules are peculiar in that they do not stain with some mucus-specific dyes. Nuclei are situated toward the bases of the cells, and the supranuclear region is occupied by spherical, discrete mucin granules. As the epithelium extends into the mouths of foveolae, fewer mucin granules are present. Adjacent to the nucleus, but usually on the apical side, is a Golgi apparatus, and the subnuclear region is occupied by mitochondria. Terminal bars and apical microvilli are present. The mortality rate of the surface epithelial cells is high, and they are replaced by mitosis of less differentiated cells situated in the deeper parts of the foveolae and upper regions of the gastric glands. Indeed, there is evidence that the entire surface epithelium is replaced every three to four days.

Gastric Glands

As just outlined, these are branched tubular in type, are densely packed, and occupy the entire thickness of the mucosa, opening in small groups into the bottom of a gastric pit by which their secretions are carried to the surface. Each gland is surrounded by a basal lamina. They number some 35 million.

Cardiac Glands. These closely re-

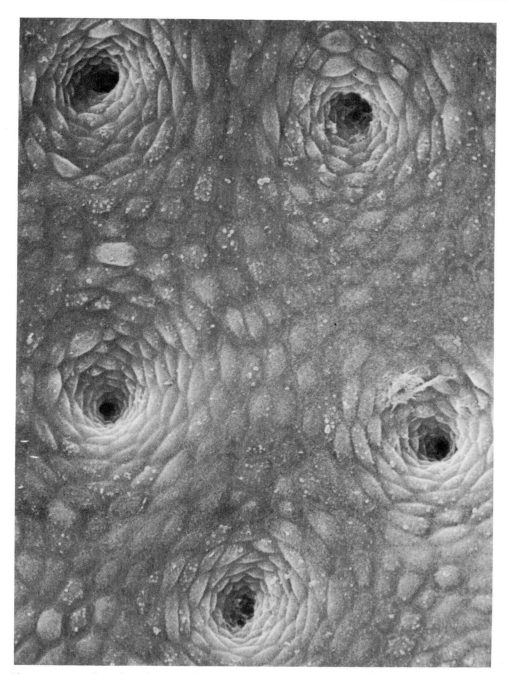

Figure 11–28. Scanning electron micrograph of the luminal surface of the stomach showing the orifices of gastric pits and the surface epithelium. × 800. (Courtesy of P. M. Andrews.)

semble the superficial mucosal glands of the lower esophagus; they are compound or simple tubular in type, extending over the deeper half of the mucosa, and several open into the base of a single gastric pit, the gastric pits occupying the superficial half of the depth of the mucosa. The cells of the cardiac glands are mucus-secreting, pale columnar cells interspersed with a few parietal cells. Their functional significance is not known.

Fundic Glands. These are the most important glands of the stomach and

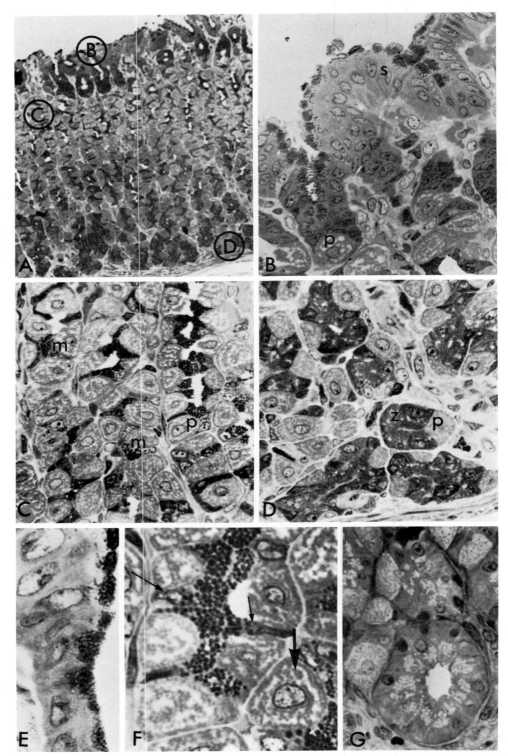

Figure 11–29. A series of photomicrographs of the fundus of bear stomach. Plastic sections, stained with toluidine blue and saffranin. *A,* Survey picture of the full thickness of the mucosa. The circled letters indicate regions from which following pictures were taken. × 125. *B,* Surface, showing surface epithelium (s) with mucin droplets, and parietal cells (p) in the isthmus of glands. × 450. *C,* The neck region, showing mucous neck cells (m) and parietal cells (p) with clear, unstained intracellular canaliculi. × 450. *D,* The bases of glands with parietal (p) and chief or zymogenic (z) cells. Part of the muscularis mucosae is shown at the bottom. × 450. *E,* Surface epithelial cells with apical mucin droplets. × 750. *F,* Thin arrows indicate mucous neck cells, of irregular outline, seemingly squashed between parietal cells; the broad arrow shows a parietal cell with an extensive intracellular canaliculus. × 1250. *G,* Cross section through the base of a gland lined totally by chief cells with apical, unstained zymogen granules. × 750.

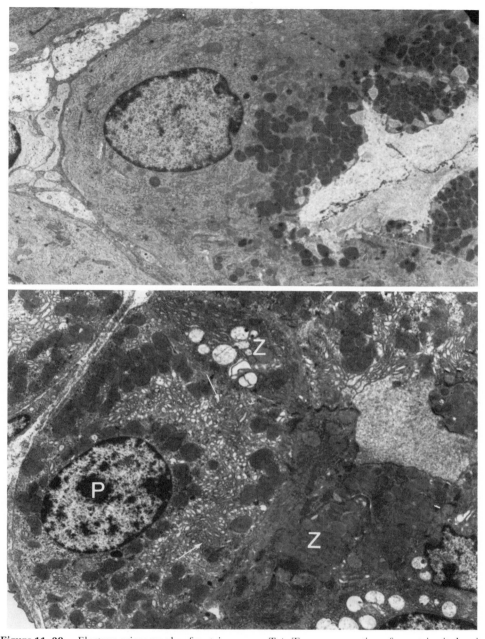

Figure 11–30. Electron micrographs of gastric mucosa. *Top:* Transverse section of a gastric pit showing surface mucous cells with apical secretory droplets. ×6500. *Bottom:* Transverse section through the base of a gastric gland showing a parietal cell (P) with canaliculi (arrows) and parts of chief (zymogenic) cells (Z). ×6500.

produce the majority of the enzymes and hydrochloric acid and some mucin. The pits are not as deep as those in the pylorus, extending for only a quarter to a third of the mucosal thickness. The glands thus are long and straight, although they may be slightly coiled in their upper extent. Usually in a section they are cut lengthwise. Each gland is said to have three parts: a base, a middle region or neck, and an upper isthmus which continues into a pit. Four cell types are present. In the isthmus, only surface epithelial cells and parietal cells are present. The main cell type in the neck is the mucous neck cell, between which are scattered parietal cells. The base is composed mainly of chief or zymogenic cells with some parietal and a few enterochromaffin cells.

Chief (Zymogenic) Cell. Chief cells are situated in the lower portions of fundic glands, extend from the basal lamina to the lumen, and in a cross section of a gland, are pyramidal in shape and bear close similarities to pancreatic acinar and to salivary serous cells. The nucleus is spherical and situated toward the base of the cell, and the cytoplasm shows basal mitochondria and chromidial substance. The apical cytoplasm contains granules which do not preserve well and in a fixed preparation may be dissolved leaving a vacuolated appearance. By electron microscopy, the cells are cuboidal to pyramidal and show apical microvilli, a supranuclear Golgi complex, and numerous profiles of granular endoplasmic reticulum with some free ribosomes concentrated mainly at the base. Mitochondria are also basally located and in the apical cytoplasm are numerous, spherical, membrane-bound granules of low electron density. These appearances, of course, are consistent with a protein-secreting function, and this cell secretes pepsinogen.

Parietal Cell. Parietal or oxyntic (i.e., acid-forming) cells are scattered singly and in small groups between the other cell types from the isthmus to the base of gastric glands, although they are most numerous in the neck and isthmus regions. They are characteristically spherical or pyramidal, of large size, and located peripherally in a gland so that their broad bases appear to bulge into the underlying lamina propria. Often their apices appear not to reach the lumen. The nucleus is spherical and central in position, and the cytoplasm appears clear and stains readily with acidic dyes. An unusual feature is the presence of an intracellular canaliculus. This is a network of canals formed by infolding of the luminal surface which may be so extensive as to reach almost to the base of the cell. In ordinary preparations it appears as an irregular, unstained area. By electron microscopy it is obvious that these canaliculi are invaginations of the apical surface and not a true intracellular system. Numerous microvilli project both into the glandular lumen and into the secretory canaliculi, where they may be so closely packed and interdigitated as to virtually occlude the lumen. The cytoplasm of parietal cells contains numerous mitochondria and the Golgi apparatus is small and often located in an infranuclear position. Free ribosomes are present; granular endoplasmic reticulum is sparse. A prominent feature of the cytoplasm is the presence of closely packed tubulovesicles, particularly near intracellular canaliculi. These tubulovesicles are bounded by a unit membrane similar if not identical to the surface plasmalemma, and probably these elements are not to be considered as part of the agranular reticulum. In a resting cell, viz., one not actively producing hydrochloric acid, the tubulovesicles are numerous and canaliculi are dilated with few microvilli. During active secretion, tubulovesicles are less numerous, and microvilli at the surface and in association with canaliculi become much more prominent. These elements are thus considered important in hydrochloric acid secretion, probably by actively transporting chloride and hydrogen ions across the cell. In this process, membrane may interchange between microvilli at the surface and tubulovesicles in the cytoplasm. No secretory granules are present in parietal cells. Recently radioautographic studies have shown that parietal cells also are the site of intrinsic factor production (necessary for vitamin B_{12} absorption).

Mucous Neck Cell. These cells are relatively few in number and located only in the necks of fundic glands. They tend to be of irregular shape, as though deformed by the cells which surround them. The nuclei are ovoid, flattened, and basally located, and the apical cytoplasm contains pale, secretory granules which stain well with mucicarmine. Other staining reactions differentiate these cells from mucus-secreting cells of oral glands and from the gastric surface epithelial cells. By electron microscopy, these cells show stubby, apical microvilli with a characteristic "fuzz" owing to the presence of very fine filaments attached to the surface. The secretory granules are dense and of varying shape. Mucous neck cells produce acid mucopolysaccharides and have a life-span of about six days.

Enterochromaffin Cells. Throughout the gastrointestinal tract are mucosal cells that have been termed enterochromaffin cells in that these cells, usually small and granular, are stained strongly by bichromate salts. They also have been termed *argentaffin cells,* as their granules reduce silver nitrate or *argyrophil* cells if the reduction occurs only in the presence of a reducing agent. While some variation in morphology occurs, they contain small cytoplasmic granules, membrane-limited, that are located in basal cytoplasm and probably are secreted into the lamina propria and thus into the vascular system. Other cytoplasmic components are sparse, and the cells always lie adjacent to the basal lamina. Their morphology and secretory mechanism make it appropriate to regard them as *endocrine*

cells (enteroendocrine cells) of the gastrointestinal tract. It is apparent that these cells have the characteristics of the so-called APUD cells (amine precursor uptake and decarboxylation) that are widespread in the body and concerned in the production and release of polypeptides and proteins with hormonal activity. In the stomach, one argentaffin cell type produces serotonin; another perhaps releases a morphine-like substance called endorphin. Others probably produce gastrin (in the pylorus) and glucagon, while, within the gut tract, others possibly are concerned with the formation of cholecystokinin and somatostatin. Most of the hormones produced by this group of endocrine cells have local, or regional, rather than general effects; viz., the target organ is not far removed from the producing cell. Thus, the digestive system is under the general control of the nervous system, modified and supported by local formation and secretion of hormones.

Pyloric Glands. Here the foveolae

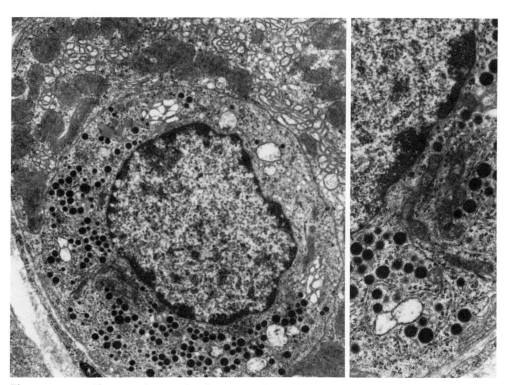

Figure 11–31. Electron micrographs of an enterochromaffin (argentaffin) cell in the base of a gastric gland. Most of the dense secretory granules lie in basal cytoplasm (to the left), viz. infranuclear (right, below). In the left micrograph, part of a parietal cell is seen above. Left, × 9,000; right, × 18,000.

are deep, extending to half of the thickness of the mucosa. The pyloric glands thus are short and are simple or branched tubular, but they are of greater diameter than those of the fundus and coiled so that rarely are they sectioned along their lengths. With the exception of a few argentaffin and parietal cells, only one cell type is present. This is very similar to the mucous neck cell, has a pale cytoplasm with indistinct granulation and a flattened basal nucleus, and produces mucin.

Lamina Propria

The lamina propria is scanty and consists of a delicate meshwork of collagenous and reticular fibers and a few fibroblasts or reticular cells. Scattered in the meshes are some lymphocytes, plasma cells, mast cells, and white blood cells, the lymphocytes occasionally being present in small, local accumulations, these being more obvious at cardiac and pyloric regions. Thin slips of smooth muscle pass from the muscularis mucosae between the gastric glands. The lamina propria, as explained earlier, owing to the masses of cardiac glands, is not extensive, being limited to the narrow, slitlike spaces between adjacent glands. The lamina is more obvious toward the surface of the mucosa where spaces are more extensive between foveolae.

Muscularis Mucosae

This is not thick and the smooth muscle of which it is composed is arranged into inner circular and outer longitudinal laminae. In some regions there is a third external coat which is circular or oblique. Slips from the muscularis mucosae extend into the lamina propria between gastric glands.

Submucosa

This tunic or coat, of fibroconnective tissue with collagenous, reticular, and elastic fibers, extends into the rugae or longitudinal folds present in the con-

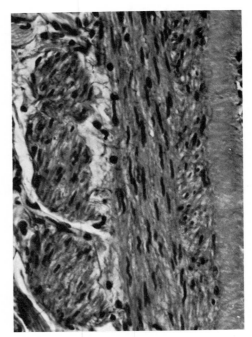

Figure 11–32. Photomicrograph of the muscularis mucosae of the cat stomach, showing three layers of smooth muscle. Aldehyde fuchsin, light green stain. × 250.

tracted stomach. In addition to fibroblasts, macrophages, plasma cells, and lymphocytes, some fat cells usually are present. Contained in the layer are blood and lymph vessels and peripheral nerves of the submucous nerve plexus.

Muscularis

There are three layers of smooth muscle, each oriented in a different plane. The outermost layer is longitudinal and continuous with that of the esophagus. The middle layer is circular, continuous with the inner layer of the esophagus, and greatly thickened at the pylorus to form the *pyloric sphincter*, where it is the thickest and most obvious layer. The innermost layer is oblique and takes the form of loops of muscle extending from the cardiac orifice around the fundus and corpus. It is not a complete layer.

Serosa

This consists of a layer of loose areolar tissue in which vessels and nerves are present, external to the muscularis and covered by a mesothelial layer, the peritoneum. At greater and lesser curvatures of the stomach, it is continuous with the greater and lesser mesenteries (omenta). The *greater omentum* hangs down from the greater curvature, is covered by peritoneum, and consists of areolar connective tissue which usually becomes increasingly adipose with age. The major blood vessels to and from the stomach course in the omenta.

THE SMALL INTESTINE

The small intestine extends from the pyloric orifice, where it is continuous with the stomach, to the ileocecal junction, where it continues into the large intestine. It is about 720 cm in length, is much coiled within the abdominal cavity, and is divided into three parts. The first part, the *duodenum*, is only 20 cm long and is relatively fixed to the posterior abdominal wall as it has no mesentery throughout the greater part of its length. The remainder of the small intestine is divided into the *jejunum*, the next two-fifths of the length, and the *ileum*, the remaining three-fifths. The jejunum and ileum are suspended from the posterior abdominal wall by the *mesentery* although the terminal ileum again is fixed to the posterior abdominal wall. The functions of the small intestine are to transport food material (chyme) from the stomach to the large intestine, to complete digestion by the secretion of enzymes from its wall and from accessory glands, to absorb the final products of digestion into blood and lymph vessels

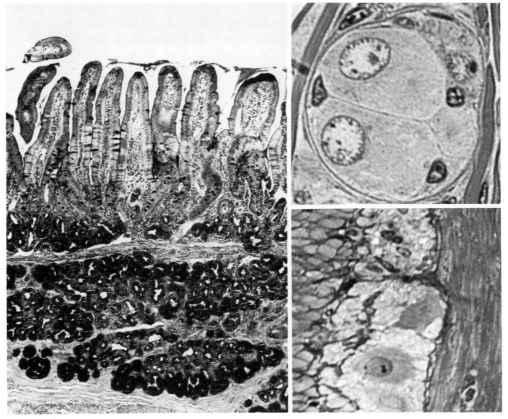

Figure 11–33. Photomicrographs of duodenum. *Left:* Longitudinal section showing mucosa with villi and intestinal glands, and submucosa with submucosal glands of Brunner. × 75. *Top right:* Part of the submucosa showing ganglion cells of Meissner's plexus. Plastic section. × 700. *Bottom right:* Ganglion cells of Auerbach's intermyenteric plexus between smooth muscle of the inner circular (left) and outer longitudinal layers of the muscularis. Plastic section. × 400.

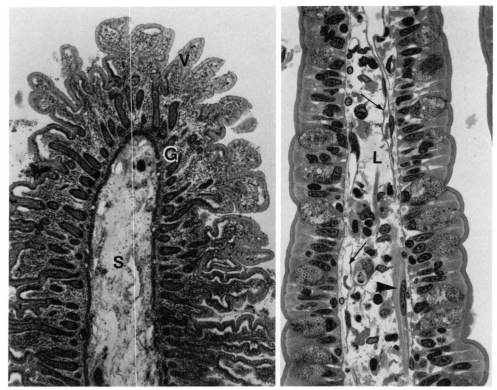

Figure 11–34. *Left:* Photomicrograph of upper jejunum to show a plica circularis with a core of submucosa (S), the mucosa showing villi (V) and intestinal glands (G). ×40. *Right:* Part of a villus from the ileum, with a core of lamina propria (L) containing capillaries (arrows), and a slip of smooth muscle (arrowhead). The lining epithelium is simple columnar with a brush border and contains numerous goblet cells. × 400.

in its wall, and to secrete certain hormones.

To subserve these functions, particularly of absorption and digestive secretion, the small intestine shows certain specializations that increase the surface area of its mucosa.

Mucosal Surface Specializations

Plicae Circulares (Valves of Kerckring). These are permanent circular or spiral folds of the entire thickness of the mucosa with a core of submucosa. Any one fold may extend two-thirds or more around the circumference of the intestine, but rarely do the folds completely encircle the lumen. Branching of some plicae occurs. The plicae commence in the duodenum within 2.5 to 5 cm of the pylorus, reach their maximum development in terminal duo-

denum and proximal jejunum, and thereafter diminish, disappearing in the distal half of the ileum.

Villi and Crypts. Villi are small finger- or leaf-like projections of the mucous membrane, 0.5 to 1.5 mm in length, found only in the small intestine. The length of villi varies and is reduced by distention of the intestine. They, of course, are covered by epithelium and have a core of lamina propria, but, unlike plicae, the muscularis mucosae and submucosa do not extend into them. In the duodenum, they are broad, spatulate structures but become cylindrical or finger-like in the ileum. Crypts or intestinal glands (of Lieberkühn) are tubelike structures opening between the bases of villi, 0.3 to 0.5 mm in depth, and extending deeply through the thickness of the mucous membrane nearly to reach the muscularis mucosae. They are not packed so closely as the gastric glands, the spaces

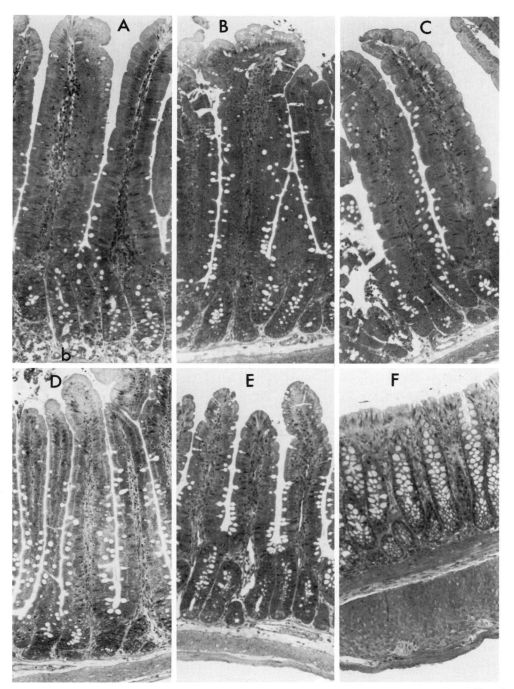

Figure 11–35. Photomicrographs of guinea pig intestinal mucosa at various levels, showing villi and glands. *A*, Upper duodenum (with Brunner's glands (b) below). *B*, Lower duodenum. *C*, Upper jejunum. *D*, Lower jejunum. *E*, Ileum. *F*, Colon. Note that villi decrease in length, goblet cells (pale staining) increase in number from above down and that the colon shows only glands. All × 100.

between them being filled with connective tissue of the lamina propria. Crypts also are present in the large intestine although villi are not, and thus it is important for identification of sections that the student be able to recognize differences between villi and crypts when cut in cross section. Villi appear as circular or oval profiles with a core of connective tissue (lamina propria) covered by epithelium. A crypt in cross section appears as a central lumen lined by epithelium, the whole embedded in connective tissue of the lamina propria.

Microvilli. To further increase surface area, the columnar absorptive cells covering villi and lining crypts have a brush or striated border composed of numerous microvillous processes. Each microvillus is covered by an extension of the plasma membrane, the outer lamina of which is associated with a feltwork of fine filaments giving a fuzzy appearance. This filamentous coat, which occupies the spaces between microvilli and at their tips, forming a continuous surface layer, contains an acid mucopolysaccharide and is resistant to proteolytic and mucolytic agents. In the cores of microvilli are thin, longitudinally oriented filaments which at the bases are continuous with the filaments of the terminal web (see later).

To the food material in the lumen of the small intestine are added the secretions of many glands. These are of three main types: the intestinal glands, the submucosal glands, and the glands situated outside the digestive tract but passing their secretions into its lumen by a duct system. Intestinal glands, as just explained, are found in both small and large intestines. Submucosal glands are located in the duodenum, are compound tubular in type, and are termed the *duodenal glands* (of Brunner). Usually, they are more extensive in the first part of the duodenum near the pylorus. Glands situated outside the digestive tract are the liver and pancreas, and both deliver their exocrine secretions into the duodenum.

Epithelium

The epithelium of the intestinal mucosa is simple columnar in type but differs from the surface epithelium of the stomach in that more than one cell type is present. There are columnar cells with a striated border, Paneth cells, goblet cells, enterochromaffin cells, and others.

Columnar (Absorptive) Cells. These tall, cylindrical cells rest upon a thin basal lamina. Nuclei are elongated

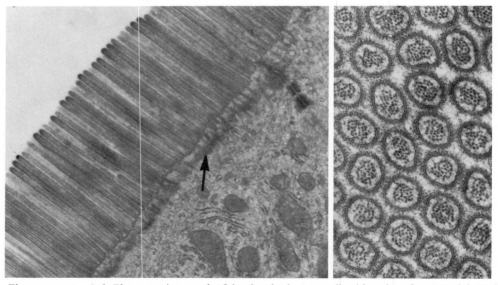

Figure 11–36. *Left:* Electron micrograph of duodenal columnar cells with an interface (top right) and apical microvilli of the brush border. Filaments in the microvilli extend into apical cytoplasm to mesh with the terminal web (arrow). × 16,000. *Right:* Microvilli in transverse section with a "fuzz" of glycocalyx on the external surface of their plasmalemmae and bundles of filaments in their cores. × 88,000.

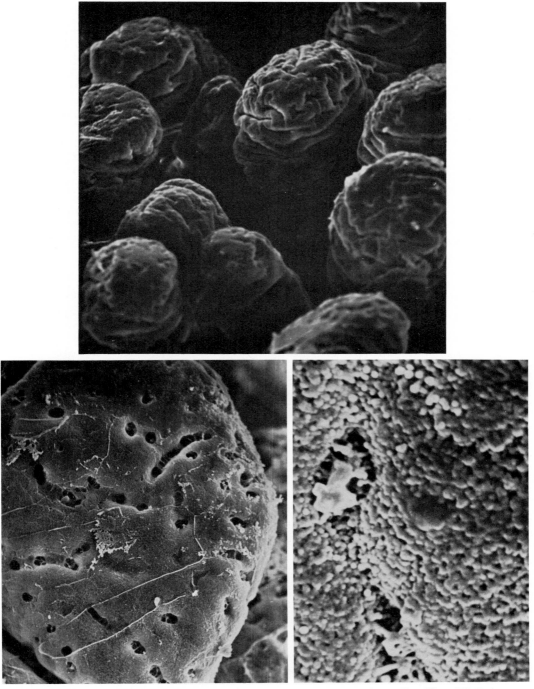

Figure 11–37. Scanning electron micrographs. *Top:* Low power showing finger-like villi. × 536. *Bottom left:* A single finger-like villus to show goblet-cell orifices with interconnecting troughs and strands of mucus (white) on the surface. × 1070. *Bottom right:* Cell surface showing microvilli and two goblet cells with mucus. × 10,300. (Courtesy of Doctors N. M. Marsh, J. A. Swift, and E. D. Williams.)

and ovoid and are located toward the base with extensive apical cytoplasm. Prominent terminal bars and a terminal web are present, and each cell has a striated (brush) border. This striated border is formed by numerous, closely packed, parallel microvilli which are longer on cells near the tip of a villus than they are on cells at the base. Each microvillus contains a bundle of parallel filaments in its core which penetrate into apical cytoplasm where they blend into the terminal web. The plasma membrane covering microvilli is covered with a glycocalyx or cell coat, and between microvilli at their bases are slender pits or invaginations of the cell surface associated with caveolae intracellulares or pinocytotic vesicles. These structures all are associated with absorption, particularly of macromolecules. Indeed, the glycocalyx contains glycoproteins that are hydrolytic enzymes. Enzymes such as disaccharidases and peptidases are localized here and concerned in the digestion of carbohydrates and proteins. Mitochondria are numerous throughout columnar cells, and lysosomes also are present, particularly in older cells near a villus tip. Granular reticulum, ribosomes, and a little agranular reticulum are present with a Golgi apparatus in a supranuclear position. These surface epithelial cells are involved in the absorption of carbohydrates, proteins, and lipids from the lumen of the small intestine.

Undifferentiated Cells. These cells are found in the bases of intestinal glands (crypts) and are the source of replacement of other cells both in crypts and on villi. They are columnar, but irregular in shape, with numerous free ribosomes, and they undergo frequent mitoses. The daughter cells migrate up the crypt and onto a villus to become absorptive cells. They resemble the absorptive cells of a villus, although while present in a crypt they are more slender, have fewer organelles, and fewer, shorter microvilli. Columnar cells in a crypt are capable of mitosis, while those on a villus do not divide. Radioautography has shown that a columnar cell in a crypt reaches a villus tip in about three days and then is shed; thus, there is a constant renewal of the intestinal epithelium and a constant migration of cells from the bases of intestinal glands up to villi.

Paneth Cells. These cells are found only in the bases of intestinal glands, scattered between undifferentiated cells, and are found throughout the small intestine. They are absent in the large intestine. Paneth cells are pyramidal in shape with a broad base resting against the basal lamina and a narrow apex. They show all the features of exocrine (protein) secretion with basal, extensive, granular reticulum, a large supranuclear Golgi complex, and apical secretory droplets or granules, which stain bright pink in a hematoxylin-eosin preparation. These cells contain zinc and secrete peptidase and, possibly, lysozyme, an enzyme which breaks down bacteria. While only a few cells of Paneth are found in the base of each intestinal gland, collectively throughout the small intestine they constitute a relatively large mass of cells.

Mucous (Goblet) Cells. On intestinal villi, goblet cells are scattered between columnar cells, and their numbers increase from duodenum to terminal ileum. In the bases of intestinal glands, in the region where Paneth cells are found, are so-called *oligomucous cells.* These cells arise by differentiation of some of the undifferentiated cells and contain a prominent Golgi apparatus and a few mucous droplets. Probably, at this stage they can divide, but with the accumulation of more mucous droplets they lose this capacity for mitosis. As they migrate up the gland and onto a villus, they accumulate more and more mucous droplets and acquire the distended or goblet shape, and like columnar cells, they are shed from the tips of villi, although their rate of replacement is slower than that of columnar cells.

Endocrine (Enterochromaffin) Cells. These cells, described previously in relation to fundic (gastric) glands, are found both in intestinal glands and on villi. As many as five different types have been described, and all are spherical or pyramidal in shape with basal granules. Some have a slender apical prolongation reaching the lumen. The various types produce gastrin (in the stomach glands only), serotonin, secretin (a hormone which stimulates the

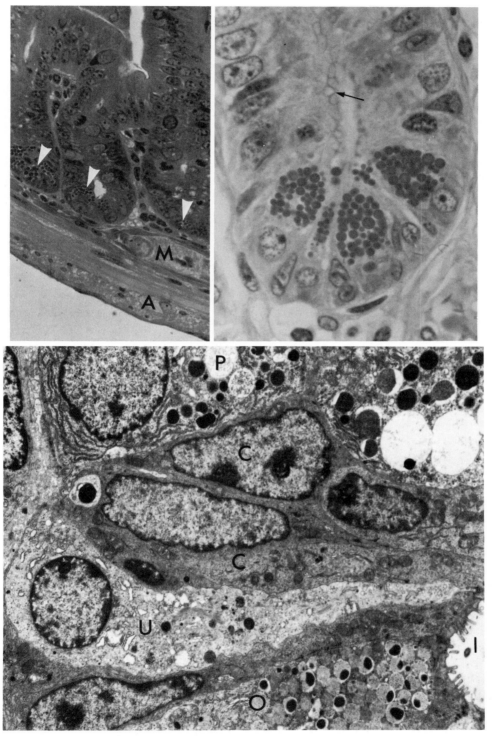

Figure 11–38. Illustration of Paneth cells in the bases of intestinal glands. *Top left:* The arrowheads indicate Paneth cells in three glands; note also ganglion cells of Meissner's (M) and Auerbach's (A) plexuses. × 200. *Top right:* Plastic section with discrete apical granules in Paneth cells of the base of one gland. Note also the terminal bars (arrow) of enterocytes. × 900. *Bottom:* Electron micrograph of the base of a jejunal gland, with lumen (1) to the right. At top is a Paneth cell (P) with prominent granular reticulum and apical secretory granules. In addition to columnar (C) cells or enterocytes, one cell probably is a young columnar or undifferentiated (U) cell and at bottom is an oligomucous (O) or early goblet cell. × 3500.

exocrine pancreas), norepinephrine, and possibly cholecystokinin (which stimulates bile secretion).

Caveolated Cell. Caveolated cells are rare and are characterized by thick, stubby, apical microvilli containing thick bundles of filaments extending deeply into cell cytoplasm and by irregular tubules (caveolae) passing as invaginations from the apical surface between microvilli. They also are found in the respiratory tract (alveoli and small bronchial tubes). Their function is unknown, although it has been suggested that they are chemoreceptors.

Migrating Cells. Lymphocytes and other cells of blood origin are found commonly migrating through the intestinal epithelium.

Lamina Propria

The lamina propria extends between intestinal glands and into the cores of villi. Its character is quite distinctive with a network of reticular fibers and many features of loose lymphatic tissue. It is best described, perhaps, as a loose, areolar connective tissue with lymphoid tendencies. Present in the meshwork of reticular fibers are primitive reticular cells with large, oval, pale-staining nuclei, lymphocytes, macrophages and plasma cells. Eosinophil leukocytes, in particular, are evident, these having migrated from blood vessels. Single smooth muscle cells oriented lengthwise in the cores of villi usually are related closely to lymphatic capillaries. These start blindly in villi, contain absorbed fat after a meal, and thus appear white in fresh or living tissue. They are called *lacteals*.

In addition to scattered lymphocytes, there are present in the lamina propria large numbers of *solitary follicles* or isolated lymphatic nodules, more numerous distally in the intestine. If large, they may occupy the entire thickness of the mucosa and bulge the surface. There are no villi and may be no crypts on the surface of large follicles which are then separated from the lumen only by a simple columnar epi-

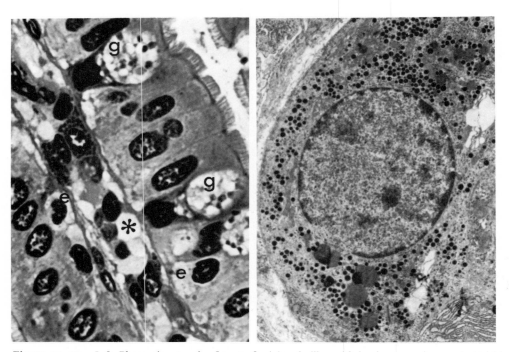

Figure 11–39. *Left:* Photomicrograph of part of a jejunal villus with lamina propria core (asterisk), columnar cells with a microvillus (striated) border, goblet cells (g) and enterochromaffin cells (e). × 900. *Right:* Electron micrograph of an enterochromaffin cell showing basal granules toward the lamina propria (left). × 9000.

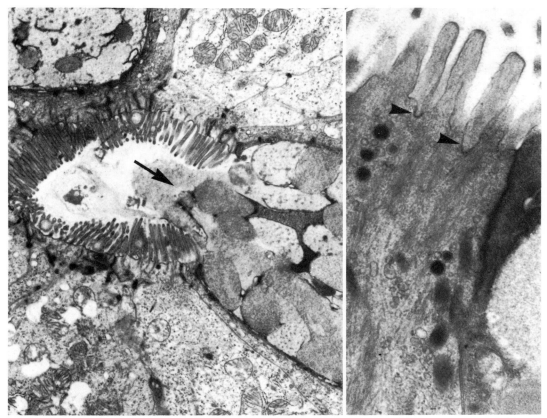

Figure 11–40. *Left:* Electron micrograph of a transverse section of an intestinal gland bordered by columnar cells with microvilli and prominent junctional complexes and by a goblet cell discharging mucus (arrow). × 7500. *Right:* The apical portion of a caveolated cell with thick, stubby microvilli, prominent clumps of cytoplasmic fibrils, and two caveolae opening between microvilli (arrowheads). On the right is part of a goblet cell. × 13,000.

thelium. In many regions, but mainly in the ileum, follicles may be so numerous and close together as to aggregate into large masses of lymphoid tissue visible to the naked eye. They vary in size from 12 to 20 mm long, and 8 to 12 mm wide, the longer axis lying along the length of the intestine. Always they are situated on the antimesenteric border, i.e., on the side away from the attachment of the mesentery. These are the *Peyer's patches* or aggregated nodules.

The muscularis mucosae, submucosa, muscularis, and serosa do not merit a separate description, although it should be noted that the submucosa usually is infiltrated with lymphocytes in the region of Peyer's patches.

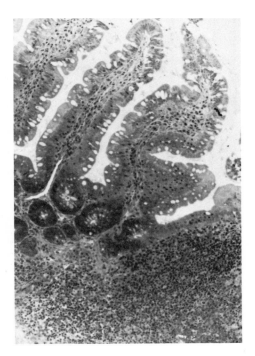

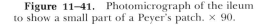

Figure 11–41. Photomicrograph of the ileum to show a small part of a Peyer's patch. × 90.

Duodenal Glands (of Brunner)

These submucosal glands of the duodenum are composed of tall cuboidal cells with dark, flattened, basal nuclei and a clear, vacuolated cytoplasm. The glandular portions continue into ducts lined by low cuboidal cells, and these penetrate the muscularis mucosae to open into intestinal glands. Often, the muscularis mucosae does not form a complete layer over the glands, and slips of smooth muscle extend in the connective tissue between the glandular units. Occasionally, Brunner's glands extend into the upper part of the jejunum, and, more commonly may be found in the pyloric region of the stomach. These glands secrete an alkaline mucus. The acidic gastric secretion could cause erosion of the duodenal mucosa, and the secretion of the submucosal glands protects against this by its mucus, by its alkalinity, and presumably by the buffering capacity of its bicarbonate content.

THE LARGE INTESTINE

The large intestine is about 180 cm in length and consists of the *cecum*, continuous with the ileum at the ileocecal valve, the *appendix*, a small diverticulum from the cecum, the *colon*, continuous with the cecum and divided into the ascending, transverse, and descending parts, and then the *rectum* and *anal canal*, terminating as the *anus* at the body surface. Food material enters the cecum in a semifluid state; it becomes semisolid, the consistency of feces, in the colon. Thus, one function of the large intestine is absorption of fluid. Other functions are secretion of mucus (lubrication becomes more important as fluid is absorbed and the fecal mass becomes harder and thus more likely to damage the mucosa) and digestion, ac-

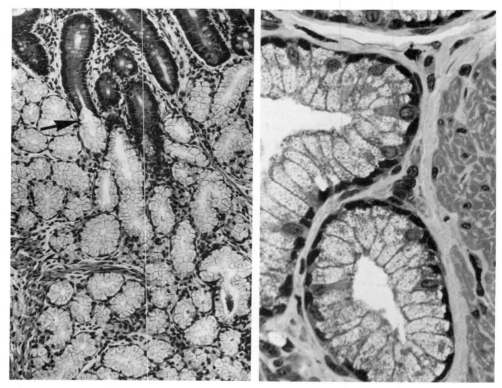

Figure 11–42. Photomicrographs of the duodenal glands (of Brunner). *Left:* The mucous glands lie in the submucosa (below) and their ducts penetrate the muscularis mucosae to open into bases of intestinal glands (arrow). × 100. *Right:* The glands at higher magnification. Smooth muscle of the muscularis mucosae is seen at right. × 400.

complished by enzymes present in the food material and by putrefaction by bacteria always present in the large intestine. No digestive enzymes are secreted by the large intestine.

The large intestine lacks plicae and villi and thus the surface epithelium is more obvious than it is in the small intestine. Intestinal glands or crypts are present and are longer than those of the small intestine and more closely packed. Epithelial cell types are identical to those of the small intestine but the goblet (mucus-secreting) cells are more numerous.

Ileocecal Junction

At the ileocecal junction there is an abrupt change in the character of the mucosa, which is thrown into anterior and posterior folds to form two *valves*. These folds consist of mucosa and submucosa supported by a mass of circular smooth muscle, a thickening of the inner layer of the muscularis, and because of their position the ileocecal orifice has the form of a vertical slit.

The ileocecal junction is located at the lower right side of the abdomen and is fixed to the posterior abdominal wall; i.e., the terminal ileum has no mesentery. The cecum is a small blind pouch hanging down from the ileocecal junction and has a structure identical to that of the colon.

Appendix

The appendix is a small, slender, blind diverticulum of the cecum arising about 2.5 cm below the ileocecal valve. In cross section, the lumen is small and usually of irregular outline, often contains cellular debris, and may be completely occluded. Villi are absent and intestinal glands are few and of irregular length. The surface epithelium is composed of columnar, striated border cells mainly, with only a few goblet cells. In the crypts there are a few Paneth cells, and enterochromaffin cells are numerous. The lamina propria is occupied by a mass of lymphoid tissue similar to that of the palatine tonsil. The muscularis mucosae usually is in-

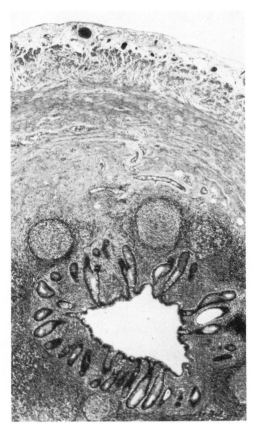

Figure 11–43. Photomicrograph of a cross section of the human appendix. Note the intestinal glands and infiltration of the lamina propria by lymphatic tissue, with lymphatic nodules. × 40.

complete. The submucosa is thick and contains blood vessels and nerves, and the muscularis is thin but shows the usual two layers. The serous coat is identical to that covering the remainder of the intestine.

The appendix so commonly is the site of acute and chronic inflammation that it is difficult to obtain a completely normal appendix. Usually, some eosinophils and neutrophils are present in lamina propria and submucosa. If present in large numbers, they are evidence of chronic and acute infection respectively.

Cecum, Colon, and Rectum

The intestinal glands are of greater depth in the large than in the small intestine and are packed more closely. They increase in depth to 0.75 mm in

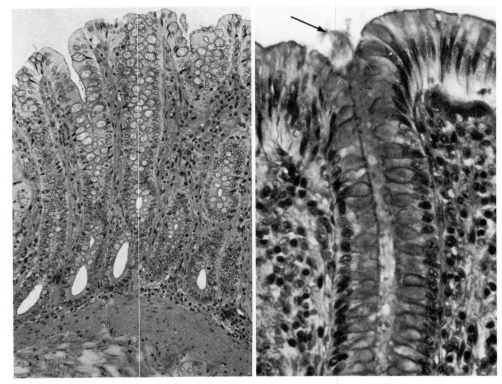

Figure 11–44.   Photomicrographs of the colon to show the mucosa. No villi are present, intestinal glands are straight tubules, and goblet cells are abundant. The arrow indicates mucus discharged from one gland. Left, Plastic section, × 125; right, × 300.

the rectum, being 0.5 mm in the colon. Goblet cells are numerous and enterochromaffin cells are occasional in the depths, but Paneth cells usually are not present. Most of the cells in the depths of the glands are undifferentiated epithelial cells which undergo rapid mitosis. These cells contain some secretory granules which are discharged before the cells reach the surface of the mucosa. The secreted material forms part of the glycocalyx. The lamina propria between glands is similar in appearance to that of the small intestine and contains scattered lymphatic nodules which extend deeply into the submucosa. The muscularis mucosae is well developed but may be irregular or deficient at the sites of lymphatic nodules. In the cecum and colon, the outer longitudinal coat of the muscularis is not a complete layer and is present as three longitudinal bands, the *taeniae coli.* In the rectum, it again becomes a complete layer. The serous

coat shows, on the surface not attached to the posterior abdominal wall, small, taglike protuberances composed of adipose tissue, the *appendices epiploicae.* In the transverse colon there is a true mesentery.

Rectoanal Junction

In the lower end of the rectum, the intestinal glands become short and disappear in the anal canal. Here, the mucous membrane is thrown into a series of longitudinal folds termed the *rectal columns of Morgagni.* In this region, the muscularis mucosae becomes broken up into a series of bundles and finally disappears so that there is no distinction between lamina propria and submucosa. In this region there are numerous longitudinal, thin-walled veins which, if dilated and convoluted, cause protrusion of the mucous membrane over them. Such a condition constitutes *internal hemorrhoids*

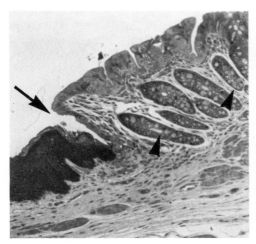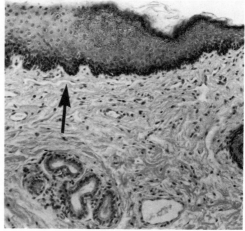

Figure 11–45. *Left:* Photomicrograph of the rectoanal junction (arrow) where the simple columnar epithelium changes abruptly to stratified squamous and intestinal glands (arrowheads) disappear. × 100. *Right:* Photomicrograph of the mucocutaneous junction (arrow) where the stratified squamous epithelium of the anal canal (left) blends into keratinized epithelium (right). Note circumanal (apocrine) glands at lower left. × 100.

or *piles*. About 2.5 cm above the anal orifice, the columnar epithelium abruptly changes to a stratified squamous epithelium which extends downward for a short extent only as a transition zone between intestinal epithelium and skin. At the anus, the epithelium is keratinized and beneath it are branched tubular glands termed the *circumanal glands*.

The muscularis at the rectoanal junction shows certain modifications. In the lower rectum, the longitudinal layer appears to be shorter than the length of the rectum and thus causes the mucosa to bulge into the lumen as transverse shelves termed the *plicae transversae*, there being two such shelves on the right and one on the left. These may aid in the support of feces but also are thought to help the separation of feces from flatus. In the lower rectum and anal canal the internal layer of the muscularis is thickened as the *internal sphincter* of the anus. Surrounding the anal canal are bundles of striated muscle, the external sphincter of the anus.

Intestinal Absorption

The digestion of food material within the intestinal lumen involves the reduction of foodstuffs to molecular size. This is accomplished by the secretions of the major digestive glands (pancreas and liver) and by secretions of intestinal juice, produced mainly by the intestinal glands (of Lieberkühn). Bile from the liver reduces lipid to triglycerides, while pancreatic juice contains lipolytic, proteolytic, and carbohydrate-splitting enzymes. Intestinal juice contains lipase, maltase, and peptidase, possibly located in the microvillous border. In the adult, amino acids resulting from the intraluminal digestion of proteins are absorbed by the intestinal epithelium. The majority of lipid is absorbed as micelles of fatty acids and monoglycerides which are re-esterified to triglyceride in the agranular reticulum of apical cytoplasm. The triglyceride then is combined with protein to form *chylomicrons*, which later enter the lacteals by an as yet unknown mechanism.

Blood Vessels

Generally throughout the digestive tract the arrangements of blood and lymph vessels are similar. Basically, arteries entering the tract pass through the muscularis to form an extensive submucous plexus. From this plexus, branches pass toward the lumen and supply capillaries to the muscularis mucosae and capillary networks throughout the mucosa and around the glands. Venous return commences superficially, from the mucosal capillary plexus, as large caliber vessels which form an extensive venous plexus just internal to the muscularis mucosae. From here, veins pass outward into the submucosa where there is a second extensive plexus which is drained by large veins passing through the muscularis to the serosa. These large veins run with the entering arteries.

In the small intestine, the arterial pattern is more extensive than that just described. In addition to capillary networks around the intestinal glands, other arterioles originate in the submucous plexus and are destined specifically to supply villi, each villus receiving one or more such arterioles. Having entered the base of a villus, these arterioles break up into a dense capillary network situated adjacent to the basal lamina of the epithelium. Small veins arise from this superficial capillary network at the tip of a villus and pass outward to join the venous plexus internal to the muscularis mucosae.

Lymphatic capillaries form an extensive system surrounding glands in the superficial layers of the mucosa, and in the small intestine this plexus is joined by lacteals. Lacteals start blindly in the apices of villi, and run axially in the cores of villi. From the mucosal plexus, branches pierce the muscularis mucosae and form a plexus of lymphatics in the submucosa from which larger lymphatics pass outward through the muscularis and follow blood vessels to the retroperitoneal tissues. In the muscularis, lymphatics receive many tributaries from another lymphatic plexus located in the muscularis.

SECTION III. THE MAJOR DIGESTIVE GLANDS

There are two large abdominal organs which connect to the digestive tract by duct systems. These are the pancreas and the liver.

THE PANCREAS

The pancreas is a large, elongated organ lying in the concavity of the duodenum and extending behind the peritoneum of the posterior abdominal wall toward the left to reach the hilum of the spleen. It is both an exocrine and an endocrine organ, the two functions being performed by different cell types.

In the fresh condition, it is pale pink or white and has no definite fibrous capsule, but is covered by thin, areolar tissue from which thin septa extend into the gland to divide it into obvious lobules. Fine, delicate reticular tissue surrounds individual acini.

Exocrine Portion

The pancreas can be classified as a large, lobulated, compound, tubuloacinar gland.

Acini

Acini or alveoli are tubular or pear-shaped, surrounded by a basal lamina and composed of five to eight pyramidal cells arranged around a small central lumen. Myoepithelial cells are not present. Between acini is delicate connective tissue containing blood vessels, lymphatics, nerves, and excretory ducts. The acini are packed in an irregular fashion, and thus in any section, they will be cut in every possible plane. Obviously, the lumen of all will not be sectioned, and in addition, the caliber of the lumen varies with the secretory phase and may contain small cells. These, the *centroacinar cells*, belong to the duct system, which often commences not from the terminations but from the central parts of acini.

In an acinar cell, the nucleus is spherical, lies toward the base, and contains abundant chromatin and one to three large nucleoli. The basal cytoplasm is basophil and may show a longitudinal striation owing to the presence of numerous elongated mitochondria. The apical cytoplasm contains acidophil secretion (zymogenic)

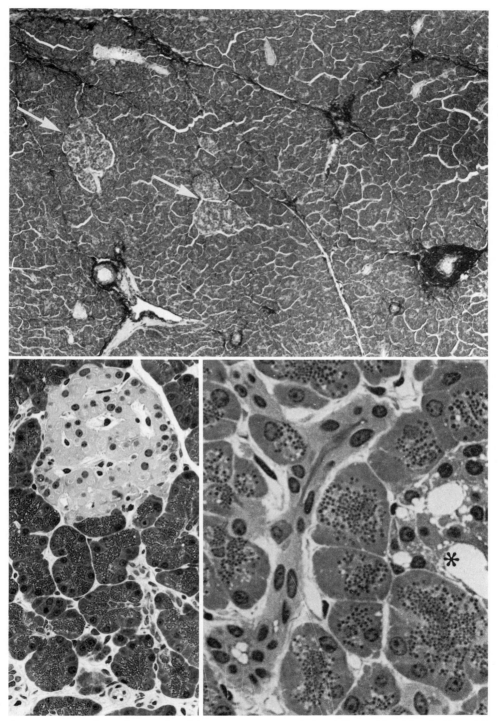

Figure 11–46. Photomicrographs of the pancreas. *Top:* Lobules delineated by thin, darkly staining slips of connective tissue, with numerous serous (exocrine) acini and two islets of Langerhans (lightly staining, arrows). × 60. *Bottom left:* Serous acini below with apical droplets or granules, an islet above with many capillary vessels between cells. Plastic section. × 250. *Bottom right:* Serous acini with small, branching intralobular duct and part of an islet (asterisk) on the right. Plastic section. × 500.

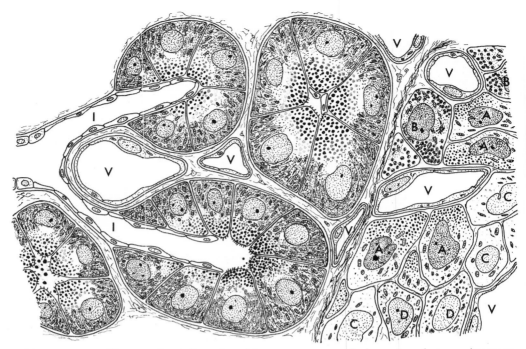

Figure 11–47.   Diagram of a small portion of the pancreas as seen by low-power electron microscopy. In the exocrine portion (left) parts of four acini are illustrated. Two are drained by intercalated ducts (I) and one (top center) shows two centroacinar cells. In a typical exocrine cell, identify the following features: nucleus with nucleolus, basal ergastoplasm and mitochondria, supranuclear Golgi zone (clear space) and apical zymogen and prozymogen droplets. In the endocrine islet of Langerhans (right), A, B, C, and D cells are labeled. Note the variation in type of secretory granules and their relation to capillary blood vessels (V). × 1500 approximately.

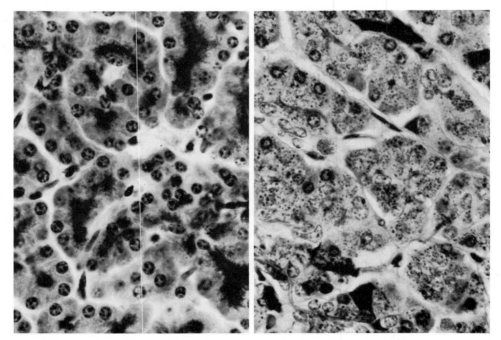

Figure 11–48.   Photomicrographs of the pancreas stained to show secretion (zymogen) granules, *left*, before a meal, and *right*, after a meal. Note that the majority of the granules have been secreted after feeding. Iron hematoxylin, osmic acid. × 350.

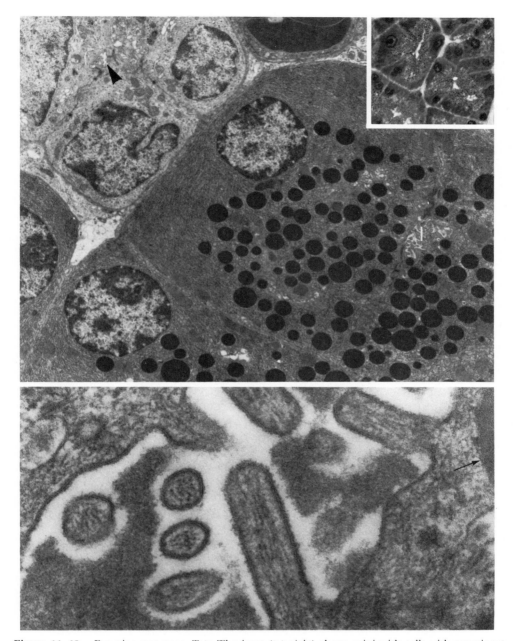

Figure 11–49. Exocrine pancreas. *Top:* The inset (*top right*) shows acini with cells with prominent nucleoli, cytoplasmic basophilia, and apical secretory droplets. × 250. The electron micrograph shows part of an acinus with lumen (1), masses of granular endoplasmic reticulum, and spherical, dense, apical secretory droplets. A small intralobular duct is seen at top left with its lumen (arrowhead) and lined by small cuboidal cells. × 4500. *Bottom:* A higher magnification of part of an acinar lumen showing microvilli in transverse and longitudinal section, the lumen containing dense secretory material. Part of a secretory droplet is indicated by arrow. × 84,000.

droplets or granules which are highly refractile. In a supranuclear position also is an extensive Golgi apparatus, sometimes visible as a clear area among the zymogen granules. By electron microscopy, acini are seen to be enclosed by a thin basal lamina supported by reticular fibers. The nucleus of each acinar cell is large and dense, and nucleoli commonly are seen. The main features of these cells are the specializations for protein secretion (see Chapter

1). The cytoplasm largely is filled with flattened sacs of granular endoplasmic reticulum (ergastoplasm), particularly prominent in the basal region but extending also into the supranuclear zone. Mitochondria are quite numerous, usually elongated, and mainly oriented perpendicularly in the basal cytoplasm. A well-developed Golgi zone is located in a supranuclear position, and the vacuoles of this zone have a content of varying density representing formative stages of zymogen granules. Zymogen granules are large, spherical, and homogeneously dense with a limiting membrane. Some with a less dense matrix have been termed prozymogen granules. A few short microvilli are present at the apex.

The formation and secretion of zy-

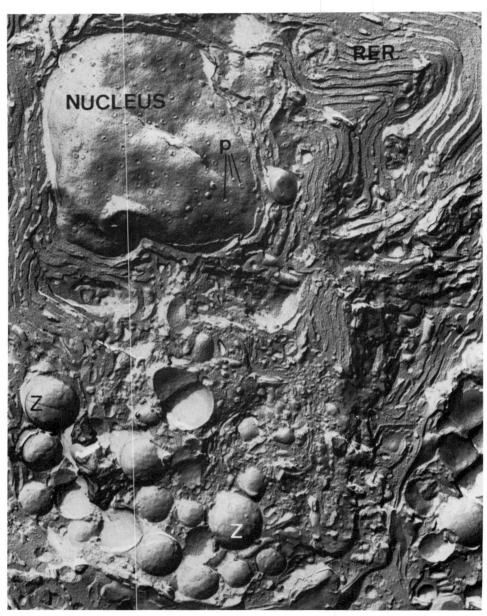

Figure 11–50. Freeze-etch micrograph of part of a pancreatic acinar cell showing nuclear pores (p). The lumen lies below. × 15,000. (Courtesy of L. Orci.)

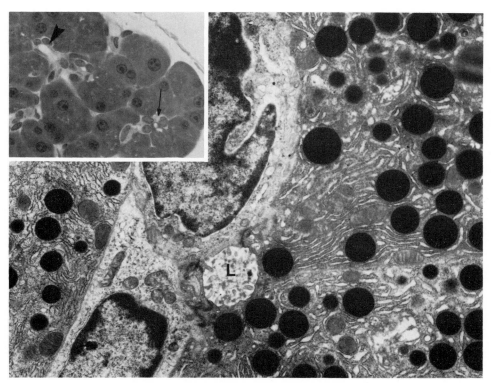

Figure 11–51. *Inset, top left:* Photomicrograph of pancreatic acini with centroacinar cells in one acinus (arrow) and an intercalated duct (arrowhead). × 250. Electron micrograph (*below*) shows an acinar lumen (1) bordered by two acinar (right) and two centroacinar (left) cells. × 9000.

mogen granules have been studied by radioautography after injection of tritiated leucine, glycine, and methionine. Such studies confirm the theory of protein secretion as explained in Chapter 1. Radioautographic label appears rapidly in the endoplasmic reticulum (about five minutes after injection) and later appears in the Golgi zone (in about 10 to 12 minutes) where protein is built into prozymogen granules, and later in zymogen granules (in 30 to 40 minutes). The life span of a zymogen granule in an acinar cell is estimated at about 50 minutes only. These figures give some indication as to the extreme activity of the pancreatic acinar cells. Thus, in summary, it is believed that the digestive enzymes of the pancreas are synthesized in the basal region of the cytoplasm, and accumulate in the canals of the endoplasmic reticulum. From here, the enzymes pass to the Golgi region where they are segregated in membrane-bound vesicles and concentrated into typical zymogen drop-

lets, which later pass to the cell surface where they are discharged by a process of exocytosis. In exocytosis, the membrane bounding the zymogen droplet fuses with the luminal plasmalemma, thus permitting extrusion of the contents of the droplet.

The pancreatic juice contains proteolytic enzymes, e.g., trypsin and chymotrypsin, which split proteins; carboxypeptidase, which cleaves peptides; ribonuclease and deoxyribonuclease, which break down RNP and DNP; amylase, which hydrolyzes starch and other carbohydrates; and lipase, which hydrolyzes neutral fat to glycerol and fatty acids.

Ducts

Three regions of the duct system are described, the cells of all three showing close similarities. They are, in order: centroacinar or centroductular, intercalated (intercalary) ductules, and intralobular to interlobular to main or accessory ducts. The transitions from one region to the next are gradual, the epithelium increasing in height from squamous through cuboidal to columnar. By light microscopy, in all regions cytoplasm is pale-staining and nuclei show little chromatin. Organelles are not prominent. Main features by electron microscopy are a thin basal lamina, lateral plasma membrane interdigitations with desmosomes and junctional complexes, indented nuclei, and apical microvilli. The interlobular and larger ducts lie in fibroconnective tissue, only fine reticular tissue surrounding intercalated and intralobular ducts. The relation of centroacinar cells and intercalated ducts is illustrated in Figure 11–47.

Secretion. While vagal stimulation induces some pancreatic secretion, control of secretion appears to be mainly hormonal by two hormones secreted by the duodenal mucosa and triggered by the passage of stomach contents into the duodenum. One, secretin, causes release of abundant, nonenzymatic, bicarbonate-rich fluid, presumably from ductal cells, while the other, pancreozymin, acts on acinar cells with release of enzyme-rich pancreatic juice.

Endocrine Portion

The endocrine portion of the pancreas, the *islets of Langerhans,* is scattered throughout the pancreas as irregular, spheroidal masses of pale-staining cells with a very rich blood supply. Islets are delineated incompletely from surrounding exocrine acini by a thin "capsule" of reticular fibers, but reticular fibers are few within islets. Islet cells are arranged in irregular cords between which are capillaries, the cells are pale-staining, and no granules are seen in an ordinary H and E preparation. Stains such as Mallory-azan show small cytoplasmic granules. Two main cell types are present: the *alpha (A) cells,* containing granules that are insoluble in alcohol, and the *beta (B) cells,* whose granules are soluble in alcohol. Also present are *delta (D) cells* and a few agranular (C) cells. All are of an irregular, polygonal

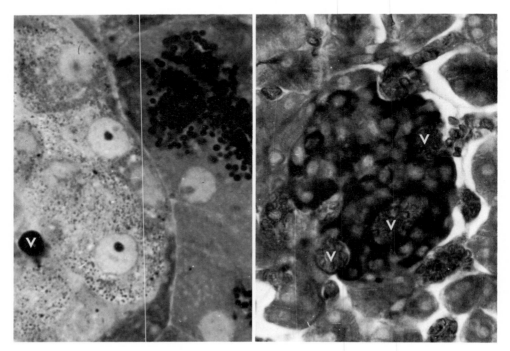

Figure 11–52. Photomicrographs of islet of Langerhans. *Left:* The islet cells contain discrete, dustlike granules (left), much smaller than zymogen granules of acinar cells (right). *Right:* An islet stained to demonstrate B cells. Note the extreme vascularity of islets (blood capillaries labeled v). Left, × 1000; right, aldehyde-fuchsin stain, × 450.

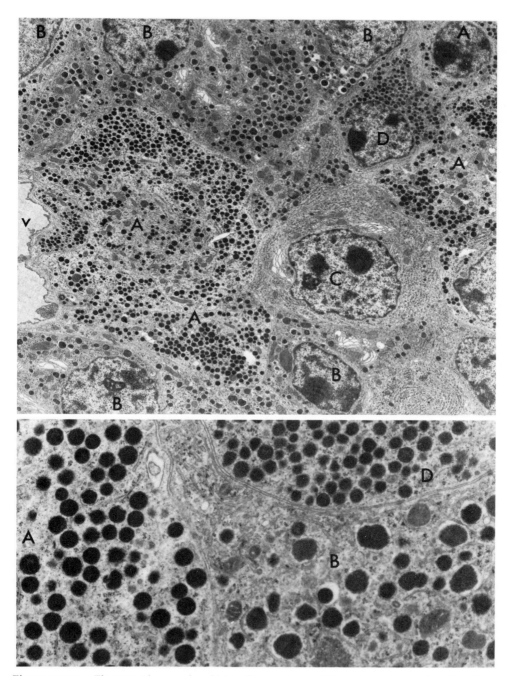

Figure 11–53. Electron micrographs of islet of Langerhans of the guinea pig showing all cell types labelled A, B, C, and D with their characteristic granules and a capillary blood vessel (v, left in upper figure). Top, × 3,000; bottom, × 28,000.

shape with central, spherical nuclei showing well-marked chromatin, small rodlike mitochondria, and a small Golgi apparatus. By electron microscopy, marked differences in the cell types, particularly in respect of their granules, are apparent, although there is considerable species difference.

Within islets, beta cells usually are more numerous and centrally located, while alpha cells tend to be peripheral and usually are adjacent to delta cells. Recent work suggests that islets vary in their cell content with differences between those located in the tail, body and upper portion of the head of the pancreas (main or dorsal) and those in the lower part of the head (distal or ventral).

Alpha cells secrete glucagon, usually number about 20 per cent of the total, and contain numerous homogeneous, dense, spherical granules that are about 300 nm in diameter and membrane bound. Often, the peripheral portion of the granule may be less dense. Secretion of glucagon from alpha cells is stimulated by low blood sugar levels, and this polypeptide hormone causes glucose release from the liver, thus raising blood sugar levels.

Beta cells secrete insulin, usually number about 66 to 80 per cent of the total and, as indicated, lie centrally in an islet. Their granules, usually less numerous and somewhat smaller (about 200 nm in diameter) than those of alpha cells, show distinct species variation. They are spherical, homogeneous, and membrane bound and usually show an electron-lucent periphery in rodents, but in man and other species they contain one or more dense crystals of rectangular, platelike form. The beta cells synthesize proinsulin that then is cleaved proteolytically, probably in the Golgi apparatus, to form insulin and C-peptide. Insulin promotes the transfer of glucose across cell membranes, particularly those in muscle and liver, with a subsequent lowering of the blood sugar level. Insulin release is stimulated by a raised blood sugar level.

Delta cells, peripherally located among A cells in an islet, have homogeneous spherical granules usually larger than those of other cell types but of varying size and density. These cells secrete somatostatin and are relatively few in number, approximately 4 per cent of the total. C cells are pale-staining, lack granules or occasionally contain a very few, and lie centrally among B cells. Their function is unknown, but they may represent a reserve or resting cell.

All endocrine cell types tend to show a polarity with respect to capillaries, with the majority of their granules adjacent to the capillaries.

Blood Vessels and Nerves

The pancreas receives a very rich arterial supply from branches of the celiac and superior mesenteric arteries. Venous return is directly or indirectly to the portal system. Major vessels run in interlobular connective tissue with fine vessels passing into the lobules. As stated previously, capillaries in the islets of Langerhans are large and numerous. Nerves to the pancreas are from the sympathetic (celiac ganglion) and parasympathetic (vagus) parts of the autonomic nervous system. Some ganglion cells are present in interlobular connective tissue.

Development

The pancreas arises from two diverticula, ventral and dorsal, from the junction of fore- and midgut. The diverticula fuse, the epithelial lining branching to form acini connected to the primary outgrowths by a duct system. Some epithelial buds lose their connection to the duct system and differentiate into islet tissue. However, it has been suggested that some of the islet cell types may arise from cells of the neural crest that migrate into the pancreas early in development. During development, the duct systems of the two diverticula become interconnected so that although the dorsal diverticulum forms the bulk of the pancreas, its secretion passes to the ventral outgrowth, the duct of which becomes the main pancreatic duct. The proximal part of the duct of the dorsal diverticulum remains as the accessory pancreatic duct, which opens into the duodenum at a higher level than the main duct. The latter has a common opening into the duodenum with the common bile duct from the liver.

THE LIVER

The liver is the heaviest gland in the body, weighing 3 or more pounds (1.5 kg), is of soft consistency, and is situated beneath the diaphragm in the upper abdomen. It is dark red or reddish-brown in the fresh condition, the color being caused mainly by a very rich blood supply. Not only does it receive an arterial supply from the celiac artery, but it also receives blood from the intestinal tract via the portal vein. Its venous drainage returns to the inferior vena cava, and thus it lies interposed along the venous drainage of the intestinal tract. It receives all the material absorbed from the intestinal tract with the exception of lipid, most of which is transported in the lymphatic system. In addition to the digested and absorbed material which is assimilated and stored in the liver, the portal blood also carries to the liver various toxic materials which then are detoxicated in, or excreted by, the liver. Bile from the liver drains via a duct system into the duodenum and is partly a secretion in that it contains bile salts which are important in digestion and partly an excretion in that it contains waste and even harmful materials for ultimate evacuation in the feces. The portal vein and hepatic artery enter and the hepatic (bile) ducts leave the liver at a region called the *porta hepatis*, a transverse fissure on the inferior surface. The remainder of the liver is covered by a fibroconnective tissue capsule (of Glisson) from which thin connective tissue septa enter the substance of the liver at

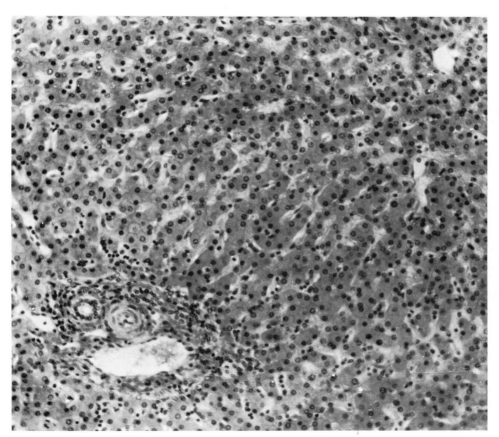

Figure 11–54. Photomicrograph of the human liver, showing a portal area (lower left), a central vein (top right), and plates of liver parenchymal cells of part of a classic lobule extending between the two. × 175.

the porta hepatis to divide it into lobes and lobules. In some animals, e.g., the pig, the content of connective tissue is much greater than it is in the human. Over a great area, the capsule is covered by peritoneum although there is an area (the "bare area") in direct contact with the diaphragm and viscera of the posterior abdominal wall.

General Histological Plan

In a section examined under low power, the liver is seen to be composed of masses of epithelial, parenchymal cells (hepatocytes) arranged in anastomosing and branching plates which form a three-dimensional lattice. Between plates are sinusoidal blood spaces. In this respect, the liver has the structure of an endocrine gland. Also present are areas termed the *portal areas* or *portal canals*, each comprising branches of the portal vein, hepatic artery, and bile duct, often also with a lymphatic vessel, lying in a small amount of connective tissue. The portal areas are so arranged as to delineate lobules of liver tissue. Such a

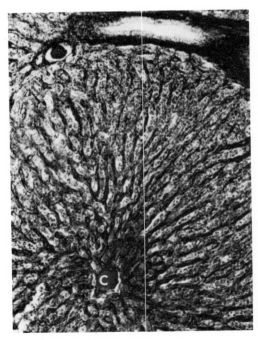

Figure 11–55. Photomicrograph to demonstrate vasculature of the liver, the blood vessels injected with colored gelatin. A portal area lies above, a central vein below, with radial sinusoids draining into the central vein (c). × 75.

lobule, the *classical* or *hepatic lobule*, has several portal canals at its periphery, and in its center is a central vein, a tributary of the inferior vena cava, from which radiate plates of parenchymal cells like the spokes of a wheel from a central hub. This unit of structure is repeated thousands of times. With the afferent vessels (portal vein and hepatic artery) at the periphery of the lobule and the efferent vessels (the central vein) at the center of the lobule, it is obvious that blood flow is from the periphery through the sinusoidal channels between plates of liver cells to the central vein. Bile secretion, on the other hand, is from the liver cells to the small bile ducts at the periphery. Closer examination of a section at higher magnification reveals that each cord or plate of liver cells is composed of one to two rows of liver cells, between which are tiny channels, the bile canaliculi, which drain peripherally in a lobule to bile ducts. These bile canaliculi are simply spaces between adjacent liver cells and have no other lining epithelium. The sinusoidal spaces between liver plates are lined by reticuloendothelial cells, cells lying in a meshwork of fine reticular fibers. Thus, cells in a liver lobule are either parenchymal (hepatic) cells, cells associated with the walls of hepatic sinusoids, or blood cells in the lumina of sinusoids.

Lobulation

The *classical* or *hepatic lobule* has just been outlined. It is a polygonal prism measuring about 1 by 2 mm, and usually appears hexagonal in cross section with a central vein at its center and portal canals peripherally at the corners. It is not delineated by connective tissue in man although it is in some mammals, e.g., the pig. Rarely in man are portal canals found at each of the six corners of the hexagon. It is obvious that such a lobule does not correspond to, for example, a lobule of an exocrine gland in which a lobule is that collection of tissue which drains into a duct, or that which clearly is demarcated by fibrous tissue. However, the classical liver lobule is of some functional significance in that it is a unit of structure from which the blood supply drains to

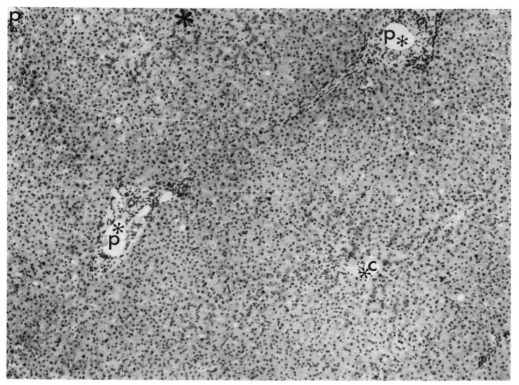

Figure 11–56. Photomicrograph of the liver to illustrate hepatic lobules. Three portal areas (p) and one central vein (c) are seen. Another central vein would be present just above the large asterisk (top) and if lines were drawn connecting the four asterisks, a liver acinus would be outlined (see Figure 11–57). × 75.

a lobular (central) vein. In that its morphological determination is made by its vascular supply, it will be obvious to the student that the peripheral parts of a lobule, i.e., those nearest the portal vein and hepatic artery, will be supplied best with food materials and oxygen. The central area will not be supplied so well.

Other criteria have been used for demarcating functional units in the liver. A *portal lobule* has as its center a portal canal and consists of the tissue draining bile into the bile duct of that portal area. Such a unit is triangular in

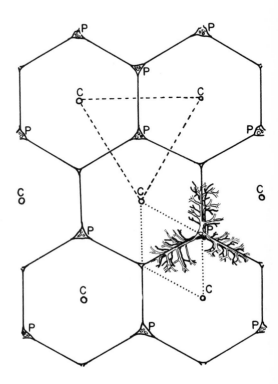

Figure 11–57. Diagram of hepatic lobules. The classic hepatic lobule is outlined with solid lines, the portal lobule with an interrupted line, and the liver acinus or functional unit with a dotted line. The branches of a portal vein and a hepatic artery (solid) from one portal area are shown at lower right. Portal areas are labeled "P," central veins "C." × 40.

cross section, contains parts of three adjacent classical lobules, and has a central vein peripherally at each corner. Pathologically, however, liver damage usually is related to blood supply and a smaller unit of liver structure now is recognized on this basis. This is the *liver acinus* or the *functional unit*. Its dimensions are illustrated in Figure 11–57. As just explained, it is rare to find a portal canal at each corner of the classical lobule. Such deficiences are supplied by branches from an adjacent area which leave parent vessels at a right angle and course along the border between adjacent classical lobules. The vessels supply and the bile ductule drains an area of diamond shape in cross section with two central veins at two opposite corners and the portal canal branches coursing transversely between them.

Parenchyma (Hepatic Cells)

The parenchymal or hepatic cells (hepatocytes) are arranged in a series of branching and anastomosing perforated plates or laminae to form a spongework or labyrinth between which are the sinusoidal spaces. These plates extend from the periphery of the classical lobule to the central vein at its center in a radial fashion. Except at the sites of anastomosis and branching, the plates usually are only one cell thick, although obviously any single parenchymal cell is bordered by several others within a plate. Around portal areas, the liver cells are arranged as a sheet, one cell thick, lying against the periportal connective tissue and termed the limiting plate. The limiting plate is composed of cells somewhat smaller than hepatic cells in the center of the lobule and is

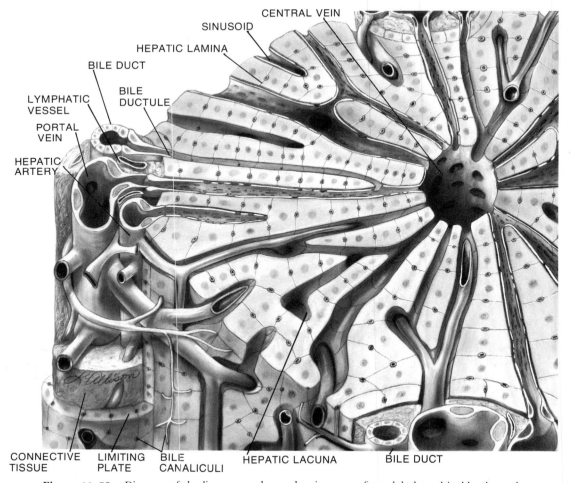

Figure 11–58. Diagram of the liver parenchyma showing part of one lobule and its blood supply.

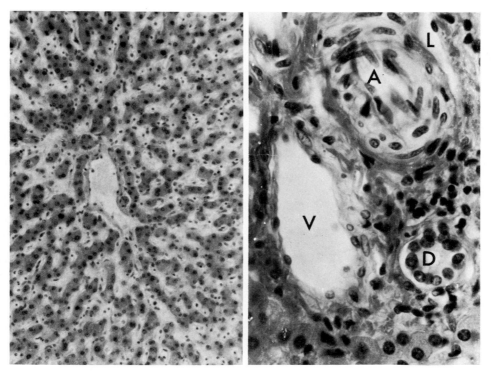

Figure 11–59. Photomicrographs of the human liver to show, *left,* the central area of a classical lobule with a central vein (× 250) and, *right,* the portal area with a branch of the hepatic artery (A), a branch of the portal vein (V), a small bile duct (D), and a lymphatic vessel (L). × 750.

perforated by blood vessels (branches of the hepatic artery and the portal vein) and by branches of the bile ducts.

Hepatic cells are polygonal with six or more surfaces, usually 20 to 35 microns (μm) in size, and with a clearly defined cell membrane. The surfaces are either external and related to a sinusoidal space, closely applied to the surface of an adjacent liver cell, or partially separated from an adjacent cell to form a bile canaliculus. Nuclei are spherical or ovoid with a regular surface and show considerable variation in size from cell to cell, a variation associated with the condition of polyploidy. Occasionally, binucleate cells are present. Each nucleus is vesicular in type with prominent, scattered chromatin granules and one or more nucleoli. Mitosis is rare in adult liver cells, but numerous mitotic figures can be found during repair following injury.

The cytoplasm of hepatic cells shows considerable variation dependent upon functional activity, particularly in gly-

cogen and fat storage. Both of these substances usually are removed during routine section preparation but are indicated by a lacelike appearance with spaces of irregular outline and by spherical vacuoles respectively. Present in all cells are clumps of basophil material, usually of such an extent as to give the cytoplasm a slightly basophil reaction. Mitochondria are small but numerous throughout the cytoplasm, and the Golgi apparatus usually is demonstrable, situated either near the nucleus or peripheral and adjacent to a bile canaliculus.

While all parenchymal cells show a similar structure, there are distinct variations in different regions and at different times in relation to feeding. This is dependent upon blood supply. The peripheral cells in a lobule have a good blood supply, but those near the central vein are farthest removed from their blood supply. After feeding, glycogen is deposited first in the peripheral zone. Only after a very heavy carbohydrate meal do the central cells show evidence

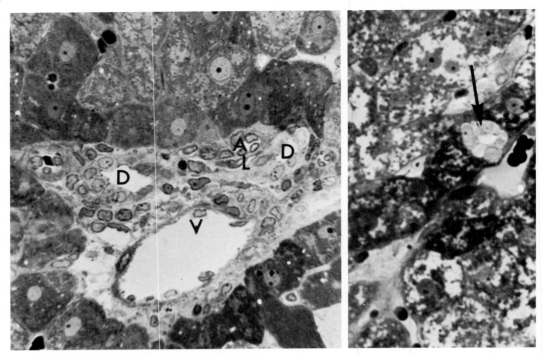

Figure 11–60. *Left:* Photomicrograph of a plastic section to show a portal area and associated parenchymal tissue. Labeling as in Figure 11–59 (right). × 550. *Right:* A small area of liver parenchyma in the region of the limiting plate to show a bile ductule or cholangiole (arrow, see page 392). Note that the parenchymal cells contain extensive unstained areas of glycogen. × 850.

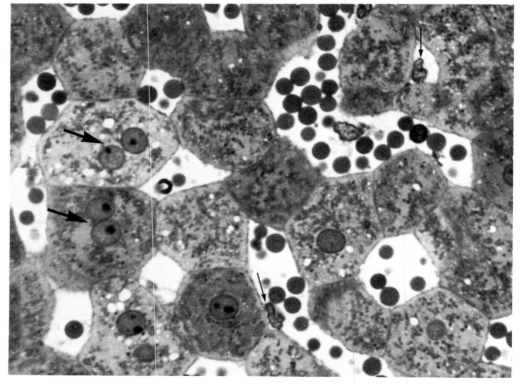

Figure 11–61. Photomicrograph of liver parenchyma showing plates of liver cells, some binucleate (large arrow), and with numerous mitochondria (dark dots) and some lipid vacuoles. Between them are sinusoids containing erythrocytes and lined by reticuloendothelium (small arrows). × 600.

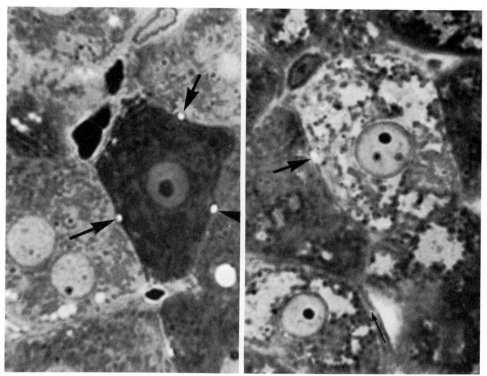

Figure 11–62. Photomicrographs of plastic sections of liver. *Left:* The dark parenchymal cell at center right shows five surfaces, two short ones adjacent to sinusoids containing red blood corpuscles, and three longer sides adjacent to surrounding parenchymal cells. On each of these three interfaces is a bile canaliculus (arrow). (Compare this cell with Figure 11–63 which has five similar surfaces.) Note also the binucleate cell (bottom left). × 1500. *Right:* The central parenchymal cell here shows extensive unstained areas of glycogen and one bile canaliculus (broad arrow). At bottom center, the perisinusoidal space between a parenchymal cell and a sinusoid lining is visible (narrow arrow). × 1500.

of glycogen storage. Similarly, when glycogen is removed to increase a falling blood sugar level, glycogen first is removed from the central cells. Under certain conditions, fat too is deposited in parenchymal cells, and it always appears first in cells adjacent to central veins of lobules. These variations between cells in a lobule are not restricted to inclusions, for mitochondria show distinct morphological changes associated with glycogen storage, being small and spherical in peripheral cells and more slender and elongated in central cells.

Fine Structure

Hepatocytes show no special nuclear features although, as already noted, there is marked variation in size, this being an expression of polyploidy, with up to 25 per cent of cells being binucleate. Both granular and agranular endoplasmic reticula are prominent in the cytoplasm, with regions of continuity between the two types. Granular reticulum usually occurs as groups of 3 to 15 parallel cisternae, the ends of which tend to expand. In addition to ribosomes attached to these membranes, polysomes are present, both free and associated with the membranes. The smooth reticulum appears as a meshwork of branching and anastomosing tubules, often continuous with granular reticulum, and may contain globules of 30 to 40 nm diameter composed of low density serum lipoprotein. The Golgi apparatus is usually multiple and located near the nucleus and adjacent to bile canaliculi, each formed by a few closely packed lamellae. Near bile canaliculi are membrane-limited, dense peribiliary bodies, about 0.2 to 0.5 μm in diameter,

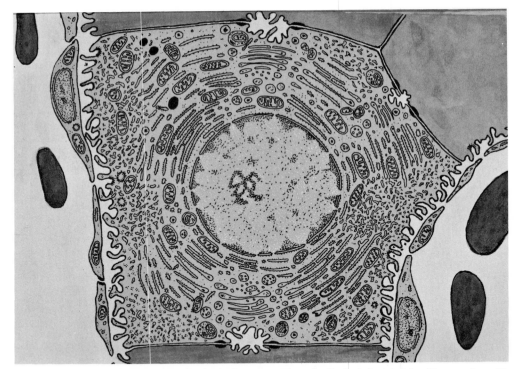

Figure 11–63. This diagram is of a single liver parenchymal cell. On left and right sides are sinusoids, lined by reticuloendothelial cells. The parenchymal cell in this section shows five surfaces, two adjacent to sinusoids and separated from reticuloendothelium by the perisinusoidal space, and three opposed to other parenchymal cells. Irregular microvilli protrude into the perisinusoidal space, and on the other three surfaces, three bile canaliculi are illustrated, each limited laterally by desmosomes (maculae adherentes). In the parenchymal cell, the nucleus and its components are shown. In the cytoplasm, note the stacks of cisternae of granular endoplasmic reticulum (ergastoplasm). In some cisternae there are terminal dilatations containing granules in relation to the Golgi apparatus. This illustrates the mechanism of protein secretion in the endoplasmic reticulum and transport to the Golgi apparatus for packaging. In other areas associated with particulate glycogen. Other organelles include mitochondria, lysosomes, and microbodies.

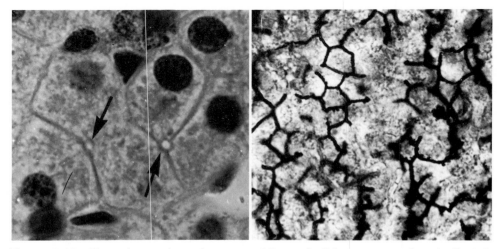

Figure 11–64. Photomicrographs to demonstrate bile canaliculi between parenchymal cells. *Left,* × 1500; *right,* silver injection, × 500.

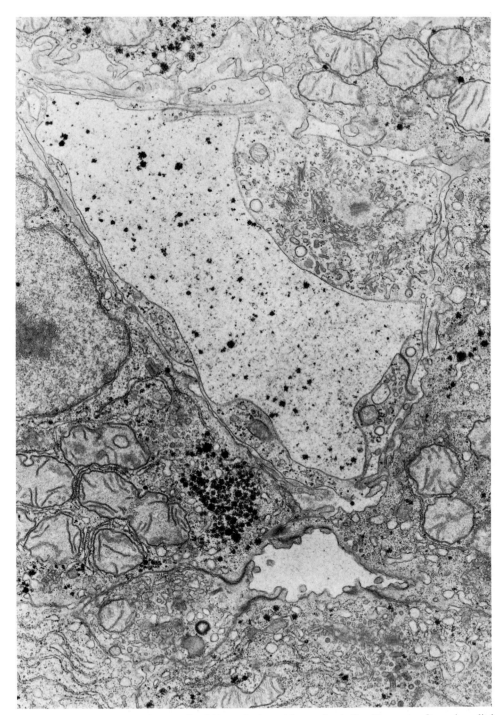

Figure 11–65. Electron micrograph of a hepatic sinusoid completely lined by parts of two sinus-lining cells. A narrow space (of Disse) separates it from surrounding parenchymal cells between which a bile canaliculus is shown below the sinusoid. The small, very dense particles are glycogen, some of which are present also in the lumen of the sinusoid. × 17,000. (Courtesy of J. Steiner and Anne-Marie Jezequel.)

containing acid hydrolases. Peroxisomes or microbodies occur in the same area. These are spherical, 0.2 to 0.8 μm in diameter, and membrane-bound; in many species (but not man) they contain a crystalline structure containing uricase and enzymes concerned with oxidation of fatty acids. Lysosomes, which also are present, vary in appearance and may contain lipofuscin. Mitochondria are numerous and usually filamentous in form. Associated with smooth reticulum are glycogen particles, usually in aggregates or rosettes (alpha particles) up to 0.1 μm diameter, composed of individual 20 to 30 nm diameter beta particles. Lipid may be present as osmiophilic, spherical droplets of varying size.

The plasma membrane of the hepatocyte, about 7.5 nm thick, shows specializations in certain regions. Adjacent to a sinusoidal blood space, the hepatocyte is separated from the wall of the vascular channel by a narrow *perisinusoidal space* (the space of *Disse)*, and here the plasmalemma shows numerous long microvilli with vacuoles and vesicles in subjacent cytoplasm. This provides a large surface area for absorption and secretion. In some regions, where connective tissue fibers are present in the perisinusoidal space, microvilli are lacking. Plasmalemmae of adjacent hepatocytes at an interface show some irregularity with occasional spot desmosomes. At the so-called "biliary pole," the two membranes of an interface separate to form an intercellular canal, the bile canaliculus, usually 1 to 2 microns (μm) across. Microvilli protrude from plasma membranes into the lumen of the canaliculus, and at each lateral border the interface usually is reinforced by a desmosome.

The union of bile canaliculi with the bile duct system is not easily demonstrated. At the periphery of a lobule, bile canaliculi drain into diverticula at the ends of the smallest bile ducts. These diverticula are located against parenchymal cells of the limiting plate, and then continue as small tubules with very thin walls. These short tubules, called bile ductules or *cholangioles,* pass in turn to bile ducts found in portal areas. The bile ducts have much more substantial walls and a wider lumen than the ductules.

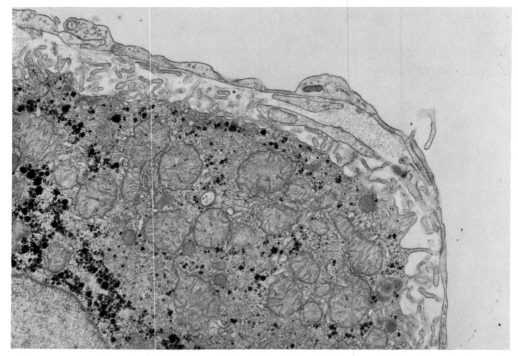

Figure 11–66. Electron micrograph to show the perisinusoidal space of Disse. Note the irregular microvilli of a parenchymal cell protruding into the space which separates the parenchymal cell from reticuloendothelium lining sinusoids. There are a few collagen fibrils in the space. × 15,000. (Courtesy of J. Steiner and Anne-Marie Jezequel.)

Bile Canaliculi

Bile canaliculi can be seen occasionally in routine H and E preparations as
tiny cavities between adjacent hepatic
cells but can be better demonstrated by
special staining methods, e.g., Gomori's
reaction for alkaline phosphatase or
silver impregnation. They form a three-
dimensional network between liver cells,
the walls of the canaliculi being adjacent
parenchymal cells as just described. The
junctions of bile canaliculi with bile
ducts at the periphery of a lobule are
not demonstrated easily. The junctions
occur by means of an intermediate
structure called the *ductule* or *canal of*
Hering. At the periphery of a lobule, the
parenchymal cells which form the wall
of the bile canaliculus are replaced gradually by smaller, lighter-staining cells
with dark nuclei and poorly developed
organelles. These cells, the ductule
cells, are underlain by a distinct basal
lamina. The lumen of such a ductule
eventually joins that of a bile duct in a
portal area.

Blood Channels Within the Lobule

Sinusoidal Spaces. As previously
explained, the blood supply of the liver
lobule is via the sinusoids which form a

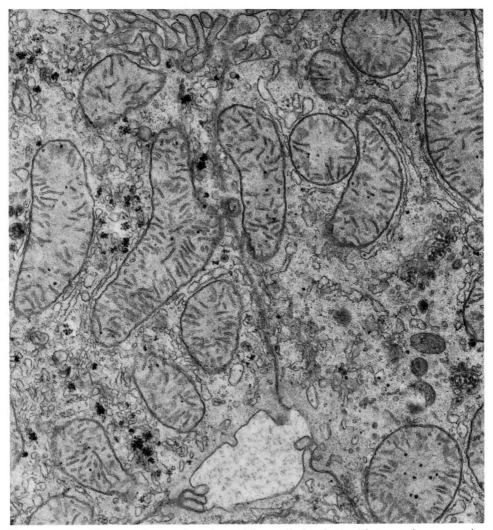

Figure 11–67. Electron micrograph to show a bile canaliculus (bottom) between three parenchymal hepatic cells. Microvilli at top center are in the space of Disse. × 28,000. (Courtesy of J. Steiner and Anne-Marie Jezequel.)

very extensive spongework between the plates of hepatic cells. Blood enters the sinusoidal meshwork at the periphery of the lobule from interlobular branches of portal vein and hepatic artery and passes in a radial fashion through sinusoidal spaces to drain from the lobule by the central vein.

Sinusoidal spaces differ from capillaries in that they are of greater diameter (9 to 12 microns or μm) and their lining cells are not typically of endothelium. The basal lamina around sinusoids is incomplete. Two main types of cell, with intermediate forms, are present in the sinusoidal lining of the adult liver.

"Endothelial" Type. This cell has a small, elongated, darkly staining nucleus and greatly attenuated cytoplasm. The cytoplasm may interdigitate with, or even overlie, cytoplasmic processes of adjacent cells of the same or other type. Organelles are few and small, although numerous micropinocytotic vesicles are present. The endothelial lining of the sinusoids appears to be incomplete, with gaps between adjacent cells and fenestrations in the attenuated cytoplasm. These fenestrations occur in groups to give areas that are sievelike. The fenestrae are larger than those found in Type II endothelium of capillaries (about 100 nm diameter) and are not closed by a diaphragm.

Phagocytic (Stellate) Cell of Kupffer. This cell has a larger, paler nucleus and more extensive cytoplasm with processes that may extend into or even across a sinusoidal space. The cells are actively phagocytic and frequently contain engulfed and degenerating erythrocytes, pigment granules, and iron-containing granules. This property of phagocytosis can be demonstrated by intravital injections of dyes such as trypan blue and particulate matter, e.g., India ink.

Although not all sinusoid lining cells are phagocytic, in time of need the stellate cells of Kupffer are increased in number, perhaps by differentiation of the more primitive endothelial cells.

At the terminations of sinusoids into a central vein or a larger sublobular tributary of a hepatic vein, there is some evidence for a contractile, sphincteric mechanism that controls blood flow through the lobules.

One question concerning sinusoids is

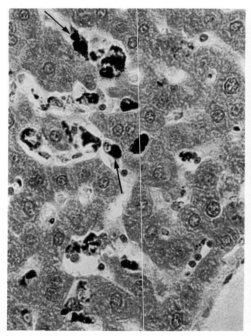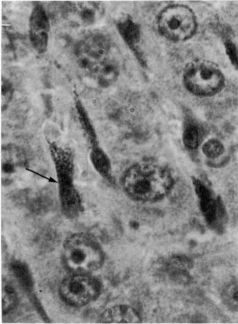

Figure 11–68. Photomicrographs of rat liver to demonstrate phagocytosis by the cells of Kupffer. *Left:* After intravital injection of India ink, carbon particles (black) are present in Kupffer cells (arrows). *Right:* After intravital injection of dye, dye particles are present (arrow). Left, × 450; right, × 1100.

whether or not the lining is discontinuous. Discontinuities in the sinusoidal lining have been demonstrated by the electron microscope using a variety of preparative techniques, and particulate material of small diameter (following injection into the portal vein) rapidly passes into the perisinusoidal space. As just noted, the basal lamina around sinusoids is incomplete and thus there is no morphological barrier between sinusoids and the perisinusoidal space. There is direct access of plasma to the surface of the liver cell, a structural feature of great functional importance for active metabolic exchange between the liver and the blood. The perisinusoidal space itself is not a true lymph channel, for it is not lined by endothelium and is to be regarded as an interstitial space containing some formed reticular and collagenous fibers but in which fluid may circulate freely. Probably it plays an important role in lymph production. Also contained in the perisinusoidal space are a few mesenchymal cells referred to as "pericytes," "fat storing cells," or "extravascular reticular cells." This cell in the adult liver is closely associated with reticular and collagenous fibers and probably is responsible for their formation. In fetal liver, this primitive mesenchymal cell probably is the stem cell for hemopoiesis. It differs from the two types of sinusoid lining cell not only in location but in that it does not become phagocytic toward particulate material.

Central Veins. These are centrally located in the lobules and are the smallest radicles of the hepatic veins. They drain into larger sublobular veins which in turn join to form collecting veins, which themselves are tributaries of hepatic veins. The last drain directly into the inferior vena cava. Sinusoids normally drain into central veins although a few probably open directly into sublobular veins.

Portal Canals (Portal Areas). These are surrounded by small amounts of fibroconnective tissue and contain the "portal triad" of hepatic artery, portal vein, and bile duct, usually with a lymphatic vessel. The largest structure usually is the branch of the portal vein and is thin-walled; the smallest is the artery or arteriole, a branch of the

hepatic artery; the bile duct is intermediate in size and recognized by its lining of cubical epithelial cells. In that a portal area is a region of branching, commonly multiples of the triad are seen. Lymphatic vessels appear as slitlike spaces lined by endothelium. All components of a portal canal increase in size and are surrounded by stronger fibroconnective tissue nearer the hilum. The larger bile ducts are lined by a columnar epithelium.

In small portal areas, the portal vein gives off smaller venules with lateral branches lying between lobules. From these arise the terminal twigs which penetrate the limiting plate of hepatic cells and open directly into sinusoids. The terminal branchings of the hepatic artery are similar, although some are said to penetrate deeply into a lobule before opening into a sinusoid. Direct communications between terminal branches of hepatic artery and portal vein also are said to exist but probably they are few in number and unimportant.

The lymphatic drainage of the liver via the large vessels in the porta hepatis is profuse. The fine lymphatic channels in small portal areas appear to commence blindly in the connective tissue, and no direct communication with the perisinusoidal spaces has been established. However, the fluid of these spaces is discharged into interstitial spaces of the connective tissue and thus passes indirectly into the lymphatic capillaries. Presumably, flow in the perisinusoidal spaces is toward the periphery of the lobule, but this must be exceedingly sluggish and perhaps intermittent consequent upon variations in blood pressure in the sinusoidal spaces.

A few fine unmyelinated nerve fibers of the autonomic nervous system accompany the portal canals.

Stroma

Connective tissue of the liver, a large organ, is sparse. Over the liver surface, covered in most areas by the mesothelium of the peritoneum, is the relatively dense fibroconnective tissue of Glisson's capsule, which at the porta hepatis is continuous with that around the portal canals. By this means, the entire organ is permeated by a fibroconnective tissue skeleton composed of collagenous fibers with relatively few cells, the majority of which are fibroblasts. Within the lobule, there is a fine meshwork of reticular and collagenous fibers around the sinusoids and within the perisinusoidal spaces, but no fibroblasts. The fibers here are elaborated and maintained by the sinus-lining cells and the pericytes of the perisinusoidal spaces. This fine meshwork is continuous at the periphery of the lobule with the connective tissues surrounding the terminal branches of the components of the portal canals.

Regeneration

After injury the liver shows quite a remarkable degree of regeneration. The organization of the repair process depends upon the nature of the injury, but remaining hepatic cells are capable of both hypertrophy and hyperplasia. Bile ducts also actively proliferate, and it is possible that new hepatic cells may arise from this source also.

Functions

The liver is essential to life and, because of its unique position interposed in the venous drainage of the digestive tract, it is susceptible to damage from absorbed toxic materials. It subserves several functions. It is important in the maintenance of blood glucose concentration. Parenchymal cells take up blood glucose and store it as glycogen: glycogen also is formed from other compounds such as lactic and pyruvic acids. The liver also is important in lipid metabolism in that lipid is transported in the blood as lipoprotein, this substance being formed in the liver. It stores also vitamins A and B and heparin (originating in mast cells). It secretes bile salts into the biliary system and fibrinogen (an antianemic factor) and plasma albumins into the blood. Also, it synthesizes cholesterol, excretes bile pigments from the breakdown of hemoglobin of damaged erythrocytes, and produces urea (a by-product of protein metabolism). Detoxication of various toxic materials circulating in the blood,

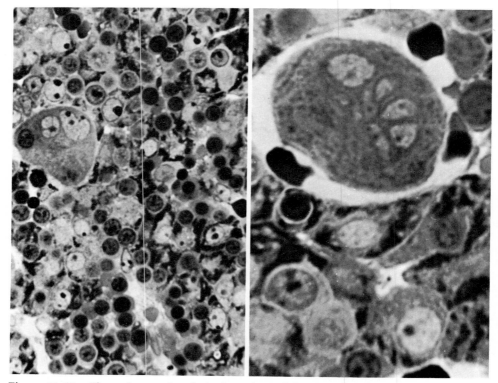

Figure 11–69. Photomicrographs of plastic sections of fetal liver to show hemopoiesis. *Left:* The normal liver structure is obscured by masses of cells of the red blood cell and granulocyte series. One megakaryocyte is shown. × 650. *Right:* A similar area showing a megakaryocyte. × 1250.

phagocytosis of particulate material by the cells of Kupffer, and hemopoiesis in the fetus and newborn are additional functions.

Development

The liver develops as a ventral diverticulum (endoderm) of the fore- and midgut junction and extends anteriorly into the mesenchyme of the septum transversum. Proliferation of the endodermal cells gives rise to the cords and plates of hepatic cells, which at first are tubular in arrangement with cells arranged around a central lumen. The sinusoids develop from vascular tissue associated with the vitelline veins, which themselves form the portal vein. Mesenchyme associated with the portal vein and that of the septum transversum develops into the connective tissue and capsule of the organ.

The original diverticulum of the gut and its main branches remain tubular as the bile and hepatic ducts. The gallbladder and cystic duct develop as a diverticulum from the main duct.

The liver, as stated before, is one of the main blood-forming organs in the fetus and retains this potentiality in the adult.

The Extrahepatic Biliary Passages

The arrangement of the major biliary passages is illustrated in Figure 11–70.

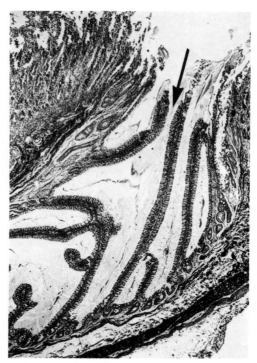

Figure 11–71. Photomicrograph of a section through the opening of combined common bile duct and main pancreatic duct into the duodenum (the ampulla of Vater). The mucosa lining the duct shows valvelike folds (arrow), with the lumen of the duodenum at top. × 40.

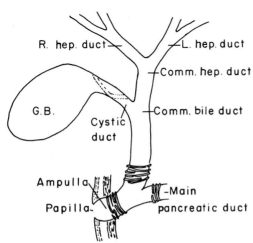

Figure 11–70. Diagram of the main bile duct system. The sphincter muscles and the spiral valve of the cystic duct are indicated.

Extrahepatic Ducts. These all are lined by a tall columnar epithelium which is mucus-secreting. There is a layer of subepithelial connective tissue with a preponderance of elastic fibers and a marked lymphoid tendency. Many lymphocytes and occasional granulocytes are found migrating through the epithelium into the lumen. In the subepithelial layer there may be accumulations of tubuloacinar glands, mostly mucous in type, and blood vessels and nerves are prominent. In the common bile duct, there is in addition a layer of smooth muscle, at first composed of isolated bundles of smooth muscle fibers but near the duodenum forming a complete investment of oblique and transverse fibers. This layer, particularly the circular fibers, is thickened at the termination of the common bile duct (the sphincter of Boyden) and around the ampulla of the conjoined bile and pancreatic ducts just proximal to the ampullary opening into the duo-

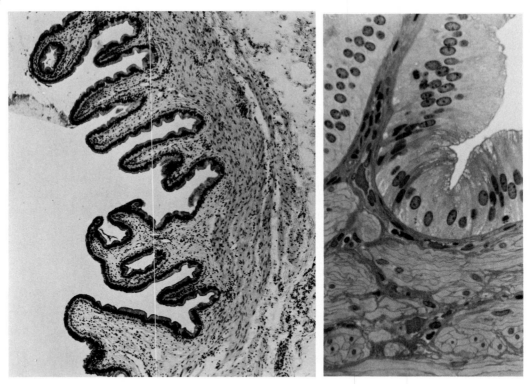

Figure 11–72. Photomicrographs of the gallbladder. Note bundles of smooth muscle (right) beneath the simple columnar epithelium. *Left*, × 40; *right*, plastic section, × 250.

denum (the sphincter of Oddi). At the opening into the duodenum (the ampulla of Vater), the mucosa shows valve-like folds protruding into the lumen. Because the common bile duct traverses the lesser omentum, it is covered also by peritoneum.

THE GALLBLADDER

The gallbladder is a blind, pear-shaped diverticulum of the common hepatic duct to which it is connected by the *cystic duct*. The gallbladder is approximately 3 inches (8 cm) in length and 1.5 inches (4 cm) in diameter but is capable of considerable distention. Its wall is composed of three layers:

Mucous Membrane

When empty, the mucosa is thrown into many folds or rugae and thus is irregular in section, often with the ap-

pearance of simple glands. All epithelial cells are similar, tall, columnar cells, with basally located nuclei. Electron microscopy demonstrates a fine, microvillous apical border. The cells are supported by a fine basal lamina and a lamina propria of delicate, reticular connective tissue with numerous small blood vessels. Occasional small lymph nodules are present with a few mucous glands at the neck of the gallbladder.

Muscularis

There is no submucosa in the gallbladder and external to the mucosa is a layer of smooth muscle, irregular in thickness and orientation of its component bundles. In any section, smooth muscle will be cut in all possible planes, for the muscularis is a meshwork of interlacing bundles of smooth muscle fibers between which are collagenous, reticular, and some elastic fibers.

Adventitia or Serosa

The gallbladder lies on the inferior surface of the liver, and its outer coat of dense fibroconnective tissue blends in some regions with that of Glisson's capsule. Elsewhere the adventitia is covered by peritoneum.

The neck of the gallbladder continues into the cystic duct, and here the mucous membrane is thrown into a spiral fold with a core containing smooth muscle. This is termed the *spiral valve of Heister* and is believed to prevent sudden changes in capacity of the gallbladder following changes of pressure. The gallbladder itself functions as a reservoir for bile, secreted continuously by the liver but discharged intermittently into the intestine. In the gallbladder bile is concentrated by absorption of fluid by the epithelium.

REFERENCES

Baltens, D., Malaisse-Lagae, F., Perrelet, A., and Orci, L.: Endocrine pancreas: three-dimensional reconstruction shows two types of islets of Langerhans. Science, *206*:1323, 1979.

Beidler, L. M., and Smallman, R. L.: Renewal of cells within taste buds. J. Cell Biol., *27*:263, 1965.

Bevelander, G.: Atlas of Oral Histology and Embryology. Philadelphia, Lea & Febiger, 1967.

Blackwood, H. J. J. (editor): Bone and Tooth, Proceedings of the First European Symposium. Oxford, Pergamon Press, 1964.

Boyden, E. A.: The sphincter of Oddi in man and certain representative mammals. Surgery, *1*:25, 1937.

Cardell, R. R., Jr., Badenhausen, S., and Porter, K. R.: Intestinal triglyceride absorption in the rat. An electron microscopical study. J. Cell Biol., *34*:123, 1967.

Caro, L. G., and Palade, G. E.: Protein synthesis, storage, and discharge in the pancreatic exocrine cell. An autoradiographic study. J. Cell Biol., *20*:473, 1964.

Cheng, H., and Leblond, G. P. (with the collaboration of G. Trigelydes, A. Grignon, and W. W. Chang): Origin, differentiation and renewal of the four main epithelial cell types in the mouse small intestine. I. Columnar cell. Am. J. Anat., *141*:461, 1974.

Elias, H.: A re-examination of the structure of the mammalian liver: I, Parenchymal architecture. Am. J. Anat., *84*:311, 1949.

Elias, H., and Selkurt, E. E.: Hepatoportallienal circulation. *In* Blood Vessels and Lymphatics, edited by D. I. Abramson. New York, Academic Press, 1962.

Grube, D., and Forssmann, W. G.: Morphology and function of the enteroendocrine cells. Horm. Metab. Res., *11*:589, 1979.

Ito, S.: The fine structure of the gastric mucosa. *In* Gastric Secretion Mechanisms and Control. Proceedings of the Symposium at The Faculty of Medicine, University of Alberta, Edmonton, Canada, September 13–15, 1965. New York, Pergamon Press, 1967.

Jamieson, J. D., and Palade, G. E.: Intracellular transport of secretory proteins in the pancreatic exocrine cell. I. Role of the peripheral elements of the Golgi complex. J. Cell Biol., *34*:577, 1967.

Jamieson, J. D., and Palade, G. E.: Intracellular transport of secretory proteins in the pancreatic exocrine cell. II. Transport to condensing vacuoles and zymogen granules. J. Cell Biol., *34*:597, 1967.

Leeson, C. R.: Structure of salivary glands. *In* Handbook of Physiology of the Alimentary Canal. Bethesda, Md., American Physiological Society, 1967, Vol. 2, pp. 463–495.

Leeson, T. S.: The rat parietal cell: canaliculi and tubulovesicles. Can. J. Zool, *52*:15, 1974.

Mall, F. P.: A study of the structural unit of the liver. Am. J. Anat., *5*:227, 1906.

Mooseker, M. S.: Brush border motility. Microvillar contraction in Triton-treated brush borders isolated from intestinal epithelium. J. Cell Biol., *71*:417, 1976.

Nabeyama, A., and Leblond, C. P.: "Caveolated cells" characterized by deep surface invaginations and abundant filaments in mouse gastrointestinal epithelia. Am. J. Anat., *140*:147, 1974.

Rappaport, A. M.: The structural and functional unit in the human liver (liver acinus). Anat. Rec., *130*:673, 1958.

Risnes, S.: The prism pattern of rat molar enamel: a scanning electron microscope study. Am. J. Anat., *155*:245, 1979.

Schofield, G. C., Ito, S., and Bolender, R. P.: Changes in membrane surface areas in mouse parietal cells in relation to high levels of acid secretion. J. Anat., *128*:669, 1979.

Sedar, A. W.: Uptake of peroxidase into the smooth-surfaced tubular system of the gastric acid-secreting cell. J. Cell Biol., *43*:179, 1969.

Selkurt, E. E.: Gastrointestinal circulation. Microscopic anatomy. *In* Blood Vessels and Lymphatics, edited by D. I. Abramson, New York, Academic Press, 1962.

Shibasaki, S., and Ito, T.: Electron microscopic study on the human pancreatic islets. Arch. Histol. Jap., *31*:119, 1969.

Travis, D. F., and Glimcher, M. J.: The structure and organization of, and the relationship between the organic matrix and the inorganic crystals of, embryonic bovine enamel. J. Cell Biol., *23*:447, 1964.

Walls, E. W.: Anorectal anatomy. Sci. Basis Med. Ann. Rev., 113, 1963.

Weinstock, A., and Leblond, C. P.: Elaboration of the matrix glycoprotein of enamel by the secretory ameloblasts of the rat incisor as revealed by radioautography after galactose-^{3}H injection. J. Cell Biol., *51*:26, 1971.

Wisse, E.: An electron microscopic study of the

fenestrated endothelial lining of rat liver sinu-soids. J. Ultrastruct. Res., *31*:125, 1970.

Wisse, E.: Ultrastructure and function of Kupffer cells and other sinusoidal cells in the liver. *In* Kupffer Cells and Other Liver Sinusoidal Cells, edited by E. Wisse and D. L. Knook. Amsterdam, Elsevier/North Holland Biomedical Press, 1977.

Wisse, E., and Knook, D. L.: The investigation of sinusoidal cells: a new approach to the study of liver function, *In* Progress in Liver Diseases, Vol. VI, edited by H. Popper and F. Schaffner. New York Grune and Stratton, Inc., 1979.

Yamada, E.: The fine structure of the gall bladder epithelium of the mouse. J. Biophys. Biochem. Cytol., *1*:445, 1955.

Zetterquist, H.: The ultrastructural organization of the columnar absorbing cells of the mouse jejunum. Stockholm, Karolinska Institutet, Aktiebolaget Godvil, 1956.

THE RESPIRATORY SYSTEM

The main function of the respiratory system is to provide for an intake of oxygen by the blood and to eliminate carbon dioxide. *Respiratory tissue*, where these gaseous exchanges occur, is located in the lungs, which lie within the thoracic cavity. This cavity virtually is a closed space. The lungs are connected to the exterior by a series of passages—the nose, the pharynx, the larynx, the trachea, and the bronchi. These passages are relatively rigid structures and are constantly patent, and together they comprise the *conducting* portion of the respiratory system. Thus, if the capacity of the thoracic cavity is increased, air will be drawn through the conducting tubes into the lung. Such inspiratory movements can be effective in drawing air into the

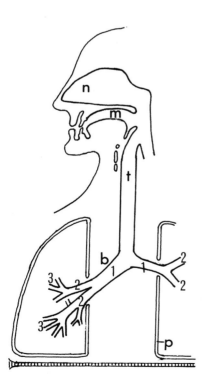
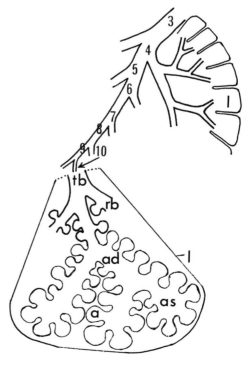

Figure 12–1.   Diagram of the respiratory system. The numbers indicate the divisions of the bronchial tree; n = nasal cavity; m = mouth; t = trachea; b = bronchus; p = pleural cavity; tb = terminal bronchiole; rb = respiratory bronchiole; ad = alveolar duct; as = alveolar sac; a = alveolus; l = lobule.

401

lungs only if the passages to the exterior remain open, which explains why the conducting part of the respiratory system is rigid. This part also has other functions—it strains out particulate matter in the inspired air, washes and humidifies the air, and either warms or cools the air dependent upon the ambient temperature.

THE NOSE

The nose is a cavity divided by a midline septum into right and left nasal cavities. Each communicates anteriorly with the exterior by an *anterior naris*, or nostril, and posteriorly with the upper part of the pharynx, the nasopharynx, by a *posterior naris*. With the exception of the anterior naris, each nasal cavity has a rigid wall of bone and hyaline cartilage. The wall of the anterior naris is of fibroconnective tissue and cartilage, and its dimensions can be varied by muscular action. Each nasal cavity is divided into a *vestibule*, the wider part immediately behind the anterior naris,

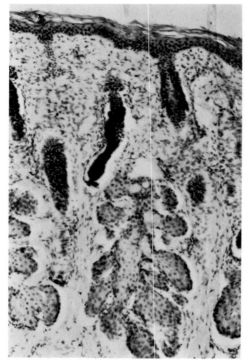

Figure 12–2. Section of the vestibule of the nose, showing large, lobulated sebaceous glands in the dermis. × 70.

and a *respiratory* part, which comprises the remainder.

The skin covering the external surface of the nose, which is characterized by some large sebaceous glands, extends into the anterior part of the vestibule where it contains some sebaceous and sweat glands and hair follicles with stiff, thick hairs. These hairs function to strain out coarse particles from the inspired air. Deeper in the vestibule, the stratified squamous epithelium becomes nonkeratinizing, and this type of epithelium gives way in the respiratory part of the nasal cavity to a pseudostratified ciliated columnar epithelium with goblet cells.

The epithelium which lines the respiratory passages lies upon a basal lamina which separates it from the underlying fibroconnective tissue, the lamina propria, in which are both mucous and serous glands. The deepest layer of the lamina propria blends into, and is continuous with, the periosteum or perichondrium of bone or cartilage in the wall of the nasal cavity. Accordingly, the mucous membrane of the nose often is termed a *mucoperiosteum* or a *mucoperichondrium* (the schneiderian membrane). The lamina propria contains both collagenous and elastic fibers, and fibroblasts, macrophages, lymphocytes, plasma cells, and granular leukocytes. Small collections of lymphatic tissue are characteristic, especially posteriorly near the nasopharynx.

In a frontal section, the nasal cavity is pear-shaped and is divided by the median nasal septum. Protruding into the cavity from the lateral wall are three curved plates of bone covered by the mucous membrane. These bones are the superior, middle, and inferior *conchae* (concha is a shell) or *turbinate* (scroll-like) bones. Of these, the inferior is the largest and it is covered by a thicker mucous membrane. In the lamina propria here, and elsewhere to a lesser degree, are numerous thin-walled, venous sinuses. This tissue has been termed *cavernous* or *erectile* tissue, but differs from the true erectile tissue of the penis in that it is venous in nature and that the smooth muscle which is present is located in the walls of the venous spaces and not in the septa between cavernous spaces.

The surface of the respiratory pas-

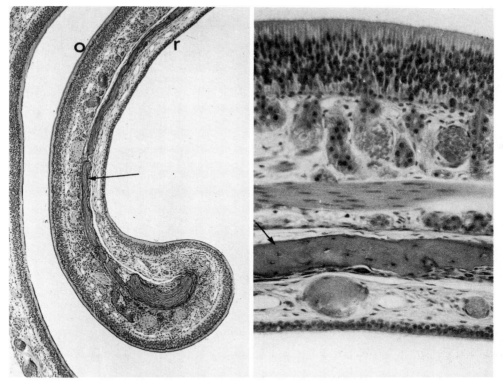

Figure 12–3. *Left:* Section through the superior turbinate bone (concha) (arrow) showing olfactory mucosa (o) and respiratory mucosa (r), the former much thicker with a taller epithelium and glands, nerves and venous sinuses in its lamina propria. × 35. *Right:* A higher magnification with olfactory epithelium at top and respiratory epithelium at bottom. The arrow indicates the superior turbinate. × 175.

sage epithelium is covered with a layer of mucus produced by its goblet cells and by the glands in the lamina propria. The cilia of the ciliated cells in the epithelium constantly move this mucus backward to the nasopharynx whence it is either swallowed or expectorated. The mucous layer serves to pick up particulate matter in the air, which thus is eliminated from the inspired air. The fluid secretions from serous and mucous glands humidify the inspired air, which also is warmed by blood temperature in the dilated venous sinuses of the erectile tissue.

Organ of Smell

In the roof of each nasal cavity and extending down over the superior concha and the adjacent part of the septum is a region where the fresh mucous membrane is yellowish-brown in contrast to the pink color of the ordinary respiratory area. This specialized area contains the receptor organs for smell, and is called the *olfactory region* or *olfactory mucosa.*

The olfactory epithelium is pseudostratified columnar, lacks goblet cells, and has no distinct basal lamina. It is very tall, being about 60 microns (μm) in height. Three types of cell comprise the epithelium.

Supporting or Sustentacular Cells. These are tall, slender, cylindrical cells relatively broad at their apices and tapering basally. Nuclei are ovoid and situated centrally and form a row lying more superficially than nuclei of the sensory cells. Apically, the cells bear many slender microvilli protruding into the overlying film of mucus and show a terminal web of filamentous material associated with junctional complexes between the supporting cells and adjacent sensory cells. A small Golgi apparatus lies superficial to the nucleus with pigment granules similar to lipo-

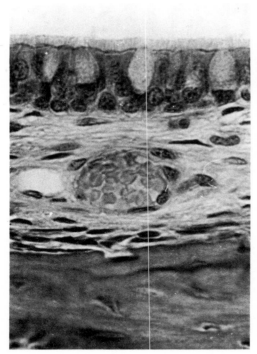

Figure 12–4. Section of the respiratory muco-sa of the nasal cavity with pseudostratified, ciliated, columnar epithelium with goblet cells (top) and a venous sinus in the lamina propria (center). Bone of a nasal concha appears at bottom. × 600.

fuscin and responsible for the yellowish brown coloration of the mucosa.

Basal Cells. These are small, coni-cal cells with dark, ovoid nuclei and branching cytoplasmic processes, lying between the bases of supporting cells. They are believed to be stem cells cap-able of differentiating into sustentacu-lar cells.

Olfactory or Sensory Cells. These are distributed evenly between the supporting cells and are modified bi-polar cells with a cell body, a dendrite extending to the surface, and an axon passing deeply into the lamina propria. Their nuclei are spherical and lie more basally than those of sustentacular cells. Apical dendrites are slender and pass between supporting cells to the surface to terminate in small bulblike swellings called *olfactory vesicles,* from each of which radiate six to ten *olfacto-ry cilia* or hairs, each with a basal body in apical cytoplasm of the vesicle. These cilia are long and nonmotile and function as the actual receptive el-ements. The proximal (basal) part of each sensory cell tapers to a slender, cylindrical process about 1 μm in di-

ameter that passes into the underlying lamina propria as the axon. In the lamina propria, olfactory nerve fibers or axons are collected into small bun-dles, the *fila olfactoria,* which then pass superiorly through the fine canals of the cribriform plate of the ethmoid bone to enter the olfactory bulb of the brain. Also within the lamina propria are lymph and venous plexuses, the former communicating with the sub-arachnoid space via capillaries running with the fila olfactoria.

Within the lamina propria of the ol-factory epithelium are branched tubulo-acinar serous glands (the *glands of Bowman)* from which a watery secretion is carried to the surface by narrow ducts. The secretion of Bowman's glands moistens the surface of the ol-factory epithelium and serves as a sol-vent for odoriferous substances. Its continuous secretion serves to freshen the surface film of fluid and prevents

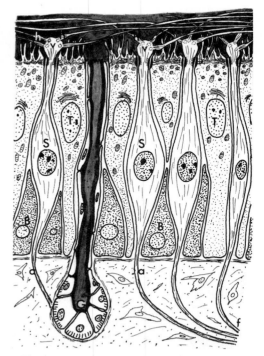

Figure 12–5. Diagram of the olfactory epithe-lium. Ganglion or sensory cells (S) show an olfacto-ry vesicle (v) with olfactory hairs (h) at the luminal surface, and basal axons (a) grouped into fila olfac-toria (f). Sustentacular cells (T) and basal cells (B) also are seen with a gland of Bowman (G) in the underlying lamina propria. Microvilli of sustentac-ular cells and olfactory hairs lie in a surface fluid film (dark).

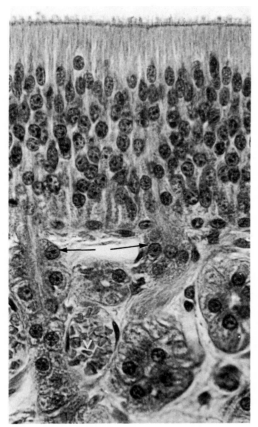

Figure 12–6. Photomicrograph of the olfactory epithelium. Note, in its lamina propria, the serous glands (of Bowman) with their ducts (arrows) and a venous sinus (v). × 425.

repetition of stimulation of the olfactory hairs by a single odor. Repeated exposure of the sensory cells to trauma from infection and other causes results in frequent damage to, and loss of, some sensory cells. Consequently it is usual for the sense of smell to be diminished in the elderly, who show an atypical olfactory epithelium.

PARANASAL AIR SINUSES

The paranasal air sinuses are connected with the nasal cavities and are air-filled cavities within the bones of the skull. They are four in number and are termed the maxillary, frontal, ethmoidal, and sphenoidal sinuses. The epithelium lining them is continuous with that of the nose and also is of the pseudostratified ciliated columnar type.

However, it is thinner and shows fewer goblet cells, and the basal lamina is poorly developed. The lamina propria too is thinner and contains fewer glands than that of the nose, and erectile tissue is not present. Like the mucosa of the nose, its deeper layers are continuous with periosteum, from which it cannot be separated.

THE NASOPHARYNX

The pharynx is a chamber, flattened anteroposteriorly, through which both food and air pass. It is subdivided into the *nasopharynx*, situated below the base of the skull, behind the posterior nares of the nose, and above the soft palate; the *oropharynx*, behind the oral cavity and posterior surface of the tongue; and the *laryngopharynx*, behind the larynx.

The lateral and posterior walls of the pharynx are muscular, and thus the chamber can dilate or, by muscular contraction, be occluded. The nasopharynx, however, although its dimensions can change, cannot be closed completely. By apposition of the soft palate and the posterior wall of the pharynx, the nasopharynx can be isolated completely from the oropharynx. This movement occurs in swallowing, for normally no food material is permitted to enter the nasopharynx.

The epithelium lining the nasopharynx is either pseudostratified ciliated columnar or stratified squamous, the latter occurring in regions where the surface is subject to attrition, e.g., over the posterior edge of the soft palate and at the posterior wall of the pharynx where these two surfaces come into contact during the movement of swallowing. Elsewhere, a respiratory passage type of epithelium with some goblet cells is present. The lamina propria in this region contains much elastic tissue, especially externally where it is in contact with the striated pharyngeal constrictor muscles. A loose submucosa is present only in the lateral parts of the nasopharynx. In the lamina propria, glands are present, mainly of the mucous type, but serous and mixed glands also are found. Lymphatic tissue is abundant throughout the pharynx, and true lymphatic follicles are present posteriorly in the nasopharynx (the adenoids or pharyngeal tonsil), laterally on each side at the junction of oral cavity and oropharynx (the palatine tonsil), and in the root of the tongue (the lingual tonsil) (see Chapter 9). Collections of lymphoid tissue laterally in the nasopharynx around the openings of the pharyngotympanic (eustachian) tubes sometimes are of sufficient size to merit the term "tubal tonsil."

THE LARYNX

The larynx is that segment of the respiratory tract which connects the pharynx and the trachea. In addition to its function as part of the respiratory conducting system it plays an important role in phonation. In its wall there is a "skeleton" of hyaline and elastic cartilages, some connective tissue, striated muscle, and mucous glands. Figure 12–7 explains the relationship of these structures. The major cartilages of the larynx (the thyroid, cricoid, and arytenoids) are hyaline, the smaller (the corniculates, cuneiforms, and tips of the arytenoids) are elastic, as is the cartilage of the epiglottis. The cartilages, together with the hyoid bone, are connected by three large, flat membranes: the thyrohyoid, the quadrates, and the cricovocal. They are composed of dense fibroconnective tissue in which many elastic fibers are present, particularly in the cricovocal membrane. As illustrated in Figure 12–7, the true and false vocal cords (vocal and vestibular ligaments) are respectively the free upper borders of the cricovocal (cricothyroid) and the free lower borders of the quadrate (aryepiglottic) membranes. Extending laterally on each side between the true and false cords are the sinus and saccule of the larynx, a small slitlike diverticulum. The cricoid cartilage has the shape of a signet ring, broader posteriorly than anteriorly, and the cavity within it is continuous below with the lumen of the trachea. Behind the cricoid and arytenoid cartilages, the posterior wall of the pharynx is formed by the striated muscle of the pharyngeal constrictor muscles, which is continuous at the lower border of the cartilage with the intrinsic musculature of the esophagus. Thus, from the larynx, the air passage extends between the vocal folds (the rima glottidis)

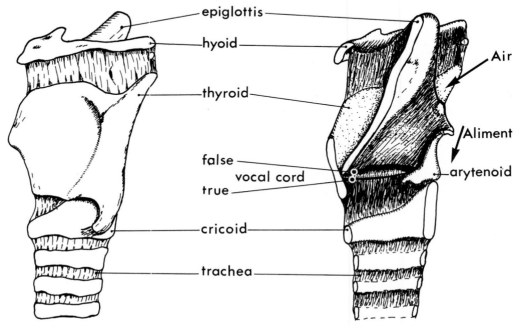

Figure 12–7. Diagrams of the larynx. *Left:* External appearance, as seen from the left side. *Right:* A sagittal section, looking toward the right half of the specimen. The rima glottidis, the narrowest part of the larynx, lies between the two true vocal cords.

through the cavity of the cricoid to the trachea, and aliment passes over the posterior surface of the cricoid into the lumen of the esophagus.

The epithelium of the mucous membrane lining the larynx varies with location. Over the anterior surface and upper one-third to one-half of the posterior surface of the epiglottis, the aryepiglottic folds (upper edges of the quadrate membranes), and the vocal cords, the epithelium is stratified, squamous, and nonkeratinizing. All these moist surfaces are subject to wear and tear. Over the remainder of the larynx, there is a pseudostratified ciliated columnar epithelium with goblet cells, i.e., a typical respiratory tract epithelium. Although the epithelium above the vocal folds mainly is pseudostrati-

fied ciliated columnar in type, patches of stratified squamous epithelium are found commonly. Over the vocal folds, the lamina propria of the stratified squamous epithelium is dense and bound firmly to the underlying connective tissue of the vocal ligament. There is no true submucosa in the larynx, but the lamina propria of the mucous membrane is thick and contains numerous elastic fibers. Within it are tubuloacinar glands, of which the majority are mucous. Some acini possess serous crescents, and some purely serous secretory units also are present. In the epiglottis, mainly mixed salivary glands are present on both surfaces, predominantly on the posterior surface, and often they lie in irregular depressions in the elastic cartilage. On the posterior or laryngeal surface, there are a few taste buds in the surface epithelium. Lymph nodules are scattered in the lamina propria.

Cilia of the laryngeal epithelium, as in all respiratory passages, beat toward the pharynx.

In any section of the larynx, striated muscle fibers will be found. In the posterior and posterolateral walls these are fibers of the constrictor muscles. In relation to the quadrate and cricovocal membranes they are fibers of the intrinsic musculature of the larynx, muscles associated with phonation, breathing, and swallowing.

THE TRACHEA

The trachea is a rigid tube about 10 to 12 cm long and 2 to 2.5 cm in diameter, continuous above with the cricoid ring. It extends down through the lower part of the neck and superior mediastinum of the thorax where it terminates by dividing into the right and left main bronchi. It has a relatively thin wall and is pliable and capable of elongation with respiratory and postural movements.

The patency of the trachea is maintained by a series of about 20 horseshoe-shaped cartilages of irregular outline oriented one above the other with the deficiencies posteriorly. These cartilages on longitudinal section of the trachea are flat externally and convex

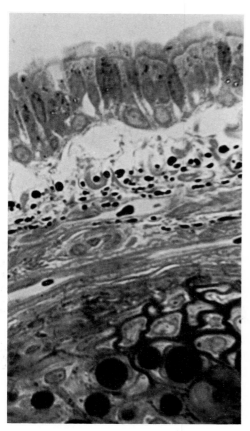

Figure 12–8. Photomicrograph of a section through part of the epiglottis to show the laryngeal surface. Note the typical respiratory tract type of epithelium (top), a loose lamina propria containing numerous elastic fibers (black), and elastic cartilage of the epiglottis (below). Plastic section. × 550.

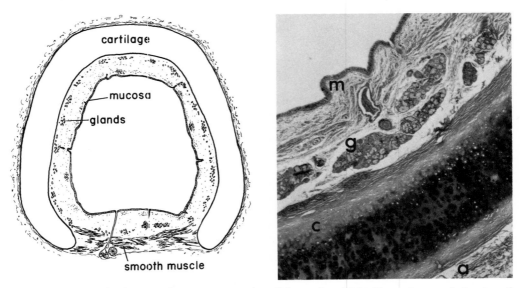

Figure 12–9. *Left:* Diagram of a transverse section of the trachea. *Right:* Photomicrograph showing all layers; a = adventitia; c = cartilage; g = glands in submucosa; and m = mucosa with its lining of pseudostratified ciliated columnar epithelium. ×40.

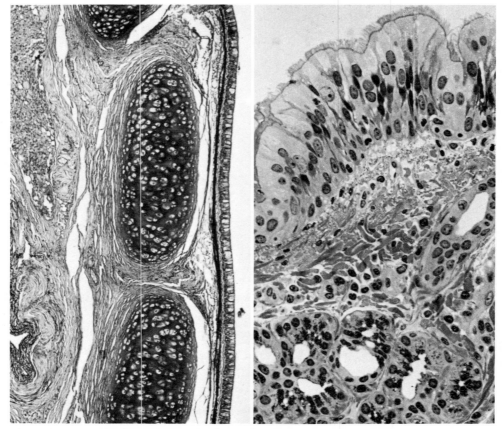

Figure 12–10. *Left:* Photomicrograph of a longitudinal section of the trachea with parts of three cartilaginous rings, respiratory (lining) epithelium to the right. × 50. *Right:* The tracheal mucosa with glands in the lamina propria (below). Plastic section. × 400.

internally. Between adjacent rings of hyaline cartilage, the relatively narrow gaps are filled by fibroconnective tissue which blends with the perichondrium of the rings. Numerous elastic fibers are present in this connective tissue and the bundles of collagenous fibers are so oriented as to give added elasticity to the tube. Posteriorly in the gaps between the ends of each horseshoe cartilage are interlacing bundles of smooth muscle fibers (the *musculus trachealis*), oriented mainly transversely and attached to the cartilages and elastic connective tissue so as to diminish the diameter of the trachea on contraction. External to the tube is loose fibroconnective tissue, termed the adventitia, containing small blood vessels and nerves (autonomic) which supply the trachea.

Internal to the cartilages is the submucosa, a layer of loose areolar fibroconnective tissue containing numerous small mixed glands and some serous secretory units. These glands lie mainly between adjacent cartilaginous rings and posteriorly, both within and external to the smooth muscle. Their ducts pierce the lamina propria of the mucosa to open on the surface. Blood and lymph capillaries are prominent in this layer.

The mucous membrane lining the trachea consists of a pseudostratified ciliated columnar epithelium with goblet cells which rests upon a thick basal lamina with a supporting lamina propria. Five cell types are distinguished in the epithelium: columnar ciliated cells, the cilia beating upward toward the pharynx; columnar (brush) cells with a microvillous or striated border; goblet mucus-secreting cells; basal cells, some of which are stem cells and some that may represent lymphocytes or macrophages migrating through the epithelium; and intermediate cells, larger than basal cells but with apices which do not reach the lumen. They repre-

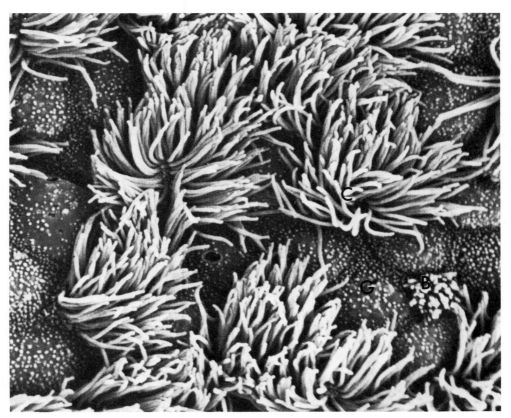

Figure 12–11. Scanning electron micrograph of tracheal epithelium showing ciliated (C), goblet (G), and brush or microvillous (B) cells. × 3600. (Courtesy of Dr. P. M. Andrews.)

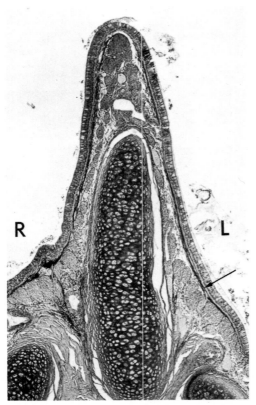

Figure 12–12. A vertical (coronal) section through the carina of the trachea as it divides into right (R) and left (L) main bronchi. Note the dense, elastic tissue (arrow, black) underlying the epithelium. × 50.

sent stages in differentiation of goblet and ciliated cells from basal cells. The lamina propria is relatively thin. There is a condensation of elastic fibers of the lamina propria to form a distinct elastic layer, the fibers of which are directed mainly longitudinally. Small accumulations of lymphocytes are common in the lamina propria. The lumen of the trachea characteristically is D-shaped in transverse section.

THE LUNGS

The Bronchial Tree

The lungs are paired organs situated one in each side of the thoracic cavity. The center of the thorax, the *mediastinum*, contains the heart and major blood vessels, the esophagus, the tra-

chea, and the remnants of the thymus gland. On each side of this, the thoracic cavity is lined by a thin, mesothelial membrane, the *parietal pleura*, which at the *hilum* or root of the lung is reflected over the lung as *visceral pleura*. The potential space between parietal and visceral pleurae is occupied by a thin film of watery (serous) fluid; this space is the *pleural cavity*. Thus the lung is connected to the mediastinum by a relatively small area termed the *lung root* in which are located all structures passing to and from the lung. The right lung has three lobes and the left two lobes, each supplied by a branch (a secondary bronchus) of a primary bronchus, the two primary bronchi (right and left) being the terminal branches of the trachea. The right primary bronchus divides into upper and lower lobe bronchi before entering the lung, the right middle lobe bronchus arising from the latter within the lung. The left primary bronchus usually does not divide into upper and lower lobe bronchi until it has entered lung tissue. In turn, the major bronchus supplying a lobe of the lung divides further, the tertiary bronchi so formed supplying *bronchopulmonary segments*. Within each bronchopulmonary segment, further orders of dichotomous branchings occur, the cross-sectional areas of the two daughter branches exceeding that of the mother branch. This means, of course, that air travels more slowly in the smaller branches of the bronchial tree and fastest within the trachea. By branching, the air passage is reduced to a size at which the duct is termed a *bronchiole*. It is the bronchiole which supplies a *lobule* of the lung. A lobule, the basic unit of the lung, is pyramidal, but often highly irregular, with a base 1 to 2 cm in diameter, a similar height, and an apex that points toward the hilum. In the human being, the lobules are poorly delineated by incomplete interlobular septa of fibroconnective tissue, but these are dense and easily seen in the pig.

In summary, the basic organization of the conducting part of the respiratory system is as follows: nasal cavity to pharynx, to larynx, to trachea, which divides into right and left primary bronchi (each supplying a lung), dividing into upper, middle (right only), and lower lobe or secondary bronchi (each supplying a lobe of a lung), dividing into tertiary bronchi (each supplying a bronchopulmonary segment, there being 10 in the right and 8 in the left lung), each continuing to divide into intrapulmonary bronchi of varying sizes, until finally a bronchiole supplies a lung lobule (about 30 to 60 lobules in each bronchopulmonary segment). Within each lobule, the terminal bronchiole continues into one to three *respiratory bronchioles*, each dividing into 2 to 11 *alveolar ducts*, from which *alveolar sacs* and *alveoli* arise. It has been estimated that there are 300 million to 500 million alveoli in the lung. From respiratory bronchiole to alveoli, gaseous exchange occurs.

The histology of each segment now will be described.

Bronchi

The extrapulmonary bronchi closely resemble the trachea in structure and differ from it only in being of smaller diameter. In the main bronchi, carti-

lage rings still are incomplete, the posterior deficiency being occupied by smooth muscle.

Intrapulmonary bronchi, however, differ from extrapulmonary bronchi in several basic features. First, the intrapulmonary bronchi are rounded in outline and so do not show a posterior flattening, as is seen in the trachea and extrapulmonary bronchi. This is due to the presence not of C-shaped cartilaginous rings but of irregular plates of hyaline cartilage, some of which completely encircle the lumen. These are so irregular that on cross section the appearance of several small areas of cartilage around the circumference is common, each small piece of cartilage being a protuberance from a large plate. The hyaline cartilage plates are surrounded by dense fibroconnective tissue containing many elastic fibers. Internal to the ring of cartilage and connective tissue is a submucosa composed of loose connective tissue with some lymphoid tendencies, and contained within it are mixed mucoserous and mucous glands. The ducts of these glands pass through the more superficial layers to open on the surface. At the junction of submu-

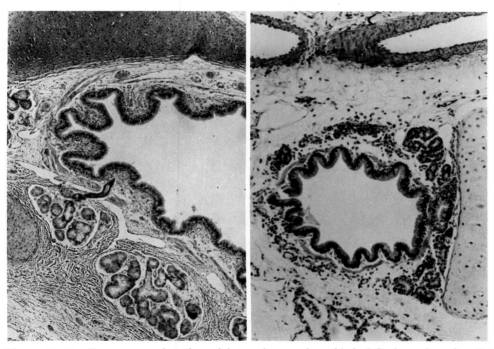

Figure 12–13. Transverse sections through intrapulmonary bronchi, the left a larger bronchus. Both show longitudinal folds of the mucosa, slips of smooth muscle at the junction of mucosa and submucosa, glands in the submucosa, and plates of hyaline cartilage. Left, × 50; right × 60.

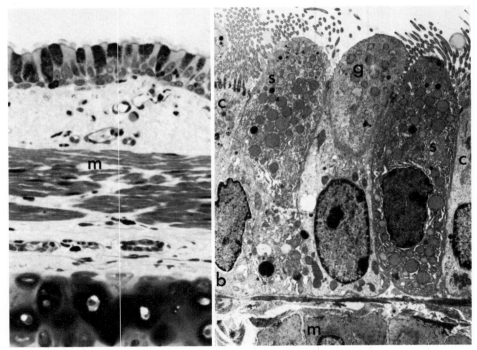

Figure 12–14. *Left:* A bronchus showing respiratory epithelium with ciliated and epithelial serous cells (dark, granular cytoplasm) with a band of smooth muscle (m) and cartilage (below). × 250. *Right:* Electron micrograph of a bronchus showing ciliated (c), goblet (g), serous epithelial (s), and a basal (b) cell; smooth muscle (m) cells below. × 3800. (The epithelial serous cells may contribute to the serous fluid found around cilia and beneath the mucous layer.)

cosa and mucosa, the condensation of elastic tissue seen in the trachea and extrapulmonary bronchi is reinforced by an outer sheet of smooth muscle fibers. These are not arranged in definite layers, as they are in the digestive tract, for example, but take the form of interlacing bundles of fibers arranged in open spirals around the bronchus, some with a left-handed and some with a right-handed twist. Intermingled with the bundles of smooth muscle fibers are numerous elastic fibers. The innermost layer is the mucosa, comprising an epithelium continuous with, and identical to, that of the trachea, and a well-defined basal lamina supported by a lamina propria of reticular and longitudinally oriented elastic fibers. Characteristically in sections, the mucosa shows numerous longitudinal folds owing to contraction of the smooth muscle.

Bronchi become smaller with successive divisions of the bronchial tree, but the basic structure as just described remains unchanged. However, the smallest bronchi contain less cartilage, that no longer forms complete rings, and the lining epithelium now is a ciliated columnar epithelium with goblet cells and is of less depth than the pseudostratified ciliated columnar epithelium lining the large bronchi. All bronchi are contained in connective tissue continuous with that of the hilum, and blood vessels are related closely to them and embedded in the same connective tissue.

Bronchioles

The term bronchiole in the past was applied to a conducting tube less than 1 mm in diameter. We regard a bronchiole as a small tube embedded in little or no connective tissue and surrounded by respiratory tissue. Thus a bronchiole may be compared with an intralobular duct of a gland. In larger bronchioles, the epithelium is ciliated columnar with some goblet cells, but with further divisions into smaller bronchioles (about 0.3 mm in diameter) it becomes ciliated

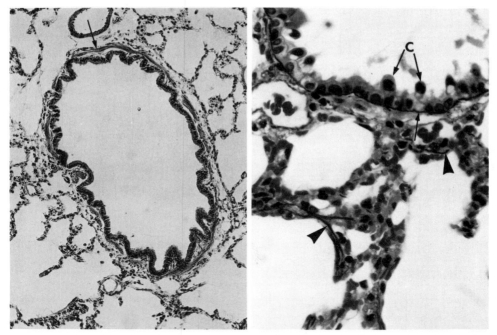

Figure 12–15. *Left:* Section through a large bronchiole lined by ciliated, low columnar epithelium and with prominent smooth muscle (arrow). × 120. *Right:* A smaller bronchiole lined by ciliated cuboidal epithelium with Clara cells (c) and with prominent, dark-staining elastic tissue (arrow). Note also the elastic tissue in interalveolar septa (arrowheads). × 350.

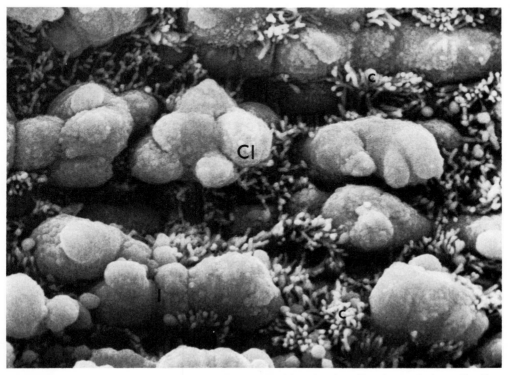

Figure 12–16. Scanning electron micrograph of bronchiole showing ciliated (c) and Clara (Cl) cells. × 2000. (Courtesy of Dr. P. M. Andrews.)

cuboidal with no goblet cells. Scattered among ciliated cells are a few nonciliated cells characterized by an apical convexity protruding into the lumen and a few apical microvilli. These cells, called Clara cells, contain some dense granules and are presumed to be secretory, the secretion probably being surfactant (see later discussion). Other characteristic features are the relative prominence of the smooth muscle, mingled with elastic fibers, and the absence of cartilage, glands, and lymph nodes. A thin adventitia of connective tissue is present. The smallest or *terminal bronchiole* is the finest part of the conducting system, its branches being within the respiratory tissue, and here the epithelium shows only patches of ciliated cells, the remainder being nonciliated.

Functional Correlations of the Conducting System. As explained previously, rigidity in the conducting tubes is essential to maintain patency, and this is achieved by the presence of cartilage from trachea to the smallest bronchi. The tubes, however, are capable of changes in length and diameter. Variation in diameter is achieved by the smooth muscle which is supplied by the autonomic nervous system. The abundance of elastic tissue in the walls of the bronchi and throughout lung tissue generally permits expansion of the lung with inspiration, and its elastic recoil aids contraction of the lung with expiration. As in the nose, mucus and cilia trap particulate matter and eliminate it from the system, and secretions aid also in humidifying inspired air. It should be noted that cilia extend further down the respiratory tree than do goblet cells and submucosal glands, thus preventing the respiratory tissue from becoming waterlogged or occluded by mucus. Cilia virtually constitute an internal drainage system for the respiratory tissue. In the smallest bronchioles, where cilia are absent, macrophages (by phagocytosis of material) take over the function of internal drainage.

Respiratory Bronchioles

Respiration, i.e., gaseous exchange, can occur only where blood in capil-

laries is separated from air by a very thin mass of material. Such an arrangement occurs from the respiratory bronchioles to the alveoli. Respiratory bronchioles are short, branching tubes, 1 to 4 mm long, the diameter being less than 0.5 mm. Usually, two or more arise from each terminal bronchiole, and they themselves can branch. The lining epithelium is cuboidal with occasional cilia only in the larger respiratory bronchioles. Cilia are lost in the smaller ones and the epithelium becomes low cuboidal or squamous, many of the cuboidal cells being Clara cells. No goblet cells are present. External to the cuboidal epithelium, the wall is formed by interlacing bundles of smooth muscle and

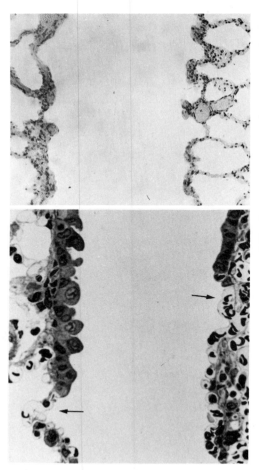

Figure 12–17. *Top:* Longitudinal section through a respiratory bronchiole. × 75. *Bottom:* Plastic section showing change in lining epithelium from cuboidal (nonciliated) to squamous with outpocketing alveoli (arrows) in a respiratory bronchiole. × 350.

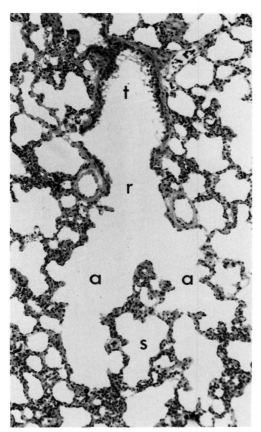

Figure 12–18.   This section shows a terminal bronchiole (t) leading into a respiratory bronchiole (r), which divides into two alveolar ducts (a). Also seen are an alveolar sac (s) and alveoli. × 75.

elastic fibers embedded in fibroconnective tissue. No cartilage is present. In that respiratory bronchioles are part of the respiratory tissue, a few alveoli are present and appear as small diverticula or outpouchings extending from the lumen of the bronchiole through deficiencies in its walls. The structure of these alveoli is identical to that of the main mass of alveoli in the lung (*vide infra*), and their number increases in the smaller bronchioles. Respiratory bronchioles terminate by branching into several alveolar ducts (2 to 11 in number).

Alveolar Ducts

Alveolar ducts are cone-shaped, thin-walled tubes with a squamous epithelial lining which is so thin as to be difficult to resolve with the light microscope. External to the epithelium, the wall is formed by fibroelastic tissue. Opening from the alveolar duct around its circumference are numerous single alveoli and alveolar sacs (clusters of alveoli). Particularly at the orifices of alveoli and alveolar sacs, smooth muscle fibers are prominent. Indeed the openings of alveoli from alveolar ducts are so numerous that it is difficult to see the wall of the alveolar duct, although this is more obvious in thick sections where bundles of elastic, collagenous, and muscle fibers can be seen interweaving between the openings of alveoli along the wall of the alveolar duct.

Alveolar Sacs and Alveoli

The alveolar duct, the terminal part of which is of greater diameter than the proximal part, ends by branching into two to four chambers which, by some authorities, are termed *atria*, and which by others are regarded simply as the terminal alveolar ducts. From these arise single alveoli and alveolar sacs, the latter being a collection or cluster of alveoli opening into a central, slightly larger chamber.

Alveoli are polyhedral or hexagonal, with one wall lacking to permit diffusion of air from respiratory bronchiole, alveolar duct, atrium, or alveolar sac. Alveoli are packed so tightly that each does not have a separate wall. Rather, adjacent alveoli are separated by an *interalveolar septum*. However, each alveolus is lined by a squamous epithelium, that is greatly attenuated but complete. In thin sections, deficiencies in interalveolar septa can be seen, thus permitting communication between adjacent alveoli. These deficiencies are termed *alveolar pores*. Contained within alveolar septa is an extremely rich capillary plexus. Thus an interalveolar septum is covered on each surface with attenuated epithelium lining alveoli, and contains blood capillaries in its supporting connective tissue framework.

The Interalveolar Septum

It is obvious that interalveolar septa must resist the pressures of air in the

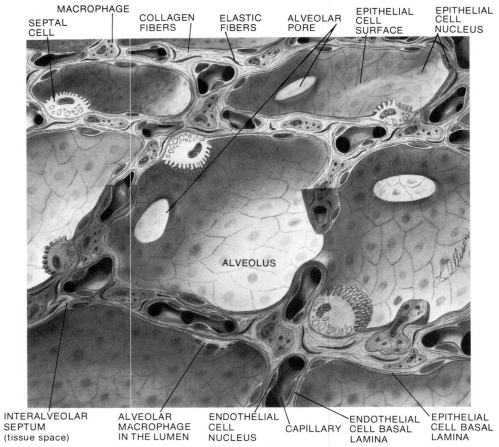

MACROPHAGE

SEPTAL
CELL

COLLAGEN
FIBERS

ELASTIC
FIBERS

ALVEOLAR
PORE

EPITHELIAL
CELL
SURFACE

EPITHELIAL
CELL
NUCLEUS

ALVEOLUS

INTERALVEOLAR
SEPTUM
(tissue space)

ALVEOLAR
MACROPHAGE
IN THE LUMEN

ENDOTHELIAL
CELL
NUCLEUS

CAPILLARY

ENDOTHELIAL
CELL BASAL
LAMINA

EPITHELIAL
CELL BASAL
LAMINA

Figure 12–19. Diagram of alveoli and interalveolar septa in the lung.

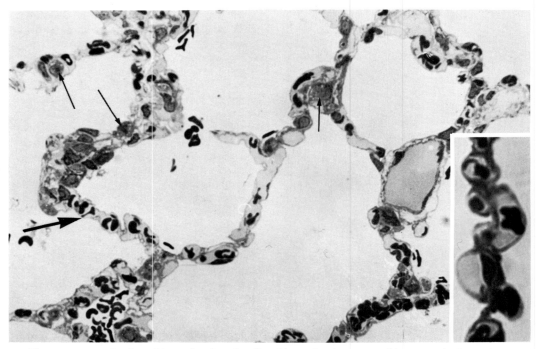

Figure 12–20. Section of lung showing alveoli and interalveolar septa. Thin arrows indicate alveolar phagocytes, and the thick arrow points to an interalveolar septum where blood capillaries are particularly prominent. Plastic section, × 300. *Inset, lower right:* A single interalveolar septum, showing blood capillaries containing red blood corpuscles. × 800.

alveoli, a pressure which varies with the phase of respiration. The support of the septa is provided in the main by a framework of reticular and elastic fibers, only a little collagen being identifiable on light microscopy. By electron microscopy, the tissue space ("*zona diffusa*") of the septum is seen to contain unit fibrils of collagen, some fine elastic fibers, and small microfibrils. This space is limited by basal laminae underlying alveolar epithelium and covering blood capillaries. In many regions, the capillaries are related so closely to the alveolar epithelium that their respective basal laminae are separated by an interval of only 15 to 20 nm, and in some regions the two basal laminae of epithelium and endothelium may fuse. These basal laminae virtually are complete but are traversed by alveolar or septal cells. Between the basal laminae is an amorphous type of ground substance in which the septal cells and fibers are embedded. Elastic fibers are randomly distributed throughout septa and show a concentration at the orifices of alveoli from alveolar ducts. Smooth muscle cells are seen only in these same regions at the openings of alveoli.

Several distinct cell types can be recognized in interalveolar septa, lining alveoli, and even lying free within alveolar spaces.

Pulmonary (surface) epithelial cells, also termed small alveolar cells or type I pneumocytes, form a complete but very thin layer (only about 0.2 μm thick) lining all alveolar spaces. By light microscopy, the flattened nuclei can be recognized, but the cytoplasm is attenuated so greatly as to be beyond resolution. Adjacent cells show tight junctions and organelles are sparse.

Septal or great alveolar cells, also termed type II pneumocytes, occur singly or in small groups of two or three cells between the surface squamous cells, with which they make tight junctions. They are globular in shape, may bulge into alveolar spaces between surface cells, but often lie in crevices in the alveolar wall. At the surface are a few microvilli and the cytoplasm contains granular reticulum, mitochondria, a Golgi apparatus, and multivesicular bodies. However, the most prominent organelle is the lamellar body or cytosome, 0.2 to 1 μm

diameter, osmiophilic and with a multilamellated appearance. These bodies contain dipalmitoyl phosphatidylcholine and it is believed they are discharged into alveolar spaces by exocytosis, the contents spreading over the surface to form a thin layer lining alveoli. This layer contains *surfactant* (discussed later). Some authors regard the cytosomes as lysosomes.

Endothelial cells line the numerous blood capillaries within interalveolar septa. Their nuclei usually are larger and less densely staining than those of surface epithelial cells. The cytoplasm, as in all capillaries, is attenuated and the cells are identified by their relationship to capillary blood spaces.

Blood cells of all types — erythrocytes, granulocytes, lymphocytes, and monocytes — can be found in septa. When located within capillary lumina, they present no problem in identification, but several of the cell types are migratory and may be found outside capillaries and in tissue spaces ("*zona diffusa*")

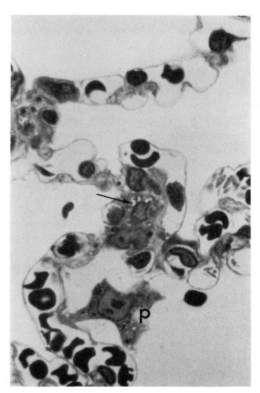

Figure 12–21. This section shows the extensive capillary network in interalveolar septa, a free alveolar phagocyte (p) containing granular material, and a septal cell (arrow). × 1100.

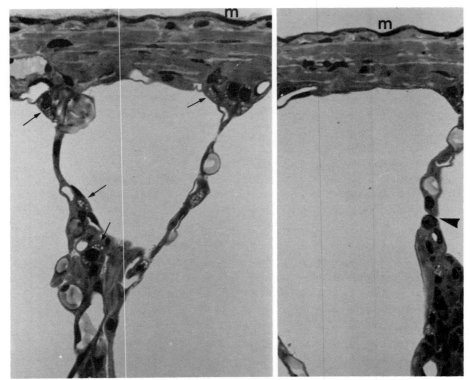

Figure 12–22. Sections to illustrate pleura (above) with flattened mesothelial cells (m) and interalveolar septa. In the left figure, septal or great alveolar cells (type II pneumocytes) are indicated by arrows and in the right figure, an alveolar pore (arrowhead) appears as a deficiency in a septum. Plastic sections, both × 400.

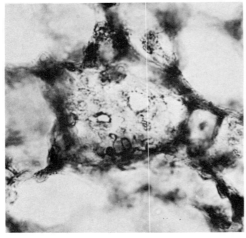

Figure 12–23. Interalveolar septum in which two interalveolar pores are present. Silver stain. × 370.

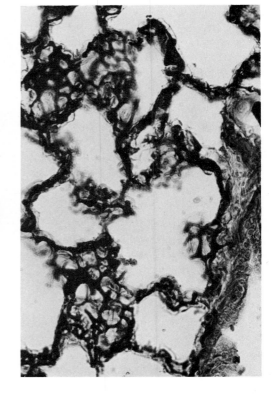

Figure 12–24. Capillary networks in interalveolar septa. Capillaries injected with colored gelatin. A bronchiole appears at lower right. × 180.

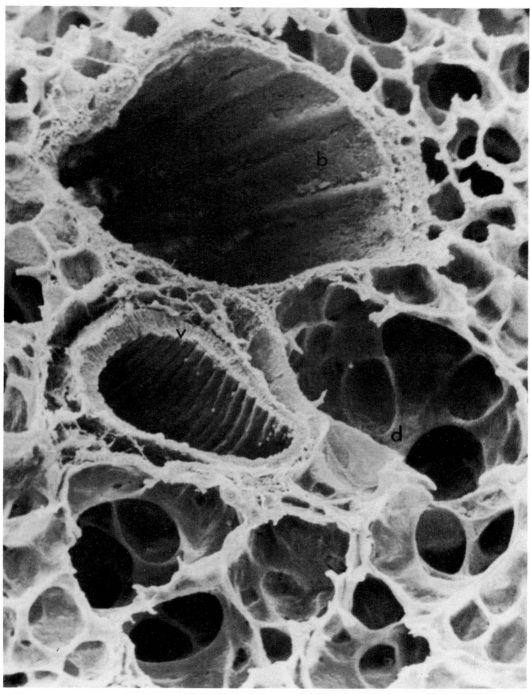

Figure 12–25. Scanning electron micrograph of rat lung showing a small bronchiole (b), a small artery (v), and an alveolar duct (d) with alveoli opening from its wall. Numerous alveoli with interalveolar septa occupy most of the field. × 200. (Courtesy of P. M. Andrews.)

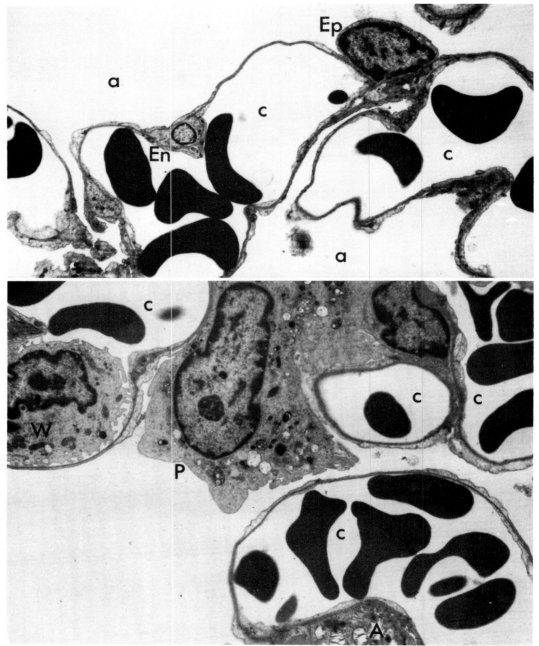

Figure 12–26. *Top:* Electron micrograph of interalveolar septum, in which are capillaries (c) containing erythrocytes. Alveoli are indicated by "a." The two nuclei are of surface epithelial or type I (Ep) and endothelial (En) cells. × 4200. *Bottom:* This micrograph shows a white blood cell (W) in the lumen of one alveolar capillary, an alveolar phagocyte (P) with phagocytosed material, and part of an alveolar type II cell (A) containing lamellated bodies. × 4500.

from which they may migrate further through epithelium into alveolar spaces.

Alveolar phagocytes or macrophages are present in interalveolar septa and often show evidence of phagocytosis. One type is vacuolated and contains numerous cytoplasmic lipid droplets, the lipid being dissolved by routine preparative techniques to give a foamy or vacuolated appearance to the cytoplasm. The lipid material may be choles-

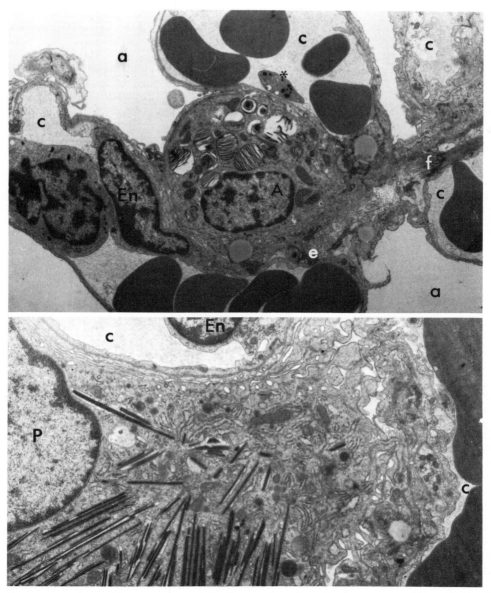

Figure 12–27. *Top:* Electron micrograph of part of an interalveolar septum with capillaries (c) containing erythrocytes and a platelet (asterisk), alveoli (a), an endothelial nucleus (En), and a septal cell or type II pneumocyte (A) with its lamellated bodies. In the septum are a few collagen microfibrils (f) and small clumps of elastin (e). × 5000. *Bottom:* Part of an alveolar phagocyte (P) occupies most of the field with numerous rodlike bodies in its cytoplasm. These are probably asbestos fibers. × 8500.

terol. Other phagocytes have a granular appearance, often containing particulate carbon material phagocytosed from inhaled air ("dust cells"), while others contain hemosiderin, the iron-containing pigment formed from disintegrating erythrocytes. These so-called "siderophages" or "heart failure cells" are numerous when there is stasis of pulmonary blood flow, e.g., in heart failure. These phagocytes undergo a rapid cell turnover and are derived from monocytes that pass through the endothelium of blood capillaries to enter tissue spaces and then pass into alveolar spaces as free cells, from which they are eliminated eventually by passing up the bronchial tree in the sputum, to be expectorated or swallowed.

Blood-Air Barrier

This comprises the structures interposed between air in alveoli and blood in pulmonary capillaries, i.e., the structures through which gaseous exchange occurs. They are the greatly attenuated cytoplasm of the pulmonary epithelial cells, the basal lamina of this epithelium, the capillary basal lamina, and the attenuated cytoplasm of the capillary endothelium.

Interposed between the basal laminae is the tissue space (zona diffusa) of varying extent. In some places it is practically nonexistent, and in other regions the two basal laminae may fuse into one. One further layer must be considered and that is a fluid film lining alveoli. This thin fluid film on the surface of squamous alveolar cells would tend, by surface tension, to cause collapse of alveoli, but it contains phospholipids including dipalmitoyl phosphatidylcholine. This surfactant, produced by type II pneumocytes, reduces surface tension in the fluid film, preventing collapse of alveoli and facilitating inflation of alveoli on inspiration. It functions as an anticollapse factor and can be seen occasionally in electron micrographs as membranous whorls and grids (see Fig. 12–29). Surfactant is especially important in the newborn. Infants suffering from the respiratory distress syndrome, with failure of alveoli to expand on inspiration and collapse of alveoli on expiration, have deficient surfactant. Full maturation of type II cells normally occurs about the twenty-fourth week of gestation with formation and release of the surface-active agent. There appears to be a constant renewal of surfactant in the surface fluid film, with the phospholipids passed by pinocytosis from the surface through squamous alveolar cells to lymph vessels in interalveolar septa.

The Lung Lobule

As explained previously, the lung lobule is the unit of structure of the lung, and is pyramidal, usually with the base at the pleural surface of the lung and the apex directed toward the hilum. At the apex, a terminal bronchiole, to be compared with an intralobular duct, enters the lobule accompanied by a branch of the pulmonary artery carrying venous blood to the respiratory tissue. In man, lobules are poorly and incompletely differentiated by connective tissue, continuous on the

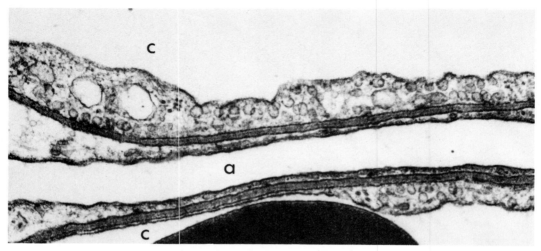

Figure 12–28. Electron micrograph to show the blood-air barrier, with a slender alveolar space (a) between two alveolar septa, each with a capillary (c). Note a single basal lamina, in each case, between endothelium and epithelium, both greatly attenuated, and the former containing micropinocytotic vesicles. × 45,000.

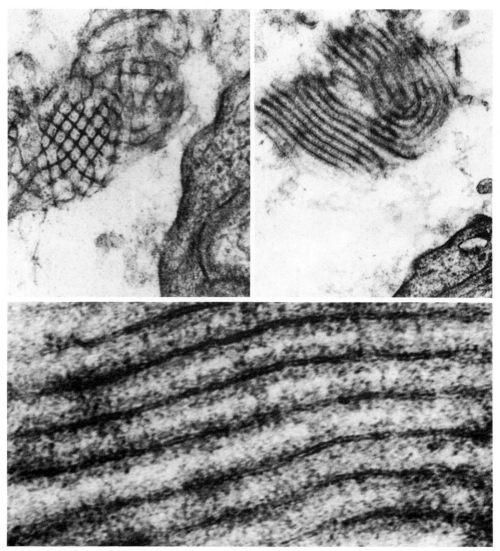

Figure 12–29. Electron micrographs of phospholipid material (surfactant) lying free in alveolar spaces. In both top figures, a small part of a pulmonary surface epithelial cell appears at lower right. Top left and top right, × 42,000; bottom, × 114,000.

one hand with the deeper connective tissue layers of the pleura, and on the other with connective tissue around major vessels and bronchi and thus with connective tissue of the hilum. Branches of the pulmonary vein run alone in connective tissue of the poorly developed interlobular septa and, at the apex of the lobule, run in company with the bronchiole and branch of the pulmonary artery. Lymphatic capillaries also travel in interlobular septa and are continuous with vessels beneath the pleura and with others around major vessels at the hilum and

its extensions. Lymphatics are important in the spread of carcinoma of the lung. Cancerous cells may break through from lymphatics in interlobular septa to adjoining pulmonary veins and thus into the systemic circulation, resulting in widespread metastases or secondary growths in, for example, bone.

Blood Vessels

There is a double blood supply to the lungs. Deoxygenated blood from the

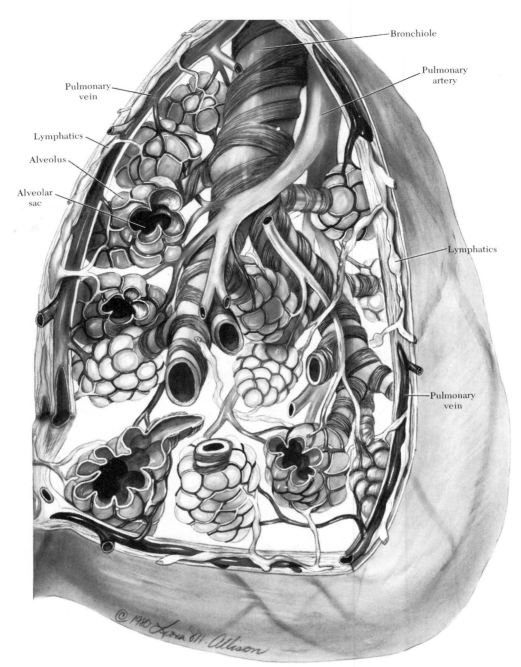

Bronchiole

Pulmonary
artery

Pulmonary
vein

Lymphatics

Alveolus

Alveolar
sac

Lymphatics

Pulmonary
vein

© 1980 Leona M. Allison

Figure 12–30. Diagram of a lung lobule.

right ventricle enters the lungs by the pulmonary arteries, which are elastic arteries of large caliber. Their branches accompany those of the bronchial tree as far as respiratory bronchioles where terminal arterioles break up into a rich capillary network around alveoli, situated in interalveolar septa. Venules from these plexuses join with others draining the pleura and travel alone in the connective tissue of interlobular septa, finally running with branches of the companion artery at the apices of lobules. In addition to this system of pulmonary arteries and veins, there are bronchial arteries and veins. The former arise from the aorta and supply the tissues of the bronchi and the connective tissue of the lung with oxygenated blood. There are communications between the terminal branches of the bronchial arteries and the pulmonary arteries, and most of the blood in the former returns in the pulmonary veins. Some, however, is drained into bronchial veins which are tributaries of the azygos system.

Lymphatics

Two sets of lymphatic vessels, with interconnections, exist in the lung. The superficial or pleural set is situated in the pleura. Relatively large lymphatics demarcate the lung lobules on the surface of the lung. They often are blackened by inhaled carbon, particularly in city dwellers, and thus are visible to the naked eye. Smaller lymphatics form delicate meshworks within the outlines of the lobules. This set is drained around the periphery of the lung to the hilum. The deep or pulmonary set of lymphatics runs with the bronchus, pulmonary artery, and pulmonary vein. The latter start in interlobular septa; those with the pulmonary artery and the bronchi extend peripherally only to the alveolar ducts. All drain centrally to the hilum where they communicate with efferent channels of the superficial set. Lymphatic nodules are prominent at the hilum.

Nerves

Small nerve fibers can be found in the lung, particularly in the region of the hilum and related to major bronchi and large vessels. Those associated with the bronchial tree are from the pulmonary plexus, formed by branches of the vagus (bronchoconstrictor), and by branches of the thoracic sympathetic ganglia (bronchodilator). Both sympathetic and parasympathetic fibers run with the pulmonary vessels. In addition, small collections of nerve cells (parasympathetic ganglia) can be found in bronchial walls.

Pleura

This comprises a thin layer of fibro-connective tissue with collagenous and elastic fibers and few cells (principally fibroblasts and macrophages), covered by a layer of mesothelium. Contained within the connective tissue layer are numerous lymph and blood capillaries and a few small nerve fibers. The pleura is responsible for the secretion of the small quantity of pleural fluid which permits friction-free movement between the parietal layer lining the thoracic cavity and the visceral layer covering the lung surface.

DEVELOPMENTAL ORIGIN OF THE RESPIRATORY SYSTEM

In the embryo, the respiratory system originates as a ventral outgrowth from the floor of the primitive pharynx, the anterior part of the foregut. The outgrowth then extends inferiorly and divides into right and left bronchial buds, each of which undergoes repeated dichotomous branchings. The primary outgrowth becomes the trachea, each bronchial bud a main bronchus, and the orders of branchings the smaller bronchi, bronchioles, and terminal alveoli. Thus, the entire system has a lining which is of endodermal origin, being derived from the lining of the foregut. Respiratory tissue initially has a glandlike appearance of

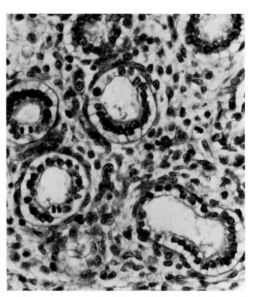

Figure 12–31. Section of developing lung of the rat. Cross sections of epithelial (endodermal) tubules lie in a cellular mesenchyme. × 240.

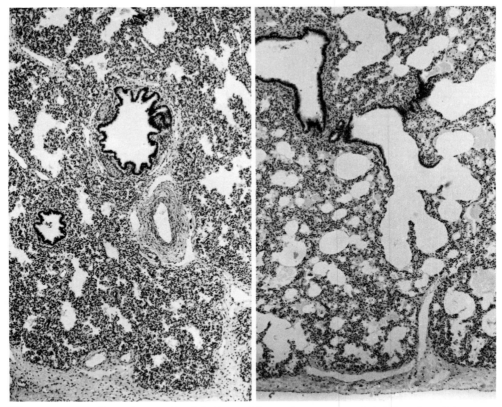

Figure 12–32.   Photomicrographs of the lung of the newborn unexpanded *(left)* and partially expanded *(right)* after the first few respirations. In both, small bronchi are visible also. Both × 50.

epithelial (endodermal)-lined alveoli embedded in mesoderm. The mesoderm forms the accessory coats of the system, e.g., connective tissue, muscle.

FUNCTION OF THE RESPIRATORY SYSTEM

As stated previously, the main function of the respiratory system is to provide for gaseous exchange. Oxygen in dissolved form passes from alveoli to blood capillaries through the blood-air barrier and carbon dioxide passes in the reverse direction. The functions of the conducting part of the system are to filter, wash, humidify, and warm or cool the inspired air. However, the lungs also function as an excretory organ in that water is lost in expired air.

REFERENCES

Baradi, A. F., and Bourne, G. H.: Gustatory and olfactory epithelia. Int. Rev. Cytol., *2*:289, 1953.

Belton, J. C., Branton, D., Thomas, H. V., and Mueller, P. K.: Freeze-etch observations of rat lung. Anat. Rec., *170*:471, 1971.

Boyden, E. A.: Segmental Anatomy of the Lung: A study of the Patterns of the Segmental Bronchi and Related Pulmonary Vessels. New York, Blakiston Division, McGraw-Hill Book Co., 1955.

Breeze, R. G., and Wheeldon, E. B.: The cells of the pulmonary airways. Am. Rev. Resp. Dis., *116*:705, 1977.

Etherton, J. E., Conning, D. M., and Corrin, B.: Autoradiographical and morphological evidence for apocrine secretion of dipalmitoyl lecithin in the terminal bronchiole of mouse lung. Am. J. Anat., *138*:11, 1973.

Hance, A. J., and Crystal, R. G.: The connective tissue of lung. Am. Rev. Resp. Dis., *112*:657, 1975.

Leeson, T. S., and Leeson, C. R.: A light and electron microscope study of developing respiratory tissue in the rat. J. Anat., *98*:183, 1964.

Leeson, T. S., and Leeson, C. R.: Osmiophilic lamellated bodies and associated material in lung alveolar spaces. J. Cell Biol., *28*:577, 1966.

Mavis, R. D., Finkelstein, J. N., and Hall, B. P.: Pulmonary surfactant synthesis. A highly active microsomal phosphatidate phosphohydralase in the lung. J. Lipid Res., *19*:467, 1978.

Polyzonis, B. M., Kafandaris, P. M., Gigis, P. I., and Demetriou, T.: An electron microscopic study of human olfactory mucosa. J. Anat., *128*:77, 1979.

Smith, M. N., Greenberg, S. D., and Spjut, H. J.: The Clara cell: a comparative ultrastructural study in mammals. Am. J. Anat., *155*:15, 1979.

Stratton, J. C.: The ultrastructure of multilamellar bodies and surfactant in the human lung. Cell Tiss. Res., *193*:219, 1978.

Takaro, T., Price, H. P., and Parra, S. C.: Ultrastructural studies of apertures in the interalveolar septum of the adult human lung. Am. Rev. Resp. Dis., *119*:425, 1979.

Yamamoto, M.: An electron microscopic study of the olfactory mucosa in the bat and rabbit. Arch. Hist. Jap., *38*:359, 1976.

THE URINARY SYSTEM

Metabolism of food by the body for the release of energy also involves the formation of waste materials, especially nitrogenous compounds such as urea and creatinine, and some of these are extremely toxic. Such waste materials are eliminated by the urinary system. The system also is the primary regulator of water and electrolyte homeostasis, being the mechanism for excretion of excess water and electrolytes, and, in so doing, it regulates the chemical composition of blood plasma and thus also that of extracellular fluid. This is the process of osmoregulation. Excretion and urine formation involve an ultrafiltration of blood plasma to form a filtrate and then selective reabsorption of most of the filtered water and other small molecules. The system comprises the two kidneys, where the functional units or *nephrons* are located, and a system of excretory passages to temporarily store and eventually conduct excreted materials to the exterior. Proper functioning of the system is essential to life. As might be expected, the kidneys have an extremely rich blood supply; indeed, the total volume of circulating blood passes through the kidneys once every five minutes. Additionally, the kidneys are involved in the maintenance of blood pressure by the release of the hormone *renin* and in producing and releasing another hormone, *erythropoietin*, that stimulates erythrocyte production in bone marrow.

THE KIDNEY

The human kidneys are bean-shaped, about 10 to 12 cm in length and 3.5 to 5 cm thick, and are situated in the posterior part of the upper abdomen, one on each side of the upper lumbar vertebrae. Each is enclosed in a thin fibroconnective tissue capsule which may be stripped easily from the underlying parenchyma, an indication that no septa are present. On the medial aspect is a depression, the *hilum*, through which the blood vessels enter and leave, and from which the excretory duct, the *ureter* leaves. The upper part of the ureter is expanded to fill the hilum of the kidney. This part, the *pelvis*, is subdivided into large and small cups, the major and minor *calyces*, there being usually two major and eight to 12 minor calyces. Each minor calyx envelops a conical protrusion of renal substance called a renal *papilla*, which is perforated by the openings of 10 to 25 *collecting ducts*. Vertical hemisection of the kidney shows that each papilla is the tip of a pyramidal area extending from the hilum toward the capsule and which in the fresh kidney is pale and striated. Such an area is a *medullary pyramid*, and its striated appearance is due to the presence of straight tubules and parallel blood vessels. The peripheral part or base of each pyramid does not show a clear demarcation from the dark, brownish, granular *cortex* of the kidney, since medullary material extends into the cortex as fine, radially oriented rays, the *medullary rays*. The student should not be confused by this term for although these medullary rays are composed of straight tubules and blood vessels, as is the medullary pyramid itself, they are located in the cortex. The medulla can be divided grossly into inner and outer zones, this being a

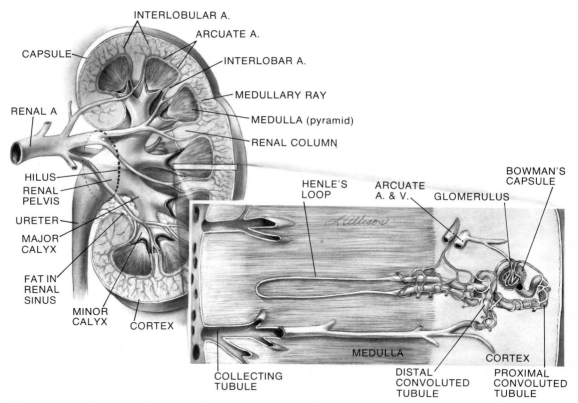

Figure 13–1. Diagram of the human kidney, sectioned vertically. A single nephron and the location of its parts is shown at lower right.

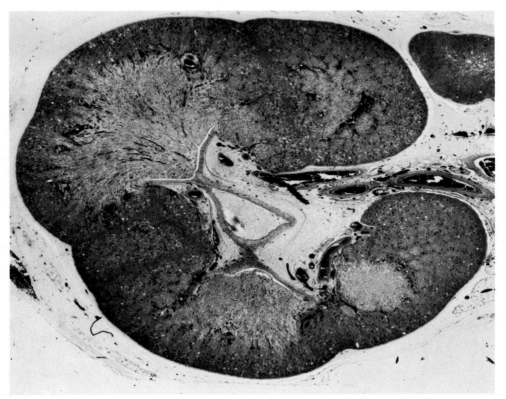

Figure 13–2. Transverse section of a human kidney. Notice the distinction between cortex and medulla, two minor calyces, and blood vessels in the hilum. Renal corpuscles are visible in the cortex as dark dots. A small portion of the adrenal gland is shown at the upper right corner. × 2.

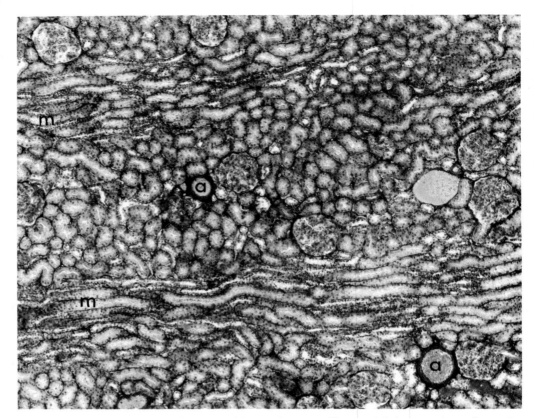

Figure 13–3.   Photomicrograph of part of the renal cortex to illustrate lobules, capsular surface to the right. Two medullary rays (m) with radially oriented tubules run from left to right and these are at the centers of two lobules. Between lobules are interlobular arteries (a). × 65.

reflection of morphological variation of the walls of the tubules within the medulla. Between adjacent medullary pyramids, cortical material extends between the pyramids to separate them and forms the *renal columns* (of Bertin). The granular appearance of the cortex is accounted for by the presence of spherical bodies, the *renal corpuscles*, and convoluted uriniferous tubules. Thus, in section, the tubules will be cut in oblique or cross fashion.

Each pyramid with its associated overlying cortex is regarded as a lobe; hence the term *multipyramidal* or *multilobar* kidney. Some of the lower mammals, e.g., rat and rabbit, have a unilobar or unipyramidal kidney. In the adult human, the lobes of the kidney are not demarcated and the kidney surface is smooth. In the fetus and young child, the kidney surface is irregular and it is described as lobulated. This term is imprecise; the term lobated is preferable since lobes, not lob-

ules, are indicated. A *lobule* of the kidney is a smaller, functional unit comprising a medullary (cortical) ray, the *kidney units* or *nephrons* which drain into it, and the continuation of the ray in a medullary pyramid. In the cortex, lobules are outlined, but not clearly demarcated, by radially oriented interlobular or cortical blood vessels, but no demarcation exists in the medulla.

Uriniferous Tubule

The kidney can be considered as a compound tubular gland which secretes urine, each kidney containing a large number of uriniferous tubules. Each tubule consists of two parts, the *nephron*, which is about 30 to 40 mm long, and the *collecting tubule*, approximately 20 mm long. The two form a continuous tubule although they have different developmental origins. The nephron is responsible for urine secretion, and the collecting tubule is the excretory duct which conveys urine to the renal pelvis.

Blood Supply of the Kidney

Each kidney receives a direct branch of the abdominal aorta, the renal artery, and in general blood passes through glomeruli before supplying the remainder of the kidney. At the hilum, the renal artery divides into three main branches, two passing anteriorly and one posteriorly to the renal pelvis, and each branch occasionally dividing further. There is little or no anastomosis between these major arteries, and each supplies three or four medullary pyramids and their corresponding cortical substance. This area of supply is termed a *renule*. In the adipose tissue around the hilum, each major branch divides into *interlobar arteries* which ascend between adjacent medullary pyramids in a column of Bertin, usually eccentrically placed to one side. There are also interlobar arteries at upper and lower poles of the kidney between the pyramids and the kidney surface.

At the corticomedullary junction, the interlobar arteries break up into several branches, the *arciform* or *arcuate* arteries, which leave the parent vessel almost at a right angle to arch over the bases of the medullary pyramids and run parallel to the surface of the kidney. From these, branches pass peripherally in the cortex in a radial fashion. These are located between medullary rays, viz., between lobules, and are termed the *interlobular arteries*. From the interlobular arteries, there are numerous side branches which enter cortical substance as *intralobular arteries* and branch into one or more afferent glomerular arterioles that supply glomeruli. The peripheral terminations of the interlobular arteries reach and supply the capillary bed of the renal capsule.

The efferent glomerular arterioles pass from glomeruli to supply the majority of other portions of the same nephrons. Those situated in the outer cortex form a cortical intertubular network of capillaries while efferent arterioles from juxtamedullary glomeruli pass into the medullary pyramids to supply them. These efferent arterioles run a straight, centripetal course and

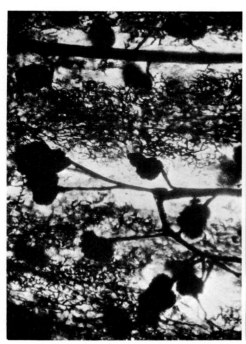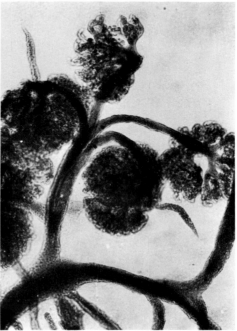

Figure 13–4. Photomicrographs to illustrate the blood supply to the kidney cortex in an injection section (*left*, × 125), and in isolated, microdissected whole glomeruli (*right*, × 350).

are called *arteriolae rectae spuriae* (false, straight arterioles), or *vasa recta*. These vessels penetrate the medulla in a radial fashion, take hairpin bends, and then return to the cortex to drain into arcuate veins. The endothelial walls of the vasa recta are very thin, the endothelium of the ascending (venous) limbs being perforated. This, together with the close proximity of the two limbs, permits rapid interchange of diffusible substances between the two limbs as a countercurrent exchange system. In the past, some investigators have claimed that the capillary networks of the medullary pyramids also are supplied by long, straight direct branches from arcuate and interlobular arteries *(arteriolae rectae verae* — true, straight arterioles), but if these do exist, they probably are so few as to be of no functional significance.

Venous drainage has a similar arrangement to the arterial supply, except, of course, that there is no venous component in the glomerulus and its arterioles. In the cortex, capillaries collect into small venules (the *stellate* veins) which then join in a starlike pattern to form *interlobular* veins, which pass toward the medulla with interlobular arteries, receiving tributaries from all levels of the cortex. These join to form *arcuate* or *arciform* veins which also receive straight vessels (the *venulae rectae*) ascending from medullary pyramids. Arcuate veins drain into interlobar veins, which pass toward the hilum and finally join to form the renal vein, which in turn drains to the inferior vena cava.

THE NEPHRON

There are a million or more nephrons in each kidney. Each is simply a long, epithelium-lined tube which starts blindly and terminates by joining an excretory duct, but the nephrons are so tortuous and so intermingled that histological sections of the kidney give no clear idea of their form. This can be achieved only by reconstructions from serial sections or by teasing out individual nephrons from kidneys after maceration. Each nephron consists of several segments of different structure and different function, and each segment is located in a definite position in the cortex or medulla.

The first part of the nephron, located in the cortex, is blind, dilated, and lined by a very thin epithelium. The expansion is invaginated into the form of a cup by a tuft of capillaries. This entire structure is called a *renal corpuscle* (of Malpighi); the expanded part is called *Bowman's capsule*, and the tuft of capillaries is known as the *glomerulus*. In the renal corpuscle an ultrafiltrate of plasma is formed from blood. This ultrafiltrate passes into the renal tubule, where later it is altered to form urine, both by secretions from tubule cells and by reabsorption of many of its filtered products. Connected to the renal corpuscle are convoluted and straight portions of the proximal tubule, a thin segment, and straight and convoluted portions of the distal tubule. The proximal convoluted tubule (convoluted part of the proximal tubule) and the distal convoluted tubule (convoluted part of the distal tubule) lie adjacent to the renal corpuscle in the cortex (see Figure 13–1). Between the tubules the remaining parts of the nephron form the *loop of Henle* which extends for a varying distance from the cortex into the medulla. The loop has descending and ascending limbs, running radially and parallel to each other and connected by a sharp bend. The descending limb comprises a thick portion (the straight part of the proximal tubule) and a thin portion, which continues round the loop as the thin part of the ascending limb. The thick remaining part of the ascending limb is the straight part of the distal tubule. Loops of Henle of nephrons located in the outer (subcapsular) cortex are short, extending only into the outer zone of the medulla; those of nephrons in the inner or juxtamedullary part of the cortex have long descending and ascending limbs with an extensive thin segment penetrating deeply to the inner zone of the medulla, and loops of Henle of nephrons with glomeruli located in midcortex show a morphology intermediate between subcapsular and juxtamedullary nephrons. The distal convoluted tubule continues into a collecting tubule or excretory duct.

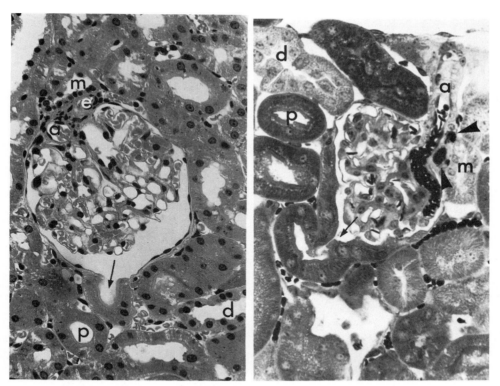

Figure 13–5. *Left:* Photomicrograph of a single renal corpuscle showing vascular pole above with afferent (a) and efferent (e) arterioles and macula densa (m), and urinary pole below (arrow). Proximal (p) and distal (d) convoluted tubules also are present. × 300. *Right:* Similar, but note juxtaglomerular (JG) granulated cells (arrowheads) in the wall of the afferent arteriole in relation to the macula densa (m). × 250.

Renal Corpuscle

Bowman's capsule, the epithelium-lined dilatation of the nephron, is invaginated by a tuft of capillaries, the glomerulus, thus acquiring a cup shape which is double walled. There is a narrow slitlike space, the capsular space, between the outer or parietal layer (capsular epithelium) and the inner or visceral layer (glomerular epithelium) which closely invests the capillary tuft. The entire renal corpuscle, i.e., Bowman's capsule plus the glomerulus of capillaries, is roughly spherical. It has a

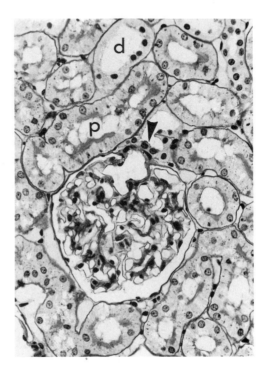

Figure 13–6. Photomicrograph of renal cortex, section stained with the PAS technique, to show basal laminae (black) of glomerulus, renal corpuscle, and surrounding proximal (p) and distal (d) convoluted tubules. In proximal tubules, the brush border also stains positively. A macula densa (arrowhead) and vascular pole of the renal corpuscle are present. × 250.

vascular pole where afferent and efferent arterioles enter and leave the glomerulus and where the parietal layer of the capsule is reflected onto the vessels as the visceral layer. The renal corpuscle also has a *urinary pole* at the opposite side of the corpuscle where capsular space is continuous with the lumen of the proximal convoluted tubule and where the parietal (squamous) epithelium is continuous with the cuboidal or low columnar epithelium of the proximal convoluted tubule.

In size, renal corpuscles vary from

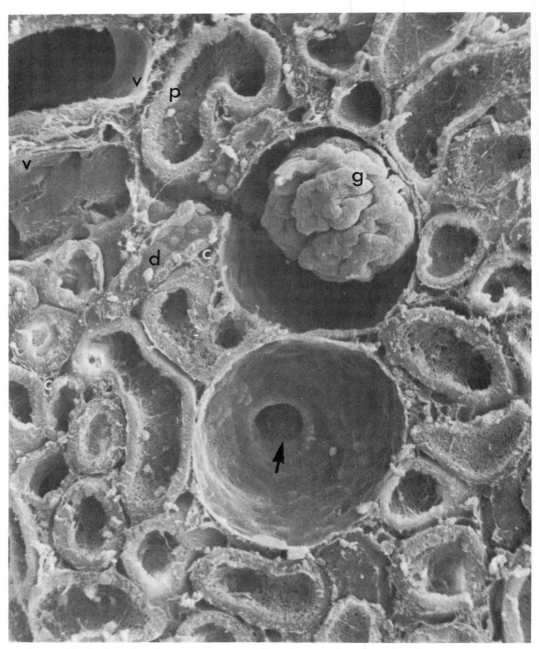

Figure 13–7.   Scanning electron micrograph of renal cortex of rat showing two renal corpuscles, the top one containing a glomerulus (g), the lower showing parietal epithelium of Bowman's capsule with a urinary pole (arrow) opening to a proximal convoluted tubule. Proximal (p) and distal (d) convoluted tubules, intertubular capillaries (c), and major blood vessels (v) are seen also. × 750. (Courtesy of P. M. Andrews.)

150 to 250 microns (μm) in diameter; those in the deeper areas of the cortex adjacent to the medulla are larger than those situated peripherally beneath the capsule of the kidney. The larger, juxtamedullary corpuscles are the first to differentiate during development.

The parietal layer of Bowman's capsule is composed of a simple squamous epithelium with nuclei which protrude slightly into the capsular space. Cytoplasmic organelles are poorly developed. At the urinary pole, these squamous cells increase in height over four or five cells to become continuous with the low columnar epithelium lining the proximal convoluted tubule. The visceral layer of epithelium closely invests glomerular capillaries with nuclei of these epithelial cells on the capsular side

of the basal lamina, but they do not form a complete sheet and the cells are extensively modified.

These cells are called *podocytes* and are basically stellate in form with their cell bodies rarely in close contact with basal laminae of glomerular capillaries but situated one or two millimicrons away. From the cell body, several *major* or *primary processes* extend from the perikaryon in the manner of the tentacles of an octopus or the limbs of a starfish toward one or more capillary loops and from the primary processes extend numerous small secondary footlike processes or *pedicels* that attach to the outer (capsular) surface of capillary basal laminae. Pedicels of adjacent podocytes and podocytic processes interdigitate in a complex manner with an extensive

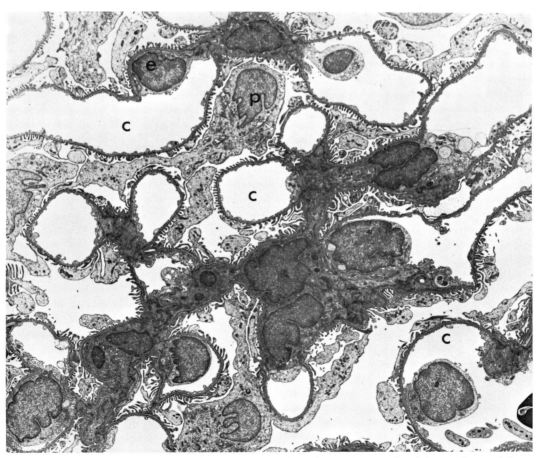

Figure 13–8. Survey electron micrograph of a portion of a renal corpuscle of the rat. Some of the capillary loops are labeled (c) and are lined by attenuated endothelium, one nucleus of which is indicated (e). Covering capillary loops are pedicels and cytoplasmic processes of the visceral epithelial cells or podocytes, one of which is labeled (p). × 3000. (Courtesy of Dr. Ruth Bulger; labeling added. See also Figure 5 in the Introduction.)

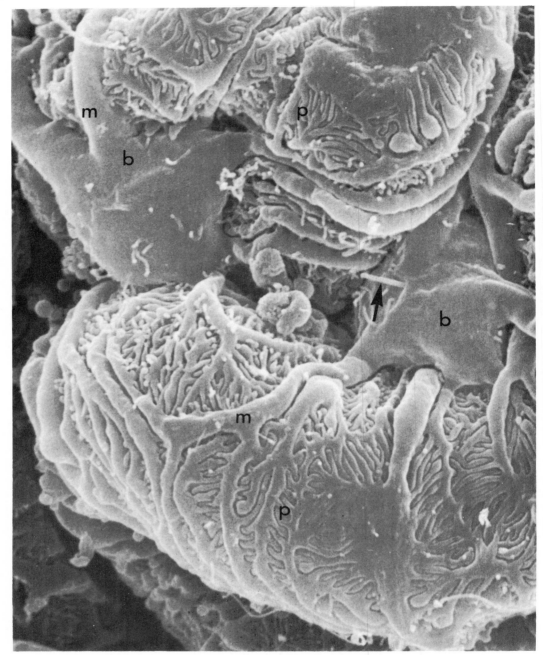

Figure 13–9.   Scanning electron micrograph of the visceral epithelium (podocytes) of monkey kidney, showing podocyte cell bodies (b), one with a single cilium (arrow), major processes (m), and pedicels (p). × 7000. (Courtesy of P. M. Andrews.)

system of clefts called *filtration slits* or *slit pores* between pedicels. These spaces are freely continuous with larger spaces beneath and between major processes and eventually all drain to the capsular space and thus into the lumen of the proximal convoluted tubule. Electron microscopy shows that podocyte nuclei are often irregular with deep infoldings and in the cytoplasm adjacent to the nucleus is a well-formed Golgi apparatus, granular endoplasmic reticulum, and some free ribosomes. Cytoplasmic filaments and microtubules are found not only in

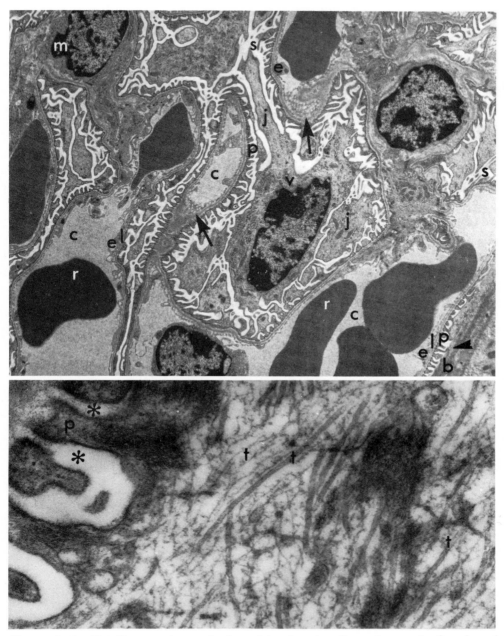

Figure 13–10. *Top:* Electron micrograph of a peripheral portion of a renal corpuscle of a guinea pig showing capillary lumina (c) containing erythrocytes (r), endothelium (e) showing pores or fenestrae where cut tangentially (arrows), basal laminae ("lamina densa", l), podocytes (v) and their major processes (j) and pedicels (p), a mesangial cell (m), and capsular (urinary) space (s). Parietal epithelium (arrowhead) and the basal lamina (b) of Bowman's capsule is seen at lower right. × 7,000. *Bottom:* Part of a major process of a podocyte showing microtubules (t) and cytoplasmic filaments (F), with pedicels (p) at left and filtration slits (asterisks) between them. × 50,000.

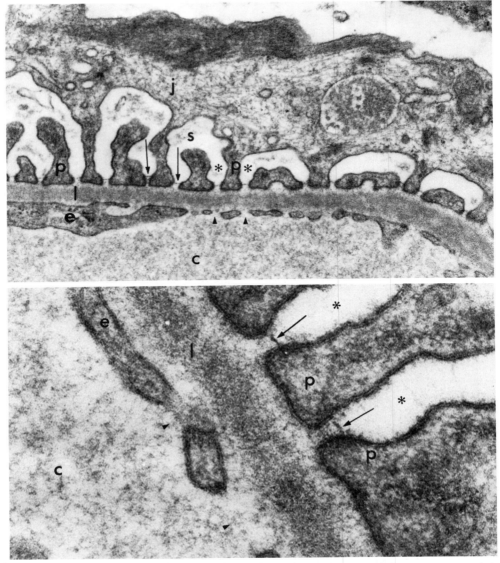

Figure 13–11. Electron micrographs to show the "filtration barrier": capillary lumen (c) containing plasma, endothelium (e) with pores (arrowheads), lamina densa (l), pedicels (p) with filtration slits (asterisks) between them, closed by slit membranes (arrows), urinary (capsular) space (s), and major process of a podocyte (j). Top, × 32,000; bottom, × 90,000.

the perikaryon but extend into primary and secondary processes. Where pedicels extend to the basal lamina of a capillary they are not in contact but are separated by slits about 25 nm wide with the outer leaflets of plasma membranes of adjacent pedicels connected by thin membranes, *the slit membranes,* only 5 to 6 nm thick. These membranes are considered to be similar to the diaphragms closing pores of fenestrated (type II) capillaries.

Beneath the pedicels, the basal lamina is about 0.3 μm thick, considerably thicker than is usual in capillaries, and is composed of an amorphous material embedded in which is a feltwork of fine filaments. The basal lamina shows a central, electron-dense lamina called the *lamina densa,* about 0.1 μm thick, with an

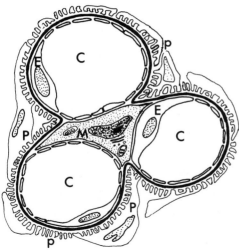

Figure 13–12. Diagram of a "lobule" of glomerular capillaries to illustrate the relationship of a mesangial cell (M) to endothelium (E) of capillaries (C), basal lamina (thick dark line), and podocytes (P) and their pedicels (p).

electron-lucent layer on external and internal aspects. Internally, the endothelium of glomerular capillaries is greatly attenuated with numerous pores or fenestrae of about 80 nm diameter, these pores not closed by pore diaphragms as are found elsewhere in the body in other fenestrated or type II capillaries.

The glomerulus is a mass of tortuous capillaries located along the course of an arteriole with an afferent arteriole running to the glomerulus and an efferent arteriole away from it. The afferent is of greater diameter than the efferent arteriole, and consequently the glomerulus is a relatively high pressure system, aiding the formation of tissue fluid in the capillary bed. On entering the renal corpuscle, the afferent arteriole branches into three to five main branches from which capillaries arise and drain to primary branches or tributaries of the efferent arteriole. A group of capillaries thus can be termed a lobule of the glomerulus, with some anastomoses between capillaries of a lobule and even between capillaries of adjacent lobules. Parietal epithelium, i.e., podocytes, surround small groups of capillaries and between the capillary loops near afferent and efferent arterioles are "stalks" with areas of adjacent capillary basal laminae not lined by endothelium. In such areas lie *mesangial* cells. These

are stellate in form, similar to pericytes found elsewhere, with cytoplasmic processes that sometimes extend between endothelium and the basal lamina. They provide some support for the capillaries and are believed to be phagocytic, removing any macromolecular substances that enter the space between capillaries. There are similarities too between mesangial and juxtaglomerular cells (vide infra), both structurally and functionally.

It has been shown that there is a turnover of basal lamina material, i.e., it is not static. New basal lamina material is added to the epithelial (outer) surface and older material is removed from the inner endothelial surface, probably by phagocytic action of mesangial cells. The overall thickness of the basal lamina thus remains constant. The older basal lamina material that is removed may contain filtration residues, and thus, the mesangial tissues probably recondition the basal lamina.

The Juxtaglomerular Complex. Adjacent to the glomerulus, smooth muscle cells in the media of the afferent arteriole are "epithelioid" in character. Their nuclei are spherical and the cytoplasm contains granules, although the granules are not visible with routine H and E staining. These are the juxtaglomerular (JG) cells. In the afferent arteriole, the internal elastic lamina is absent so that the JG cells lie adjacent to endothelium and thus to blood in the lumen. The cells also are closely related to the *macula densa,* a specialized region of the distal convoluted tubule at its commencement where it lies between afferent and efferent arterioles. The macula densa lacks a basal lamina. Associated with the granulated JG cells are some lightly staining cells called *lacis* or extraglomerular mesangial cells. Their function is not clear, but they may produce erythropoietin, a hormone that stimulates erythropoiesis in bone marrow. By electron microscopy, the JG cells contain granular endoplasmic reticulum, a well-developed Golgi apparatus, and secretory granules of 10 to 40 nm diameter, spheroidal or oval, membrane bounded, and with a granular or crystalline content.

The JG cells produce an enzyme

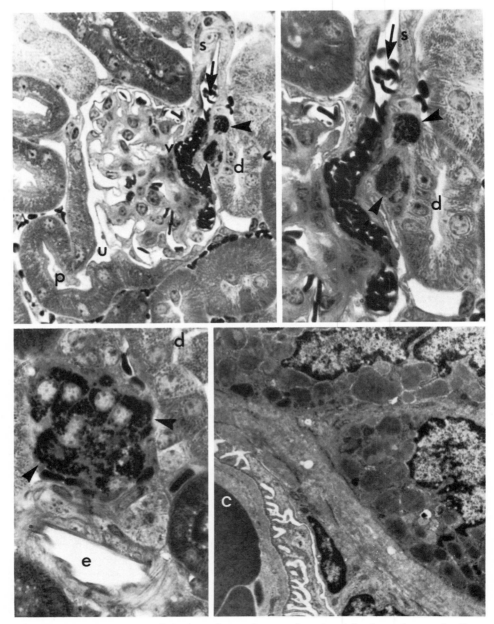

Figure 13–13.   Illustrations of the juxtaglomerular complex. *Top: left,* photomicrograph of a renal corpuscle with urinary pole (u) continuous with proximal convoluted tubule (p), vascular pole (v) and afferent arteriole (arrow) passing to the glomerulus with smooth muscle cells (s) in its wall changing to granulated JG cells (arrowheads), related on the outer (right) aspect to a macula densa (d) of the distal convoluted tubule; *right,* a higher magnification of the vascular pole. *Bottom: left,* a JG complex (arrowheads) sectioned obliquely (as in a vertical cut down the page in top left figure) to show its extent: the efferent arteriole (e) and macula densa (d) also are seen; *right,* electron micrograph showing portions of two JG cells adjacent to a glomerular capillary (c). Top left, × 450; top right, × 1000; bottom left × 1000; bottom right, × 7500.

called *renin*. In the blood stream, renin acts on angiotensinogen, a plasma globulin, to produce angiotensin I. Angiotensin I is inactive but is converted to angiotensin II, a potent vasoconstrictor substance. Angiotensin II raises blood pressure by constriction of arterioles and by increasing release of aldosterone from adrenal cortex, aldosterone increasing sodium reabsorption, and therefore water, from the distal convoluted tubules to expand plasma volume and thus increase blood pressure. The basic mechanism thus is that the JG cells release renin when the blood pressure falls, the renin ultimately acting to increase blood pressure.

Filtration Barrier

The filtration barrier is a term applied to the structures that separate blood in glomerular capillaries from filtrate in the capsular space of the renal corpuscle. The barrier comprises the fenestrated, attenuated endothelium, the basal lamina, and pedicels of the podocytes connected by slit membranes. The only continuous layer of the three is the basal lamina and it is regarded as the main filter preventing passage of large molecules, although the slit membranes may also be significant. Experimentally, large particulate tracers such as ferritin pass through endothelial pores but are held up for some time by the basal lamina; smaller particles such as horseradish peroxidase pass through into the capsular space. The functional pore size of the filtration barrier is approximately the molecular size of plasma albumin (mol. wt. 70,000); i.e., molecules smaller than this pass through, but larger molecules do not.

Functional Correlation

Ultrafiltration through the barrier is dependent upon hydrostatic pressure of blood in glomerular capillaries, usually about 75 mm Hg. As explained, the glomerulus is a relatively high pressure system and the tunica media of circularly arranged smooth muscle fibers is thick in the efferent arteriole. By con-

traction, it can regulate pressure in the glomerulus. Thus, physiologically, the renal corpuscle is regarded as an ultrafilter with tissue fluid leaving blood along the entire extent of the glomerular capillary bed. In man, the total glomerular filtrate in 24 hours is from 170 to 200 liters, of which some 99 per cent will be resorbed by the uriniferous tubules, with 1.5 to 2 liters being excreted as urine. (The term "uriniferous tubule" encompasses the tubular part of the nephron and the collecting duct.)

Proximal Convoluted Tubule

The proximal convoluted tubule, commencing at the urinary pole of a renal corpuscle, is approximately 14 mm long with an outside diameter of 50 to 60 microns (μm). As the name suggests, it follows a tortuous course and always takes one large loop toward the capsular surface of the kidney in addition to numerous minor twists and turns. It terminates by straightening out and passing into the nearest medullary ray where it becomes continuous with the loop of Henle. As the longest and widest part of the nephron, it constitutes the bulk of the cortex, appearing in sections as oblique and transverse profiles. In it, glomerular filtrate begins its transformation into urine by the absorption of some constituents and the addition of others.

At its commencement, there is a narrow zone termed the *neck* where there is a rapid transition from the squamous type of epithelium of the parietal cells of Bowman's capsule to the simple low columnar type of the proximal convolution. The cells are truncated pyramids, with cell interfaces which are defined poorly because cell membranes are irregular and cells interdigitate with their neighbors. The cytoplasm is abundant and usually intensely eosinophilic, the nucleus being large, spherical, and pale staining. Although there may be six to twelve cells around the circumference of a proximal convoluted tubule, rarely are more than four or five nuclei seen, the cells being considerably greater in width than the thickness of the section. The height of the epithelial cells, and thus the diameter of the

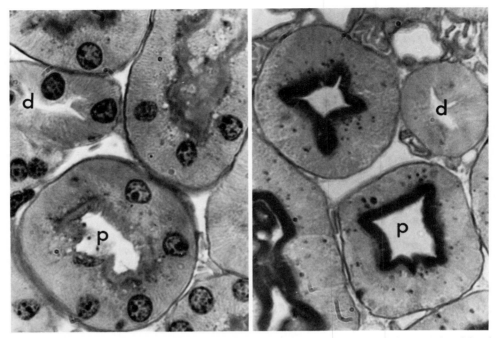

Figure 13–14.   Photomicrographs of proximal (p) and distal (d) convoluted tubules. Note brush border in proximal tubules that stains positively with the periodic acid–Schiff technique (*right*), as do basal laminae. Both × 1200.

lumen, varies to some extent with functional activity although the lumen is never occluded completely in well-fixed tissue.

In material well fixed immediately after death, the basal cytoplasm is striated by long, parallel mitochondria, and a brush border is obvious on the luminal surface. The brush border is alkaline phosphatase positive. A Golgi apparatus is located in a supranuclear position.

As evident by electron microscopy, the lumen is relatively wide, each cell having long, thin, closely packed microvilli on its apical surface. Between the bases of microvilli are tubular pits or small apical canaliculi, and the apical cytoplasm also contains numerous small vesicles, some of which appear to bud off from apical canaliculi. This represents a mechanism for absorption of protein from the glomerular filtrate. The basal cytoplasm shows interesting specializations. The basal plasma membrane exhibits numerous infoldings, between which are elongated mitochondria. In addition, there is a complex interdigitation of adjacent cells, processes

from one cell lying in basal pockets of adjacent cells. There also are complex intercellular interdigitations of lateral cell interfaces. Beneath the basal plasma membrane is a continuous basal lamina, separating the epithelial cells from surrounding capillaries, which are lined by a fenestrated (type II) endothelium.

The cytoplasm of proximal tubule cells contains a few, free RNP granules, a poorly developed granular endoplasmic reticulum, a prominent Golgi zone in a supranuclear position, and a few lysosomes and peroxisomes.

The morphological appearance is similar in cells along the length of the proximal convoluted tubule although regional differences have been recognized in many species. In the straight portion of the proximal tubule (in the descending limb of the loop of Henle), the cells are not as tall, and they show fewer basal infoldings and interdigitations, smaller mitochondria, and shorter and less numerous microvilli.

Functionally, the proximal tubule resorbs 85 per cent or more of the water and sodium chloride in the glomerular filtrate, and while this reduces the *volume* of the filtrate, the osmolarity is unchanged. The cells actively transport sodium, and the chloride and water follow passively to maintain osmotic equilibrium. Normally, all glucose also is resorbed but if the level of glucose in the blood is excessively high, the capacity for resorption is exceeded and glucose appears in the urine. This occurs, for example, in diabetes. Other substances also are resorbed, e.g., amino acids, protein, vitamin C, and inorganic ions. In addition, cells of the proximal tubule pass materials into the lumen, a process of excretion. Some examples are creatinine and various dye materials, such as Diodrast and phenol red,

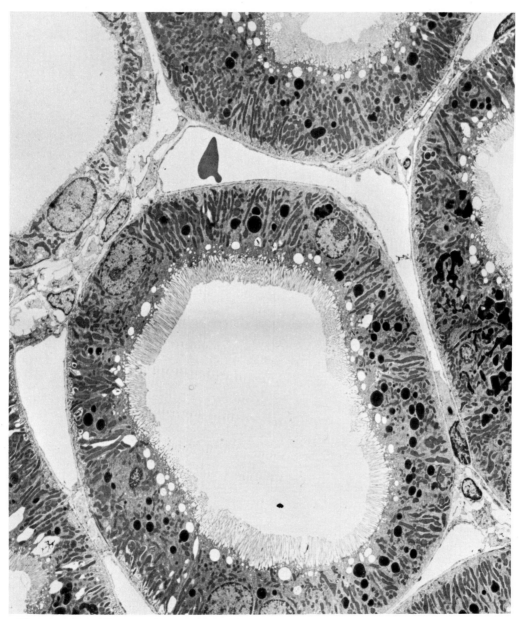

Figure 13–15. Electron micrograph of renal cortex showing proximal convoluted tubules and one distal convoluted tubule (top left). Note the elongated mitochondria and apical microvilli of the former, and the capillaries between the tubules. × 3300. (Courtesy of Dr. A. B. Maunsbach.)

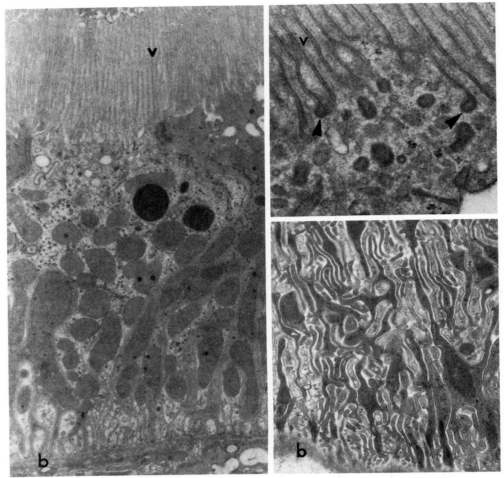

Figure 13–16.   Electron micrographs of proximal convoluted tubule. *Left:* Apical microvilli (v), basal infoldings of plasma membrane, and basal interlocking of cytoplasmic processes of adjacent cells (b is the basal lamina) and numerous mitochondria. × 18,000. *Top right:* Apical canaliculi or tubular pits (arrowheads) between microvilli. × 45,000. *Bottom right:* Oblique section through the base of a tubule showing the complex interlocking of cytoplasmic processes. × 24,000.

which are used clinically to assess tubular function.

Loop of Henle

The loop of Henle consists of the straight part of the proximal tubule in the descending limb, a thin segment in the descending and ascending limbs, and the straight part of the distal tubule in the ascending limb. The two limbs lie close together and are oriented radially in the kidney. There is some variation in loops of Henle in the human, as mentioned previously. Those of juxtamedullary nephrons are long

with the loops formed by the thin limb (as shown in Figure 13–1) which may extend nearly to the apex of the medullary papilla. Loops of Henle of subcapsular nephrons are much shorter with the bend formed by the thick ascending limb, and the thin descending limb being very short. These loops extend only into the outer part of the medulla. This arrangement accounts for the zonation seen in the medulla.

The transition from straight portion of proximal tubule to descending thin limb occurs abruptly over a few cells. The epithelium changes from low columnar or cuboidal to squamous, the thin limb having an outside diameter of only 12 to 15 μm. Nuclei of the squamous cells protrude into the lumen and only three to five are seen in a cross section of a thin limb. They resemble those of capillaries except that the nuclei protrude more and are closer together than those of endothelial cells. The cytoplasm is less eosinophilic than that of proximal tubule cells. By electron microscopy, the cells show only a few short apical microvilli and an occasional single cilium, small basal infoldings of the plasma membrane, and few organelles. Characteristically, there are numerous interdigitations of processes of adjacent cells with many lateral interfaces (extending from base to lumen).

Thus, around the circumference of a thin segment in cross section there may be up to 20 or more portions of cells, only a few of which contain a nucleus.

The transition from thin segment to ascending thick limb (the straight part of the distal tubule) also is abrupt, the cells increasing in height from squamous to cuboidal. The ascending limb has an outside diameter of 30 to 50 μm and ascends from the medulla to cortex in a radial fashion to reach the glomerulus of origin at the vascular pole. Here, it lies between afferent and efferent arterioles and is specialized as a *macula densa* (dense spot) (discussed later). In the ascending limb, cells show numerous interdigitations and basal in-

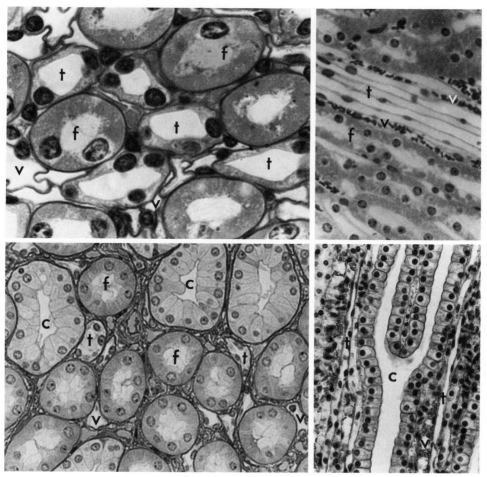

Figure 13–17. Photomicrographs of the renal medulla to illustrate collecting ducts (c) and thin (t) and thick (f) segments of the loop of Henle and vasa recta (v) in transverse (*left*) and longitudinal (*right*) section. Note the union of two collecting ducts (*lower right*). Top, left, × 700; right, × 200. Bottom, left, × 250; right, × 150.

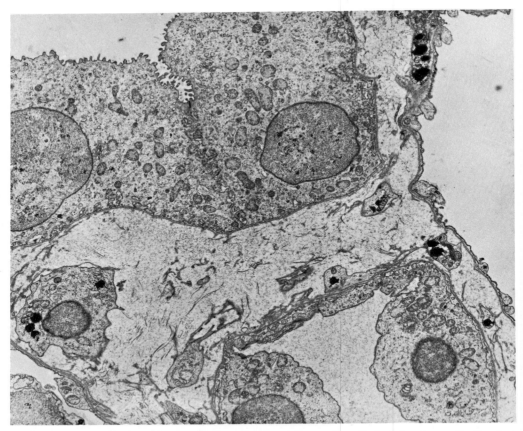

Figure 13–18.   Electron micrograph of a section through a renal papilla (rat) showing a collecting duct (top left), a thin limb of the loop of Henle (bottom right), and a blood capillary (top right). × 4500. (Courtesy of Dr. Ruth Bulger.)

foldings of the plasmalemma with elongated mitochondria between the infoldings.

Functionally, the loop of Henle is essential for the production of urine which is hypertonic to blood plasma. This is discussed further below.

Macula Densa. Where the ascending limb of the loop of Henle (straight part of the distal tubule) contacts the parent renal corpuscle between afferent and efferent arterioles, there is a specialized region of the distal tubule called the macula densa. The epithelial cells of the tubule, where they are immediately adjacent to an arteriole, show dense packing in a palisade manner. This is closely adjacent to the juxtaglomerular apparatus of the afferent arteriole, but a large macula densa also may be present in relation to the efferent arteriole. The tubule cells of the macula densa show less speciali-zation and infolding of the basal plasma membrane, fewer mitochondria, and a Golgi zone which is subnuclear, i.e., near the arteriole. In addition, the basal lamina here is thin or absent. The close relation between the JG cells and the cells of the macula densa suggests a role in regulation of blood flow to the glomerulus. That role is unclear but it is theorized that cells of the macula densa detect changes in sodium ion concentration, a decrease occurring with decreased glomerular filtration consequent upon a lowered blood pressure. This decrease perhaps results in release from JG cells of renin into the afferent arteriole.

Distal Convoluted Tubule

From the region of the macula densa, the nephron continues as the

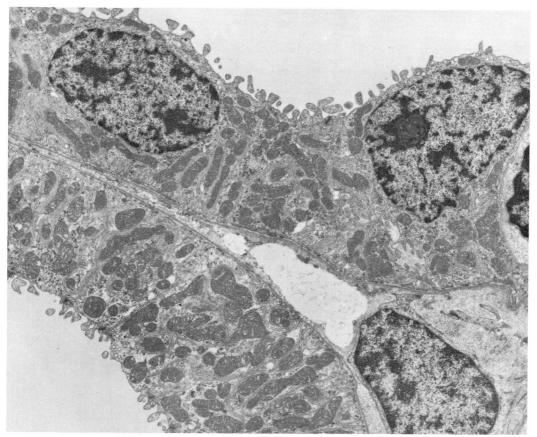

Figure 13–19. Electron micrograph of distal convoluted tubules from the kidney of a spider monkey. Note the complex infolding and interdigitation of the basal plasmalemma. × 4000. (Courtesy of Dr. Ruth Bulger.)

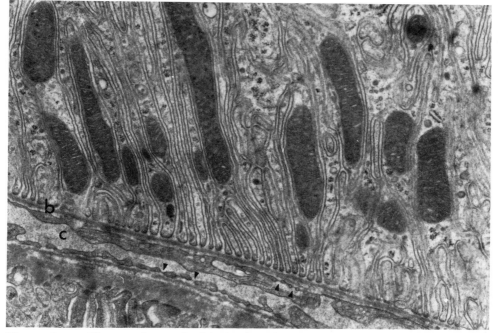

Figure 13–20. Electron micrograph of the basal portion of a distal convoluted tubule showing basal infoldings and interdigitation of the basal plasmalemma with elongated mitochondria in the cytoplasmic compartments. Note the peritubular capillary (c) with fenestrated endothelium (pores indicated by arrowheads) and basal lamina (b) of the tubule. × 24,000.

447

distal convoluted tubule, which follows a short, tortuous course in the cortex and terminates near a medullary ray by continuing into a collecting duct. The distal convoluted tubule is shorter than the proximal convoluted tubule, and thus in a section appears in smaller numbers, its overall diameter is less, and the cells are cuboidal, smaller, and have no brush border. Usually six to eight nuclei are seen in a cross section. Generally the cells stain less intensely than those of the proximal convoluted tubule. As seen by electron microscopy, the cells are cuboidal with a clear cytoplasm and central, spherical nuclei. A few, short, apical microvilli are present. Mitochondria are elongated, and most of them are in basal cytoplasm between infoldings of the basal plasma membrane. These infoldings are developed more highly than in the proximal convoluted tubule.

Each distal convoluted tubule drains by a short connecting duct into a small collecting tubule. Developmentally, the nephrons and the excretory or collecting ducts have different origins.

Collecting Tubules

The collecting tubules, or excretory ducts, are not considered parts of the nephron. Each distal convoluted tubule connects to a collecting tubule via a short side branch of the latter located in a medullary ray, there being several such branches. The collecting tubule passes in a medullary ray and down into the medulla. In the more central parts of the medulla, several collecting tubules join at acute angles to form large ducts which open onto the apex of a papilla. These are the *papillary ducts* of Bellini and have a diameter of 100 to 200 μm or more. Their openings onto the surface of a papilla are so large, so numerous, and so closely packed as to give the papilla the appearance of a sieve (the *area cribosa*).

The cells lining these excretory ducts vary in size from low cuboidal in the proximal parts to tall columnar in the main papillary ducts. Cell borders are regular with few interdigitations, and cells generally are pale-staining with few organelles. In the large collecting ducts,

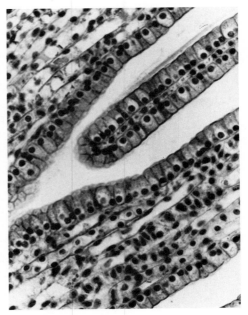

Figure 13–21. Photomicrograph of collecting ducts uniting to form ducts of Bellini. × 250.

free ribosomes are prominent and there are widened intercellular spaces into which protrude pseudopodium-like processes from adjacent cells. The collecting tubules conduct urine from the nephrons to the ureteric pelvis, with some absorption of water which is under the control of the antidiuretic hormone (ADH).

Concentration and Dilution of Urine. It is possible for the body to conserve water by excreting a concentrated urine or to produce a dilute urine and eliminate excess water. This occurs in the kidney and involves a countercurrent multiplier system in the loop of Henle and a countercurrent exchange system in the vasa recta and collecting ducts.

As noted above, urine is concentrated in the proximal convoluted tubule (about 85 per cent of water and sodium chloride being resorbed), but while the volume is reduced, the osmolarity is unchanged. Unlike the cortex, interstitial fluid in the papillae and outer renal medulla is hyperosmotic to blood plasma, sodium ions being "trapped" in the medulla. In the loop of Henle, the wall of the descending limb (thin segment) is permeable to so-

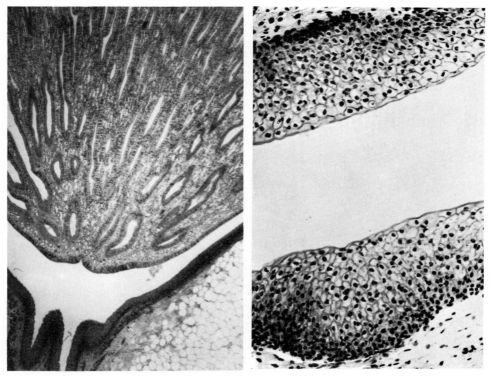

Figure 13–22. Photomicrographs of, *left,* the apex of a medullary pyramid showing ducts of Bellini that perforate the pyramid at the area cribrosa with transitional epithelium lining the renal pelvis (below), and, *right,* the transitional epithelium covering a medullary pyramid. Left, × 40; right, × 550.

dium and water while the ascending limb (thick segment) actively transports sodium from the urine to the interstitium (a "sodium pump"), thus increasing the osmotic concentration of the interstitium. However, water is retained in the ascending limb so that, with the loss of sodium, the fluid in the ascending limb becomes increasingly hypotonic as it ascends to the distal convoluted tubule. The descending limb passes through the medullary interstitium, which is hyperosmotic, and loses water to the interstitium, and sodium passes into it by passive diffusion with consequent concentration of the urine. Thus, urine becomes increasingly hypertonic as it passes down the descending limb, but as it ascends in the ascending limb, it first becomes isotonic and then hypotonic. In the distal convoluted tubule, urine entering it thus is hypotonic, although reduced in volume, but here, under the influence of ADH, water is resorbed and the urine again becomes isotonic. As it passes into

the collecting duct, more water passes out to the hypertonic interstitium of the medulla, and thus urine leaving collecting ducts is hypertonic. If ADH is low, the permeability of the distal convoluted tubule and collecting duct is low, and little water is removed. Thus, a large volume of dilute urine will be excreted.

The straight blood vessels (vasa recta) of the renal medulla are arranged with parallel ascending and descending vessels connected by a sharp bend so that blood runs in opposite directions in the two limbs. This allows equilibration of concentration of blood in ascending and descending vessels which thus does not disturb the osmotic gradient in the medulla.

Lymphatics of the Kidney

There are networks of lymphatic capillaries in the capsule and in association with the renal vessels, and the two

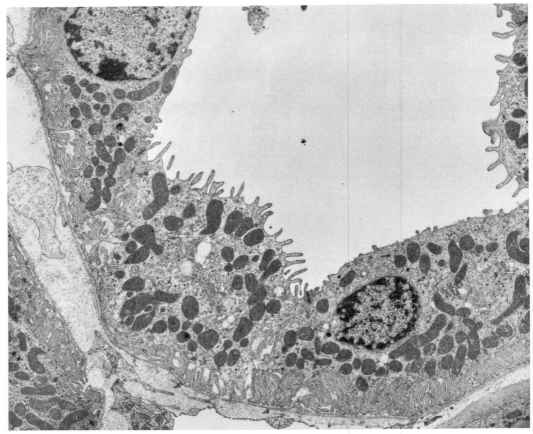

Figure 13–23.   Electron micrograph of a portion of a collecting duct from the kidney of a spider monkey. × 4500. (Courtesy of Dr. Ruth Bulger.)

groups are connected by a few anastomotic channels. There is considerable disagreement on the extent of the lymphatic channels in cortical and medullary substance, but certainly none are found in glomeruli. Small longitudinal channels are present in medullary pyramids. They commence blindly near apices and drain toward the cortex terminating in lymphatic vessels accompanying arcuate vessels. There are said to be extensive networks also between uriniferous tubules in the cortex. All vessels leave the kidney at the hilum.

Nerves

Nerves from the celiac sympathetic plexus enter the kidney with the arteries. They terminate in relation to large vessels and probably extend to glomeruli. The renal pelvis and capsule are innervated by sensory fibers also.

Embryology

During development the kidney arises from intermediate mesoderm situated in the posterior abdominal wall. Primitive nephrons develop from the cords of mesenchymal cells and acquire a lumen, and the blind dilated end of the nephron (the future Bowman's capsule) is invaginated by a tuft of capillaries. The ureteric bud, a diverticulum arising from the mesonephric or wolffian duct, grows into the mass of developing kidney or metanephros. The mesonephric duct later becomes associated with the genital system, and by differential growth, the ureteric bud originating from it is taken up into the developing urinary bladder. When the growing end of the ureteric bud reaches the metanephros, it undergoes a series of divisions, each terminal branch becoming continuous with a developing nephron. The fine branches

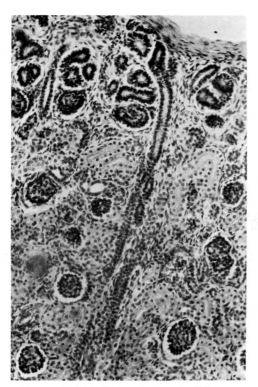

Figure 13–24. Photomicrograph of the cortex of developing human kidney of four months gestation. Note that the cortical renal corpuscles (top) are less well developed than those near the medulla (bottom). × 125.

of the ureteric bud thus become the various orders of collecting or excretory ducts, and its main branches become the minor and major calyces of the renal pelvis; the ureteric bud itself becomes the ureter. As just indicated, the first nephrons to develop are those in the deeper layers of the cortex. At birth the kidney is irregular in outline (fetal lobulation), and the outer cortical region consists of undifferentiated mesenchyme from which additional nephrons will develop for some months or even years after birth. When development is complete, the kidney outline becomes smooth.

Developmental abnormalities of the kidney and excretory passages are not uncommon. Early division of a ureteric bud before it reaches the metanephros can result in conditions such as bifid or double ureter, and double kidney. Failure of individual nephrons to connect with terminal divisions of the ureteric bud results in cysts, usually multiple (multicystic kidney).

EXCRETORY PASSAGES

The excretory passages convey urine from the kidney to the exterior. Essentially they are simple ducts, but they do add some mucus to the urine and may function to a limited extent to absorb a small amount of fluid. All parts have a relatively thick muscularis which on contraction aids the expulsion of urine.

Pelvis and Ureter

As noted, the upper expanded portion of the ureter, the pelvis, is situated in the hilum of the kidney and splits into major and minor calyces, each minor calyx fitting like a cup around a medullary papilla. The wall of the pelvis is thinner than that of the ureter itself, and, indeed, the thickness of the wall gradually increases from the start to the termination of the excretory ducts. The ureter is 10 to 12 inches (25 to 30 cm) in length, is situated in the posterior abdominal wall behind the peritoneum, and terminates by perforating obliquely the wall of the urinary bladder.

Mucosa. In the pelvis and ureter, the lining mucosa consists of transitional epithelium supported by a lamina propria, the epithelium being only two to three layers of cells in the pelvis and four to five layers in the ureter. As described in Chapter 2, the surface cells present a convex border to the lumen, may be binucleate, and may show specializations. The apical plasma membrane has an outer leaflet (of the trilaminar membrane) that is thicker than the inner leaflet, with some associated extracellular filamentous material. It is assumed that this membrane serves as a barrier to the passage of ions from the cell cytoplasm to the hypertonic urine in the lumen. The epithelium rests upon a thin basal lamina, and the lamina propria is a relatively dense fibroconnective tissue in which elastic fibers are prominent. Some loose lymphatic tissue is present, and the outer layer of the lamina propria is looser: this is regarded by some as a submucosa. No glands are present in the lamina propria. In transverse section, the lumen has a stellate outline due to longitudinal

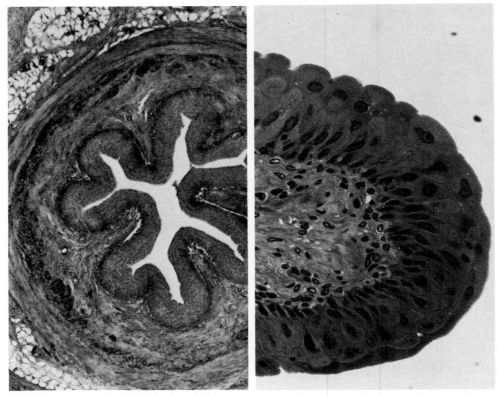

Figure 13–25. *Left,* photomicrograph of a transverse section through the ureter showing all layers, and, *right,* plastic section of the transitional epithelium lining the ureter. Left, × 40; right, × 400.

folds of the mucosa; these folds result from the looseness of the outer layer of the lamina propria, the presence of elastic tissue, and the muscularis. The folds are "ironed out" when the ureter is distended.

Muscularis. The muscularis is thick and consists of bundles of smooth muscle cells separated by strands of connective tissue. This smooth muscle is arranged as an inner longitudinal coat and an outer circular coat (the opposite orientation to that of smooth muscle in the intestine), but the layers are not clearly distinct and a third, outer longitudinal or oblique layer is present at the lower end of the ureter. In the pelvis, the muscle mainly is oriented in a circular pattern around papillae and possibly has a sphincteric action, perhaps squeezing or "milking" the papillae and thus expressing urine from the ducts of Bellini. At the lower end of the ureter, circularly arranged smooth muscle disappears, but the two longitudinal layers, now not separated by the circular layer, are prominent and continue down to the ureteric orifice. Reflux of urine from the bladder up the ureter is prevented by a flap of bladder mucous membrane and by internal distention of the bladder. Urine does not flow continuously down the ureter but enters into the bladder in spurts, the longitudinal muscle fibers contracting to dilate the orifice.

Adventitia. External to the muscularis is a coat of fibroelastic connective tissue, which at the pelvis blends with the capsule of the kidney, and which is continuous with surrounding connective tissue of the posterior abdominal wall along the length of the ureter. The anterior surface of the pelvis and ureter is covered loosely by peritoneum.

The ureter has a rich arterial blood supply, with vascular and lymphatic plexuses in muscularis and lamina propria. Nerves, associated with some ganglion cells, are present and they supply motor fibers of the autonomic system to the muscularis. Sensory fibers extend through the muscularis to penetrate between the cells of the epithelium.

Bladder

The urinary bladder has a similar appearance to the ureter in sections. The transitional epithelium is thicker, consisting of six to eight layers of cells in the empty bladder, and only two to three layers in the distended bladder. The surface cells show, by electron microscopy, in their apical cytoplasm a collection of flat vesicles bounded by an asymmetrical, trilaminar membrane identical to the surface plasmalemma. These may represent a reservoir of surface membrane material which can be mobilized rapidly for expansion of the surface during distention of the bladder. A few small glands of clear mucus-secreting cells, with simple or branched ducts, are present in the lamina propria, particularly near the ureteric and

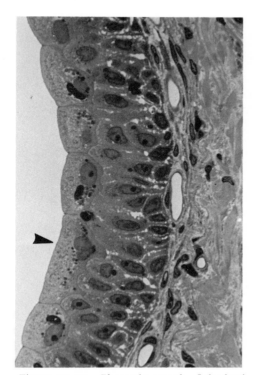

Figure 13–26. Photomicrograph of the lamina propria and transitional epithelium lining the distended bladder. One surface cell is binucleate (arrowhead). Plastic section, × 400.

internal urethral orifices. The lamina propria is thick with a loose external layer, sometimes called the submucosa, which permits the mucous membrane to become folded in the contracted bladder. The muscularis is of moderate thickness and consists of three layers, the middle circular layer being the most prominent and highly developed as a sphincter around the internal urethral orifice and, to a lesser extent, around the ureteric orifices. The adventitia is of fibroelastic tissue, with peritoneum covering only the superior surface of the bladder, where it is attached loosely.

The terminal urinary excretory passage connecting the bladder to the exterior is the urethra. That of the male differs markedly from that of the female.

Male Urethra

The male urethra is 15 to 20 cm in length and for descriptive purposes is divided into three regions. The first part passes inferiorly from the internal urethral orifice of the bladder to traverse the prostate gland. This is the *pars prostatica,* and opening into it are the two ejaculatory ducts and the ducts from prostatic glands. The second part, the *pars membranacea,* is short and passes from the apex of the prostate between striated muscles of the pelvis to perforate the perineal membrane and terminate in the bulb of the corpus cavernosa urethrae. The terminal urethra traverses the corpus spongiosum to open at the glans penis. This is called the *pars cavernosa* or *spongiosa,* or, simply, the penile portion of the urethra.

In the prostatic urethra, the lining epithelium is transitional in type but changes to a stratified or pseudostratified columnar epithelium in the remainder of the urethra, with patches of stratified squamous epithelium. The terminal dilatation of the penile urethra, the fossa navicularis, is lined by stratified squamous epithelium. A few mucus-secreting goblet cells are present. A loose, fibroelastic connective tissue lamina propria underlies the epithelium. The entire urethral

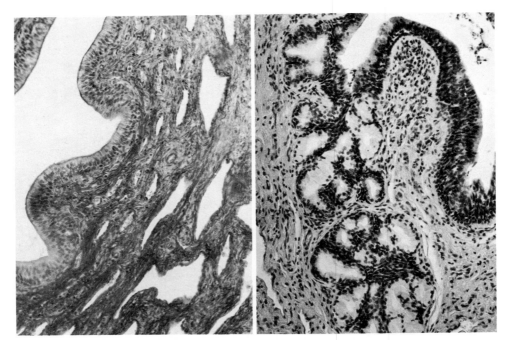

Figure 13–27. Photomicrographs of the penile portion of the male urethra. *Left:* The lining epithelium is stratified columnar. Note the surrounding cavernous tissue. × 125. *Right:* The lining epithelium is irregular and extends into the underlying lamina propria as a branching tubular gland of Littre. × 100.

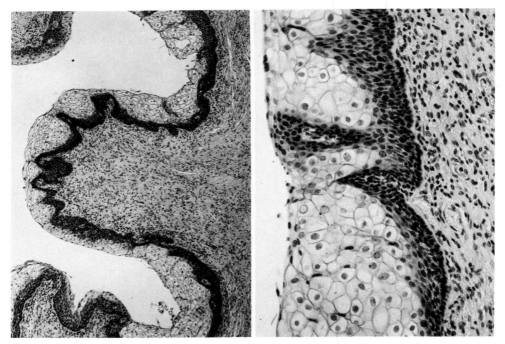

Figure 13–28. Photomicrographs of the epithelium lining the terminal urethra of the male *(left)* and female *(right),* both stratified squamous in type. Left, × 50; right, × 125.

mucous membrane is irregular with small depressions or pits extending deeply as branching tubular glands (of Littre). These are more numerous on the dorsal surface of the penile urethra, and are oriented obliquely with their bases situated proximal to their orifices. These glands are lined by epithelium similar to that lining the urethra and are mucus secreting.

Female Urethra

The female urethra is much shorter than that of the male, being only about 4 cm in length. It has a muscularis of two layers of smooth muscle oriented in a manner similar to those of the ureter, but reinforced by a striated muscle sphincter at its orifice. The lining epithelium is mainly stratified squamous in type, with patches of pseudostratified or stratified columnar epithelium. Glandular outpocketings, similar to the glands of Littre of the male, are present. The lamina propria is a loose fibroconnective tissue characterized by the presence of numerous venous sinuses resembling cavernous tissue.

REFERENCES

Andrews, P. M.: Scanning electron microscopy of the kidney glomerular epithelium after treatment with polycations in situ and in vitro. Am. J. Anat., 153:291, 1978.

Andrews, P. M., and Porter, K. R.: A scanning electron microscopic study of the nephron. Am. J. Anat., 140:81, 1974.

Barajas, L.: The ultrastructure of the juxtaglomerular apparatus as disclosed by three-dimensional reconstructions from serial sections. The anatomical relationship between the tubular and vascular components. J. Ultrastruct. Res., 33:116, 1970.

Brenner, B. M., and Rector, F. C. (eds.): The Kidney, Vol. 1. Philadelphia, W. B. Saunders Co., 1976.

Burg, M. B.: The nephron in transport of sodium, amino acids, and glucose. Hosp. Prac., 13:99, 1978.

Chapman, W. H., Bulger, R. E., Cutler, R. E., and Striker, G. E.: The Urinary System. An Integrated Approach. Philadelphia, W. B. Saunders Co., 1973, p. 263.

Christensen, J. A., Meyer, D. S., and Bohle, A.: The structure of the human juxtaglomerular apparatus. Arch. Pathol. Anat. Histol., 367:83, 1975.

Farquhar, M. G., Wissig, S. L., and Palade, G. E.: Glomerular permeability. I. Ferritin transfer across the normal glomerular capillary wall. J. Exp. Med., 113:47, 1961.

Fujita, T., Tokunaga, J., and Edanaga, M.: Scanning electron microscopy of the glomerular filtration membrane in the rat kidney. Cell Tiss. Res., 166:299, 1976.

Karnovsky, M. J., and Ryan, G. B.: Substructure of the glomerular slit diaphragm in freeze-fractured normal rat kidney. J. Cell Biol., 65:233, 1975.

Lacy, E. R., and Schmidt-Nielsen, B.: Ultrastructural organization of the hamster renal pelvis. Am. J. Anat., 155:403, 1979.

Latta, H., and Maunsbach, A. B.: The juxtaglomerular apparatus as studied electron microscopically. J. Ultrastruct. Res., 6:547, 1962.

Latta, H., and Maunsbach, A. B.: Relations of the centrolobular region of the glomerulus to the juxtaglomerular apparatus. J. Ultrastruct. Res., 6:562, 1962.

Leeson, T. S.: An electron microscope study of the postnatal development of the hamster kidney, with particular reference to the intertubular tissue. Lab. Invest., 10:466, 1961.

Leeson, T. S., and Leeson, C. R.: The rat ureter. Fine structural changes during its development. Acta Anat., 62:60, 1965.

Orci, L., Humbert, F., Amherdt, M., Grosso, A., de Sousa, R. C., and Perrelet, A.: Patterns of membrane organization in toad bladder epithelium: a freeze-fracture study. Experientia, 31:1335, 1975.

Pricam, C., Humbert, F., Perrelet, A., and Orci, L.: Gap junctions in mesangial and lacis cells. J. Cell Biol., 63:349, 1974.

Roesinger, B., Schiller, A., and Taugner, R.: A freeze-fracture study of tight junctions in the pars convoluta and pars recta of the renal proximal tubule. Cell Tiss. Res., 186:121, 1978.

Waugh, D., Prentice, R. S. A., and Yadav, E.: The structure of the proximal tubule: A morphological study of basement membrane cristae and their relationships in the renal tubule of the rat. Am. J. Anat., 121:775, 1967.

THE ENDOCRINE SYSTEM

The endocrine system is composed mainly of glands which have lost connection with the parent epithelium. They possess no ducts and their secretions (hormones) are passed directly into the blood or lymph circulation; hence these glands are designated as *ductless glands* or *glands of internal secretion*. They have a rich and intimate blood supply which serves not only for the metabolic needs of the tissue but also for the transport of the secretory products. Most endocrine glands are separate entities, for example, hypophysis and thyroid. Some, however, are present as scattered masses within an exocrine gland, for instance, pancreatic islets, interstitial cells (of Leydig) of the testis, and corpora lutea of the ovary. These combined organs are called *mixed glands.* The liver also is a mixed gland, but here each hepatic cell exhibits both exocrine and endocrine functions. It secretes bile into the duct system and also passes internal secretions directly into the blood vessels.

Endocrine glands, as a group, have a very simple microscopic structure; they consist of either cords, plates, or clumps of cells separated by sinusoids or capillaries and supported by delicate connective tissue. The parenchyma is usually, although not invariably, composed of cells of epithelial or epithelioid character. The glands vary in their embryological derivation; as a group they are derived from all three germ layers in the embryo. The hypophysis, suprarenal medulla, and chromaffin bodies are of ectodermal origin. The ovaries, testes, and suprarenal cortex are derived from mesoderm. Parenchymal cells of thyroid, parathyroid, and islets of Langerhans arise from endoderm. The placenta possesses both maternal and fetal components.

Each endocrine gland secretes one or more specific substances called *hormones.* Hormones are discharged from cells of endocrine glands into the blood or lymph circulation and eventually are distributed to the tissue fluids everywhere. A hormone has an effect upon a particular tissue or organ or upon the body as a whole. Some hormones affect certain tissues and organs specifically; the organs affected are termed *target organs* or *receptors.* Only a minute quantity of hormone is required to produce an effect, usually an arousal or activation, occasionally an inhibitory type of response. Hormones comprise a regulatory system that is superimposed upon existing controls of cellular metabolism. The endocrine glands interact to regulate themselves in numerous, complex ways that as yet are not completely understood. Additionally, many hormones produce an effect upon the nervous system, and some endocrine glands are regulated by neural mechanisms. This overlapping regulatory control, which involves both endocrine and nervous components, is regarded by many authorities as a single system termed the *neuroendocrine system.* Hormones differ greatly in their chemical composition; some are steroids, other polypeptides or proteins.

In some endocrine glands secretion accumulates within the cells of origin, e.g., pancreatic islets. In others the secretory product is stored in a central mass surrounded by secretory cells thus forming a follicle, e.g., thyroid. In the suprarenal cortex, however, secretion is released almost as rapidly as it is formed.

This chapter deals with those endocrine glands which are separate organs. Other endocrine tissues, which are contained within organs of a wholly different type such as the pancreas and the gonads, will be described with the major organs of which they form a part.

HYPOPHYSIS

The hypophysis (pituitary gland) is the most complex of the endocrine glands. It is composed of two different tissues. The *adenohypophysis* (glandular portion) is derived from oral ectoderm, which migrates dorsally as *Rathke's pouch* to surround partially the *neurohypophysis* (nervous portion), a ventral evagination from the floor of the diencephalon (forebrain). The hypophysis is buried in a bony fossa of the sphenoid bone, the sella turcica, and is covered by an extension of the dura mater, the *diaphragma sellae*. There is a small aperture in the diaphragm through which passes the hypophyseal stalk.

The hypophysis is about the size of a small, flattened grape. It is approximately 1 cm in length, 1 to 1.3 cm in width, and 0.5 cm in height. It weighs about 0.5 to 0.6 gram in adults. It undergoes some enlargement during pregnancy and may weigh a gram or more in women who have borne children.

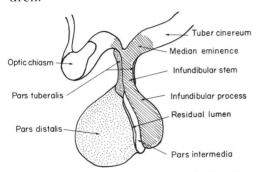

Figure 14–1. Diagram of midsagittal section of hypothalamus and hypophysis to show the various divisions.

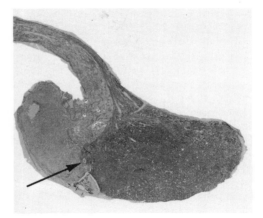

Figure 14–2. Low-power photomicrograph of a midsagittal section of human hypophysis. The pars nervosa, which lies toward the left, is continuous above with the infundibular stem. The latter is in direct relationship anteriorly with the pars tuberalis. The pars distalis (darkly staining) is separated from the pars nervosa by the pars intermedia, represented here by a few vesicles (arrow). × 5.

The adenohypophysis, which is pinkish in color in the fresh condition, is subdivided by the *residual lumen* of Rathke's pouch into two unequal portions. Anterior to the cleft is the *pars distalis*. An extension of this, the *pars tuberalis*, surrounds the neural stalk (see Figure 14–1). The third component of the adenohypophysis is the *pars interme-*

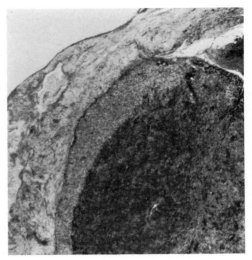

Figure 14–3. Midsagittal section of human hypophysis. The narrow pars intermedia is interposed between the pars nervosa (left) and the pars distalis (right). Aldehyde fuchsin-trichrome stain. × 20.

dia, which forms a thin cellular partition behind the cleft. The neurohypophysis, which appears white and fibrous in the fresh condition, consists of three parts. The major portion is the *pars nervosa* (infundibular process), which lies immediately posterior to the pars intermedia. Above, the pars nervosa is continuous with the *infundibular stem* and the *median eminence* of the tuber cinereum. The latter two together constitute the *infundibular (neural) stalk*. The *hypophyseal stalk* is composed of the infundibular stalk and the pars tuberalis.

The terms *anterior lobe* and *posterior lobe* are well established in the clinical and endocrinological literature; the anterior lobe refers to the portion anterior to the residual lumen, i.e., pars distalis and pars tuberalis, and the posterior lobe includes the parts posterior to the lumen, pars intermedia and pars nervosa.

Pars Distalis

The pars distalis constitutes about 75 per cent of the hypophysis, and is enclosed almost completely in a dense fibrous capsule. The parenchyma is in the form of anastomosing cords and clusters of epithelial cells supported by a network of reticular fibers continuous at the periphery with component fibers of the capsule. Between the parenchymal cells are sinusoidal capillaries.

The parenchyma is composed of two main categories of cells, *chromophils* and *chromophobes*. The former are subdivided into *acidophils* and *basophils* on the basis of the staining reactions of their cytoplasmic granules. However, the dyes used to distinguish these cells are acid dyes and do not distinguish acidic and basic properties of the cells. Many workers have adopted the noncommittal terms *alpha* and *beta cells* for the two

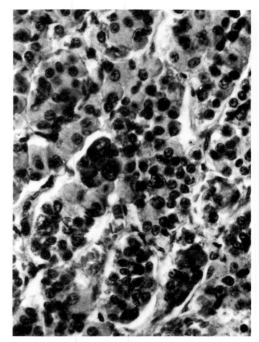

Figure 14–4. Representative area of pars distalis. Numerous acidophils are scattered throughout the field. A group of chromophobes (right center) and a small cluster of densely staining basophils (left center) also are present. × 300.

types of chromophils. The chromophobe cells, which have little affinity for dyes, sometimes are referred to as *chief* or *C cells*. The relative proportions of the cells vary markedly in man. Chromophobes constitute approximately 50 per cent of cells, acidophils 35 per cent, and basophils 15 per cent. The proportions may be altered considerably by castration, thyroidectomy, or other experimental procedures. Additional cell types may be demonstrated within the alpha and beta groups by special staining techniques and histochemical methods.

Chromophobes (C Cells). These faintly staining cells in the past were known as *reserve cells*. They are small,

TABLE 14–1. Terminology of the Pituitary Gland

Adenohypophysis (glandular lobe)	⎰ Pars distalis ⎱ Pars tuberalis ⎰ Pars intermedia	Anterior lobe
Neurohypophysis	⎰ Pars nervosa ⎱ Infundibular stem ⎰ Median eminence	Posterior lobe

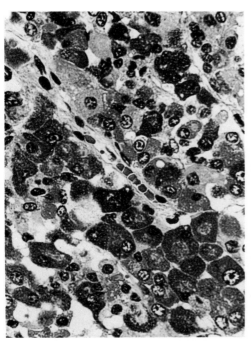

Figure 14–5. Pars distalis. Note the distinct granulation within chromophils. Beta chromophils constitute the majority of cells in this micrograph and tend to be somewhat larger than alpha chromophils. × 500.

rounded or polygonal cells with relatively little cytoplasm. The cells' boundaries are not easily visible in ordinary preparations and generally on light microscopy the cytoplasm lacks specific granules. On electron microscopy, however, many cells exhibit small secretory granules. It appears that most chromophobes are partially degranulated chromophils and that only a small percentage of them should be considered reserve or nonsecretory cells. The chromophobes often appear in groups in the center of the cords.

Acidophils (Alpha Cells). The acidophils stain readily and are identified easily in ordinary preparations. They are larger than chromophobes and their cell boundaries are distinct. The cytoplasm is crowded with small specific granules which are stained by numerous dyes, such as eosin, acid fuchsin, orange G, and azocarmine. The affinity of the granules for the latter two dyes is used to differentiate two types of acidophils. Those whose granules take up the orange G of an azan stain are called *orangeophils* or *alpha*

acidophils; those in which the granules stain intensely with azocarmine are *carminophils* or *epsilon acidophils.* The orangeophils are thought to be the cells responsible for the secretion of growth hormone, known as *somatotropin* (STH). Thus they are termed *somatotrophs* by some authors. These cells on electron microscopy show an extensive development of granular endoplasmic reticulum and contain a population of electron-dense granules which range from 3000 Å (300 nm) to 3500 Å (350 nm) in diameter. Somatotropin stimulates general body growth, particularly growth at the epiphyses of bones. Hypophysectomy causes a cessation of growth which can be restored to normal by administration of the hormone. Undersecretion leads to dwarfism in certain animals, and oversecretion, as in certain tumors of the anterior lobe, causes *gigantism* in children. If oversecretion occurs after closure of epiphyseal discs, a condition known as *acromegaly,* in which the bones become thicker and the hands and feet broader, results.

In carminophils, granules are much larger (up to 7000 Å, or 700 nm, in diameter) than in orangeophils and are more scattered within the cytoplasm. Granular endoplasmic reticulum is sparse. These cells, also termed *mammotrophs,* are concentrated in the posterolateral regions of the pars distalis and are greatly increased in number during and after pregnancy. They secrete a *lactogenic hormone (prolactin, luteotropic hormone,* or LTH), which initiates and maintains the secretion of milk after pregnancy and stimulates the corpus luteum of the ovary to secrete progesterone.

Basophils (Beta Cells). The basophils tend to be appreciably larger than the acidophils. The granules are less numerous than in acidophils and are smaller (about 150 to 200 mμ [nm] in diameter). They stain rather poorly with hematoxylin but are stained deeply with methylene blue. Basophils are best identified by the periodic acid–Schiff (PAS) technique where they are strongly positive owing to the concentration of glycoproteins in their secretory granules. In most mammals at least two types of basophils can be dis-

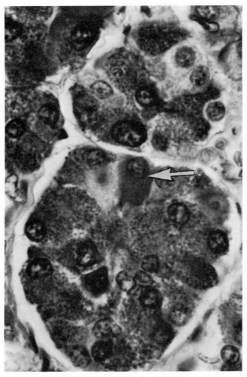

Figure 14–6. Human pars distalis. Basophils are the principal cell type present in this micrograph. Note the discrete granulation of their cytoplasm. One acidophil, in which discrete granules are not apparent, occupies the center of the field (arrow). Aldehyde fuchsin-trichrome stain. × 625.

tinguished. One type stains with aldehyde fuchsin (*beta basophil*), whereas the other (*delta basophil*) does not.

Beta basophils, or *thyrotrophs*, secrete thyrotropic hormone (thyroid-stimulating hormone, TSH). The cells are relatively large and contain numerous granules principally concentrated within the peripheral cytoplasm. The granules are dense and small, and range in size from 1000 Å (100 nm) to 1500 Å (150 nm) or more. TSH maintains and stimulates the thyroid epithelium. Hypophysectomy results in atrophy of the thyroid which may be restored to activity by administration of hormone extracts. Injections of TSH in normal animals produce all the symptoms of hyperthyroidism. Thyroidectomy results in an increase in the percentage of basophils within the pars distalis.

Delta basophils, or *gonadotrophs*, secrete two hormones: the *follicle-stimulat-*

ing hormone (FSH) and the *luteinizing hormone* (LH). At present, it is not known if this population of cells consists of two distinct cell types or only one which secretes both hormones. The cells are large, with a well-developed Golgi zone and concentrations of granular endoplasmic reticulum. Secretory granules are numerous, electron-dense, and vary from 1000 Å (100 nm) to 3000 Å (300 nm) in diameter. FSH promotes growth of ovarian follicles in the female and activates the seminiferous epithelium of the testes to produce spermatozoa in the male. In the female, FSH acts usually in association with LH, which ensures final maturation of the follicle, ovulation, and subsequent formation of the corpus luteum. Atrophy of the sex organs occurs after hypophysectomy. They may be restored nearly to normal by administration of FSH, but complete recovery requires some LH in addition to FSH. LH alone has no direct action on the ovary of a hypophysectomized animal. It acts only after prior stimulation of follicles by FSH. LH is necessary for the conversion of the ruptured follicle into a corpus luteum. In the male the luteinizing hormone (also termed *interstitial cell–stimulating hormone* or ICSH) stimulates the interstitial (Leydig) cells of the testes to produce an androgen, presumably testosterone, which in turn maintains the accessory reproductive organs and the secondary sex characteristics. The effect is augmented by the administration of FSH. After castration, the rat hypophysis contains increased amounts of gonadotropic hormones and the basophils become enlarged and vacuolated (*castration cells*).

In man, certain basophils also may be responsible for the secretion of *adrenocorticotrophic hormone* (ACTH) and of the *melanocyte-stimulating hormone* (MSH). The intensely PAS-positive granules in the cytoplasm of some basophils, termed *corticotrophs*, have been shown to stain immunocytochemically for ACTH, which promotes growth of the suprarenal cortex and stimulates secretion of glucocorticoids. The atrophy of the suprarenal cortex which follows hypophysectomy can be prevented by the administration of ACTH. The site of production of MSH still is in doubt, but

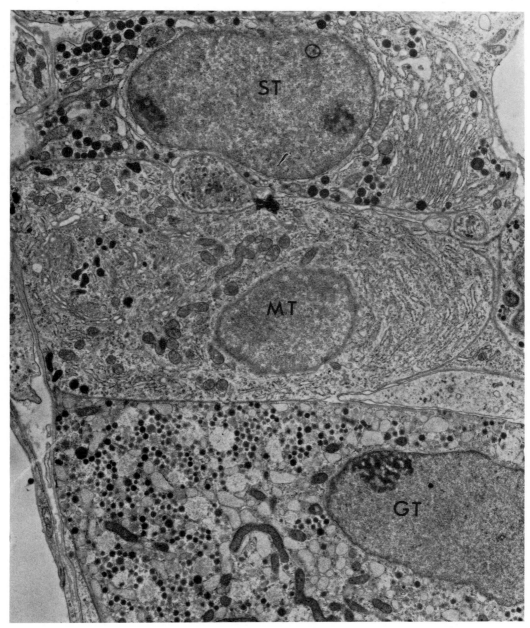

Figure 14–7. Electron micrograph of rat pars distalis. Note the varying appearance of the different cell types. In the anterior lobe of the rat pituitary, there are thought to be four morphologically distinct functional cell types: somatotrophs (ST), mammotrophs (MT), gonadotrophs (GT), and thyrotrophs (TT), so named to denote their association with the production of growth, mammotropic (lactogenic), gonadotropic (GT), and thyrotropic hormones, respectively. With the light microscope, cell types are distinguished by differences in staining affinities of their secretion granules, somatotrophs and mammotrophs being acidophil, and gonadotrophs and thyrotrophs basophil. With the electron microscope, secretory granule size is the most useful criterion for identification of cell types. In the rat pituitary, maximum granule diameters are: ST, 350 mμ(nm); MT 600 to 900 mμ(nm); GT, 200 mμ(nm); TT, 150 mμ(nm). × 7000. (Courtesy of M. G. Farquhar.)

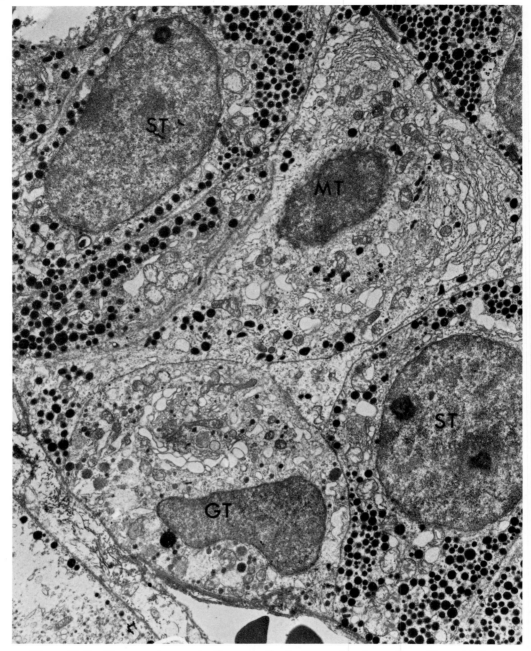

Figure 14–8.   Electron micrograph of rat pars distalis. For explanation, refer to Figure 14–7. A portion of a capillary is shown lower center. × 7000 (Courtesy of M. G. Farquhar.)

antisera raised against MSH appear to react with corticotrophic cells and with some cells of the pars intermedia, particularly in animals in which this lobe is well developed.

In the chromophils, it is believed that the granules are actual precursors of the secretion. The degree of granularity is correlated with the physiological state of the cell when fixed. The cells are thought to secrete cyclically rather than continuously. Mitoses are seen rarely in any of the cell types, and it is certain that few if any of the cells are destroyed

TABLE 14–2. Summary of Current Views on Cellular Origin and Site of Action of Anterior Pituitary Hormones

Hormone	Cell Type		Site of Action
	General	Specific	
Growth hormone or somatotropin (STH)	Acidophil	Somatotroph	Skeletal tissues
Lactogenic or luteotropic hormone, prolactin (LTH)	Acidophil	Mammotroph	Breast
Thyrotropic hormone (TSH)	Basophil	Thyrotroph	Thyroid
Follicle-stimulating hormone (FSH)	Basophil	Gonadotroph	Ovary and testis
Luteinizing hormone (LH) or Interstitial cell–stimulating hormone (ICSH)	Basophil	Gonadotroph	Ovary / Testis
Adrenocorticotropic hormone (ACTH)	(Basophil)	Corticotroph	Suprarenal cortex
Melanocyte-stimulating hormone (MSH)	(Basophil)	Corticotroph	Skin

when the secretory product is released. It appears that some chromophobes represent reserve or inactive cells which give rise to the chromophils. As the chromophobes become active, granules form within their cytoplasm. The granules are specific for the different cell types. Engorged cells then secrete and the cells revert to an inactive state.

Pars Intermedia

In man the pars intermedia is less well developed than in many other animals and usually is poorly defined. It forms only about 2 per cent of the hypophysis. It is composed of a thin layer of cells and of vesicles which contain colloid. It lies in close relation to the residual lumen, which virtually is obliterated in most adults. Some component cells, polygonal in shape, are small and pale staining; others are somewhat larger and granular, and stain deeply with basic dyes. The cells which are basophil frequently extend as cords for a short distance into the pars nervosa. The cells lining the colloid-containing vesicles commonly are ciliated, and some are mucus-secreting.

In certain species, e.g., amphibia, the pars intermedia is well developed and produces *intermedin* or the *melanocyte-stimulating hormone* (MSH), which is a polypeptide that influences the production of melanin. In man, the normal function of the hormone is obscure and

it is not clear at present whether MSH is synthesized by the basophils of the pars intermedia or by corticotrophs within the pars distalis.

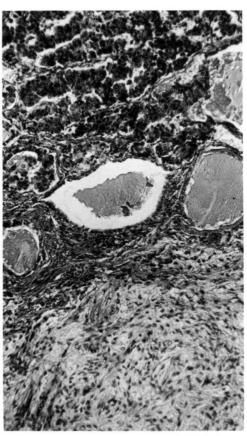

Figure 14–9. Pars intermedia. Follicles of the latter are interposed between the pars distalis (above) and the pars nervosa (below). × 100.

Pars Tuberalis

The pars tuberalis forms a collar of cells around the infundibular stalk. The cells, in close association with numerous blood vessels, are arranged in groups or short cords longitudinally oriented. They are cuboidal and the cytoplasm, which is weakly basophil, contains fine granules and some glycogen. Small vesicles, which contain colloid, are seen occasionally.

The function of the pars tuberalis, if any, is unknown.

Neurohypophysis

The neurohypophysis includes the median eminence of the tuber cinereum, the infundibular stem, and the infundibular process (pars nervosa). All three portions have the same characteristic cells and the same nerve and blood supply and contain the same active hormonal principle. Some 100,000 unmyelinated nerve fibers, constituting the *hypothalamo-hypophyseal tract*, pass into the neurohypophysis. Their cell bodies lie in the supraoptic

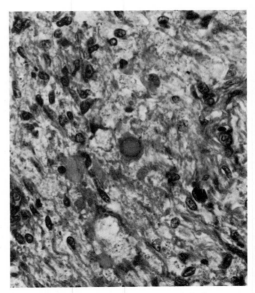

Figure 14–11. Pars nervosa. A distinct Herring body is present in the center of the field. × 250.

and paraventricular nuclei of the hypothalamus.

The cells of the neurohypophysis, *pituicytes*, resemble neuroglia cells elsewhere in the central nervous system. Pituicytes are small cells with short branching processes which end in relation either to blood vessels or to connective tissue septa. Within the cytoplasm are fatty droplets, granules, and pigment. Pituicytes are present throughout the neurohypophysis and are especially abundant in the pars nervosa. The cells can be blackened by silver and, according to their morphological appearance in silvered preparations, four types are distinguished: *reticulopituicytes, micropituicytes, fibropituicytes,* and *adenopituicytes*.

A feature of the neurohypophysis is the presence within it of granules of varying size which stain deeply with chrome alum hematoxylin. These are the so-called *Herring bodies*, which are particularly abundant in the pars nervosa. The earlier view that Herring bodies represented extracellular accumulations of secretory material has been disproved. Electron micrographs reveal granules in the cytoplasm of cells of the supraoptic and paraventricular nuclei, in the nerve fibers of the hypothalamo-hypophyseal tract, and in

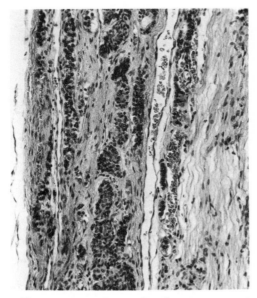

Figure 14–10. Pars tuberalis. Groups and cords of small cells lie in relation to blood vessels, here sectioned longitudinally. A small portion of the infundibular stem lies to the right of the figure. × 100.

the nerve terminals. The secretory material is not elaborated in the pituicytes. Nerve cells of the supraoptic and paraventricular nuclei are neurosecretory and elaborate material which passes along the unmyelinated nerve fibers to the neurohypophysis where the secretion is stored. Herring bodies represent marked accumulations of neurosecretory material in the nerve terminals, which lie in close proximity to the capillary network. After sectioning of the hypophyseal stalk, there is a disappearance of neurosecretory material distal to the lesion and an accumulation of granules in relation to the severed nerve fibers in the stump.

The neurosecretory material is believed to be a protein which is associated with the actual hormones. The hormones of the neurohypophysis are *oxytocin* and *vasopressin*, both polypeptides. Oxytocin causes the smooth muscle of the uterus to contract. It also induces contraction of the myoepithelial (basket) cells of the alveoli and ducts of the mammary gland. Vasopressin is also known as the antidiuretic hormone (ADH), which influences the kidney tubules to reabsorb water from the provisional urine. Pharmacologically, it also raises blood pressure by stimulating contraction of smooth muscle in the walls of blood vessels. Both hormones appear to be released by exocytosis from the nerve terminals that contain granules. At present, it is not known if the hormones are synthesized by the same cell or by different cells but there are indications of at least two different types of granules within the nerve terminals.

Blood and Nerve Supply of the Hypophysis

The blood supply of the hypophysis has unusual features and plays an important role in the secretory activity of the gland.

The anterior lobe is supplied by several *superior hypophyseal arteries* which arise from the internal carotids and the circle of Willis. Some arteries pass directly to the anterior lobe where they empty into sinusoidal capillaries. Others anastomose freely in the region of the median eminence and the infundibular stem and pass into a capillary network in the median eminence. The capillaries of this network drain into veins which run downward around the hypophyseal stalk to reach the sinusoidal capillaries of the anterior lobe. This system of venous connections between the capillaries of the median eminence and the sinusoidal capillaries of the adenohypophysis constitutes the *hypophyseal portal system.* The system appears to represent a connection by which neurohumoral substances ("hormone-releasing factors") from the median eminence may pass to the anterior lobe. It is an important pathway in the regulation of adenohypophyseal function.

The posterior lobe receives blood from the *inferior hypophyseal arteries,* branches of the internal carotids. Veins from anterior and posterior lobes drain into the cavernous sinuses.

The capillaries of the posterior lobe are smaller than the sinusoidal capillaries of the anterior lobe. Electron micrographs show an attenuated type of endothelium, with fenestrations, both in the capillaries and in the sinusoids. The deficiencies within the endothelial lining presumably facilitate passage of secretory material into the vessels.

The principal innervation of the neurohypophysis is the hypothalamo-hypophyseal tract, which originates mainly from the supraoptic and paraventricular nuclei. The unmyelinated nerve fibers of the tract course down the infundibular stalk to the infundibular process where they end in close relation to the fenestrated capillaries. It is questionable if any of the fibers extend into the anterior lobe.

Histogenesis of the Hypophysis

The hypophysis arises from two separate sources. One portion arises as an evagination of the ectoderm of the primitive buccal cavity which extends as *Rathke's pouch* toward the floor of the diencephalon. The pouch comes in close relationship with a downgrowth, the *infundibulum,* from the floor of the

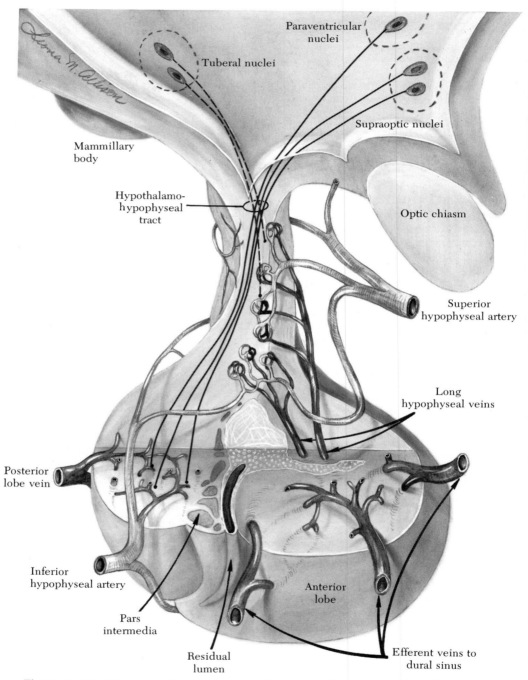

Figure 14–12. Diagram to illustrate the principal vascular and nervous relations of the hypophysis.

diencephalon. The infundibulum gives rise to the neural stalk and the pars nervosa. Rathke's pouch loses its attachment to the pharyngeal roof by rupture of its original stalk and develops into the adenohypophysis. The cells of its anterior wall proliferate actively and reduce the lumen of the pouch to a narrow cleft. This proliferation forms the pars distalis and from its upper part cells extend around the neural stalk to form the pars tuberalis. The posterior wall of the original pouch, lying between the residual cleft and the pars nervosa, remains thin and becomes the pars intermedia.

THYROID GLAND

The thyroid gland, which is situated in the anterior region of the neck, consists of two *lateral lobes* connected by a narrow *isthmus*. The isthmus lies over the second to the fourth tracheal cartilages, and the lateral lobes lie in relation to the superior part of the trachea and to the inferior part of the larynx. Frequently a median *pyramidal lobe*, which extends upward anterior to the larynx, is present in addition.

The gland is enveloped externally by a connective tissue capsule which is continuous with the deep cervical fascia. Under this there is an inner, true capsule which is thinner and which adheres closely to the gland. Delicate continuations of the inner capsule extend as septa into the gland, dividing it into indefinite *lobes* and *lobules.*

Follicles, the structural units of the gland, compose the lobules. They vary greatly in size, depending upon the degree of distention by secretion. They also vary in shape but usually are irregularly spheroidal. The follicles are embedded within a delicate meshwork of reticular fibers which also supports a close net of capillaries.

A follicle consists of a layer of simple epithelium enclosing a cavity which usually is filled with a stiff jelly called *colloid.* The shape of the component cells varies but commonly is cuboidal. The cells are low when the gland is hypoactive, high when the gland is hyperactive. Cell height in any one follicle is uniform and the arrangement is reg-

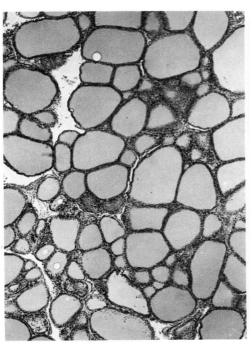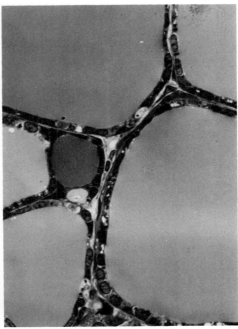

Figure 14–13. Microphotographs of the thyroid gland. Follicles, each lined with a simple epithelium, are filled with colloid. Left, × 50; right, plastic section, × 400.

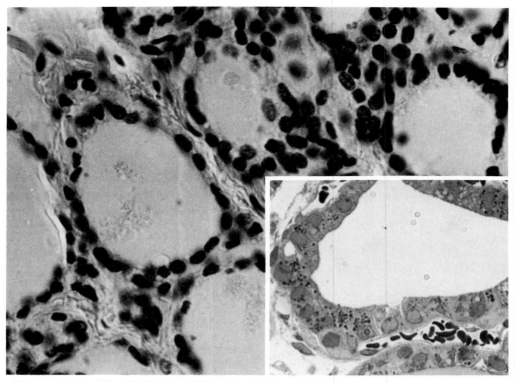

Figure 14–14. Thyroid gland. Follicles are closely packed and are separated only by a delicate connective tissue. They are lined by a cuboidal epithelium and contain colloid which appears almost homogeneous. × 450. *Inset:* Plastic section. × 550.

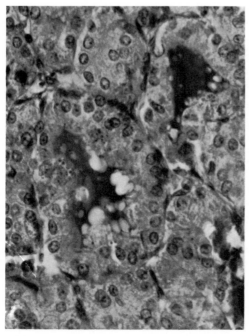

Figure 14–15. Thyroid follicles. Colloid stains deeply owing to the staining method used. Darkly staining granules are present in the apical cytoplasm of some follicular cells. PAS reaction. × 350.

ular. The bases of the cells rest upon a delicate basal lamina. The large, vesicular nuclei lie centrally or toward the base. The cytoplasm is finely granular and basophil and contains numerous mitochondria, abundant granular endoplasmic reticulum, and lysosomes. The Golgi apparatus and centrioles are located above the nucleus. Lipid droplets and other inclusions, principally *colloid droplets,* are found in the cytoplasm of some cells. Junctional complexes are a feature of the interface between cells, and the free border is provided with small microvilli, visible only with the electron microscope. Some cells possess true cilia.

Colloid fills the follicular lumen. Fresh colloid is homogeneous, clear, and viscous. However, it undergoes shrinkage during the procedures employed in the preparation of microscopic sections and may show irregularities. Spaces often are present between the colloid and the epithelium, and vacuoles may occur within the colloid. The irregularities are indications of the state of the colloid and

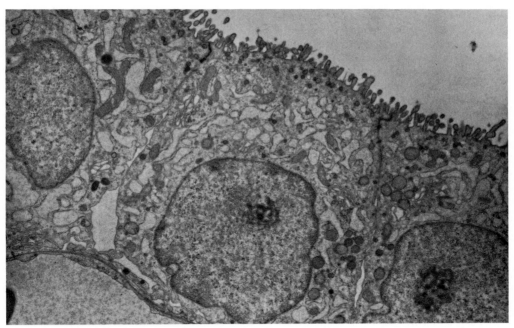

Figure 14–16. Electron micrograph of thyroid follicular cells. The cytoplasm contains dilated profiles of endoplasmic reticulum and scattered elements of the Golgi apparatus. The apical border is provided with small microvilli. A perifollicular capillary is present in the lower left corner of the figure. × 7200. (Courtesy of S. L. Wissig.)

are most common in activated glands. Colloid stains basophil in active follicles, whereas in inactive follicles it is weakly basophil or acidophil.

Colloid, which represents a reserve of secretion, is rich in nucleoproteins (hence its basophilia) and contains *thyroglobulin* and enzymes. Thyroglobulin is a glycoprotein containing several iodinated amino acids, the proportions of which vary from follicle to follicle. Thyroglobulin stains deeply with the PAS reaction.

The secretory process is complex and difficult to follow. It involves synthesis of the thyroid hormone, temporary storage, and release into the perifollicular capillaries. Both synthesis and release may occur at the same time. Thyroid cells remove iodine rapidly from the blood stream and concentrate it. The major part of the iodine is incorporated in follicles in an organic form. The incorporation of iodine in follicular cells and in colloid can be followed by the use of radioactive iodine (^{131}I). The iodine within the colloid is present in the form of *diiodothyronine, triiodothyronine,* and *tetraiodothyronine (thyroxine),* bound to a globulin. These are components of thyroglobulin. The release of the active

component also is difficult to follow. It is thought that thyroglobulin first is recovered from the colloid by a process of pinocytosis at the apical surface of follicular cells. Hydrolytic enzymes from lysosomes then break down thyroglobulin into smaller molecules (principally thyroxine and triiodothyronine) which pass through the bases of follicular cells into the underlying capillary plexuses.

The thyroid contains, in addition to the principal cells of the follicles, a small population of *parafollicular cells (C, clear, or light cells).* These cells, which lie adjacent to the follicles but within the basal lamina, do not abut on the follicular cavity. Generally they are larger than follicular cells and their nuclei are placed eccentrically. They are characterized by the presence of numerous membrane-bound dense granules throughout the cytoplasm. Immunofluorescent studies have shown that these cells are the site of production of *thyrocalcitonin* (or *calcitonin*).

Function of the Thyroid Gland

The most striking effect of the thyroid secretion is its regulation of the metabolic rate. Thyroxine increases cell metabolism and thus is concerned with development, differentiation, and growth. *Hypothyroidism* in the infant leads to *cretinism;* hypofunction in the adult causes *myxedema.* Symptoms in both conditions are due to a reduction in the metabolic rate and may be removed by the administration of thyroid. *Hyperthyroidism* leads to overactivity and sometimes is complicated by the development of *exophthalmic goiter.* In hyperthyroidism some follicles become enlarged and follicular cells increase in height. Surgical removal of a part of the thyroid or the administration of antithyroid drugs or radioiodine reduces the metabolic rate.

The thyroid gland elaborates, in addition to the thyroid hormone, thyrocalcitonin, a product of the parafollicular cells. This hormone is a polypeptide that actively lowers the concentration of calcium in the plasma by a direct action on bone, inhibiting bone resorption. Hypercalcemia is the stimulus for secretion of the hormone and hypocalcemia inhibits secretion. It appears therefore that secretion is controlled by a feedback mechanism operating through the plasma calcium level in a manner similar to that of control of the secretion of the parathyroid hormone, but in the reverse direction.

The thyroid gland has certain interrelations with the anterior pituitary gland. Thyrotropic hormone (thyroid-stimulating hormone, or TSH) stimulates release of thyroxine. Thyroidectomy results in hypertrophy of the anterior lobe with degranulation of alpha cells and the appearance of beta cells which morphologically exhibit certain alterations (so-called *thyroidectomy cells*). Secretion of thyrocalcitonin by parafollicular cells is dependent on blood calcium levels and is not related to pituitary, thyroid, and parathyroid functions.

Blood Vessels and Nerves

Blood and lymph capillaries form intimate plexuses about the thyroid follicles. The blood capillaries are of the fenestrated type, an arrangement that is thought to aid the passage of the hormone into the capillary lumen. Arteriovenous anastomoses are common. The architecture of the blood vessels indicates that there are fluctuations in the amount of blood supplied to different regions of the gland.

Numerous unmyelinated nerve fibers are present in the walls of the thyroid arteries. Most of these are vasomotor in function. A few fibers end in relation to the bases of some thyroid cells, but no definite secretory function has been ascribed to them.

Histogenesis of the Thyroid

The thyroid gland develops as a median downgrowth of the base of the tongue. The foramen cecum of the adult tongue is a vestige that indicates the site of origin. The thyroglossal duct, which connects the developing gland with the foramen cecum, usually becomes obliterated. Remnants of the duct may give rise to cysts or to the pyramidal lobe, a cranial extension of the isthmus. The thyroid gland may include also derivatives of the branchial pouches, such as the *ultimobranchial body.* Thyrocalcitonin has been isolated from ultimobranchial tissue in lower vertebrates, and some authors consider this body to be the origin of parafollicular cells.

The primordium of the gland initially is a compact mass of epithelial cells which later splits to form a network of solid cords or plates. These break up into small cellular groups, in each of which a lumen develops. As the lumen enlarges, the cells surrounding it become arranged into a single layer to form the definitive follicle.

PARATHYROID GLANDS

There are usually two pairs of parathyroid glands in man, but accessory glands occur frequently. The glands are small, brownish, oval bodies which lie in close relation to the thyroid gland. The upper parathyroids lie on the posterior surface of the thyroid about midway between the upper and lower poles of the lobes, whereas the lower ones are in relation to the lower poles of the thyroid lobes. The parathyroid glands develop from the endo-

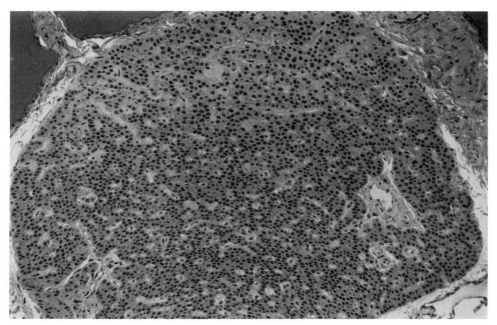

Figure 14–17. Low-power microphotograph of the parathyroid gland. The parenchymal cells are arranged in irregular cords. Portions of the thyroid gland (top right and top left) also are shown. Plastic section. × 125.

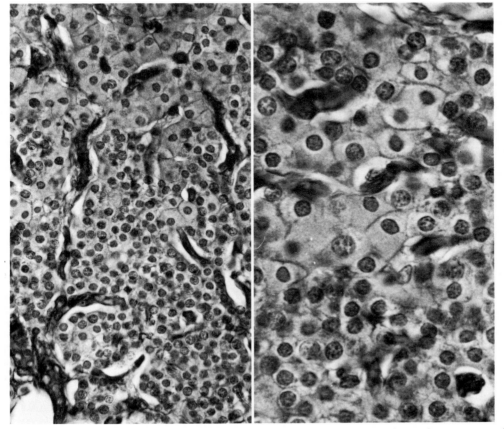

Figure 14–18. Parathyroid gland. The parenchymal cells, arranged in irregular cords, are separated by a network of capillaries. Note the difference in size between chief (principal) cells (below) and oxyphil cells (above). Left, × 250; right, × 600.

derm of the pharyngeal pouches; the superior parathyroids from the fourth pouch, and the inferior parathyroids from the third pouch. In their development, the latter are closely associated with the developing thymus, and they are drawn down with it during its caudal migration. Normally, they migrate only as far as the lower poles of the thyroid gland.

Each parathyroid gland is covered by a thin capsule which separates it from the thyroid. Delicate septa, which pass inward from the capsule, carry blood vessels and a few nerve fibers into the gland. The connective tissue of the capsule and of the septa contains fat cells, which increase in number with age. A network of reticular fibers supports the parenchyma, which is composed of masses and cords of epithelial cells. The epithelial cells are of two types, *chief* or *principal cells* and *oxyphil cells.* Chief cells, which are more abundant than oxyphil cells, sometimes are divided into clear and dark forms. Clear chief cells have large vesicular nuclei and a clear, pale staining cytoplasm which contains few granules. Dark chief cells have smaller nuclei and a finely granular cytoplasm. The granules are electron-dense and are bounded by a membrane. Both forms are rich in glycogen.

Oxyphil cells are larger than chief cells and characteristically are present in small or large groups. They have small, darkly staining nuclei, and the cytoplasm is acidophil and contains fine granules and numerous mitochondria. They are not present in man until about five to seven years of age, and thereafter they increase in number, especially after puberty. Cells with features intermediate between those of chief and oxyphil cells also are seen in many preparations for light microscopy.

Small colloid follicles are seen occasionally and are more noticeable in old age. The material they contain has no functional relation to the colloid of the thyroid gland.

Function

The parathyroid glands elaborate the parathyroid hormone, a protein con-

sisting of a single polypeptide chain. It is thought that the hormone is produced principally by the dark chief cells and that the light chief cells represent a stage of secretory inactivity. The function of the oxyphil cells is uncertain. The parathyroid hormone (*parathormone*) is important in the regulation of calcium metabolism. A lowering of the plasma concentration of calcium is followed by an increased output of the hormone, which in turn withdraws calcium from the bones. It is claimed that the action of the hormone is due to its ability to stimulate the transformation of osteogenic cells into osteoclasts. Atrophy or removal of the parathyroids causes a fall in blood calcium, which is accompanied by nervous hyperexcitability and muscular spasms, leading to death due to tetany. Administration of calcium or parathyroid extract relieves the symptoms. Hypertrophy of the glands occurs in conditions such as rickets, when there is a calcium deficiency. *Hyperparathyroidism* may result from tumor or hyperplasia and is associated with an elevated blood calcium level and extensive bone resorption.

Blood Vessels and Nerves

The parathyroids have a rich vascular supply, the larger vessels following the septa into the interior of the gland. A fine net of capillaries lies in relation to the parenchyma.

Unmyelinated nerve fibers, probably vasomotor, are scanty.

SUPRARENAL GLANDS

The suprarenal, or adrenal, glands are roughly pyramidal, flattened organs, one at the cranial pole of each kidney. The hilum is an indentation on the anterior surface. A sectioned, fresh gland shows two regions, an outer *cortex* which is yellow externally and reddish-brown internally and a thin inner *medulla* which is gray. These regions are distinct structurally, developmentally, and functionally. The cortex develops from epithelium (mesothelium) lining the primitive body cavity (coelom) and the medulla from the neural crest and presumptive autono-

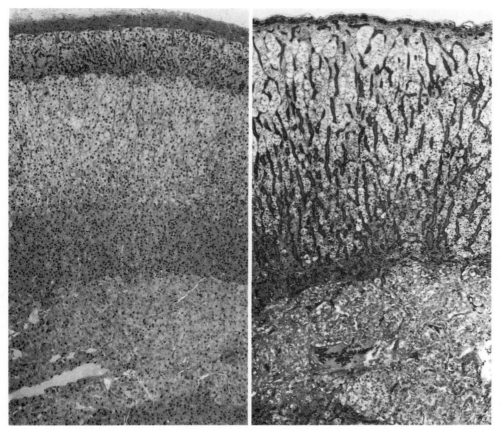

Figure 14–19. Low-power micrographs of sections through the suprarenal gland, with the capsule above and the medulla occupying the lower third of each micrograph. If the left figure, the darkly staining cells in immediate relationship to the medulla constitute the inner portion of the zona fasciculata and the zona reticularis. In the right figure, note the wide sinusoidal capillaries within the cortex. Left, plastic section, × 55; right, Mallory-Azan stain, × 50.

mic ganglion (*sympathochromaffin*) tissue. In lower vertebrates the two tissues are not united into a single organ.

Each gland is surrounded by a tough connective tissue capsule which sends radial trabeculae, consisting principally of reticular fibers, into the cortex. Capillaries penetrate into the gland along the delicate trabeculae.

Cortex

The cortex, the major part of the gland, is divided into three ill-defined layers: a thin, outer zone, the *zona glomerulosa;* a thick middle zone, the *zona fasciculata;* and an inner zone, the *zona reticularis*, directly in relation to the medulla.

The zona glomerulosa consists of columnar epithelial cells arranged in ovoid groups which normally show no central lumen. Nuclei stain deeply and the cytoplasm contains basophil material.

The zona fasciculata, the thickest layer, is composed of large, irregularly cuboidal cells arranged in long, radial cords, usually two cells wide. Nuclei are vesicular and frequently cells are binucleate. The cytoplasm is basophil and contains lipid droplets, composed of cholesterol, fatty acids, and neutral fat. Lipid droplets are most numerous in cells of the outer two-thirds of the zone. Since lipids are removed by the usual technical procedures, the cells here appear vacuolated and have a spongy appearance; hence sometimes they are called *spongiocytes*. The inner third of the zone is relatively free of lipid material and is more basophil.

In the zona reticularis, the cell cords

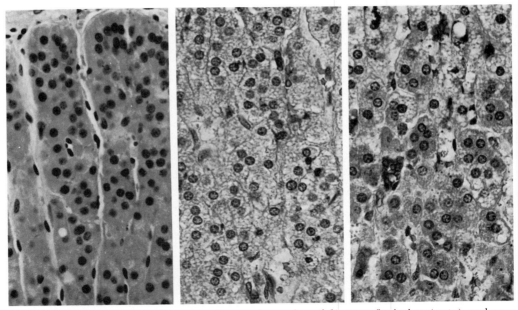

Figure 14–20. Representative areas of zona glomerulosa (*left*), zona fasciculata (*center*), and zona reticularis (*right*). Note the vascuoladed appearance of the cytoplasm of component cells (spongiocytes) of the zona fasciculata. × 250.

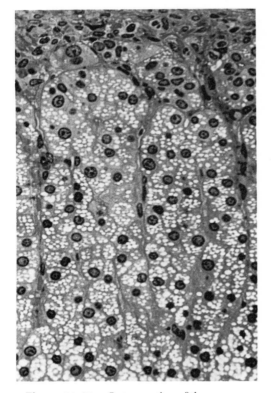

Figure 14–21. Outer portion of the suprarenal cortex. Note the ovoid groups of cells in the zona glomerulosa (above) and the vacuolated cytoplasm of these cells and of those of the zona fasciculata (below). Plastic section. × 350.

form an anastomosing network. Near the zona fasciculata, component cells differ little from those of that zone; in general the cytoplasm contains fewer lipid droplets. Near the medulla the cells appear "light" or "dark" depending upon their staining affinities. Many cells have shrunken nuclei and deeply staining cytoplasm and contain pigment granules. Both light and dark cells show evidence of degeneration.

The zonation just considered is based upon the general arrangement and organization of cells in the cortex. On the basis of cell structure, however, the cortex can be divided into four zones. The outer zone corresponds to the zona glomerulosa. The second zone is the outer two-thirds of the zona fasciculata, consisting of spongiocytes. The inner third of the zona fasciculata and the outer half of the zona reticularis comprise the third zone, a region poor in lipids. The fourth zone is the inner half of the zona reticularis (the juxtamedullary portion), in which many component cells are senescent and contain pigment. Previously it was thought that new cells were produced in the zona glomerulosa, migrated inward to the zona fasciculata, and finally degenerated in the zona reticularis. The ob-

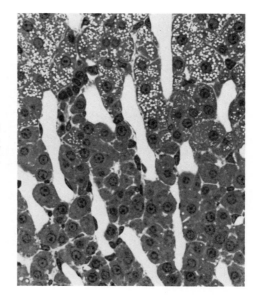

Figure 14–22. Inner portion of the suprarenal cortex. Note the vacuolated cells of the zona fasciculata (above) and the deeply staining cytoplasm of cells of the zona reticularis (below). Wide sinusoidal capillaries occur between the cells. Plastic section. × 250.

servation of mitotic figures in all zones, particularly in the outer region of the zona fasciculata, and of degenerating cells in zones other than the reticularis has thrown doubt upon this hypothesis.

On electron microscopy, the most characteristic feature of component cells of the outer two zones is the well-developed, smooth-surfaced endoplasmic reticulum. In cells of the zona glomerulosa, this appears as an anastomosing network of tubules, and the extent of this network is even more marked in cells of the zona fasciculata. The cells of all zones contain numerous mitochondria with tubular cristae. In the zona reticularis, the Golgi apparatus is large, and lysosomes and pigment granules (secondary lysosomes) also are prominent features.

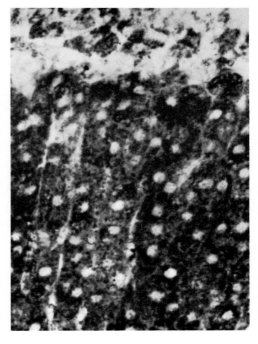

Figure 14–23. Zona fasciculata of suprarenal gland in a frozen section stained specifically to show lipid material, which appears as darkly staining droplets within the cytoplasm. The empty spaces represent the nuclear areas. A portion of the zona glomerulosa is present above. Sudan black B. × 375.

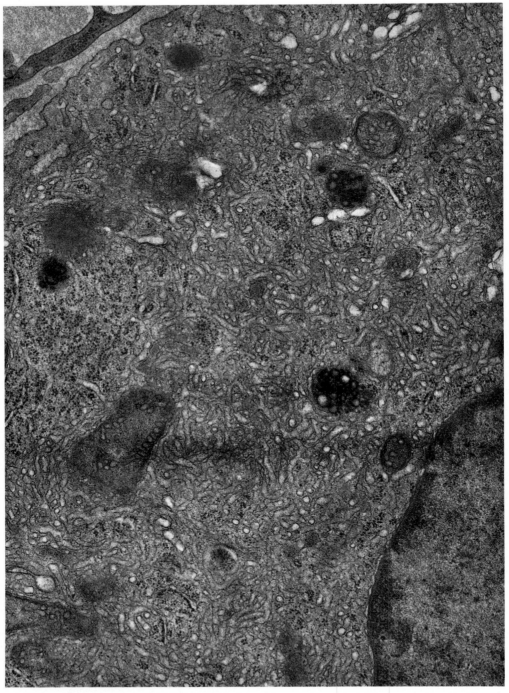

Figure 14–24. Electron micrograph of a zona fasciculata cell of human adrenal cortex. Note the extensive development of smooth-surfaced endoplasmic reticulum (center). The dark masses are pigment granules. × 18,600. (Courtesy of J. A. Long.)

Medulla

The boundary between cortex and medulla usually is irregular in man, although in many other animals the boundary may be sharp. Cells of the medulla are ovoid or polyhedral and occur in groups or short, anastomosing cords, surrounded by venules and capillaries. Medullary cells have large vesicular nuclei, and their cytoplasm contains fine granules which become brown when oxidized by potassium bichromate. This is the *chromaffin reaction,* and the cells therefore are called *chromaffin* (or *pheochrome*) *cells.* The reaction is due in large part to the presence of the *catecholamines epinephrine* and *norepinephrine.* The granules also stain green with zinc chloride and brown with

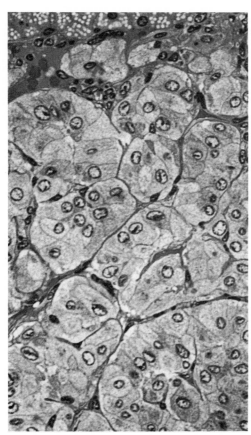

Figure 14–25. Suprarenal medulla. Component cells occur in groups, surrounded by capillaries and delicate connective tissue. The boundary between the medulla and the cortex is present above. Plastic section. × 300.

osmic acid. On electron microscopy, the cells show a well-developed granular endoplasmic reticulum, mitochondria, and Golgi complex. The cytoplasmic granules are of two types: some are of medium electron density and contain epinephrine; others, containing norepinephrine, exhibit a marked electron density. In most mammals two kinds of medullary cells occur, each containing only one of the granule types. Each chromaffin cell is said to be oriented with one end abutting on a capillary, the other on a venule. In addition to chromaffin cells, the medulla contains a few autonomic ganglion cells.

Functions of the Suprarenal Glands

The cortex and medulla are functionally distinct. The cortex is essential to life. Cortical destruction by tuberculosis (Addison's disease) or removal is fatal unless averted by administration of cortical extract. The cortex is necessary to man in a variety of essential factors. It maintains *water and electrolyte balance* in the body. After ablation of the cortex, there is concentration of the plasma, excessive excretion of sodium, and a shift of water from extracellular spaces to tissue cells. The cortex also maintains *carbohydrate balance.* If control is lost, glycogen stores in liver and muscle are depleted and *hypoglycemia* results. *Maintenance of the intercellular substances* of connective tissue is an additional function of the cortex.

More than forty steroid compounds have been isolated from the cortex, at least seven of which have been shown to possess physiological activity. In general, the active compounds can be divided into three categories as judged by their type of activity. Those of the first group are called *mineralocorticoids (aldosterone* and *deoxycorticosterone*), and they control electrolyte and water balance. Those of the second category participate in carbohydrate metabolism and are known as the *glucocorticoids (hydrocortisone* and *cortisone*). The latter compounds also affect connective tissues. Steroid hormones of the third category include both female sex hormones (estrogen and progesterone) and several androgenic hormones. Some tumors that arise in the cortex have a masculinizing or a feminizing effect.

There is some evidence pointing to a functional specialization of the various cortical zones. It appears that the mineralocorticoids are produced primarily in the zona glomerulosa, the glucocorticoids in the zona fasciculata, and the sex hormones in the zona reticularis.

The normal activity of the suprarenal cortex is partially under the control of the adrenocorticotropic hormone (ACTH) of the adenohypophysis, which affects principally the zona fasciculata.

Marked changes occur in the human suprarenal cortex after birth. Within two weeks after birth, most of the inner or *boundary zone* of the cortex *(fetal cortex)* has disappeared, leaving only *subcapsular (permanent) cortex.* The latter consists of zona glomerulosa and zona fasciculata. Zona reticularis becomes established by the end of the third year. The significance of the fetal cortex is poorly understood, but its development is thought to be dependent upon hormones elaborated by the placenta.

The suprarenal medulla is not essential to life. It produces *epinephrine* and *norepinephrine,* which are *catecholamines.* Their presence in the cytoplasmic granules can be detected by the chromaffin reaction. The number of chromaffin granules in a cell is an index of its secretory state. The two hormones are closely related chemically and norepinephrine may be a precursor of epinephrine, but they have somewhat different effects. Epinephrine has a marked effect on metabolism, increasing oxygen consumption and mobilizing glucose from liver glycogen stores. It increases cardiac output and prepares the body to meet emergency situations. Norepinephrine has little general metabolic action, and its chief

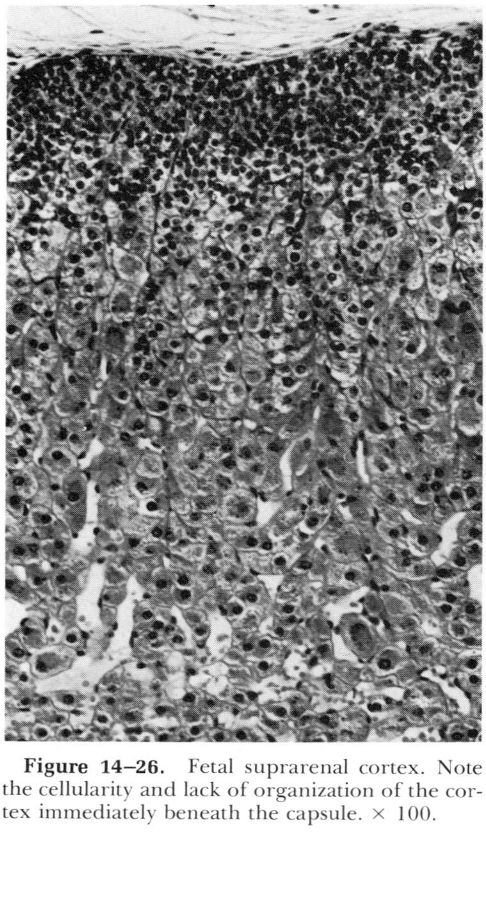

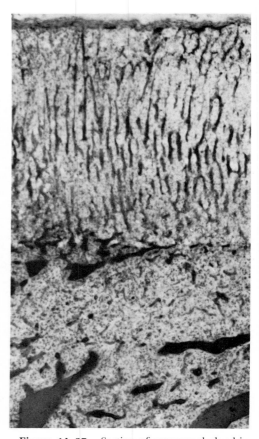

Figure 14–26. Fetal suprarenal cortex. Note the cellularity and lack of organization of the cortex immediately beneath the capsule. × 100.

Figure 14–27. Section of suprarenal gland in which the blood vessels were injected with red gelatin. Note the longitudinally oriented cortical sinusoidal capillaries and the large veins in the medulla. × 60.

function is as the principal transmitter substance or mediator of adrenergic nerve impulses acting upon the heart and blood vessels to maintain blood pressure. Epinephrine has an additional effect upon the secretory activity of the anterior hypophysis, causing it to produce increased amounts of ACTH.

Blood Vessels and Nerves

The suprarenal glands receive a rich vascular supply. A variable number of arteries supplies each gland. As the arteries reach the gland, they branch into numerous arterioles which pierce the capsule. Some arterioles enter cortical sinusoidal capillaries, which possess a fenestrated endothelium. Other arterioles pass directly to the medulla where they empty into a capillary plexus. Venous blood both from the cortex and from the medulla drains into a system of venules which join to form a medullary vein.

Lymphatic vessels are found only in the capsule and in the connective tissue surrounding large veins.

Numerous unmyelinated nerve fibers from the splanchnic nerves enter the capsule in small bundles. A few fibers end in the cortex. Most fibers follow the trabeculae to the medulla and end as preganglionic fibers in relation to medullary cells. Every cell is said to be

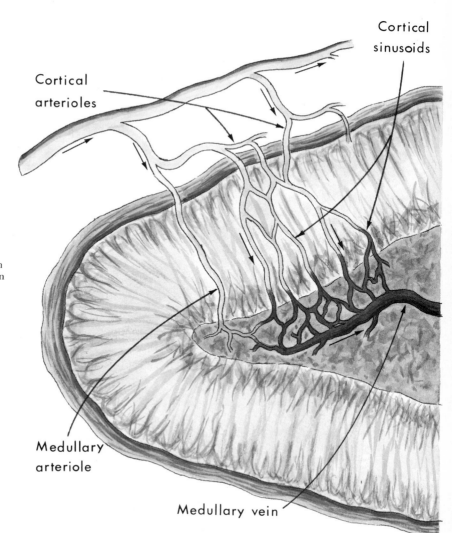

Figure 14–28. Diagram to show the vascularization of the suprarenal gland.

Cortical arterioles

Cortical sinusoids

Medullary arteriole

Medullary vein

innervated. Stimulation of the splanchnic nerves causes a heavy discharge of epinephrine, whereas section of the splanchnic nerves inhibits secretory activity of medullary cells.

THE PARAGANGLIA (CHROMAFFIN SYSTEM)

The term paraganglia embraces several widely scattered groups of cells which are similar in many ways to medullary cells of the suprarenal glands. The cell groups largely lie retroperitoneally, often in association with sympathetic ganglia. The largest groups are the paired or joined *paraaortic bodies of Zuckerkandl.*

Component cells of the paraganglia are chromaffin cells, and they stain positively with chromic and osmic acid. They lie in close association with capillaries. Because the cells are embryologically and morphologically similar to the chromaffin cells of the suprarenal medulla, it has been assumed that they secrete epinephrine, although this has not been established satisfactorily. The carotid and aortic bodies, which function as chemoreceptors, are associated with small islands of chromaffin cells.

THE PINEAL BODY

The pineal body, or *epiphysis cerebri,* is a small cone-shaped body attached by a stalk to the roof of the third ventricle. Pia mater covers the pineal body except at its attachment and forms a thin capsule which sends septa into the organ, dividing it incompletely into lobules. The lobules are composed of *epithelioid cells* or *pinealocytes* and neuroglia. The epithelioid cells are difficult to define in routine preparations but can be seen well in silver preparations, when they appear as irregularly shaped cells with long, branching processes which terminate in bulbous endings. The cytoplasm is variable in amount and may contain granules, lysosomes, and lipid droplets. In addition, it is characterized by the presence of an extensive endoplasmic reticulum, mostly smooth-surfaced, and of large numbers of microtubules.

The neuroglial cells (astrocytes and microglia) serve as supporting elements.

The epiphysis attains its maximum development by about seven years of age and thereafter shows retrogressive changes which involve principally the supporting elements. Connective tissue

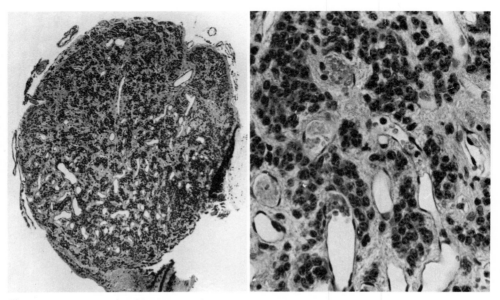

Figure 14–29. Rat pineal body. Note the groups of epithelioid cells (pinealocytes) separated by a rich vascular plexus. Left, × 40; right, × 300.

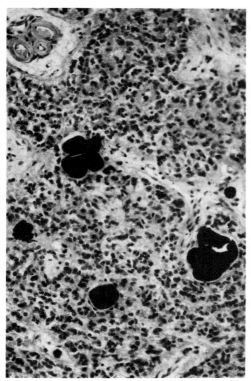

Figure 14–30. Adult human pineal body. Connective tissue separates the groups of pinealocytes into irregular lobules. The scattered dense bodies are acervuli. × 120.

been shown to contain *melatonin* and *serotonin*, compounds which have a similar molecular structure. The content of both melatonin and serotonin in the rat pineal undergoes marked circadian rhythms. Melatonin, when injected into rats, slows the estrous cycle and causes the ovaries to lose weight. The ability of melatonin to modify gonadal function suggests that its secretion may be concerned with the timing of the estrous and menstrual cycles. In man, it has been suggested that the pineal exerts an influence upon gonadal development, particularly in the period prior to sexual maturity. Pineal tumors in children commonly are associated with delayed puberty as a result of increased pineal activity.

Although the precise role of the pineal is open to question, it appears that in mammals it acts as a neuroendocrine transducer, converting a neural input (its sympathetic neurons releasing norepinephrine) into an hormonal output that ultimately modifies the functional activity of other endocrine organs and synchronizes endogenous rhythms.

increases in amount and the lobules become well delineated. *Acervuli* (*brain sand* or *corpora arenacea*) are concretions which appear mainly in the capsule and septa. They are lamellated bodies which vary greatly in size and in number.

A few blood vessels and nerve fibers, both myelinated and unmyelinated, supply the gland. The capillaries within the gland are of the thin, fenestrated type. The nerve fibers are from the sympathetic portion of the autonomic nervous system. Electron microscope studies have shown that the nerve terminals end directly upon the pineal cells, instead of on blood vessels or smooth muscle cells, as in most other organs.

The epiphysis of mammals is a vestige of the photoreceptive pineal system of lower vertebrates. In mammals the epiphysis appears to have a secretory function. The pineals of many mammals, including human beings, have

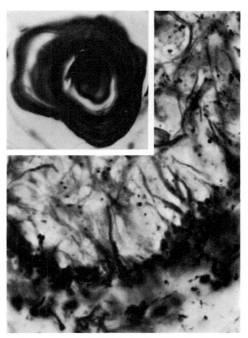

Figure 14–31. Human pineal body in which the epithelioid cells have been made visible with silver. Long branching processes of the cells terminate in bulbous endings. Del Rio-Hortega silver method. × 625. *Inset*: Acervulus ("brain sand"). × 250.

REFERENCES

Hypophysis

Bargmann, W.: Relationship between neurohypophysial structure and function. Proc. 8th Symp. Colston Res. Soc., 11, 1957.

Bergland, R. M., and Page, R. B.: Pituitary-brain vascular relations: a new paradigm. Science, 204:18, 1979.

Brownstein, M. J., Russel, J. T., and Gainer, H.: Synthesis, transport, and release of posterior pituitary hormones. Science, 207:373, 1980.

Farquhar, M. G., and Rinehart, J. F.: Electron microscopic studies of the anterior pituitary gland of castrate rats. Endocrinology, 54:516, 1954.

Farquhar, M. G., and Wellings, S. R.: Electron microscopic evidence suggesting secretory granule formation within the Golgi apparatus. J. Biophys. Biochem. Cytol., 3:319, 1957.

Green, J. D.: The histology of the hypophyseal stalk and median eminence in man, with special reference to blood vessels, nerve fibers, and a peculiar neurovascular zone in this region. Anat. Rec., 100:273, 1948.

Green, J. D.: The comparative anatomy of the hypophysis, with special reference to its blood supply and innervation. Am. J. Anat., 88:225, 1951.

Halmi, N. S.: Two types of basophils in the rat pituitary; "thyrotrophs" and "gonadotrophs" vs. beta and delta cells. Endocrinology, 50:140, 1952.

Harris, G. W.: Neural control of the pituitary glands. Physiol. Rev., 28:139, 1948.

Harris, G. W., and Donovan, B. T.: The Pituitary Gland (3 volumes). Berkeley and Los Angeles, University of California Press, 1966.

Lawzewitsch, I. von, Dickmann, G. H., Amezúa, L., and Pardal, C.: Cytological and ultrastructural characterization of the human pituitary. Acta Anat., 81:286, 1972.

Lawzewitsch, I. von, and Sarrat, R.: Comparative anatomy and the evolution of the neurosecretory hypothalamic-hypophyseal system. Acta Anat., 81:13, 1972.

Mikami, S.: Light and electron microscopic investigations of six types of glandular cells of the bovine adenohypophysis. Z. Zellforsch., 105:457, 1970.

Moriarty, G. C., and Garner, L. L.: Immunocytochemical studies of cells of the rat adenohypophysis containing both ACTH and FSH. Nature, 265:356, 1977.

Paiz, C., and Hennigar, G. R.: Electron microscopy and histochemical correlation of human anterior pituitary cells. Am. J. Pathol., 59:43, 1970.

Rosa, C. G.: New concepts in gonadotropic and mammotropic secretory activity in the adenohypophysis of the normal rat. In Biology of Reproduction, Basic and Clinical Studies, edited by J. T. Velardo and B. A. Kasprow. 3rd Pan American Congress of Anatomy, New Orleans, 1972, p. 115.

Scharrer, E., and Scharrer, B.: Neurosekretion. In Handb. Mikr. Anat. Menschen, edited by von Mollendorff. Berlin, Springer Verlag, 1954, Vol. 6, p. 953.

Turner, C. D.: General Endocrinology. 4th ed. Philadelphia, W. B. Saunders Company, 1966.

Thyroid

Bussolati, G., and Pearse, A. G. E.: Immunofluorescent localization of calcitonin in C cells of pig and dog thyroid. J. Endocrinol., 37:205, 1967.

Chan, A. S., and Conen, P. E.: Ultrastructural observations on cytodifferentiation of parafollicular cells in the human fetal thyroid. Lab. Invest., 25:249, 1971.

De Robertis, E.: Cytological and cytochemical basis of thyroid function. Ann. N. Y. Acad. Sci., 50:317, 1949.

Ekholm, R., and Sjöstrand, F. S.: The ultrastructural organization of the mouse thyroid gland. J. Ultrastruct. Res., 1:178, 1957.

Fujita, H.: Morphological aspects on the site of iodination of thyroglobulin in the thyroid gland. Arch. Histol. Jap., 34:109, 1972.

Fujita, H.: Fine structure of the thyroid cell. Int. Rev. Cytol., 40:197, 1975.

Klinck, G. H., Oertel, J. E., and Winship, T.: Ultrastructure of normal human thyroid. Lab. Invest., 22:2, 1970.

Leblond, C. P., and Gross, J.: The mechanism of the secretion of thyroid hormone. J. Clin. Endocrinol., 9:149, 1949.

Rasmussen, H., and Pechet, M. M.: Calcitonin. Sci. Am., 223:42, 1970.

Wissig, S. L.: The anatomy of secretion in the follicular cells of the thyroid gland. I. The fine structure of the gland in the normal rat. J. Biophys. Biochem. Cytol., 7:419, 1960.

Wissig, S. L.: The anatomy of secretion in the follicular cells of the thyroid gland. II. The effect of acute thyrotrophic hormone stimulation on the secretory apparatus. J. Cell Biol., 16:93, 1963.

Young, B. A., Care, A. D., and Duncan, T.: Some observations on the light cells of the thyroid gland of the pig in relation to thyrocalcitonin production. J. Anat., 102:275, 1968.

Parathyroid

Bensley, S. L.: The normal mode of secretion in the parathyroid gland of the dog. Anat. Rec., 98:361, 1947.

Fetter, A. W., and Capen, C. C.: The ultrastructure of the parathyroid gland of young pigs. Acta Anat., 75:359, 1970.

Munger, B. L., and Roth, S. I.: The cytology of the normal parathyroid glands of man and Virginia deer. J. Cell Biol., 16:379, 1963.

Nunez, E. A., Whalen, J. P. and Krook, L.: An ultrastructural study of the natural secretory cycle of the parathyroid gland of the bat. Am. J. Anat., 134:459, 1972.

Suprarenal

Baxter, J. S.: The growth cycle of the cells of the adrenal cortex in the adult rat. J. Anat., 80:139, 1946.

Bennett, H. S.: The life history and secretion of the cells of the adrenal cortex of the cat. Am. J. Anat., 67:151, 1940.

Brenner, R. M.: Fine structure of adrenocortical cells in adult male rhesus monkeys. Am. J. Anat., 119:429, 1966.

Brown, W. J., Barajas, L., and Latta, H.: The ultrastructure of the human adrenal medulla:

with comparative studies of white rat. Anat. Rec., *169*:173, 1971.

Coupland, R. E.: Electron microscopic observations on the structure of the rat adrenal medulla. I. The ultrastructure and organization of chromaffin cells in the normal adrenal medulla. J. Anat., *99*:231, 1965.

Coupland, R. E.: Electron microscopic observations on the structure of the rat adrenal medulla. II. Normal innervation. J. Anat., *99*:255, 1965.

Deane, H. W., and Greep, R. O.: A morphological and histological study of the rat's adrenal cortex after hypophysectomy, with comments on the liver. Am. J. Anat., *79*:117, 1946.

Idelman, S.: Ultrastructure of the mammalian adrenal cortex. Int. Rev. Cytol., 27:181, 1970.

Long, J. A., and Jones, A. L.: Observations on the fine structure of the adrenal cortex of man. Lab. Invest., *17*:355, 1967.

Rhodin, J. A. G.: The ultrastructure of the adrenal cortex of the rat under normal and experimental conditions. J. Ultrastruct. Res., *34*:23, 1971.

Pineal

Anderson, E.: The anatomy of bovine and ovine pineals. J. Ultrastruct. Rec., Suppl. 8, 1965.

Axelrod, J.: The pineal gland: a neurochemical transducer. Science, *184*:1341, 1974.

Clabough, J. W.: Ultrastructural features of the pineal gland in normal and light deprived golden hamsters. Z. Zellforsch., *114*:151, 1971.

Del Rio-Hortega, P.: Pineal gland. *In* Cytology and Cellular Pathology of the Nervous System, edited by Penfield. Baltimore, Williams & Wilkins Co., 1932, Vol. 1, p. 637.

Kelly, D. E.: Pineal organs: Photoreception, secretion, and development. Am. Sci., *50*:597, 1962.

Kitay, J. I., and Altschule, M. D.: The Pineal Gland: A Review of the Physiologic Literature. Cambridge, Harvard University Press, 1954.

Nir, I., Reiter, R. J., and Wurtman, R. J.: The pineal gland. J. Neural Transm., Suppl. 13, 1978.

Quay, W. B.: Pineal structure and composition in the orangutan (*Pongo pygmaeus*). Anat. Rec., *168*:93, 1970.

Quay, W. B., and Harvey, A.: Experimental modification of the rat pineal's content of serotonin and related indole amines. Physiol. Zool., *35*:1, 1962.

Reiter, R. J.: Pineal control of reproductive biology. *In* Biology of Reproduction, Basic and Clinical Studies, edited by J. T. Velardo and B. S. Kasprow. 3rd Pan American Congress of Anatomy, New Orleans, 1972, p. 105.

Tapp, E., and Huxley, M.: The histological appearance of the human pineal gland from puberty to old age. J. Pathol., *108*:137, 1972.

Wurtman, R. J., Axelrod, J., and Fischer, J. E.: Melatonin synthesis in the pineal gland: Effect of light mediated by the sympathetic nervous system. Science, *143*:1328, 1964.

Wurtman, R. J., and Axelrod, J.: The pineal gland. Sci. Am., *213*:50, 1965.

THE FEMALE REPRODUCTIVE SYSTEM

The female reproductive system comprises the ovaries, a system of genital ducts (the uterine tubes, uterus, and vagina), and the external genitalia. The mammary glands, although not one of the genital organs, are included here since they are important glands of the female reproductive system. The principal functions of the system, which are controlled by hormonal and nervous mechanisms, are production of female gametes, the ova, by a process of oogenesis; reception of male gametes, the spermatozoa; provision of a suitable environment for fertilization of ova by spermatozoa and for development of the fetus; a mechanism for the expulsion of the developed fetus into the external environment; and nutrition of the newborn.

THE OVARY

The ovaries are classified as double glands since they produce both exocrine (cytogenic) and endocrine secretions. They are slightly flattened, ovoid bodies, measuring about 4 cm in length, 2 cm in width, and 1 cm in thickness. One lies on each side of the uterus on the lateral wall of the pelvic cavity. Each is attached at one of its margins, the *hilum*, by the *mesovarium*, a fold of peritoneum, to the broad ligament of the uterus. At the hilum the vascular connective tissue of the mesovarium becomes continuous with the ovarian stroma. The peritoneal covering of the mesovarium ceases abruptly at the hilum and is replaced by a layer of cuboidal cells, the *germinal epithelium*, which covers the free surface of the ovary. This specialization of the peritoneal mesothelium rests upon a thin basal lamina. Beneath the epithelium there is a layer of dense connective tissue, the *tunica albuginea,* which increases in density with advancing age.

In sections of the ovary two zones may be distinguished, an outer layer, the *cortex,* and an inner portion, the *medulla,* which merges with the vascular connective tissue of the mesovarium at the hilum. There is no distinct line of demarcation between the two zones. The medulla consists of loose fibroelastic connective tissue containing numerous large blood vessels, lymphatics, and nerves. The stroma contains scattered strands of smooth muscle fibers.

The cortex consists of a compact, cellular stroma that contains the *ovarian follicles.* The stroma is composed of networks of reticular fibers and spindle-shaped cells, which exhibit characteristics of both fibroblasts and smooth muscle cells. These stromal cells contribute to the growth of the theca folliculi (discussed under Growing Follicles). Elastic tissue is sparse and occurs only in the walls of blood vessels. The follicles may be seen in all stages of development, and the appearance of the ovarian cortex depends upon the age of the individual and the stage of the ovarian cycle. Before puberty only *primary,* or *primitive, follicles* are seen. Sexual maturity is characterized by the presence of *growing follicles* and their end products (*corpora lutea, atretic follicles*). After the menopause

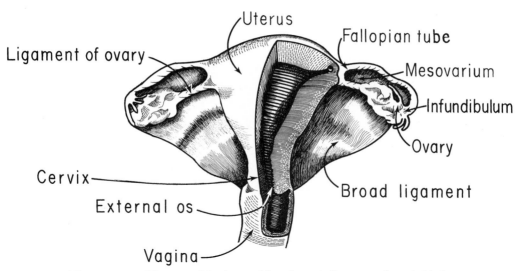

Figure 15–1. Diagram of the internal female genitalia as seen from behind.

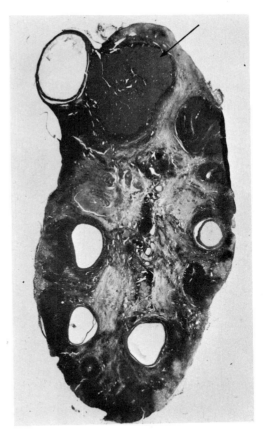

Figure 15–2. Section of the ovary from a 32-year-old woman. Follicles in various stages of differentiation and a corpus luteum (arrow) are present in the cortex. Note the large blood vessels in the loose connective tissue of the medulla. ×5.

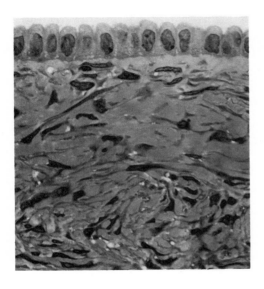

Figure 15–3. Section of the germinal epithelium of the ovary. Note the distinct cuboidal cells. Beneath the epithelium is the dense connective tissue of the tunica albuginea. Plastic section. × 400.

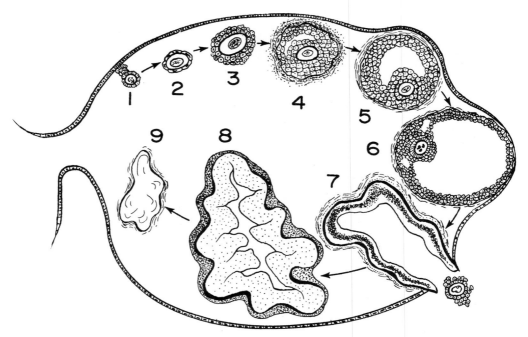

Figure 15–4. Diagram of the ovary, illustrating development and fate of ovarian follicles. (1) Oogonium, surrounded by follicular cells, the latter arising from germinal epithelium. (2) Primary follicle. (3–5) Maturing follicles. (6) Graafian follicle. (7) Ruptured follicle. (8) Corpus luteum. (9) Corpus albicans.

follicles disappear and the senile cortex eventually becomes a narrow zone of fibrous connective tissue.

Follicles

Each ovarian follicle consists of an immature ovum surrounded by epithelial cells. The immature ovum, the *oogonium*, is a spheroidal cell with a large vesicular nucleus and a prominent nucleolus. The cytoplasm is opaque and finely granular.

In the newborn infant the follicles are believed to number about 400,000. Their number decreases progressively throughout life until virtually none is left soon after the menopause. Most follicles seen are *primary follicles*, which measure about 40 microns (μm) in diameter. A primary follicle consists of an immature ovum surrounded by a single layer of flattened *follicular cells*, believed to be derived from the germinal epithelium. A thin basal lamina separates the follicle from the ovarian stroma.

Growing Follicles

The progressive development of follicles that occurs after puberty is char-

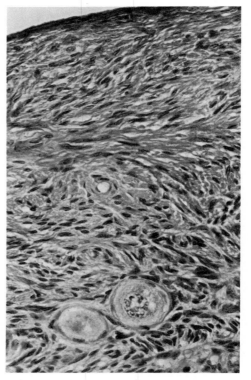

Figure 15–5. Portion of the cortex of an ovary from a 25-year-old woman. The cortical stroma, which is markedly cellular, contains two primary follicles. × 250.

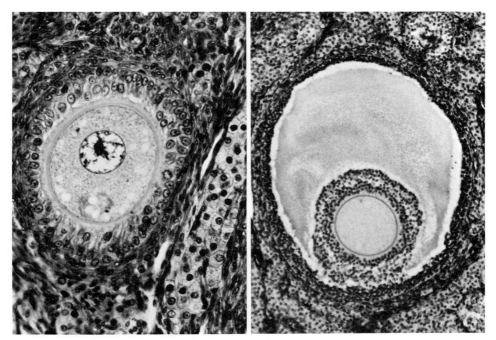

Figure 15–6. *Left:* Growing follicle, showing an immature ovum with a large vesicular nucleus and a prominent nucleolus, a zona pellucida, and a stratified layer of follicular cells. Also present is a group of large epithelioid cells, the so-called interstitial cells (right), derived from the theca interna of an atretic follicle. × 250. *Right:* A more mature follicle, showing a well-developed membrana granulosa, an antrum, and cumulus oophorus with an immature ovum. The ovum is sectioned tangentially and does not show a nucleus. × 100.

acterized by growth and differentiation of the ovum, proliferation of follicular cells, and development of a connective tissue capsule from the surrounding stroma.

The immature ovum increases in size and a refractile, deeply staining membrane, the *zona pellucida,* is formed around it. The zona pellucida contains glycoproteins and appears homogeneous in the fresh condition. It is elaborated probably by both the ovum and the surrounding follicular cells.

The flattened follicular cells become first cuboidal and then columnar in shape. They divide actively to produce a stratified layer around the ovum. The proliferation occurs more rapidly on one side of the ovum so that the follicle becomes ovoid in shape and the ovum eccentric in position. Irregular small spaces filled with a clear fluid appear within the follicular mass. An increase in the amount of this fluid causes a further increase in the size of the follicle. The fluid-filled spaces fuse to form a single cavity, the *antrum,* within the follicular layer. The ovum, surrounded

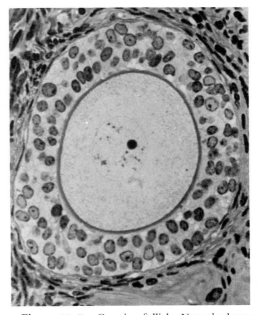

Figure 15–7. Growing follicle. Note the large immature ovum which shows a vesicular nucleus with a prominent nucleolus and a pale, granular cytoplasm. The ovum is surrounded by a densely staining zona pellucida and a stratified layer of follicular cells. The surrounding stroma shows early organization into a theca folliculi. Plastic section. × 300.

by a group of follicular cells, is pressed to one side and forms a definite projection into the antrum cavity. This eccentric mound is known as the *cumulus oophorus.* The follicular cells of the cumulus oophorus directly in relation to the ovum become radially arranged and form the *corona radiata,* separated from the ovum only by the zona pellucida. Phase and electron microscope studies have shown that processes from the corona radiata cells extend through the zona pellucida to contact the cell membrane of the ovum. Additionally, microvillous processes of the ovum pass into the zona pellucida. Elsewhere the stratified epithelium, composed of follicular cells, forms a continuous, regular layer around the antrum cavity, the *membrana granulosa.*

As the follicle increases in size, the adjacent stroma organizes into a capsule, the *theca folliculi,* separated from the membrana granulosa by a basal lamina (the *glassy membrane*). The theca folliculi differentiates into two layers,

an inner vascular layer, the *theca interna,* and an outer fibrous layer, the *theca externa.* The theca interna consists of enlarged (epithelioid) stromal cells between which are numerous capillaries. The theca externa, composed of closely packed collagenous fibers and fusiform cells, merges peripherally into the surrounding ovarian stroma.

Mature Graafian Follicles

It is believed that a follicle requires 10 to 14 days to reach maturity. A mature graafian follicle is 10 mm or more in diameter and occupies the full breadth of the cortex and indents the medulla. It bulges on the free surface of the ovary. At this point, called the *stigma,* the tunica albuginea and the theca folliculi become attenuated. The large antrum, distended with fluid, is bound by the membrana granulosa. The ovum has attained its full size, and it is surrounded by a thick zona pellucida and a conspicuous corona radiata.

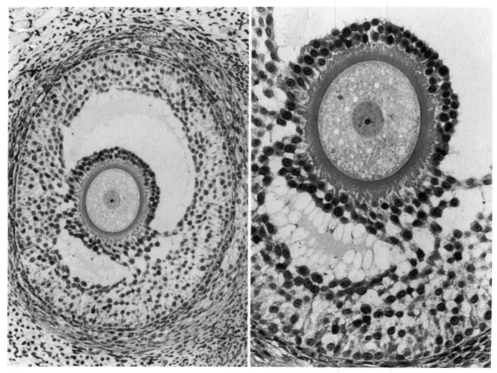

Figure 15–8.   Almost mature graafian follicle, showing cumulus oophorus and a large antrum. The corona radiata is composed of the follicular cells of the cumulus that lie directly in relation to the ovum, separated from it only by the wide zona pellucida. A well-defined theca folliculi surrounds the membrana granulosa. Plastic section. Left, × 100; right, × 250.

As follicular maturity is attained, small irregular spaces filled with fluid appear between the cells of the cumulus oophorus, thus weakening the connection of the ovum with the membrana granulosa.

Ovulation

As the follicle reaches maturity, there is increased secretion of liquor, more watery than that formed previously, which causes further expansion in diameter of the follicle. This is termed *preovulatory swelling.* The follicle, covered with thinned cortex, ruptures at the stigma, and follicular fluid oozes out into the peritoneal cavity. The ovum, which is surrounded by cells of the corona radiata, is torn away from the cumulus and discharged with the liquor. This process constitutes *ovulation.* Usually only one ovum is discharged at one time, but in some cases two or, rarely, more may be released. The free ovum retains the capacity to be fertilized only for 24 hours. In the human female ovulation occurs at intervals averaging 28 days.

Maturation of the Ovum: Oogenesis

The ovum which is released at ovulation is actually a *secondary oocyte* and technically is immature. In preparation for fertilization, the ovum passes through a series of nuclear changes similar to that described for spermatozoa (see Chapter 16). The end result is the same as with spermatogenesis, i.e., the reduction of the chromosomes to one-half the somatic (diploid) number.

Oogonia, or primitive ova, which contain the diploid number of chromosomes, divide mitotically to produce *primary oocytes* in the fetal ovary. During follicular development, the primary oocyte grows and then passes through a period of maturation in which it undergoes two maturation divisions, as a result of which the chromosomes are reduced to the haploid number. The first maturation division occurs shortly before ovulation. The chromatin is divided equally between the daughter cells, but the division of cytoplasm is extremely unequal. One of the daughter cells, the *secondary oocyte,* receives practically all the cytoplasm of the mother cell; the other becomes the *first polar body,* which soon degenerates. In each the chromosome assortment is reduced to a single set of 23 chromosomes. At about this time ovulation occurs and the secondary oocyte is released. At this time, the nucleus of the secondary oocyte commences the second maturation division, which stops in the metaphase and remains in this condition until fertilization. Penetration of the spermatozoon head into the oocyte activates it to complete the second maturation division. Again the cytoplasm is divided unequally. The majority of cytoplasm is retained in the mature *ovum.* The other daughter cell is the *second polar body.* Thus only one daughter cell of a primary oocyte becomes functional.

The Corpus Luteum

After ovulation there is sometimes a little bleeding into the cavity of the follicle. The wall of the follicle collapses and is thrown into folds. The follicular wall becomes transformed into a temporary glandular structure, the *corpus luteum.* The granulosa cells of the follicle differentiate into large, pale-staining cells with large vesicular nuclei. The cytoplasm acquires an accumulation of fine lipid droplets and lipofuscin pigment granules, which are lysosomal in nature. Dispersed within the cytoplasm are numerous mitochondria with tubular cristae and abundant granular and agranular endoplasmic reticulum. The transformed granulosa cells are called *granulosa lutein cells,* and they form a thick, folded layer about the remains of the follicular cavity.

Cells of the theca interna, which prior to ovulation have increased in size, form *theca lutein cells.* They are smaller in size than granulosa lutein cells and possess compact, dark-staining nuclei. They aggregate peripherally, especially in the recesses between the folds of granulosa lutein cells. The theca externa retains its regular ovoid outline, and component cells here do not undergo transformation.

Numerous capillaries and connective tissue from the theca invade the lutein mass. Fibroblasts organize a delicate re-

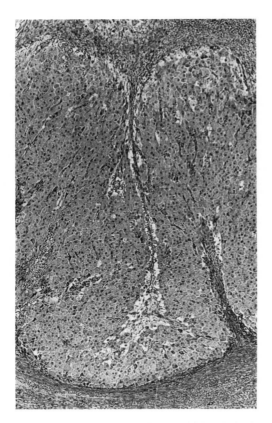

ticulum throughout the corpus luteum and form a continuous lining on the inner surface of the lutein cells in relation to the reduced follicular cavity.

If the discharged ovum is not fertilized, the corpus luteum attains its greatest development about nine days after ovulation and then begins to degenerate. This is the *corpus luteum* of *menstruation.* The former rich vascularization declines, and component cells decrease in size and undergo a fatty degeneration. Connective tissue between lutein cells increases in amount and becomes hyalinized and gradually the corpus luteum is transformed into a white scar, the *corpus albicans.*

If the ovum is fertilized, the corpus luteum increases in size and is known as the *corpus luteum* of *pregnancy.* The cells continue to grow in size until the middle months of pregnancy, and

Figure 15–9. Portion of a corpus luteum from a woman 4 months pregnant. Note the folded outline and the large size of granulosa lutein cells. × 50.

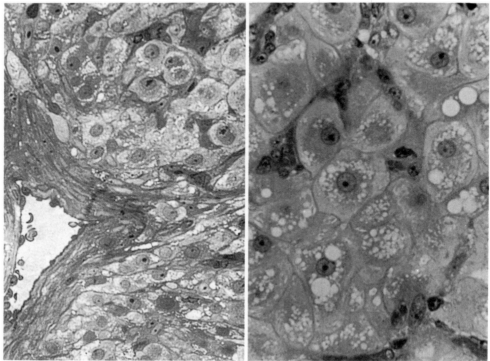

Figure 15–10. Corpus luteum of pregnancy. *Left:* Periphery of the corpus luteum showing the bases of two folds and a blood vessel within the surrounding stroma. *Right:* A group of granulosa lutein cells. The appearance is typical of a steroid-producing endocrine gland. Numerous capillaries lie between component cells. Plastic section. Left, × 250; right, × 550.

thereafter a slow involution occurs. After delivery involution proceeds rapidly. The resulting corpus albicans is large and usually causes a retraction of the surface of the ovary following contraction of fibrous tissue formed as a result of involution.

Atresia of Follicles

Only about 400 follicles reach full maturity. The period of sexual activity in the human female is about thirty years, and during this time ordinarily only one ovum is discharged each month. All unsuccessful follicles undergo degeneration, either as primary follicles or after a varying period of growth. This involution of follicles is called *atresia*. Atresia appears to occur initially in the ovum. This is followed by degeneration of the follicular cells. In atresia of primary follicles the space resulting is filled with stromal tissue. Atresia of growing follicles is a more

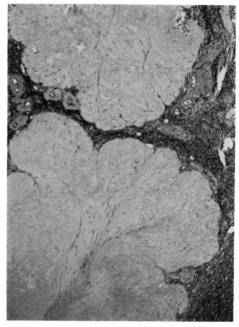

Figure 15–12. Portions of two corpora albicantia. There has been complete replacement of the corpora lutea by connective tissue. × 40.

complicated process. As in primary follicles, the first degenerative signs occur in the ovum and follicular cells. The zona pellucida swells and may persist for some time after the disappearance of the ovum and follicular cells. Cells of the theca interna develop much like those in a corpus luteum. They increase in size and become arranged in vascularized, radial strands. The glassy membrane also increases in thickness and forms a hyalinized band. After resorption of follicular cells, the theca cells degenerate and are replaced by connective tissue. The resulting masses of scar tissue are similar in appearance to corpora albicantia, but are smaller (*corpora atretica*).

Interstitial Cells

Large epithelioid cells are present in the ovarian stroma of some mammals, particularly rodents. These are the so-called *interstitial cells*, which are large spheroidal cells containing small lipid droplets. They are thought to be derived from the theca interna of follicles un-

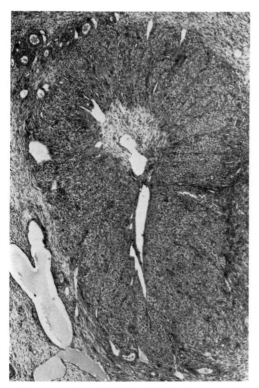

Figure 15–11. Early involution of a corpus luteum. Component cells are smaller than during the active phase, and connective tissue strands between lutein cells are prominent. × 35.

dergoing atresia. Thus they are most abundant when atresia is most marked. In the human this is in the first year of life. In the adult human ovary they either are absent or are present as small radiating cords of cells.

Hormones of the Ovary

The ovaries, in addition to producing sex cells (a cytogenic secretion), secrete the so-called female sex hormones, *estrogen* and *progesterone*. These are steroids. Estrogen (principally estradiol) is produced mainly by the growing follicles, progesterone primarily by the corpus luteum. Estrogen induces growth and development of the female reproductive tract and the mammary glands. Progesterone causes the uterine glands to secrete and renders the mucosa receptive to a nidating ovum.

Since the sequence of structural changes in the ovary is follicular growth, ovulation, and formation of a

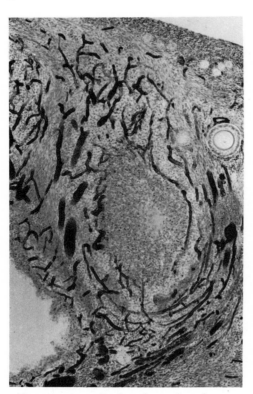

Figure 15–13. Section of a portion of an ovary in which the blood vessels had been injected with colored gelatin prior to sectioning. Note the abundant capillary networks in relation to the growing follicles. × 40.

corpus luteum, the levels of the two hormones normally exhibit regular cyclic fluctuations. Estrogen secretion is high during the preovulatory period (follicular phase); progesterone production increases rapidly during luteinization of the ruptured follicle and remains at a high level until the corpus luteum regresses (luteal phase). These rhythmic changes in ovarian secretory activity are responsible for the cyclic changes which occur in the structure of the reproductive tract, notably in the mucosa of the uterus (see Figure 15–19).

The ovarian cycle in turn is activated and governed by the gonadotropins secreted by the anterior lobe of the hypophysis. The gonadotropins, follicle-stimulating hormone (FSH) and luteinizing hormone (LH), control the maturation of follicles and the formation of corpora lutea.

Blood Vessels, Lymphatics, and Nerves

Large branches from the ovarian and uterine arteries enter the medulla and divide into a number of spiral vessels, often called *helicine arteries*. At the boundary zone between cortex and medulla these form a plexus from which smaller twigs pass into the cortex to ramify around follicles. Capillary networks are abundant in the theca interna of growing follicles. Veins, which arise from the capillary networks, accompany the arteries and leave the ovary at the hilum.

Lymph capillaries begin in the theca externa of follicles and unite to form larger vessels which pass to the medulla and leave at the hilum. There they are combined into a smaller number of lymphatic trunks that drain into lumbar lymph nodes.

Nerve fibers, mostly unmyelinated, follow the blood vessels and supply their muscular coat. Some fibers penetrate into the cortex and form delicate plexuses around the follicles and beneath the germinal epithelium.

THE FALLOPIAN TUBES

The *fallopian (uterine) tubes*, or *oviducts*, are paired structures which ex-

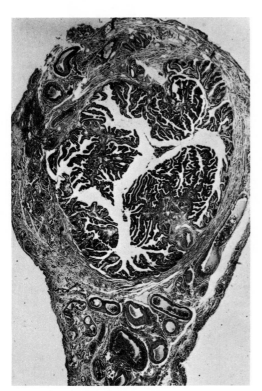

Figure 15–14. Section through the ampulla of the fallopian tube. The lumen appears markedly irregular owing to extensive folding of the mucosa. × 12.

tend from the ovary to the uterus in a fold of peritoneum, the upper free margin of the broad ligament. Each tube is 12 to 15 cm long and about 1 cm in diameter. The end of the tube in relation to the ovary opens into the peritoneal cavity; the other end opens into the uterine cavity. The uterine tube shows four regions. The *infundibulum* is the funnel-shaped opening into the peritoneal cavity. Its margins are drawn out into numerous fringed folds (*fimbriae*). The expanded intermediate segment, comprising two-thirds of the length of the tube, is the *ampulla*, which is thin-walled. It leads into the *isthmus*, slender and narrow, which connects with the uterus. The fourth part, the *intramural (interstitial) portion*, is the continuation of the canal through the uterine wall. The wall of the tube thickens progressively toward the uterus, whereas the lumen diminishes in size in this direction.

The wall of the fallopian tube consists of a *mucous membrane*, a *muscular layer*, and a *serosa*.

Mucosa

The mucosal lining is thrown into characteristic longitudinal folds. In the ampulla the folds branch in a complex manner to divide the lumen into a labyrinth of spaces. In the isthmus the folds rarely branch and in the intramural portion of the tube the folds are low.

The epithelium consists of simple columnar cells, some of which are ciliated, whereas others are not. The nonciliated cells are narrow and peg-shaped and appear to be secretory in nature. Ciliated cells occur in small groups, alternating with groups of cells that are nonciliated. The proportion of cells with cilia is greatest at the infundibulum and least at the isthmus. The cilia beat down toward the uterus. The height of the epithelium varies somewhat with the reproductive cycle, being greatest during the follicular phase and lowest during the latter part of the luteal phase. During pregnancy the epithelium is low and there is an increased number of "peg" cells.

The lamina propria of the mucosa is composed of an unusually cellular connective tissue containing a few scattered fusiform cells. It is separated from the epithelium by a thin basal lamina. At the rim of the infundibulum the mucosal lining of the tube becomes continuous with the mesothelium of the serosa.

Muscularis

The mucosa rests directly upon the muscular coat, which consists of a broad inner circular layer and a thin outer layer. The outer layer is not continuous but consists of scattered bundles of fibers, oriented longitudinally. Toward the uterus the muscularis increases in thickness. Contractions of the muscular coat, occurring in peristaltic waves, aid in the movement of the ovum down the tube to the uterine cavity.

Serosa

The uterine tube is invested with a fold of reflected peritoneum, the serosa, consisting of loose connective tissue surfaced with mesothelium. The deeper layers of the connective tissue

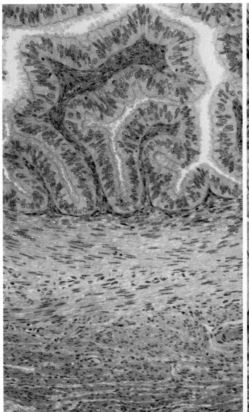

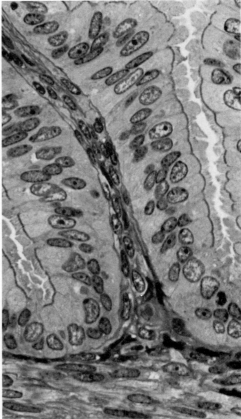

Figure 15–15. Portion of the ampullary region of the fallopian tube, sectioned transversely. Note the numerous folds of the mucosa and the ciliated epithelium. Beneath the thin, cellular lamina propria is the muscular coat, consisting of inner circular and outer longitudinal layers. Plastic section. Left, × 100; right, × 400.

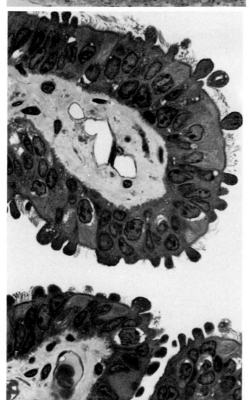

Figure 15–16. Ampullary region of the fallopian tube of a pregnant monkey. Note the "peg" cells alternating with groups of ciliated cells. Plastic section. × 400.

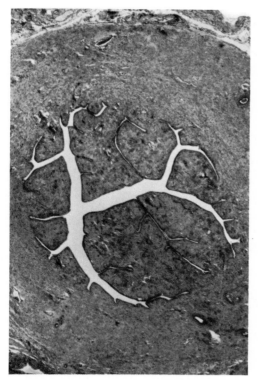

Figure 15–17. Isthmus of the fallopian tube. Folding of the mucosa is less marked than in the ampullary region, and the muscularis is increased in thickness. × 20.

contain the longitudinal bundles of the muscularis.

Blood Vessels, Lymphatics, and Nerves

Numerous blood vessels and lymphatics are present in the lamina propria and the serosa. Nerves form a rich plexus in the serosa, from which nerve fibers pass to supply muscle fibers and the mucosa.

THE UTERUS

The uterus is the thick-walled segment of the tubular female reproductive system that is interposed between the fallopian tubes and the vagina. It is a pear-shaped organ, somewhat flattened in a dorsoventral direction, and averages 7 cm in length, 5 cm in width at its broadest part, and 2 to 3 cm in thickness. Two major portions may be

recognized: the expanded upper portion, the *body* or *corpus uteri*, and the lowermost, cylindrical portion, the *neck* or *cervix*, a part of which projects into the vagina as the *portio vaginalis*. The term *fundus* refers to the rounded upper end of the body, from which the fallopian tubes extend. The *isthmus* is the narrow zone of transition between the body and the cervix.

The wall of the uterus consists of three layers: the outer—serosa or *perimetrium;* the middle—muscularis or *myometrium;* and the inner—mucosa or *endometrium.*

Perimetrium

The perimetrium is a typical serosa consisting of a single layer of mesothelial cells supported by a thin layer of connective tissue. It is continuous on each side of the organ with the peritoneum of the broad ligament and is deficient over the lower half of the anterior surface, where the urinary bladder abuts.

Myometrium

The myometrium is a massive coat of smooth muscle, about 12 to 15 mm in thickness. The muscle fibers are arranged in bundles, separated by connective tissue. Individual fibers are large and their length varies from 40 to 90 microns (μm). During pregnancy the fibers increase greatly in size and may attain a length of 600 microns (μm) or more. Three layers of muscle may be distinguished, although they are somewhat ill-defined owing to the presence of interconnecting bundles. There is an inner muscular layer consisting mostly of longitudinally oriented fibers, the *stratum subvasculare,* a thick middle layer of circular and oblique muscle fibers with numerous blood vessels, the *stratum vasculare,* and an outer thin, longitudinal muscle layer immediately beneath the perimetrium, the *stratum supravasculare.*

Endometrium

The endometrium (mucosa), which is firmly adherent to the underlying myo-

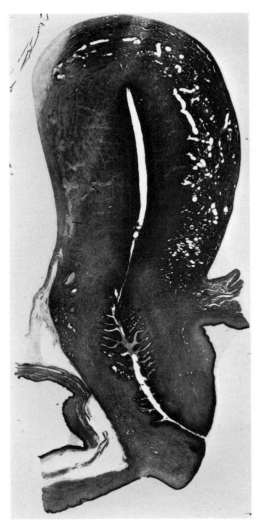

Figure 15–18.   Median sagittal section through the uterus and upper portion of the vagina. Note the thickness of the uterine wall (principally myometrium), the prominent cervical glands, the portio vaginalis, and a portion of the bladder (anterior) to the left. × 2½.

glands extend through the full thickness of the mucosa. These are simple tubules which may branch toward their basal ends. They are separated from each other by connective tissue, the *stroma*. Stromal cells are irregular, stellate cells which have large, ovoid nuclei. They lie in a framework of reticular fibers which are condensed beneath the epithelium to form a basal lamina. Wandering lymphoid cells and granular leukocytes also are present in the stroma.

Blood Vessels, Lymphatics, and Nerves

Branches from the uterine arteries penetrate to the middle layer of the myometrium and from these vessels two systems of branches arise. One system supplies the superficial layers of the myometrium. The other system supplies the remainder of the myometrium and sends two sets of vessels to the endometrium. One set of arterial extensions supplies the basal part of the endometrium. Another set spreads out into a rich capillary bed superficially. Vessels of the latter set are more or less contorted and are termed *coiled arteries*. Thus the endometrium is supplied by a basal and a superficial set of vessels. The basal set does not undergo changes during the menstrual cycle, but the coiled arteries show pronounced modifications.

Veins in the endometrium are thin-walled and form an extensive network. A plexus of large vessels is present in the middle (vascular) layer of the myometrium.

Lymph vessels are abundant and form plexuses throughout the layers of the uterus with the exception of the superficial zone of the mucosa.

Myelinated nerve fibers enter the mucosa and form a plexus beneath the epithelium. Unmyelinated nerve fibers supply blood vessels and muscle bundles.

Cyclic Changes in the Endometrium

Beginning with puberty and ending at the menopause, the endometrium

metrium, is subject to cyclic changes in response to ovarian secretory activity. These changes culminate in partial destruction of the mucosa leading to tissue necrosis and hemorrhage, an event known as *menstruation*. Menstruation occurs typically at intervals of about 28 days and lasts for three to five days. The first day of menstruation is counted as the first day of the menstrual cycle.

The body of the uterus is lined by a simple columnar epithelium which possesses scattered groups of ciliated cells. From the surface epithelium, uterine

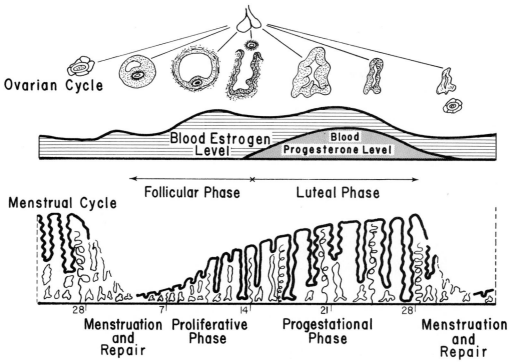

Figure 15–19. Diagram (modified from Schroder) to illustrate the interrelations of ovary and endometrium during a menstrual cycle.

undergoes periodic changes. Four stages can be recognized in a continuous cycle of events, and each stage passes gradually into the next: the *menstrual stage,* during which there is external menstrual discharge; the *proliferative (follicular) stage,* which is concurrent with follicular growth and estrogen secretion; the *progestational (luteal) stage,* usually associated with an active corpus luteum; and the *ischemic (premenstrual) stage,* when there is interruption of blood flow in the coiled arteries.

The Proliferative (Follicular) Stage. This stage begins at the end of a menstrual flow and is characterized by rapid regeneration of the endometrium from the narrow zone remaining after menstruation. Epithelial cells from the remnants of torn glands glide over the denuded surface of the mucosa. Numerous mitoses occur in cells of the glands and of the endometrial stroma. The mucosa increases in thickness from 1 mm or less to 2 mm or more. This increase coincides with growth of ovarian follicles and secretion of estro-

gen. The glands proliferate, lengthen rapidly, and become closely packed. Rebuilding of the lamina propria occurs as a result of the mitotic activity of stromal cells. Toward the end of the proliferative phase the lumina of the glands widen and they become wavy in outline. Glycogen accumulates in the basal region of the cells, but only a thin mucoid secretion is released at this stage. Coiled arteries grow into the regenerating tissue but are not found in the superficial third of the endometrium, which possesses only capillaries and venules.

The Progestational (Secretory) Stage. The endometrium increases in thickness and becomes 4 mm or more in depth. The increase is due largely to hypertrophy of gland cells and to an increase of edema fluid. The glands swell and secrete profusely. Secretory material at first is localized in the basal portions of the cells. During the latter half of the stage the secretion moves to the apical zone of the cells. The secretion is thick and rich in glycogen. The glands become serrated and their lu-

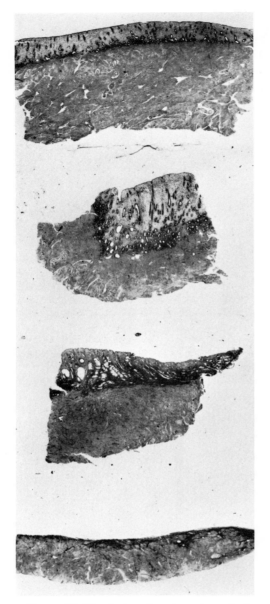

Figure 15–20. Series of sections through the uterus at various stages during the menstrual cycle. From top to bottom, early proliferative stage, late proliferative stage, late secretory stage, and late menstrual stage. Note the varying height of the endometrium and the character of the uterine glands. × 4.

mina become wider. Coiled arteries grow nearly to the surface. Toward the end of this stage, stromal cells enlarge to become *decidual cells.* Their cytoplasm contains numerous free ribosomes, abundant granular endoplasmic reticulum, and scattered glycogen.

These cells form aggregations around the coiled arteries and beneath the surface epithelium.

Once the structural changes associated with this stage become apparent, three zones of the endometrium can be distinguished. Nearest the surface is the *compact layer,* which is a relatively narrow zone. It contains the straight necks of the glands and shows little edema. Under this layer is a thick *spongy layer,* in which are the tortuous portions of glands, separated by a lamina propria that is grossly edematous. The compact and spongy layers together are termed the *functional layer,* which is lost at menstruation and at parturition. Deepest of all is the thin *basal layer,* containing the blind ends of glands. This layer participates little in the cyclic changes and is not lost at menstruation or at parturition.

The Ischemic (Premenstrual) Stage. This occurs 13 to 14 days after ovulation and is characterized by extensive vascular changes. The coiled arteries constrict intermittently. The functional layer becomes pale and shrinks as a result of anemia and anoxia. The stroma increases in density and becomes infiltrated with leukocytes.

The Menstrual Stage. The functional layer undergoes necrosis and is shed. After a number of hours the coiled arteries relax, the walls of the vessels near the surface break, and blood is added to the secretion of the glands and the necrotic endometrial tissue. Patches of tissue separate and are lost. Blood oozes from veins exposed by the shedding process. The menstrual discharge thus contains altered arterial and venous blood, disintegrated epithelial and stromal cells, and glandular secretions. Finally the whole functional layer of the endometrium is lost, leaving a raw surface. The surviving basal layer remains intact, epithelial cells glide out of the torn ends of glands, and the surface epithelium is quickly restored once the menstrual discharge ceases.

As stated previously, the uterine changes are related closely to the ovarian cyclic changes. The proliferative stage corresponds to the preovulatory period of follicular maturation. The progestational stage is associated

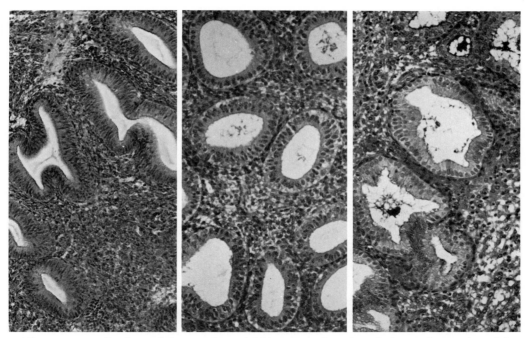

Figure 15–21. Portions of three endometrial biopsy samples taken during various stages of the menstrual cycle. *Left,* Proliferative stage; *center,* early secretory phase; *right,* late secretory phase. Note the varying character of the glands and of the stroma. In the early secretory phase, vacuolation of the basal cytoplasm of glandular cells is indicative of glycogen accumulation; in the late secretory phase, secretion is present in the apical zone of cytoplasm and in the lumina of glands, which become irregular in outline. The stroma becomes less dense in the secretory phase owing to fluid accumulation. × 100.

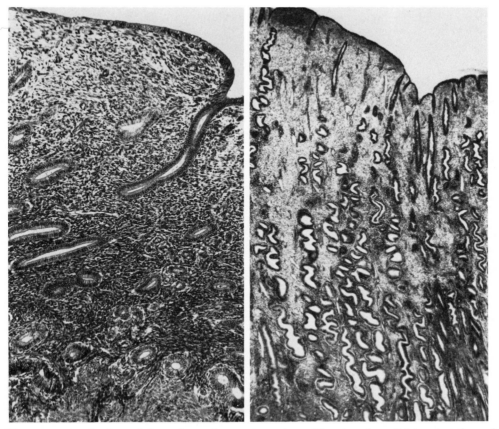

Figure 15–22. Sections of the endometrium at the early proliferative phase (*left*) and at the early secretory phase (*right*). Note the cellular stroma in the former and the increased thickness of the endometrium in the latter. Left, × 50; right, × 25.

499

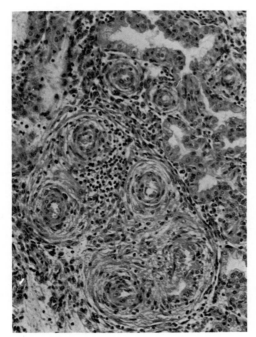

Figure 15–23. Horizontal section through the endometrium during the secretory phase of the cycle. Note the prominent coiled arteries in the stroma. × 100.

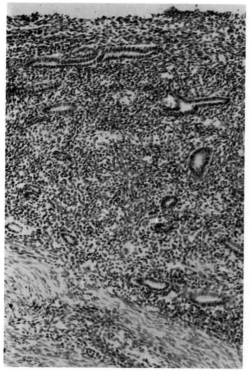

Figure 15–24. Section of the endometrium at the termination of the menstrual stage. Only the basal layer, consisting of the torn ends of uterine glands and a dense stroma, remains. Beneath is a portion of myometrium. × 100.

with the formation and activity of the corpus luteum. The time lapse between its start and the onset of bleeding is quite uniform, regardless of the length of the cycle. The onset of bleeding corresponds to the beginning involution of the corpus luteum.

In certain instances the ovary may not produce a ripe follicle in the course of a cycle. Nevertheless bleeding will occur, but from a proliferative endometrium at the expected time. Such a cycle is known as an *anovulatory cycle*.

The Uterus During Pregnancy

The fertilized ovum undergoes segmentation as it moves down the fallopian tube and enters the uterus. By this time several cell divisions have occurred, and it consists of a mass of cells. A cavity appears within the cellular mass, after which it is called a *blastocyst*. The blastocyst becomes implanted within the endometrium six or seven days after ovulation. At this time, the endometrium is in the progestational phase. It is thick and edematous and the glands are large and swollen with secretion. The site of implantation may be anywhere on the wall of the uterus but usually it is high up toward the fundus.

The blastocyst wall is composed of a single layer of cells, called the *trophoblast*, with, in the cavity of the blastocyst, an *inner cell mass*. The inner cell mass will not be considered further here since it is from this mass that the embryo is destined to form. As the blastocyst attaches to the endometrium, trophoblast cells proliferate and the trophoblast becomes several cells thick. The uterine epithelium breaks down at the point of attachment, and the blastocyst sinks into the endometrial stroma. The defect in the endometrium is closed temporarily by a plug of fibrin, but later the endometrial epithelium grows over the embedded blastocyst to restore continuity of the uterine lining.

Once the blastocyst becomes embedded within the endometrium, the trophoblast over the entire surface proliferates and by the eleventh day after ovulation it consists of two layers of cells. The inner layer of cells, the *cytotrophoblast*, is composed of cells with clearly defined cell boundaries. The outer layer is thicker and consists of a multinucleated protoplasmic mass, the *syncytial trophoblast.* From the surface of the syncytial trophoblast, epithelial cords extend out into the surrounding space. These are the *primary (primitive) villi.* Later primitive embryonic connective tissue comes into relation with the trophoblast, and the two layers together constitute the *chorion.* Connective tissue, containing fetal blood vessels, extends into the villi, which now are termed *secondary (chorionic) villi.*

Villi on the deeply embedded surface of the blastocyst grow rapidly and form the fetal component of the placenta, the *chorion frondosum.* Villi of the chorion frondosum are attached to a firm portion of the chorion, the *chorionic plate.* Villi on the surface of the chorion facing the uterine cavity do not grow as rapidly as on the deeply embedded surface, and they degenerate by the end of the third month of pregnancy. This portion of the chorion is known as the *chorion laeve.*

The endometrium also shows impor-tant structural changes during pregnancy. Since all the endometrium, except the deepest layer, is destined to be shed at parturition, the endometrium in a pregnant uterus is referred to as *decidua.* Three regions of the decidua are distinguished: overlying the blastocyst is the *decidua capsularis;* underlying it is the *decidua basalis;* all the remaining mucosa of the body of the uterus is the *decidua parietalis.* It is the decidua basalis which becomes the maternal component of the placenta. In the early part of pregnancy the endometrium increases in thickness. A characteristic feature is the presence of *decidual cells,* which are enlarged stromal cells. The cytoplasm is vesicular or finely granular and contains large amounts of glycogen. The function of these cells is obscure.

As chorionic villi grow into the decidua basalis, they destroy and erode endometrium, leaving spaces or *lacunae.* With further enlargement of villi, lacunae become interconnecting and contain blood liberated by penetration of the maternal vessels by the trophoblast.

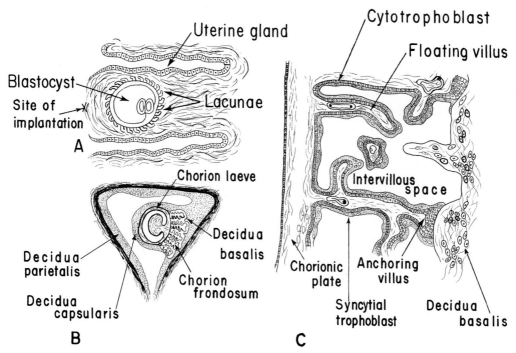

Figure 15–25. Series of diagrams, illustrating the relationships of the blastocyst to the uterus. *A,* Newly implanted blastocyst within the endometrium. *B,* Components of the decidua. *C,* Small segment of the early placenta, showing fetal and maternal contributions.

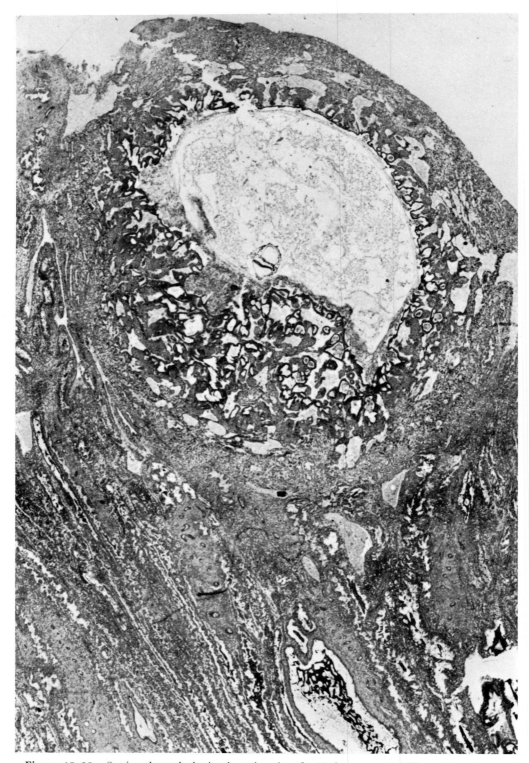

Figure 15–26.   Section through the implantation site of a 15-day ovum. A differentiating inner cell mass lies within a large trophoblast cavity. The trophoblast, which is invading the endometrium, already shows more extensive development toward the decidua basalis (chorion frondosum) than toward the decidua capsularis (chorion laeve). × 15.

Diffusion of dissolved substances now can occur between the maternal blood in the lacunae and fetal blood in the capillaries of the villi.

The Placenta

By 16 weeks, the chorion frondosum is well developed and the placenta is discoid in shape. It continues to increase in size throughout most of the gestational period owing mainly to growth of the villi. It consists of two components, a fetal and a maternal. The fetal component consists of the chorionic plate and the villi which arise from the plate. The villi lie in lacunae through which maternal blood circulates. Villi usually are classified into two types, *anchoring villi* and *free villi*. Anchoring villi pass from the chorionic plate to the decidua basalis. They give

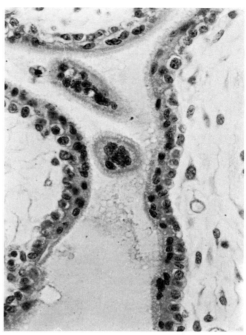

Figure 15–28. Portions of three chorionic villi during the third week of pregnancy. The trophoblast covering each villus consists of a complete layer of cytotrophoblast (cells with pale nuclei) and a layer of syncytial trophoblast, the cytoplasm of which contains numerous dark nuclei. The irregularity at the surface of the syncytial trophoblast is artifactual but is indicative of a microvillous border. × 250.

rise to branches which float in the lacunae.

Villi are alike histologically. In the loose connective tissue core of each villus there is a fetal capillary lined with typical endothelium. Large cells with large spherical nuclei (*cells of Hofbauer*) also are present in the cores; possibly they are phagocytic cells. The trophoblast covering each villus consists of two layers until approximately the tenth week of pregnancy, after which time the cytotrophoblast progressively disappears until at parturition only isolated clumps of its cells remain.

The cytotrophoblast, also called *Langhans' layer*, rests upon a basal lamina and consists of large, discrete, pale cells. The cytoplasm contains vacuoles and some glycogen. Desmosomal contacts occur between adjacent cytotrophoblast cells and between cytotrophoblast and syncytial trophoblast layers. It is generally accepted that growth and mitotic activity of the cytotrophoblast are responsible for the de-

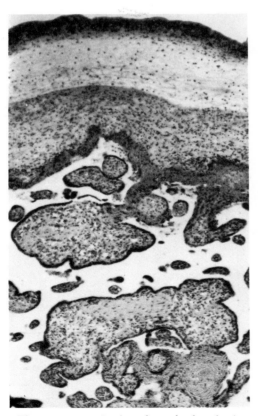

Figure 15–27. Section through the chorion frondosum during the fourth week of pregnancy. Above is a portion of the chorionic plate; below are sections through numerous villi, each containing a core of primitive mesenchyme. × 40.

velopment of the syncytial trophoblast, a dark layer of variable thickness in which numerous small dark nuclei are present. No intercellular boundaries can be distinguished. In some places the outer surface possesses microvilli. The cytoplasm is dense and contains abundant granular endoplasmic reticulum and numerous primary and secondary lysosomes. In the latter half of pregnancy the syncytial trophoblast thins out over the fetal capillaries to form a narrow layer. In other regions it often becomes aggregated into protuberances called *syncytial knots* or *sprouts.* On the surface of the villi irregular masses of an eosinophil, homogeneous substance called *fibrinoid,* are present. This becomes increasingly abundant in older placentae.

The maternal component of the placenta is the decidua basalis. The enlarged endometrial stromal cells are known as decidual cells. Epithelial cells lining the glands are rich in glycogen and lipid droplets. By the third month,

the glands of the decidua basalis become stretched and appear as horizontal clefts. Passing through the decidua basalis are spiral arteries which open into the intervillous space. The decidua is eroded more deeply opposite the anchoring villi than elsewhere, and this leaves projections of decidual tissue between the main villi. Such projections are termed *placental septa,* and they divide the placenta into lobules or *cotyledons.* From the fourth month on, the decidua basalis becomes loose in texture owing to the development of a dense venous plexus within it.

Functions of the Placenta. The placenta transfers from the maternal to the fetal circulation the nutritive and other substances necessary for the growth of the embryo. It also transfers waste products of fetal metabolism to the maternal circulation. The maternal circulation is separated from the fetal circulation only by the syncytial trophoblast, the cytotrophoblast (in the first trimester of pregnancy only), the

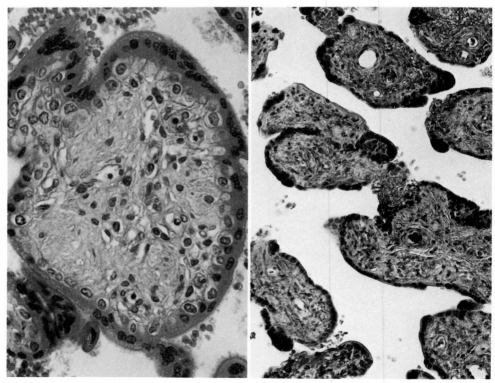

Figure 15–29. *Left:* Section of a villus during the third month of pregnancy. The dense nuclei and dense (acidophil) cytoplasm of the syncytial trophoblast are prominent. Beneath this layer the pale cells with distinct cell boundaries comprise the cytotrophoblast, which already shows evidence of discontinuity. × 250. *Right:* The appearance of villi during the eighth month of pregnancy. Cytotrophoblast is not evident and the syncytial trophoblast is thinned and forms prominent syncytial knots. × 100.

basal lamina of the trophoblast, fetal connective tissue, the basal lamina of the fetal capillaries, and the fetal endothelium. These structures comprise the so-called *placental barrier,* which is selective against particulate matter, such as microorganisms, and against chemical substances over a certain molecular size.

The placenta elaborates hormones: it secretes estrogen, progesterone, and *chorionic gonadotropin.* All these hormones are thought to be synthesized by the syncytial trophoblast. The cytotrophoblast, previously considered to be active in the synthesis of hormones, apparently functions chiefly in the formation of the syncytial trophoblast.

The Cervix

The cervix is the lowest segment of the uterus. The mucous membrane of the cervical canal, which shows branching folds on its surface, comprises an epithelium and a lamina propria. The epithelium consists of tall, mucus-secreting columnar cells. The oval nuclei lie at the bases of the cells and the cytoplasm above is pale. Some of the cells are ciliated. Numerous large, branching glands extend into the lamina propria. The glands sometimes become transformed into large cysts, the *nabothian follicles.* The lamina propria is a cellular connective tissue that contains no coiled arteries.

The portion of the cervix which projects into the vagina is covered by stratified squamous nonkeratinizing epithelium. The transition between the simple columnar epithelium of the cervical canal and the stratified squamous epithelium of the portio vaginalis is abrupt and occurs usually just inside the cervical canal. The mucosa of the cervical canal does not desquamate during menstruation, although minor

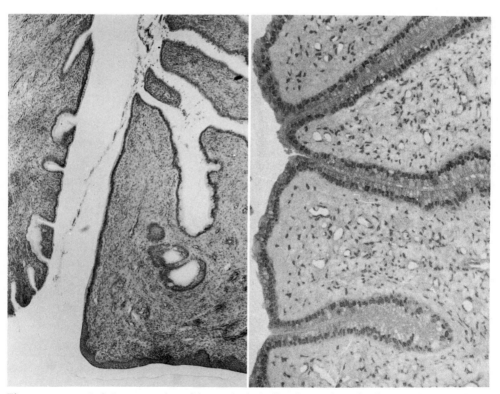

Figure 15–30. *Left:* Lower portion of the cervix, including the portio vaginalis. Note the cervical glands and the transition between the simple columnar epithelium of the cervical canal and the stratified squamous epithelium of the portio vaginalis. × 35. *Right:* The simple columnar epithelium of the cervical canal and glands. Note the basally situated nuclei within the epithelium and the delicate lamina propria. Plastic section. × 125.

changes in the structure of the cervical glands do occur. During pregnancy, the glands secrete large amounts of a more viscous secretion that forms a plug in the cervical canal.

The mucosa rests upon a myometrium which is composed chiefly of dense collagenous connective tissue. Smooth muscle present is arranged mainly in irregular bundles. The thin outer longitudinal layer continues into the vagina.

THE VAGINA

The vagina is a fibromuscular sheath lined with a mucous membrane. Under ordinary conditions it is collapsed and the anterior and posterior walls are in contact. The walls of the vagina consist of three coats: mucosa, muscularis, and adventitia.

The mucosa exhibits transverse folds,

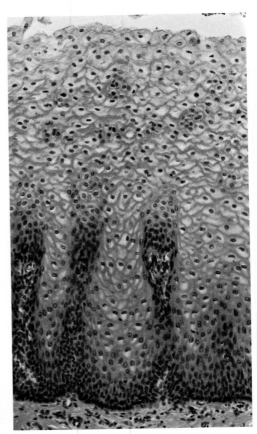

Figure 15–32. Portion of the vaginal mucosa. Note the depth of the epithelium, many component cells of which appear vacuolated, and the well-developed papillae of the lamina propria. × 100.

or *rugae*. It is lined with thick, stratified squamous epithelium which is nonkeratinizing. Component cells are loaded with glycogen and thus they appear vacuolated in most histological sections. The epithelium, which lacks glands, is lubricated by mucus which originates from the cervix. Beneath the epithelium there is a lamina propria which is a dense connective tissue containing numerous elastic fibers, polymorphonuclear leukocytes, lymphocytes, and occasional lymph nodules. Many lymphocytes and polymorphonuclear leukocytes invade the epithelium, especially around the time of menstruation.

The surface cells of the vaginal epithelium are desquamated continuously and may be studied by the smear method. In subhuman primates and many other mammals, the vaginal epithelium undergoes cyclic changes correlated with other events of the

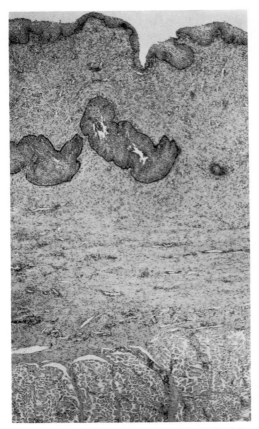

Figure 15–31. Section through the wall of the vagina, showing mucosa and a portion of the muscularis. × 25.

reproductive cycle. In the human, the epithelium varies little during the cycle, although the study of desquamated vaginal cells is useful in the diagnosis of atrophic conditions and in evaluation of the effectiveness of estrogen therapy.

The muscularis of the vagina is composed of smooth muscle fibers which are arranged in interlacing bundles. The inner portion, where most muscle bundles are circularly arranged, is thin. The thick outer portion contains longitudinal bundles which are continuous above with the myometrium of the uterus. At the introitus there is a sphincter of skeletal muscle.

The adventitia is a thin layer of dense connective tissue which blends with that of surrounding organs.

The *hymen*, a transverse fold of the mucosa, partially occludes the opening of the vagina into the vestibule.

Blood Vessels, Lymphatics, and Nerves

Blood vessels and lymphatic vessels are abundant in the wall of the vagina. Veins are particularly numerous and give the adventitia the appearance of erectile tissue.

The vagina receives both myelinated and unmyelinated nerve fibers. The latter form a ganglionated plexus in the adventitia and supply the muscularis and the walls of blood vessels. Myelinated nerve fibers terminate in special sensory endings in the mucosa.

THE EXTERNAL GENITALIA

The external genitalia, known collectively as the *vulva*, comprise the clitoris, the labia majora and minora, and certain glands which open into the vestibule.

The *clitoris* is a rudimentary and incomplete counterpart of the penis. It consists of two cavernous, erectile bodies which end in a rudimentary *glans clitoridis*. It is covered with a thin, stratified squamous epithelium that is associated with specialized sensory nerve endings.

The *labia minora* are folds of mucous

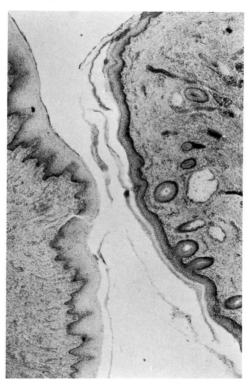

Figure 15–33. Section through portions of the labium minus (left) and the labium majus (right). The former is covered with nonkeratinized stratified squamous epithelium, the latter with cornified epidermis containing sweat and sebaceous glands. × 25.

membrane which form the lateral walls of the vestibule. They are covered with a stratified squamous epithelium and have a core of richly vascularized connective tissue. Tall papillae of connective tissue penetrate far into the epithelium. Sebaceous glands occur on both surfaces of the fold, which is devoid of hair follicles.

The *labia majora* are folds of skin that cover the labia minora externally. The inner surface is smooth and hairless. The outer surface is covered with cornified epidermis which contains numerous hairs, sweat glands and sebaceous glands. The core of each fold contains a considerable amount of adipose tissue and some smooth muscle fibers.

The *vestibule*, into which the vagina and urethra open, is lined by a typical stratified squamous epithelium and contains numerous small glands, the *minor vestibular glands*. These are located mainly around the urethral opening and near the clitoris. They resemble the urethral glands (of Littre). The *major vestibular glands (glands of Bartholin)*, analogous to the bulbourethral glands in the male, are located in the lateral walls of the vestibule. They are tubuloalveolar glands which secrete lubricating mucus. Their ducts open near the base of the hymen.

THE MAMMARY GLAND

The mammary gland is a specialized, cutaneous gland located within the subcutaneous tissue. It is a modified sweat gland and is said to have an apocrine type of secretion (*vide infra*). Mammary glands are present in both sexes and they develop only slightly during childhood. At puberty the glands enlarge rapidly in the female, principally as a result of development of adipose and other connective tissue, but very slowly in the male. The glands remain incompletely developed in the female until

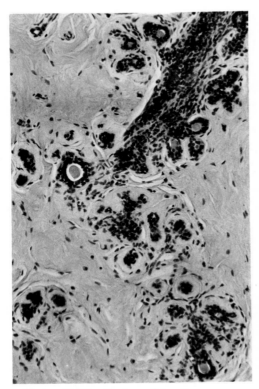

Figure 15–34. Section of inactive mammary gland. The lobules, which are composed principally of ducts, are separated by abundant interlobular connective tissue. × 100.

pregnancy occurs. After puberty there is no further development of the gland in the male.

The gland consists of 15 to 20 lobes, each of which actually is an independent gland with a duct opening at the apex of the nipple. A lobe is surrounded by interlobar connective tissue containing many fat cells. The fat and connective tissue also divide each lobe into numerous lobules. The intralobular connective tissue is loose, delicate, and cellular. Intralobular ducts drain into interlobular ducts, which join to form a single excretory duct from each lobe, the *lactiferous duct*. The lactiferous duct courses through the nipple and dilates near its termination at the summit of the nipple into a *lactiferous sinus*.

Areola and Nipple

The nipple is traversed by lactiferous ducts, each of which opens by a pore on the surface. There are fewer pores than main ducts, owing to terminal fusions. The skin of the nipple is pigmented, and the underlying dermis is characterized by the presence of tall papillae and smooth muscle fibers. Contraction of the muscle hardens and elevates the nipple. The *areola*, an area of skin extending outward from the nipple, is pigmented and contains special *areolar glands (glands of Montgomery)*, which are large, branched glands of the apocrine type. Sweat and sebaceous glands and a number of coarse hairs are present also.

Parenchyma

The parenchyma of the mammary gland shows extensive structural changes which are dependent upon the functional condition.

The Inactive Mammary Gland

The ducts are the principal epithelial tissue seen. Intralobular ducts are grouped together into lobules. The lining of the ducts changes from a simple cuboidal to a two-layered epithelium from the small to the main ducts. Alveoli, if present, are small buds. Be-

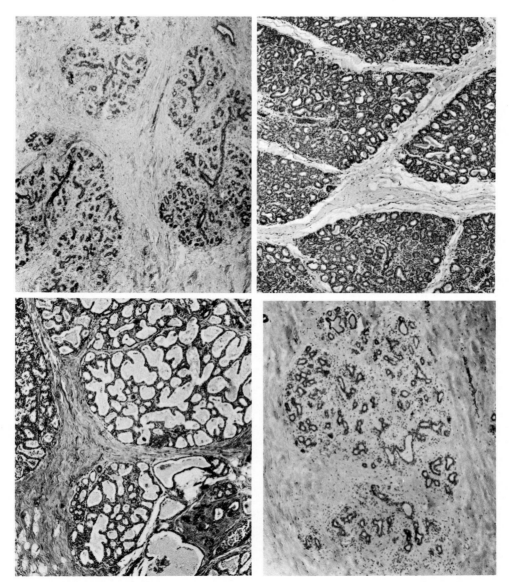

Figure 15–35. Sections of the breast, illustrating the different histological pictures during varying functional conditions. *Top left:* During the fourth month of pregnancy. *Top right:* Immediately after parturition. *Bottom left:* During lactation. *Bottom right:* After cessation of lactation. Note the degree of development of the lobules during these functional states. After cessation of lactation (bottom right) the breast does not return completely to the nulliparous state (compare with Figure 15–34). × 25.

tween the epithelium and the basal lamina there is a layer of myoepithelial cells. Intralobular connective tissue is dense and abundant and contains varying amounts of adipose tissue.

The Mammary Gland During Pregnancy

The gland exhibits extensive changes in preparation for lactation. In the first half of pregnancy, intralobular ducts undergo rapid proliferation and form buds which enlarge into alveoli. Owing to the expansion of lobules, interlobular fat and connective tissue decrease in amount and the 15 to 20 lobes become distinct entities. Intralobular connective tissue also decreases in amount and becomes infiltrated with lymphocytes. During the second half of pregnancy, alveoli enlarge and begin to elaborate some secretory material. At the end of pregnancy some cloudy, watery fluid, *colostrum,* is secreted.

During pregnancy increased pigmentation occurs in the skin of the nipple and areola.

The Mammary Gland During Lactation

Soon after parturition, the mammary gland begins active secretion of milk, which is rich in fat, sugar, and protein. Many alveoli become dilated and appear as saccules. They are distended by milk and have a low epithelial wall. Other alveoli are resting; they have a relatively tall epithelial lining and small lumina. Individual alveolar cells, which contain an extensive system of granular endoplasmic reticulum and numerous free ribosomes, undergo a cyclic process of secretion. The secretory process appears to be partly merocrine and partly apocrine. Milk proteins are synthesized within the granular endoplasmic reticulum and are condensed into small vacuoles within the Golgi complex. The granules move to the apical surface, where they are released by exocytosis. This process, which involves no loss of cytoplasm or of cell membrane, is merocrine in type. The fatty components of milk are elab-

orated and discharged in a different manner. Small fat droplets appear within the cytoplasm and later coalesce to form large fat globules at the cell apex. As these globules are released, they carry with them the apical cell membrane and a thin coating of cytoplasm. This is an apocrine type of secretion, although the extent of cytoplasmic loss is less marked than in most glands of this type. The secretory cycle is then repeated.

The lumen of each alveolus is filled with these two types of discharged cellular products suspended in a watery fluid. The alveolar epithelium rests upon a basal lamina. Between the alveolar cells and the basal lamina are stellate *basket* (myoepithelial) *cells.* These are thought to be contractile and to aid in the movement of milk from the alveoli into the ducts.

Intralobular ducts histologically appear similar to alveoli. Functionally they are true secretory ducts which also possess myoepithelial elements.

Regression

After cessation of lactation, the gland undergoes retrogressive changes and returns to a resting state. Alveoli decrease in size and some cells degen-

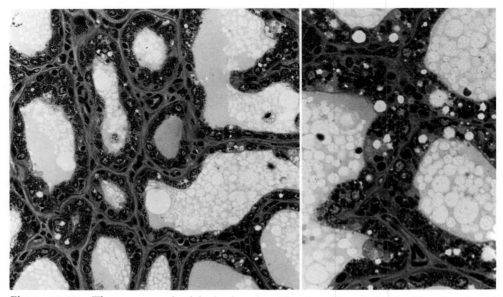

Figure 15–36. The mammary gland during lactation. Alveoli are distended with milk and are lined by a low epithelium. The cytoplasm of epithelial cells is crowded with dense granules and large lipid globules. Plastic sections. Left, × 250; right, × 400.

erate. Connective tissue and fat again become abundant. However, the gland usually does not return to the nulliparous state; many alveoli remain recognizable as such and remnants of secretory material may be retained within the ducts for a considerable time.

Involution

After the menopause, the mammary gland undergoes involution. The secretory epithelium atrophies and only a few remnants of the duct system persist. Cystic dilatation of the remaining ducts occurs frequently. The connective tissue becomes increasingly dense and homogeneous.

Hormonal Control

Growth of the duct system which occurs at puberty is influenced by estrogen and progesterone secreted cyclically by the ovaries. Further growth of the gland in pregnancy is due to continuous and prolonged production of both estrogen and progesterone by the ovaries and placenta. The initiation of secretion seems to be induced by the lactogenic hormone (prolactin) of the pars distalis of the hypophysis. Maintenance of lactation appears to depend upon a number of hormones. Oxytocin, a posterior pituitary hormone, causes contraction of the myoepithelial cells in the gland, leading to ejection of milk from alveoli and ducts. Secretion of oxytocin is initiated by nerve impulses reaching the hypothalamus following stimulation of tactile receptors in the nipple area.

Blood Vessels, Lymphatics, and Nerves

Blood vessels enter the gland from several sources, ramify in the stroma, and terminate in rich capillary plexuses around the ducts and alveoli. The vascular supply becomes much richer in the active gland. From the capillaries, veins arise which accompany the arteries.

Lymph vessels are found in the areola, around the ducts, and in the interlobular connective tissue. Collecting lymphatics pass to the axillary nodes; a few penetrate the intercostal spaces and follow the branches of the internal thoracic artery.

Afferent nerve fibers supply the tactile organs of the nipple. Some nerve fibers follow the interlobular connective tissue and form delicate plexuses around the alveoli.

EMBRYOLOGY OF THE MALE AND FEMALE REPRODUCTIVE SYSTEMS

The primordia of the gonads arise as thickenings of mesodermal epithelium, the *genital ridges,* on the mesial surface of the mesonephros. The epithelial cells of the ridge proliferate and form a band of tissue composed of two types of cells. Most cells are small, cuboidal elements and scattered between them are large, spheroidal cells, the *primitive sex cells.* The epithelial cells penetrate the underlying mesenchyme and form *sex cords.*

In the male human embryo the testis becomes recognizable at about seven weeks. The sex cords become more distinct and elongate to form the seminiferous tubules. Their peripheral ends anastomose and unite with a number of mesonephric tubules to form the rete testis. Prior to the onset of puberty component cells of the seminiferous tubules differentiate into spermatogonia and Sertoli cells.

Differentiation of the ovary does not commence until about the eighth week of gestation. The sex cords formed during the indifferent stage gradually disappear. The covering (germinal) epithelium continues to proliferate and produces the primitive cortex of the ovary. This mass of cortical cells is subdivided by strands of mesenchyme into clusters containing oogonia, probably derived from the primitive sex cells. Proliferation of cortical tissue continues into the latter half of fetal life.

Genital ducts develop in close connection with the embryonic urinary system. They are laid down initially as two paired longitudinal ducts, the *ducts of Wolff* and *of Müller,* the latter from mesoderm lining the coelomic cavity. In the male the wolffian duct is transformed into ductus epididymidis and ductus deferens. Connection of the ductus epididymidis with the rete testis is established by a number of mesonephric tubules which become the ductuli efferentes. The müllerian duct involutes, leaving only small rudiments. In the female, the wolffian ducts regress and the müllerian ducts transform into the female genital ducts. Caudally the two müllerian ducts fuse to form a single tube which opens into the urogenital sinus (cloaca). The paired upper portions form the fallopian tubes and the unpaired terminal portion becomes the uterus and vagina.

In man, as in most mammals, the XY and XX sex chromosome complements determine male and female sex, respectively. In the former, the genetic determinant on the Y chromosome is responsible for differentiation of the indifferent gonad into a testis, which otherwise develops as an ovary. The differentiating testis produces sub-stances that suppress müllerian duct development and promote wolffian duct differentiation. In the absence of a testis, müllerian ducts differentiate and wolffian ducts fail to undergo differentiation.

Vestigial Structures

Certain vestigial structures occur in relation to the ovary.

The *epoophoron* consists of several blind tubules situated in the broad ligament between the ovary and the fallopian tube. The tubules fuse into a longitudinal canal, the *duct of Gartner,* which passes along the lateral wall of the uterus.

The *paroophoron,* consisting of a few blind tubules, lies in the connective tissue of the broad ligament close to the hilum.

Both epoophoron and paroophoron are remnants of mesonephric tubules. Gartner's duct represents a remnant of the mesonephric duct.

REFERENCES

Adams, E. C., and Hertig, A. T.: Studies on the human corpus luteum. 1. Observations on the ultrastructure of development and regression of the luteal cells during the menstrual cycle. J. Cell Biol., 41:696, 1969.

Adams, E. C., and Hertig, A. T.: Studies on the human corpus luteum. II. Observations on the ultrastructure of luteal cells during pregnancy. J. Cell Biol., 41:716, 1969.

Anderson, E., and Albertini, D.: Gap junctions between the oocyte and companion follicle cells in the mammalian ovary. J. Cell Biol., 71:680, 1976.

Boyd, J. D., and Hamilton, W. J.: Development of the human placenta in the first three months of gestation. J. Anat., 94:297, 1960.

Boyd, J. D., Hamilton, W. J., and Boyd, C. A. R.: The surface of the syncytium of the human chorionic villus. J. Anat., 102:553, 1968.

Crisp, T. M., Dessouky, A. D., and Denys, F. R.: The fine structure of the human corpus luteum of early pregnancy and during the progestational phase of the menstrual cycle. Am. J. Anat., 127:37, 1970.

Enders, A. C., and Schlafke, S.: Cytological aspects of trophoblast-uterine interaction in early implantation. Am. J. Anat., 125:1, 1969.

Gregoire, A. T., Kandil, O., and Ledger, W. J.: The glycogen content of human vaginal epithelial tissue. Fertil. Steril., 22:64, 1971.

Gruenwald, P.: The development of the sex cords in the gonads of man and mammals. Am. J. Anat., 70:359, 1942.

Hertig, A. T., and Adams, E. C.: Studies on the human oocyte and its follicle. I. Ultrastructural and histochemical observations on the primordial follicle stage. J. Cell Biol., 34:647, 1967.

Hertig, A. T., and Rock, J.: Two human ova of the previllous stage, having a developmental age of about seven and nine days respectively. Contributions to Embryology No. 200, Carnegie Institution of Washington Publ. No. 557, 31:67, 1945.

Hertig, A. T., Rock, J., and Adams, E. G.: A description of 34 human ova within the first 17 days of development. Am. J. Anat., 98:435, 1956.

Kurosumi, K., Kobayashi, Y., and Baba, N.: The fine structure of mammary glands of lactating rats, with special reference to the apocrine secretion. Exp. Cell Res., 50:117, 1968.

Linzell, J. L.: The silver staining of myoepithelial cells particularly in the mammary gland, and their relation to the ejection of milk. J. Anat., 86:49, 1952.

Nilsson, O.: Electron microscopy of the glandular epithelium in the human uterus. I. Follicular phase. J. Ultrastruct. Res., 6:413, 1962.

Nilsson, W.: Electron microscopy of the glandular epithelium in the human uterus. II. Early and late luteal phase. J. Ultrastruct. Res., 6:422, 1962.

Papanicolaou, G. N.: The sexual cycle in the human female as revealed by vaginal smears. Am. J. Anat., 52:519, 1933.

Papanicolaou, G. N.: Atlas of Exfoliative Cytology. Cambridge, Mass., Harvard University Press, 1954.

Patek, E., Nilsson, L., and Johannisson, E.: Scanning electron microscopic study of the human fallopian tube. Report I. The proliferative and secretory stages. Fertil. Steril., 23:459, 1972.

Patek, E., Nilsson, L., and Johannisson, E.: Scanning electron microscopic study of the human fallopian tube. Report II. Fetal life, reproductive life, and postmenopause. Fertil. Steril., 23:719, 1972.

Pitelka, D. R., Hamamoto, S. T., Duafala, J. G., and Nemanic, M. K.: Cell contacts in the mouse mammary gland. I. Normal gland in postnatal development and the secretory cycle. J. Cell Biol., 56:797, 1973.

Rock, J., and Hertig, A. T.: The human conceptus during the first two weeks of gestation. Am. J. Obstet. Gynecol., 55:6, 1948.

Schlafke, S., and Enders, A. C.: Cellular basis of interaction between trophoblast and uterus at implantation. Biol. Reprod., 12:41, 1975.

Wimsatt, W. A.: Some comparative aspects of implantation. Biol. Reprod., 12:1, 1975.

Wislocki, G. B., and Bennett, H. S.: The histology and cytology of the human and monkey placenta, with special reference to the trophoblast. Am. J. Anat., 73:335, 1943.

Wooding, F. B. P.: The mechanism of secretion of the milk fat globule. J. Cell Sci., 9:805, 1971.

Wooding, F. B. P.: The structure of the milk fat globule membrane. J. Ultrastruct. Res., 37:388, 1971.

CHAPTER
16

THE MALE REPRODUCTIVE SYSTEM

The male reproductive system comprises the testis, the ducts of the testis, the auxiliary glands associated with them, and the penis.

THE TESTIS

The testis is a double gland since functionally it is both exocrine and endocrine. The exocrine product is chiefly the sex cells, and thus the testis may be referred to as a cytogenic gland. The endocrine product is an internal secretion elaborated by certain specialized cells. The testis is suspended within the scrotum and is immediately surrounded by the *testicular capsule*, composed of three layers. The outer component, the *tunica vaginalis*, is a

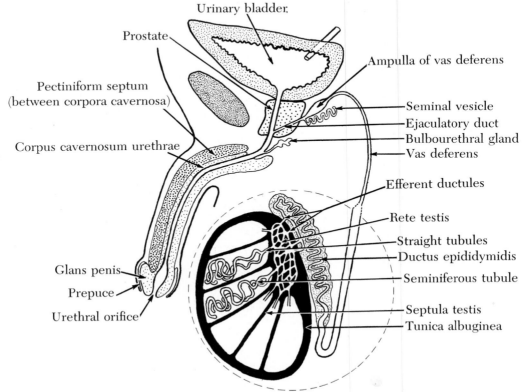

Urinary bladder.

Prostate

Ampulla of vas deferens

Pectiniform septum
(between corpora cavernosa)

Seminal vesicle
Ejaculatory duct
Bulbourethral gland
Vas deferens

Corpus cavernosum urethrae

Efferent ductules

Rete testis

Straight tubules
Ductus epididymidis

Glans penis

Seminiferous tubule

Prepuce

Urethral orifice

Septula testis
Tunica albuginea

Figure 16–1. Diagram of the male reproductive system. The portions of the system within the circle are represented as more highly magnified than the other components of the system.

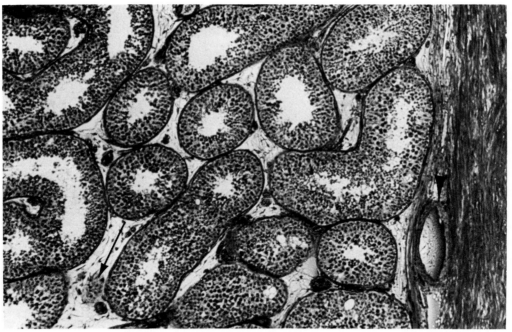

Figure 16–2. Low-power photomicrograph of a portion of a section of human testis. The seminiferous tubules, bordered by a distinct boundary (peritubular) tissue, are lined by a stratified seminiferous epithelium and are embedded within a loose, vascular connective tissue containing occasional groups of specific interstitial (Leydig) cells (arrow). Portions of the tunica albuginea and the tunica vasculosa (broad arrowhead) lie to the right. ×65.

single layer of attenuated mesothelial cells which frequently are destroyed during preparation. This layer is part of a closed serous sac that surrounds the anterior and lateral surfaces of the testis. It rests upon a basal lamina that separates it from the middle and most prominent layer, the *tunica albuginea.* In the past, the tunica albuginea has been described as a thick layer of dense fibroelastic connective tissue, but recently it has been shown to contain some smooth muscle cells also. In the human, although the smooth muscle elements are widely scattered, they are concentrated predominantly on the posterior aspect of the testis adjacent to the epididymis. The innermost layer of the testicular capsule, the *tunica vasculosa,* consists of networks of blood vessels embedded within a delicate areolar connective tissue. Recent studies indicate that the testicular capsule is not, as previously thought, an inert covering to the testis but it acts as a dynamic membrane capable of periodic contractions. The contractions probably serve to maintain the correct pressure within the testis, regulating movement of fluid out of, and back into, the capillaries, and to massage the duct system and thus aid in the movement of spermatozoa in an outward direction. Additionally, the capsule appears to posses the characteristics of a semipermeable membrane and to be involved in several aspects of testicular physiology.

The tunica albuginea is thickened along the posterior surface of the testis where it projects into the gland as the *mediastinum testis.* Thin, fibrous partitions radiate from the mediastinum testis to the capsule and divide the interior of the testis into about 250 pyramidal compartments, the *lobuli testis,* with their apices toward the mediastinum. The septa show numerous deficiencies and the lobules thus intercommunicate quite freely. Each lobule contains one to four highly convoluted *seminiferous tubules,* which are embedded in a loose connective tissue stroma containing vessels, nerves, and several types of cells, principally the specific *interstitial cells* (of

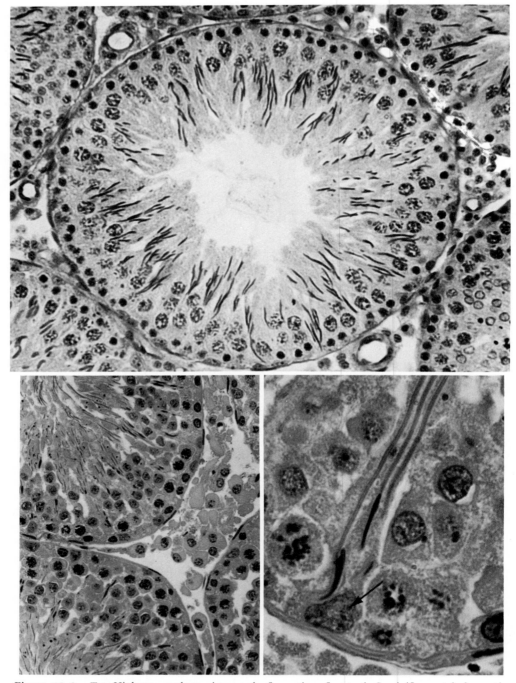

Figure 16–3. *Top*: High-power photomicrograph of a portion of rat testis. Seminiferous tubules, cut in cross section, are separated by a slight amount of interstitial connective tissue containing groups of Leydig cells. ×300. *Bottom left:* Portion of four tubules, showing component cells of the germinal epithelium. Note the interstitial cells between tubules. Plastic section. ×300. *Bottom right:* Portion of one tubule, showing boundary tissue, spermatocytes, spermatids, and spermatozoa in relationship to the cytoplasm of a Sertoli cell. The nucleus of the latter is indicated by an arrow. Plastic section. ×1300.

Leydig). These are large cells, commonly in groups, and are important because of their endocrine role.

Seminiferous Tubules

Each seminiferous tubule is highly convoluted and is about 0.2 mm in diameter and 30 to 70 cm long. The tubules commence as free blind ends or as anastomosing loops either with neighboring tubules of the lobule or, less frequently, with tubules of adjoining lobules. At the apex of a lobule, each tubule loses its convolutions and becomes a *straight tubule.* The seminiferous tubule is lined by a complex germinal or seminiferous epithelium, which is a modified stratified cuboidal epithelium. The epithelium rests upon a thin basal lamina and is covered externally by a specialized zone of fibrous tissue, the so-called boundary or peritubular tissue, which contains numerous connective tissue fibers, flattened fibroblasts, and some cells with the characteristics of smooth muscle

cells. These myoid elements exhibit junctional complexes between neighboring cells that retard, but do not entirely prevent, the passage of macromolecules from the interstitial space to the seminiferous epithelium. It is thought that the myoid cells, by their contraction, may alter the diameter of the seminiferous tubule and aid in the movement of spermatozoa along the length of the tubule. The thickness of this zone varies with age and shows a great increase in extent in many clinical conditions, particularly those associated with some chromosomal abnormalities (such as Klinefelter's syndrome). An extensive system of lymphatic capillaries lies external to the boundary tissue.

The seminiferous epithelium contains two distinct categories of cells, the nutrient and supporting elements, and the germ or spermatogenic cells. The latter form the vast bulk of the epithelium and, by proliferation and complex differentiation, give rise to the spermatozoa.

Supporting Elements. The supporting cells, or *sustentacular cells* of

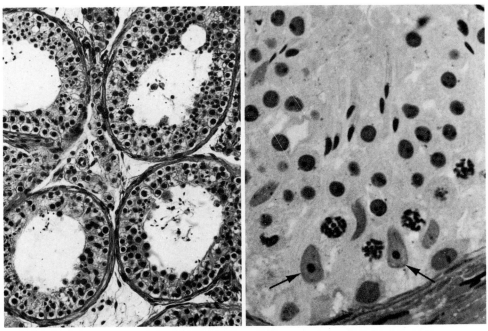

Figure 16–4. Human testis. *Left:* The wide lumina of the seminiferous tubules contain some spermatozoa. The boundary tissue around the tubules and groups of Leydig cells in the interstitial connective tissue are seen clearly. ×160. *Right:* A portion of a tubule showing dense nuclei of spermatogonia in relation to the boundary tissue (below), nuclei of Sertoli cells (arrows), nuclei of spermatocytes in division, small rounded nuclei of numerous spermatids, and heads of developing spermatozoa. Plastic section. ×550.

Sertoli, are relatively few in number and are spaced along the tubule at fairly regular intervals, crowded between the germ cells. They are tall, pillarlike cells, with their bases resting upon the basal lamina of the tubule. The cell outline is irregular, indistinct, and very complex since the heads of maturing spermatozoa lie in deep recesses of the cytoplasm. The nucleus is located some distance above the base of the cell, and is pale and ovoid with its long axis directed radially. The definite nucleolus of these cells readily distinguishes them from the spermatogenic elements within the tubule; it is prominent and of a compound nature, consisting of a central acidophil portion and smaller peripheral concentrations of basophil material. In fixed preparations, the cytoplasm has a reticular appearance and contains small fibrils, lipid droplets, small discrete granules which stain with iron hematoxylin, and small elongated mitochondria. On electron microscopy, the cytoplasm exhibits profiles of agranular endoplasmic reticulum, scattered free ribosomes, and primary and secondary lysosomes. Occasionally one can also see a tapering crystalloid body, believed to be protein in nature, near the nucleus. Where two Sertoli cells border on each other, the contiguous surfaces show complex occluding junctional specializations. Recent evidence indicates that these sites of membrane apposition and fusion, together with the peritubular tissue, constitute the morphological basis of the blood-testis barrier. The extensive junctions between Sertoli cells form a continuous barrier that is impermeable to the electron tracer, lanthanum nitrate, and in effect they define two distinct compartments within the seminiferous tubule. The basal compartment permits relatively free interchange of nutrients and other materials between the interstitial vasculature and the spermatogenic cells that lie between the junctions and the basal lamina. The adluminal compartment, beyond the level of the junctions, is isolated from such a direct interchange, and spermatogenic cells within it, which represent more differentiated stages than those within the basal compartment, must rely upon Sertoli cells for the availability of nutrients and other

substances. Additionally, the barrier prevents proteins from spermatogenic cells within the adluminal compartment from reaching the interstitial vasculature and inducing the formation of antibodies.

During their period of differentiation, spermatids (immature germ cells) attach to the sustentacular cells and apparently are nourished by them. Sustentacular cells are resistant to various noxious influences that destroy the spermatogenic cells.

Spermatogenic Cells. The germ or spermatogenic cells comprise a stratified layer of epithelium, four to eight cells deep, lining the seminiferous tubule. The cells differentiate progressively from the basal region of the tubule to the lumen. Proliferation pushes the cells toward the lumen, and those nearest the lumen transform into spermatozoa and detach from the epithelium, coming to lie free within the lumen. The sequence of events is referred to as *spermatogenesis*, which involves the two processes of cell multiplication, including reduction from the diploid to the haploid number of chromosomes, and cellular differentiation (spermiogenesis).

Spermatogenesis, a process which is thought to occupy about three weeks, commences with the *spermatogonia,** which lie immediately adjacent to the basal lamina. These are the only germ cells present until the time of puberty. Each spermatogonium contains a diploid number of chromosomes within its nucleus (44 autosomes and two sex chromosomes, XY).

Two principal types of spermatogonia are described. *Type A spermatogonia* possess ovoid nuclei with either dark or pale nucleoplasm in which chromatin granules are finely dispersed. When type A spermatogonia increase in number by a normal mitotic form of cell division, about half the daughter cells become type A spermatogonia (stem cells) and the other half become *type B spermatogonia.*

Type B spermatogonia are distinguished from type A spermatogonia by their more spherical nuclei which con-

---

*Greek: *sperma*, seed; *gonē*, generation.

tain densely stained chromatin masses in relation to the nuclear membrane. When type B spermatogonia divide by mitoses, they produce daughter cells that all eventually differentiate to become primary spermatocytes. During this process the daughter cells move away from the basal lamina, increase in size, and show a change in the character of the nucleus. More complex classifications of spermatogonia have been proposed by some authors; for example, since the number of type B spermatogonial generations in man is four, they have been designated as B_1, B_2, B_3, and B_4. However, it is convenient to consider two principal types, recognizing that type A spermatogonia constitute a reservoir of stem cells and that by mitotic activity they give rise to type B spermatogonia which further increase in number and differentiate into primary spermatocytes.

Primary spermatocytes are the largest germ cells seen within the seminiferous tubule, where they occupy the middle zone of the epithelium. Each

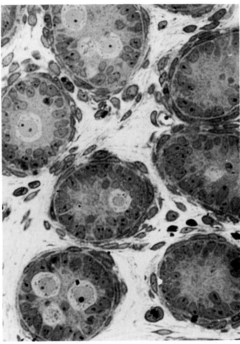

Figure 16–5. Early prepubertal testis. The seminiferous tubules appear solid and the epithelium is composed principally of Sertoli cells. The only germ cells present are spermatogonia which appear pale. The surrounding interstitium is more cellular than in the adult. Plastic section. ×325.

cell is spherical or ovoid in outline, and the nucleus is usually in some stage of karyokinesis. The cell division which occurs within primary spermatocytes is a reduction division, *meiosis*, in which whole chromosomes (synaptic mates, or the halves of the bivalent chromosomes) move to opposite poles of the spindle, unlike a somatic mitosis in which individual chromosomes split and the half chromosomes separate. As a result of the meiotic division, 23 chromosomes (22 autosomes plus one sex chromosome, either X or Y) pass into each daughter cell or *secondary spermatocyte*. The meiotic division also is peculiar in that cytokinesis is incomplete, and the two daughter cells (secondary spermatocytes) resulting from the division of a primary spermatocyte remain connected by a bridge of protoplasm. The two conjoined secondary spermatocytes later divide mitotically, and the resultant four cells (*spermatids*) remain in a syncytial cluster since cytokinesis again is incomplete.

The secondary spermatocytes are about half the volume of the primary spermatocytes and lie nearer the lumen. They are seen rarely in sections of seminiferous tubules since they are short-lived and divide quickly to produce spermatids. The division here is a somatic mitosis and a complete set of 23 chromosomes (i.e., the haploid number) is present in each spermatid. With the division, there is a further reduction in volume to half that of the secondary spermatocyte. The spermatids lie close to the lumen. No further division occurs and each spermatid is transformed by an extensive differentiation (*spermiogenesis*) into a spermatozoon. The cytoplasmic continuity between clusters of spermatids may constitute a basis for the synchrony of their later differentiation. Soon after their appearance, spermatids become closely applied to the surface of sustentacular cells, where commonly they lie in deep recesses formed by the irregular surface of sustentacular cells. In this environment they undergo metamorphosis into spermatozoa.

Spermiogenesis. The newly formed spermatid contains a centrally located spherical nucleus with a well-delineated Golgi zone nearby, numer-

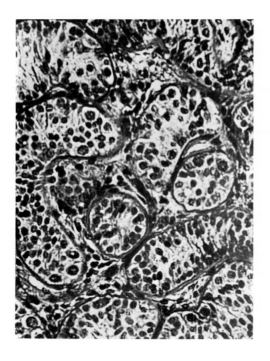

ous mitochondria, and a pair of centrioles. Spermiogenesis involves marked differentiation of all these cellular structures. Initially, several small granules appear within the numerous small vesicles of the Golgi zone. They coalesce to form a single large granule, the *acrosome*, which lies within an *acrosomal vesicle* (see Figure 16–7). This complex lies between the main components of the Golgi zone and the nucleus. The membrane bounding the acrosomal vesicle, derived from the Golgi zone, then adheres to the outer layer of the nuclear membrane. The acrosomal vesicle grows over the sur-

Figure 16–6. Photomicrograph of the human testis from a 21-year-old patient suffering from pituitary hypofunction (see page 524). The tubules show no evidence of spermatogenesis, and the appearance is similar to that of a prepubertal gland. ×275.

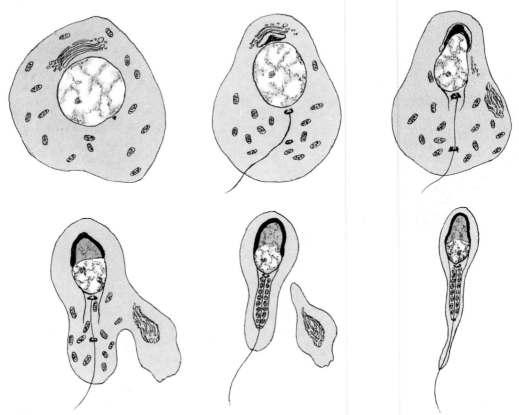

Figure 16–7. Six successvie stages in the transformation of the spermatid into the spermatozoon (spermiogenesis). The nucleus condenses to form the sperm head; the acrosome, which appears initially within the Golgi zone, gives rise to the head cap. The flagellum arises in relation to one of the centrioles, and mitochondria migrate around the flagellum to form the sheath of the middle piece.

face of the nuclear membrane and eventually covers about half of the nuclear surface. Part of the enlargement of the acrosomal vesicle and of the acrosome is contributed to by the Golgi zone, which later migrates from the region of the acrosomal vesicle and comes to lie at the opposite pole of the nucleus. With the migration of the Golgi zone, there appears to be resorption of the fluid content of the acrosomal vesicle, which collapses onto the acrosome and forms a close-fitting *head cap* over the nucleus, containing the acrosome between its layers.

As acrosome formation is in progress at one pole of the nucleus, the centrioles become associated with the nuclear membrane at the opposite pole and a slender flagellum grows out from one of them. As the flagellum grows, a thin, filamentous sheath, the *caudal tube* or *manchette,* is laid down around the axial filaments of the flagellum, and the other centriole migrates toward the cell surface and encircles the longitudinal axial filaments as a ring or *annulus.* The nucleus becomes condensed, slightly flattened, and elongated, and is displaced toward the cell membrane where it now forms the definitve sperm head. Meanwhile, there is a shift of the bulk of the cytoplasm toward the tail end of the cell. Mitochondria, until now randomly distributed in the cytoplasm, migrate to the region between the basal centriole and the annulus; there they become aligned in a spiral array or helix around the proximal portion of the flagellum as the *mitochondrial sheath,* thus delineating the *middle piece* of the future spermatozoon.

As differentiation proceeds, most of the surplus cytoplasm is cast off as the *residual body,* and only a thin layer of cytoplasm remains as a cover over the nucleus, middle piece, and tail piece of the spermatozoon. The residual bodies are thought to be phagocytosed by sustentacular cells. Their lipid content remains within the cytoplasm of sustentacular cells and probably constitutes the bulk of lipid seen in these cells to which differentiating spermatids are attached. There is some evidence to suggest that this lipid is utilized by sustentacular cells in the production of a hormone which might play an impor-

tant role in regulating spermatogenesis locally. The tail piece is similar in structure to a cilium, containing the same number and arrangement of longitudinal filaments. Upon completion of differentiation, spermatozoa are released from their intimate contact with sustentacular cells (*spermiation*) and enter the lumen of the seminiferous tubule. At this time they are mature morphologically but are immature functionally in that they are nonmotile and are limited in their ability to effect fertilization of the ovum. The final step in the maturation of spermatozoa, a process known as *capacitation,* is thought to occur after ejaculation into the female. It involves a process of activation which precedes fertilization, but the mechanism is uncertain.

In many lower mammalian orders, spermatogenesis occurs in definite cyclic waves along the length of the seminiferous tubules, but in man the waves are less distinct. On the basis of morphological changes in germ cell nuclei and the development of the acrosome during spermiogenesis, the human spermatogenetic cycle may be divided into six characteristic stages. The features of these stages are complex and will not be detailed here. However, the student should recognize that, due to the cyclic nature of spermatogenesis, not every stage can be seen at the same time at a given point along the seminiferous epithelium.

Mature Sperm

The mature human spermatozoon consists of a head, middle piece, and tail. The head comprises the condensed nucleus and a head cap, including the dense acrosome at its anterior margin. The head contains the DNA, or genetic material. The acrosome is thought to contain hyaluronidase, an enzyme that facilitates the passage of spermatozoa between the cells that surround unfertilized eggs, thereby aiding fertilization. The middle piece, which is separated from the head piece by a narrow neck, contains a core of longitudinal filaments surrounded by a mitochondrial sheath, and it is thought that it is responsible for control of movements of

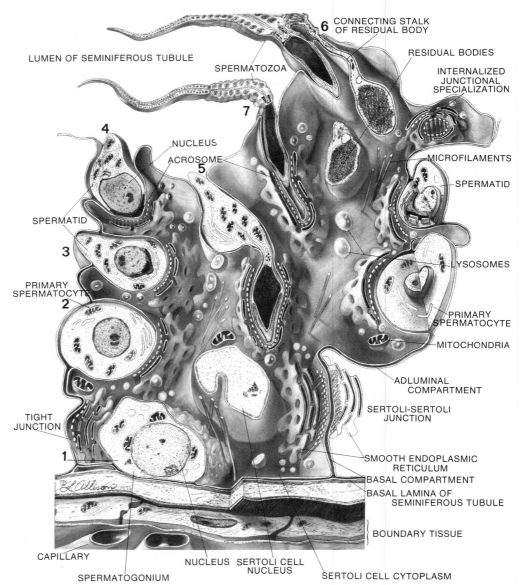

Figure 16–8.   A diagrammatic representation of a segment of a human seminiferous tubule to illustrate the process of spermatogenesis.

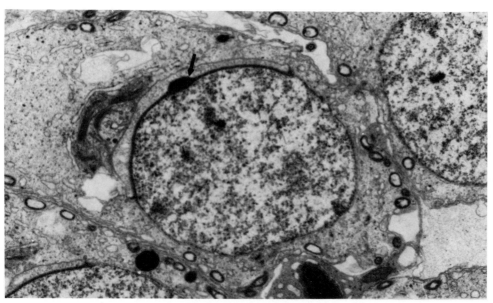

Figure 16–9. Electron micrograph of an early spermatid, showing the formation of the acrosome (arrow). Mitochondria are still dispersed throughout the cytoplasm and the nucleus is not condensed. × 22,000.

the tail. The tail has two central and nine peripheral double filaments (an arrangement essentially identical to that in a cilium), ensheathed by a thin layer of cytoplasm, except for the very tip which is naked.

The Interstitium

The interstitial tissue, within the lobuli testis, lies between the seminiferous tubules. It contains some collagenous fibers, blood and lymph vessels, nerves, and several cell types, including fibroblasts, macrophages, mast cells, and some undifferentiated mesenchymal cells. Blood vessels and nerves enter and leave at the mediastinum and form networks around the tubules. The specific interstitial cells of Leydig are a marked feature of this tissue. They lie in compact groups, usually in the angular areas created by the packing of seminiferous tubules. They are large cells in which the cytoplasm often appears vacuolated in light microscopy preparations. The nucleus contains coarse chromatin granules and a distinct nucleolus. Binucleate

cells are common. The cytoplasm is rich in inclusions such as lipid droplets and, in the human, it may contain peculiar rod-shaped crystalloids. On electron microscopy, the most striking feature of these cells is the extensive development of agranular (smooth-surfaced) endoplasmic reticulum. This appears as a fine meshwork of anastomosing tubules, to the surface of which no ribosomes are attached. Unlike the endoplasmic reticulum associated with ribosomes, which is concerned with protein synthesis, the agranular reticulum is thought to be the site of synthesis of steroid hormones.

Blood Vessels, Lymphatics, and Nerves

Branches from the testicular artery pierce the tunica albuginea at the mediastinum testis and pass to the tunica vasculosa. Smaller arteriolar branches follow the septula to the parenchyma where they terminate in networks of nonfenestrated capillaries. Venous drainage occurs principally through the mediastinum testis. Small lymphatic ves-

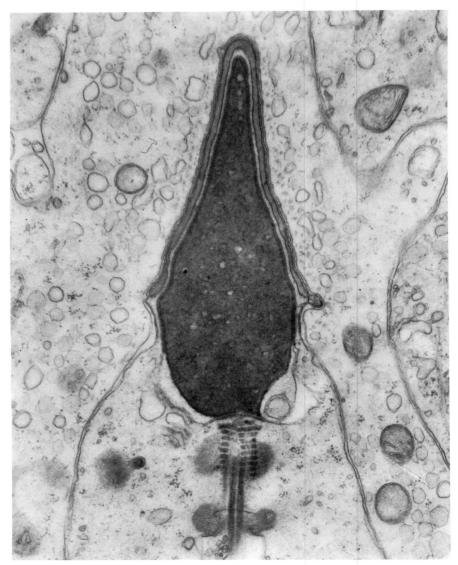

Figure 16–10.   Electron micrograph of a section of a human spermatid at an advanced stage of development. The head cap is complete, and the acrosome can no longer be identified as a separate entity. A well-developed flagellum extends from the lower pole of the nucleus. × 27,500.

sels form extensive networks within the interstitial tissue.

Nerves accompany the major blood vessels and form fine plexuses around smaller blood vessels and in relation to interstitial cells.

Functional Considerations of the Testis

The principal exocrine function of the testis, the production of male sex cells, is dependent upon numerous factors. Follicle-stimulating hormone (FSH) of the anterior lobe of the hypophysis stimulates spermatogenesis in mammals, although the effect is not so marked in man as it is in lower forms. FSH does act on Sertoli cells to stimulate the synthesis of a receptor, the *androgen-binding protein,* which combines with testosterone and is secreted into the lumina of seminiferous tubules. A suitable temperature is critical for spermatogen-

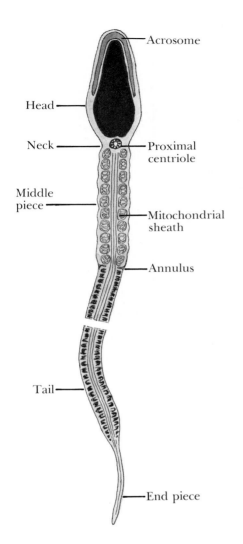

Acrosome

Head

Neck

Proximal
centriole

Middle
piece

Mitochondrial
sheath

Annulus

Tail

End piece

Figure 16–11. Diagrammatic representation of a mature spermatozoon.

Figure 16–12. *Below. Left:* Electron micrograph of longitudinal section of middle piece of a spermatozoon showing close apposition of mitochondrial sheath to outer dense fibers of the flagellum. ×26,000. *Right:* Transverse section through the proximal portion of the tail (principal piece) of a spermatozoon, showing circumferential fibers (arrowhead), outer fibers (upper arrow), and microtubules (lower arrow). ×42,000.

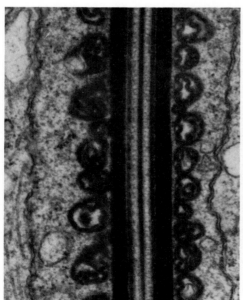

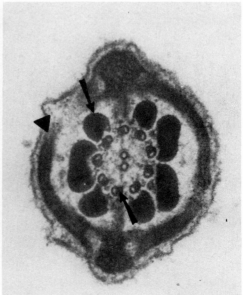

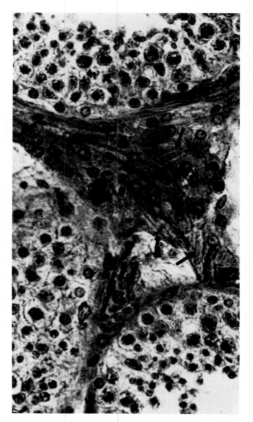

Figure 16–13. Light microphotograph of a portion of human testis. Between segments of three seminiferous tubules, the interstitium contains a large clump of Leydig cells. Within the cytoplasm of many cells are unstained crystalloids of Reinke (arrows). Iron hematoxylin. × 250.

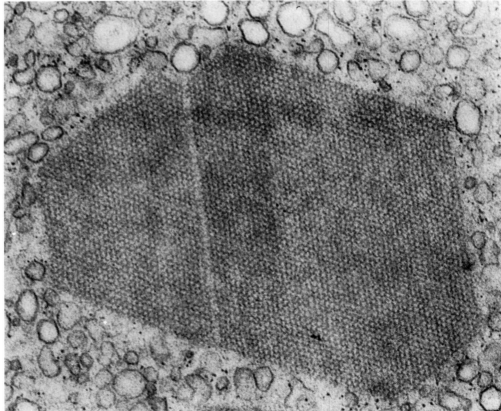

Figure 16–14. Electron micrograph of a portion of a human Leydig cell containing a crystalloid of Reinke. × 40,000.

esis. This is furnished by the position of the testis in the scrotum. In cases of cryptorchism (maldescent of the testis), spermatogenesis does not proceed to completion. In man, spermatogenesis is a continuous process throughout sexual maturity. The sex-determining role of spermatozoa is correlated with the production of two types of spermatozoa. Half of the secondary spermatocytes contain a female determining chromosome (X) and the other half a male determining chromosome (Y), this distinction continuing into daughter spermatids and into spermatozoa.

The principal endocrine secretion of the testis is testosterone, produced by the interstitial cells, which constitute a peculiar type of endocrine gland in that they do not develop from an epithelial surface, as do most glands, but from the mesenchymal stroma of the testis. In the stroma, abundantly supplied with capillaries, they have easy access for their secretory product into the vascular system. The production of testosterone by the testis depends upon stimulation by luteinizing hormone (LH) of the anterior lobe of the hypophysis. Since the target organ here is represented by the interstitial cells, luteinizing hormone often is referred to as interstitial cell–stimulating hormone (ICSH) in this context. Testosterone controls the appearance of secondary sex characteristics, the sex impulse, and the proper development and maintenance of the genital ducts and accessory glands.

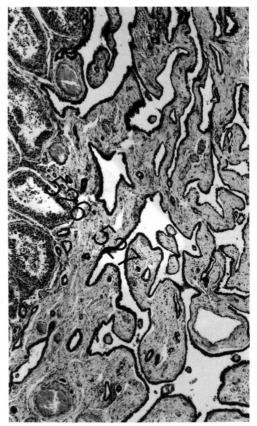

Figure 16–15. Low-power photomicrograph of a portion of the human testis and mediastinum. Straight tubules (tubuli recti) pass from the seminiferous tubules (left) into the network of the rete testis (right). × 75.

THE MALE GENITAL DUCTS

Tubuli Recti. At the apex of each lobule, the component seminiferous tubules join to form a straight tubule. Each straight tubule is short and devoid of convolutions, and has a diameter of about 25 microns (μm). At the point of continuity with the seminiferous tubules, the spermatogenic cells disappear, and only Sertoli cells remain, forming a simple columnar epithelium. Component cells contain numerous fat droplets. The epithelium rests upon a basal lamina and the surrounding loose connective tissue is devoid of smooth muscle cells.

Rete Testis. The straight tubules course to the dense connective tissue of the mediastinum testis where they enter a network of anastomosing channels, the rete testis. The lining of these irregular spaces is simple cuboidal or squamous epithelium, some component cells of which bear a single cilium. The epithelium rests upon a delicate basal lamina. Passage of spermatozoa through the tubuli recti and the rete testis is thought to occur rapidly, since in sections one rarely sees spermatozoa within the lumina.

Ductuli Efferentes. In the superior portion of the posterior border of the testis, some 10 to 15 spirally wound, efferent ductules emerge from the rete to form *lobules of the epididymis.* Each ductule is about 6 to 8 cm long and about 0.05 mm in diameter. The ductules are bound by connective tissue, and each is surrounded by a thin layer of circularly arranged smooth muscle fibers; together they constitute the major portion of the head of the epididymis. The ductuli efferentes are lined by a typical epithelium, mostly simple columnar, which rests upon a thin basal lamina. Externally each tubule has a regular outline, but internally the lumen is irregular in outline owing to the varying height of the epithelium. Groups of tall columnar cells alternate with groups of much shorter cells, the latter forming intraepithelial glands. Cells of these glands appear clear and contain pale secretory material and scattered pigment granules. Some cells bear cilia. The tall cells have a dense acidophil cytoplasm containing fat droplets and pigment granules, and many are ciliated. The cilia of both cell types beat toward the epididymis and thus help in transporting spermatozoa to the epididymis. The efferent ductules possess the only motile cilia in the entire duct system.

Ductus Epididymidis. The efferent ductules run into a single ductus epididymidis. This duct, which is surrounded by connective tissue, is highly tortuous and forms the body and the tail of the epididymis. It is a long storage duct (5 to 7 meters long) through which spermatozoa pass slowly. In their passage, they acquire motility and optimal fertilizability. The duct has a cylindrical outline both inside and outside, since the epithelium, unlike that of the efferent ductules, is uniform in height. The epithelium is pseudostratified, composed of basal cells and tall columnar cells. Lipid droplets are found in the cytoplasm of both cell types, and the tall columnar cells also contain pigment granules, lysosomes, and secretion droplets and on their free surface bear a tuft of nonmotile stereocilia (long slender cellular processes, which differ from microvilli in the repeated branching near their bases). The secretory product of the epithelium passes into the lumen through this irregular surface. The epithelium also functions in resorption of fluid. Experimental studies have indicated that more than 90 per cent of the fluid leaving the testis is resorbed in the ductus epididymidis. The duct is surrounded by a definite basal lamina, ex-

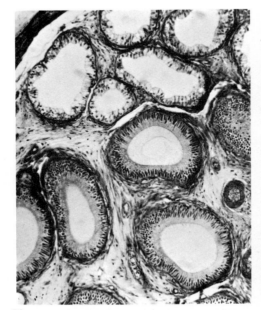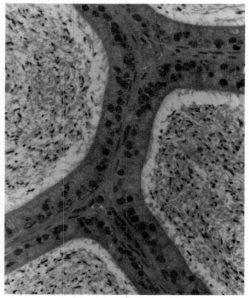

Figure 16–16. *Left:* Low-power photomicrograph of a section of the head of the epididymis. At the top of the picture are cross sections of efferent ductules and below are sections of the ductus epididymidis. Note the tall epithelial cells of the latter and the irregular height of the epithelium of the efferent ductules. *Right:* Section of efferent ductules. The tall cells, many of which are ciliated, possess a finely granular apical cytoplasm. The presence of spermatozoa within the lumina is unusual. Plastic section. × 250.

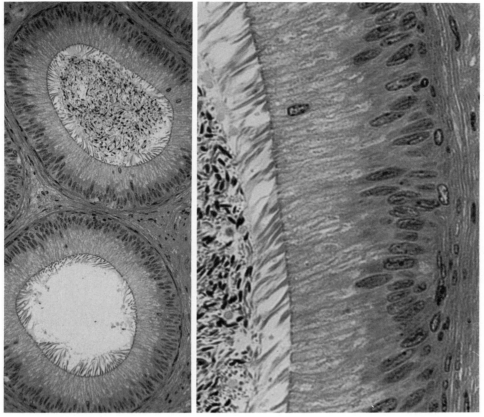

Figure 16–17. Sections of the ductus epididymidis. Note the regular height of the epithelium, tall stereocilia projecting into the lumen, and the presence of spermatozoa within the lumen. Plastic sections. Left, × 100, right, × 450.

ternal to which there is a thin layer of circularly arranged smooth muscle fibers. The muscle is thought by its contraction to aid in transporting spermatozoa down the duct.

Ductus Deferens. The ductus epididymidis straightens out at its termination and becomes continuous with the ductus deferens, which ascends from the scrotum to the inguinal region, traverses the inguinal canal, and courses down the side wall of the pelvis retroperitoneally toward the urethra. Relatively, its wall is thick and the lumen narrow. In the scrotum and inguinal canal, the ductus deferens lies within the spermatic cord, where it is easily palpable because of its thick wall. The spermatic cord contains, in addition to the ductus, arteries, veins of the pampiniform plexus, lymph vessels and nerves of the testis and epididymis, and longitudinal strands of smooth muscle.

Prior to its termination, the duct dilates into a spindle-shaped enlargement, the *ampulla.*

The epithelium of the ductus deferens is pseudostratified and many of the tall cells bear stereocilia. A delicate basal lamina intervenes between the epithelium and a thin lamina propria, which is characterized by the presence of numerous elastic fibers. The mucosa rises into longitudinal folds, which are responsible for the stellate outline of the lumen one sees in cross sections. Beneath the lamina propria there is an ill-defined submucosa, containing numerous blood vessels, which separates the mucosa from the muscular coat. This coat is thick and is composed of three distinct layers of smooth muscle. The inner layer is a relatively thin one of longitudinally oriented muscle. The middle or circular layer is markedly robust, and beyond this there is an-

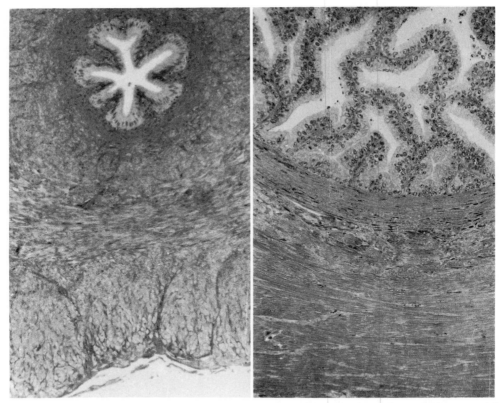

Figure 16–18. *Left:* Cross section of the ductus deferens. Note the stellate outline to the lumen and the thick muscular coat. Plastic section. × 65. *Right:* Ampulla of ductus deferens, showing the marked folding and branching of the epithelium. Plastic section. × 120.

other well-developed layer in which the muscle fibers are arranged longitudinally. A fibrous adventitia surrounds the muscular coat and blends with that of adjoining tissues.

Ampulla of Ductus Deferens. In the terminal dilatation of the ductus deferens, the lumen is wider and the mucosa much more folded than in the main portion of the ductus. Many of the epithelial folds branch and fuse with each other, producing a number of pocket-like recesses. The simple epithelium may show evidence of secretion. The musculature is much less regularly arranged than in the rest of the ductus deferens. Usually only the external longitudinal layer retains its identity.

Ejaculatory Duct. This is the short, terminal segment of each genital duct system. It is formed by the junction of the ampulla and the excretory duct of the seminal vesicle. It pierces the pros-

tate gland to open into the urethra just to the side of the prostatic utricle. The ejaculatory duct is lined by a simple columnar or pseudostratified epithelium, probably capable of secretion, which shows some mucosal outpocketings similar to those of the ampulla but less extensive. The supporting wall is fibrous connective tissue only.

THE AUXILIARY GENITAL GLANDS

The glands associated with the duct systems of the testes are the seminal vesicles, the prostate, and the bulbourethral glands.

Seminal Vesicles. Each vesicle is a tortuous, elongated diverticulum off the ductus deferens at the termination of the ampullary portion, situated posterior to the prostate gland. The wall consists of an external connective tissue

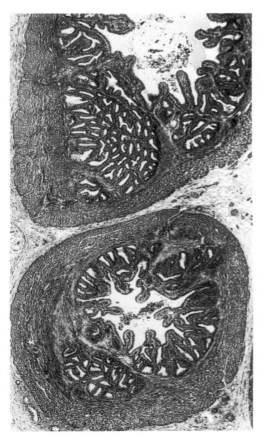

Figure 16–19. Low-power photomicrograph of the seminal vesicle. Owing to the highly tortuous nature of this gland, it appears here as two separate profiles. Note the intricate folding of the mucosa. × 40.

Component cells contain secretory granules and a yellow pigment. The secretion is a yellowish, viscid liquid which in sections appears as a deeply acidophil coagulum within the lumen. The epithelium depends upon hormonal support, testosterone, for its maintenance. Castration is followed by involution and loss of secretory function of the gland, which is promptly restored by the administration of testis extract. The seminal vesicle functions as a gland, secreting and storing the viscid component of the seminal fluid. It is not a site of storage of spermatozoa, although some spermatozoa may be seen within the lumen after death, presumably as the result of backflow.

Prostate. The prostate surrounds the urethra at its origin from the bladder. It is an aggregate of 30 to 50 small compound tubuloalveolar glands that drain into the prostatic urethra by 15 to 30 small excretory ducts. The glandular elements are distributed in three different areas, more or less concentrically arranged around the urethra. Small glands lie in the mucosa and these are surrounded by submucosal glands. The main, or principal, glandular elements lie peripherally and constitute the bulk of the gland. The whole

adventitia containing numerous elastic fibers, a smooth muscle coat thinner than that of the ductus deferens and consisting of inner circular and outer longitudinal layers, and a mucosa which is markedly folded. The high primary folds of the mucosa themselves branch into secondary and tertiary folds which project far into the lumen and merge with one another frequently. As a result, numerous compartments of different sizes are formed. All communicate with the lumen, although in sections many appear to be isolated. The lamina propria is a loose connective tissue that is richly vascularized. The epithelium typically shows many variations. It is usually pseudostratified but may be simple columnar. The height varies with the phase of secretion, age, and other influences.

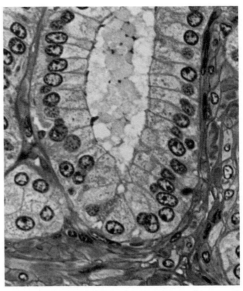

Figure 16–20. High power photomicrograph of the seminal vesicle. The epithelial cells are columnar and the apical cytoplasm contains fine granular material. Plastic section. × 450.

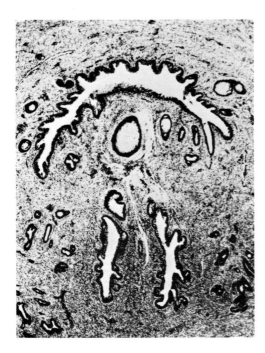

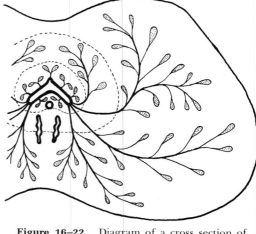

Figure 16–21. Low-power photomicrograph of the prostatic urethra and surrounding tissue. Immediately below the urethra, which is crescentic in outline, is the utriculum prostaticus and, below it, portions of both ejaculatory ducts. The surrounding stroma contains portions of some ducts of the prostate gland. × 55.

Figure 16–22. Diagram of a cross section of the human prostate. Note the distribution of the mucous, submucous, and main components of the gland.

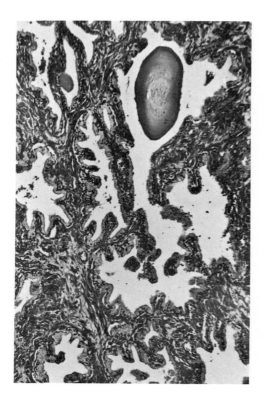

Figure 16–23. Medium-power photomicrograph of a portion of the prostate gland. Note the large concretion in the lumen of one alveolus. × 90.

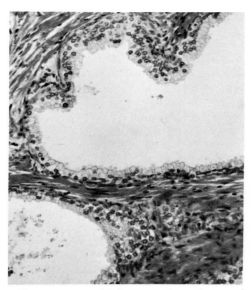

Figure 16–24. High-power photomicrograph of a small portion of the prostate gland. Note the character of the epithelium and the presence of numerous smooth muscle fibers in the stroma of the gland. × 160.

gland is surrounded by a fibroelastic capsule containing an extensive plexus of veins, and the glandular components are embedded in an abundant, dense stroma which is continuous at the periphery with the capsule. This stroma is again fibroelastic and in addition contains numerous strands of smooth muscle fibers. The secretory alveoli and tubules are very irregular and vary greatly in size and form. They branch frequently and both alveoli and tubules have wide lumina. There is no distinct basal lamina and the epithelium is very folded and cuboidal to columnar in type. The cytoplasm contains numerous secretory granules and lipid droplets. The ducts, too, have irregular lumina and resemble smaller secretory tubules.

The secretion of the prostate is a thin, milky liquid which is slightly alkaline. It contains large amounts of acid phosphatase. In prostatic carcinoma, there frequently is a pronounced discharge of

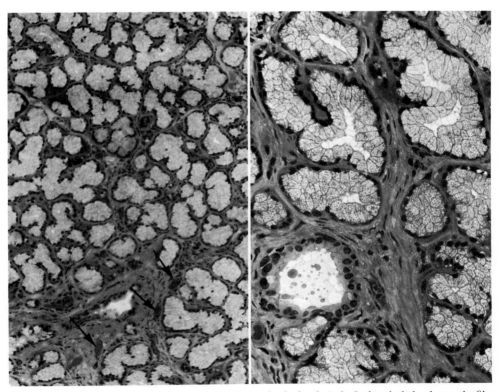

Figure 16–25. Sections of a lobule of a bulbourethral gland. *Left:* Isolated skeletal muscle fibers (arrows) are scattered in relation to the secretory end pieces. Plastic section. × 100. *Right:* High-power to show details of the secretory end pieces and of a duct (lower left). Plastic section. × 400.

this enzyme, which may result in high concentrations of it within the blood. In sections, the secretion appears as an acidophil granular mass. It frequently contains spherical or ovoid bodies, the prostatic concentrations *(corpora amylacea)* that are condensations of the secretions and may become calcified.

Bulbourethral Glands. The bulbourethral glands (of Cowper) are paired bodies, each the size of a pea, lying in the connective tissue behind the membranous urethra. Each is a compound tubuloalveolar gland whose duct enters the posterior portion of the cavernous segment of the urethra. The bulbourethral gland is surrounded by a thin connective tissue capsule, external to which are skeletal muscle fibers. Septa pass into the gland to divide it into lobules. The connective tissue septa contain numerous elastic and skeletal and smooth muscle fibers. The secretory end pieces are variable, being either alveolar, saccular, or tubular. The epithelium, too, is variable, being either cuboidal or columnar. The cyto-plasm contains mucigen droplets and some acidophil, spindle-shaped inclusions. Nuclei are basally located. The secretory ducts are lined by a pseudo-stratified epithelium resembling that of the urethra, and may contain patches of mucous cells. They are surrounded by an incomplete coat of circularly arranged smooth muscle. The secretion is clear, viscid, and mucous.

THE PENIS

The penis serves as the common outlet for urine and for seminal fluid and as the copulatory organ. It is formed by three cylinders of erectile tissue: the paired *corpora cavernosa penis* dorsally and the single *corpus cavernosum urethrae* (corpus spongiosum) ventrally. The latter encloses the cavernous portion of the urethra. The paired corpora cavernosa penis are separated from each other proximally but join beneath the pubic angle and run forward together, united by a common median partition,

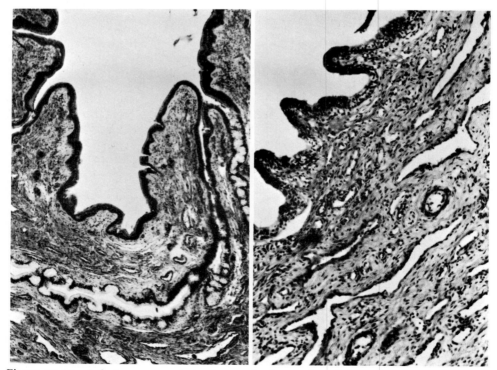

Figure 16–26. *Left:* Low-power photomicrograph of a portion of the cavernous part of the male human urethra together with the glands of Littre. × 90. *Right:* High-power photomicrograph of portion of penile urethra. Note the blood sinuses in the erectile tissue. Plastic section. × 150.

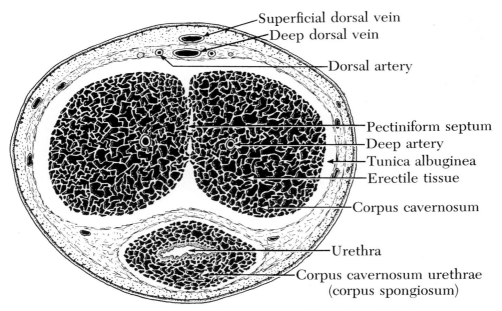

Superficial dorsal vein
Deep dorsal vein
Dorsal artery
Pectiniform septum
Deep artery
Tunica albuginea
Erectile tissue
Corpus cavernosum
Urethra
Corpus cavernosum urethrae
(corpus spongiosum)

Figure 16–27. Diagram of a cross section of the penis in midshaft.

the *pectiniform septum,* to the region of the *glans penis.* The deep groove beneath the corpora cavernosa is occupied by the corpus spongiosum. This ends in a cup-shaped enlargement, the glans penis, which forms a cap over the conical ends of the corpora cavernosa penis. The three cylinders of erectile tissue are surrounded by subcutaneous tissue which is devoid of fat but contains many smooth muscle fibers. The skin covering the organ is thin and delicate and terminally it reduplicates over the glans as a fold, the *prepuce.* The inner surface of the prepuce, in relation to the glans, is moist and nonkeratinized. The epithelium over the glans itself is firmly adhered to the fibrous tissue beneath. The skin of the penis contains small sweat glands and infrequent sebaceous glands unassociated with hair follicles, there being no hair follicles over the distal part of the penis. On the glans and on the inner surface of the prepuce there are a number of modified sebaceous glands, the *glands of Tyson.*

Each cylinder of the corpus cavernosum penis is surrounded by a thick fibrous sheath, the *tunica albuginea.* The collagenous fibers of the sheath are arranged in two layers, outer longitudinal and inner circular. The pectiniform septum, common to both cylinders, is pierced by numerous slitlike openings through which the cavernous spaces of both sides communicate. Trabeculae, continuous with the fibrous sheath, consist of collagenous, elastic, and smooth muscle fibers and form a dense internal framework. The spaces between the framework are lined by a thin squamous endothelium and constitute the blood sinuses. Owing to the arrangement of the trabeculae, the cavernous spaces are largest in the central zone of each cylinder and gradually diminish in size toward the periphery.

The sheath (tunica albuginea) of the corpus spongiosum is much thinner than that of the corpora cavernosa penis and contains many elastic and smooth muscle fibers. Trabeculae are thinner and more elastic than those present in the paired corpora. The cavernous spaces are small, almost uniform in size, and gradually pass into the small venous spaces around the urethra.

Blood Vessels and the Mechanism of Erection

The principal arterial branches within the penis are the dorsal arteries, which run in the interval between the corpora cavernosa superiorly on either side of the deep dorsal vein, and the deep arteries of the penis traversing

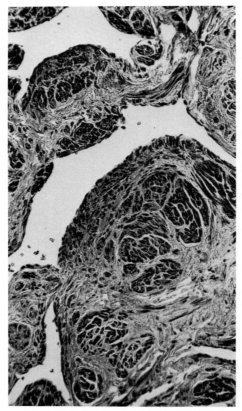

Figure 16–28. Low-power photomicrograph of the erectile tissue of the penis. The framework consists of irregular trabeculae containing connective tissue fibers (pale) and bundles of smooth muscle fibers (dark). Within the framework are irregular endothelium-lined spaces, the blood sinuses. × 150.

each of the corpora. Branches from the dorsal arteries pierce the fibrous capsule along the upper surface to enter the corpora cavernosa, especially near the distal end of the penis. On entering the cavernous spaces, all arteries divide into branches, some of which end in capillary plexuses; others are longitudinal vessels directed distally. In the quiescent state, these vessels, the *helicine arteries,* have a spiral course, their media is thick, and their intima is thrown into longitudinal folds. These vessels open directly into the sinuses of the erectile tissue. Blood from the cavernous spaces and the capillary plexuses is drained by a plexus of venules within the tunica albuginea. Some emerge from the base of the tunica and converge on the dorsum of the penis to join the deep dorsal vein. Others pass

directly out on the upper surface of the corpora cavernosa to enter the same vein. The smooth muscle of the arteries and the trabeculae is supplied both by sympathetic and by parasympathetic fibers.

Under conditions of erotic stimulation, parasympathetic stimulation produces a relaxation of the smooth muscle, and the helicine vessels straighten out and their lumina dilate. Blood flows freely from them into the cavernous spaces, which become engorged with blood. Thus there is a rerouting of blood into a greatly enlarged vascular bed. The venous drainage at the periphery of the corpora is said to be diminished owing to compression of the thin-walled veins under the tunica albuginea by the engorged trabecular spaces. The corpora cavernosa become rigid and enlarged. Since there is less compression of the venous drainage of the corpus spongiosum and a more yielding tunica, there is less rigidity here and the urethra contained within it remains patent to allow for egress of seminal fluid during ejaculation. At the termination of sexual excitement, the penis returns to the flaccid state through a process of *detumescence.* The arteries regain muscular tone owing to sympathetic stimulation, and the amount of blood supplied to the sinuses diminishes. The excess of blood in the corpora cavernosa slowly is pressed out by contraction of the muscle fibers within the trabeculae, and the ordinary route of blood flow through the organ is restored.

Seminal Fluid

Seminal fluid (semen) consists of spermatozoa together with the fluid in which they are suspended. The fluid is a product of all the auxiliary genital glands together with a minor contribution supplied by the system of genital ducts. Semen is a whitish, opaque fluid containing about 100 million spermatozoa in 1 ml, but the number varies greatly. The ejaculate averages about 3 ml, and thus contains about 300 million spermatozoa. The discharge of semen is said to occur in a definite sequence. The bulbourethral glands and the urethral glands of Littre discharge their mucous secretion during erection and lubricate the cavernous urethra. During actual ejaculation, the prostate discharges first. Its alkaline secretion reduces the acidity of the urethra which initially may contain some residual urine. This is followed by the sper-matozoa which are forced out of the ductus epididymidis and the ductus deferens by powerful contraction of the muscular walls. Finally, the thick secretion of the seminal vesicles, which contains fructose and is nutrient to the sperm, is added to the mass.

REFERENCES

Bedford, J. M., and Nicander, L.: Ultrastructural changes in the acrosome and sperm membranes during maturation of spermatozoa in the testis and epididymis of the rabbit and monkey. J. Anat., 108:527, 1971.

Brandes, D.: The fine structure and histochemistry of prostatic glands in relation to sex hormones. Int. Rev. Cytol., 20:207, 1966.

Burgos, M. H., Vitale-Calpe, R., and Aoki, A.: Fine structure of the testis and its functional significance. In The Testis, edited by A. D. Johnson, W. R. Gomes, and N. L. VanDemark. New York, Academic Press, 1970. Vol. 1, p. 551.

Camatini, M., Franchi, E., and de Curtis, I.: Sertoli junctions in human testes: a freeze fracture and lanthanum tracer study. J. Submicr. Cytol., 11:511, 1979.

Christensen, A. K.: The fine structure of testicular interstitial cells in guinea pig. J. Cell Biol., 26:911, 1965.

Christensen, A. K., and Fawcett, D. W.: The fine structure of interstitial cells of the mouse testis. Am. J. Anat., 118:551, 1966.

Clark, R. V.: Three-dimensional organization of testicular interstitial tissue and lymphatic space in the rat. Anat. Rec., 184:203, 1976.

Clermont, Y.: Renewal of spermatogonia in man. Am. J. Anat., 118:509, 1966.

Clermont, Y., and Lebond, C. P.: Spermiogenesis of man, monkey, ram and other mammals as shown by the "periodic acid-Schiff" technique. Am. J. Anat., 96:229, 1955.

Davis, J. R., Langford, G. A., and Kirby, P. J.: The testicular capsule. In The Testis, edited by A. D. Johnson, W. R. Gomes, and N. L. VanDemark. New York, Academic Press, 1970, Vol. 1, p. 282.

De Kretser, D. M., Kerr, J. B., and Paulsen, C. A.: The peritubular tissue in the normal and pathological human testis. An ultrastructural study. Biol. Reprod., 12:317, 1975.

Dym, M.: The mammalian rete testis: A morphological examination. Anat. Rec., 186:493, 1976.

Dym, M., and Cavicchia, J. C.: Functional morphology of the testis. Biol. Reprod., 18:1, 1978.

Dym, M., and Fawcett, D. W.: Further observations on the number of spermatogonia, spermatocytes, and spermatids connected by intercellular bridges in the mammalian testis. Biol. Reprod., 4:195, 1971.

Fawcett, D. W.: The mammalian spermatozoon. Dev. Biol., 44:394, 1975.

Fawcett, D. W., and Burgos, M. H.: Observations on the cytomorphosis of the germinal and interstitial cells of the human testis. In Ciba Founda-tion Colloquia on Ageing. London, J. & A. Churchill, Ltd., 1956, Vol. 2, p. 86.

Fawcett, D. W., and Burgos, M. H.: Studies on the fine structure of the mammalian testis. II. The human interstitial tissue. Am. J. Anat., 107:245, 1960.

Friend, D. S., and Fawcett, D. W.: Membrane differentiation in freeze-fractured mammalian sperm. J. Cell Biol., 63:641, 1974.

Hargrove, J. L., MacIndoe, J. H., and Ellis, L. C.: Testicular contractile cells and sperm transport. Fertil. Steril., 28:1146, 1977.

Leeson, C. R., and Leeson, T. S.: The postnatal development and differentiation of the boundary tissue of the seminiferous tubule of the rat. Anat. Rec., 147:243, 1963.

Leeson, C. R., and Leeson, T. S.: The postnatal development of the ductus epididymis in the rat. Anat. Anz., 114:159, 1964.

Leeson, T. S., and Leeson, C. R.: The fine structure of cavernous tissue in the adult rat penis. Invest. Urol., 3:144, 1965.

Mann, T.: Secretory function of the prostate, seminal vesicle and other male accessory organs of reproduction. J. Reprod. Fertil., 37:179, 1974.

Nagano, T., and Suzuki, F.: Freeze-fracture observations on the intercellular junctions of Sertoli cells and of Leydig cells in the human testis. Cell Tissue Res., 166:37, 1976.

Riva, A.: Fine structure of human seminal vesicle epithelium. J. Anat., 102:71, 1967.

Roosen-Runge, E. C., and Barlow, F. D.: Quantitative studies on human spermatogenesis. Am. J. Anat., 93:143, 1953.

Roosen-Runge, E. C., and Holstein, A. F.: The human rete testis. Cell Tissue Res., 189:409, 1978.

Ross, M. H.: The Sertoli cell specialization during spermiogenesis and at spermation. Anat. Rec., 186:79, 1976.

Russell, L. D.: The blood-testis barrier and its formation relative to spermatocyte maturation in the adult rat: A lanthanum tracer study. Anat. Rec., 190:99, 1978.

Russell, L. D., and Ross, M. H.: Characterization of Seroli cell-germ cell junctional specializations in dissociated testicular cells. Anat. Rec., 193:23, 1979.

Setchell, B. P.: The Mammalian Testis. Ithaca, N.Y., Cornell University Press, 1978.

Steinberger, E.: Hormonal control of mammalian spermatogenesis. Physiol. Rev., 51:1, 1979.

Vitale-Calpe, R., Fawcett, D. W., and Dym, M.: The normal development of the blood-testis barrier and the effects of clomiphene and estrogen treatment. Anat. Rec., 176:333, 1973.

ORGANS OF SPECIAL SENSE

SENSORY RECEPTORS

Organs of general sensibility are distributed widely in epithelium, connective tissue, muscle, and tendon, while special receptors associated with sensations of smell, taste, sight, hearing, and balance occur in limited areas. All, of course, are transducers in the sense that they convert one form of energy into another, receiving a stimulus and creating an action potential. Receptors are either nerve endings or cells specialized for this function.

Classification of receptors can be made on more than one basis. Often they are classified by the particular energy type or modality to which they are sensitive and thus there are thermoreceptors (sensitive to temperature changes), mechanoreceptors (sensitive to touch, pressure), chemoreceptors (sensitive to chemical changes), and osmoreceptors (sensitive to changes in osmotic pressure). A further classification relates to the source of the stimulus in relation to the body and on this basis there are *exteroceptors* located at the body surface and responding to external stimuli; *proprioceptors* responding to change of position and movements and mainly associated with the musculoskeletal system; and *interoceptors* located in viscera and blood vessels. On a morphological basis, receptors are classified into two main types: *free or naked* (nonencapsulated) endings unassociated with other cell types and *encapsulated* (corpuscular) endings where nonnervous elements are associated with the nerve ending. Some receptors have been described where appropriate in previous chapters.

Free Nerve Endings. Sensory afferent nerve fibers terminate as free nerve endings, often in a plexiform manner, and are distributed widely in the body. They are found in all types of connective tissue (fascia, ligaments, tendons, periosteum, joint capsules, dermis) and in most epithelia (epidermis, cornea, alimentary tract, glands). From the free terminals, nerve fibers are both myelinated and unmyelinated, but all are of small diameter and myelinated fibers lose their Schwann cell investments before terminating. In many areas, e.g., in skin and mucous membranes with a stratified squamous epithelium, the nerves form subepithelial plexuses from which branches penetrate the epithelium to end in small knoblike swellings between epithelial cells. In relation to hair follicles, there are extensive nerve branches parallel to the follicle in the dermis with naked filaments encircling the hair and terminating as free endings, mainly in the dermal root sheath but with some in the outer root sheath. These are called *peritrichial endings.* Some of these endings in relation to epithelial cells of hair follicles and in skin and oral mucosa are not truly "free" but terminate on specialized epithelial cells called *Merkel's discs.* These are large, dark-staining cells that contain numerous dense-cored granules with many spiny cytoplasmic processes extending between adjacent keratinocytes. The Merkel cells probably detect movement in adjacent keratinocytes as well as movement of the epithelial membrane in relation to the underlying connective tissue. These endings and the peritrichial ones are mechanoreceptors. While most free endings are regarded as sensitive to touch and pain, their functional significance is not clear. Certainly the peritrichial endings are the main tactile organs of hairy skin and although, for example, free nerve endings only are found in tooth pulp and cornea and therefore considered to be pain receptors, there is little evidence for this.

Encapsulated Nerve Endings. These vary greatly in shape and size but in all the terminal nerve fiber is enveloped by a capsule.

The *lamellated corpuscles* (of Pacini or

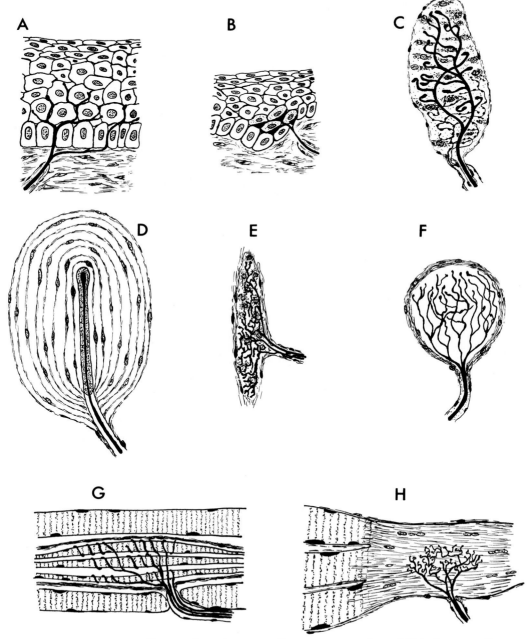

Figure 17–1. Diagram to illustrate the various types of sensory nerve endings. *A*, Naked nerve endings in cornea (pain). *B*, Merkel's disk in epidermis (touch). *C*, Meissner's corpuscle (touch). *D*, Vater-Pacini corpuscle (pressure). *E*, Ruffini's corpuscle (heat). *F*, Krause's end bulb (cold). *G*, Neuromuscular spindle (proprioception). *H*, Neurotendinous organ (proprioception).

Vater-Pacini) are found in subcutaneous tissue of the palms, soles and digits, nipples, periosteum, mesentery, tendons, ligaments, and external genitalia. They are spherical or ovoid, and large (2 mm in length, 0.5 to 1 mm in diameter), the largest being visible to the naked eye. Structurally, they resemble an onion. Each corpuscle is supplied by a large myelinated fiber that loses its Schwann cell sheath at the edge of the corpuscle and then passes through the core of the corpuscle as an unmyelinated fiber to terminate in an expanded bulb. The nerve axon contains numerous mitochondria. It is surrounded by about 60 closely packed lamellae composed of flattened cells, bilaterally arranged with two longitudinal clefts at the sides. Outside this core is an intermediate cellular zone that is only one cell thick and from which, by mitosis, cells are added either to the core or externally to the capsule. It is not conspicuous in the mature corpuscle. Externally is a capsule of up to 30 concentric lamellae of flattened, endothelium-like cells with basal lamellae and a few collagen fibrils between layers. Owing to fluid pressure between lamellae of the capsule, lamellated corpuscles exhibit turgidity and respond to pressure and vibration. In relation to joints, they register movement and position.

The *tactile corpuscles* (of Meissner) are located in dermal papillae, particularly of digits, lips, nipples, and genitalia, and are cylindrical in shape, their long axes perpendicular to the skin surface and about 80 μm long and 40 μm wide. There is a thin connective tissue capsule continuous with the perineurium of the nerve supplying the corpuscle and a central stack of transversely disposed flattened cells. A few myelinated nerve fibers supply each corpuscle from which both myelinated and unmyelinated branches ramify between cells of the corpuscle. These corpuscles are sensitive to touch and permit two-point tactile discrimination (distinguish between two closely placed pointed stimuli). The corpuscles decrease in number with age.

Bulbous corpuscles (of Krause) are found in mucocutaneous areas (lip and external genitalia), in the dermis, and in relation to hairs and are spheroidal in shape, about 50 μm in diameter, with a thick capsule continuous with endoneurium. Within the corpuscle, the myelinated fiber loses its myelin and branches, still covered by Schwann cells. The fiber may be branched or coiled, and it terminates in clublike endings. These corpuscles decrease in number with age. Much doubt exists about these bulbous corpuscles. They may be mechanoreceptors or be sensitive to cold but have been considered by some to represent a degenerative process in nerve terminals and not true receptors.

The corpuscles of Ruffini are found in connective tissues, including dermis and joint capsules, and have a thin connective tissue capsule containing a spraylike nerve ending with terminal swellings. They may be heat receptors or mechanoreceptors, being similar to Golgi tendon organs. The *neurotendinous endings* (of Golgi) are located in tendons near the junctions with muscle (see also Chapter 6). About 500 μm long and 100 μm wide, they consist of small bundles of tendon fibers (the intrafusal fasciculi) enclosed in a lamellated capsule with free, nonmyelinated nerve endings arborizing around the tendon bundles. They are stimulated by stretching or contraction of the associated muscles.

Neuromuscular spindles (also noted in Chapter 6) are found in muscles, often near a tendon, and consist of several small muscle cells (intrafusal fibers) with motor and sensory nerve fibers, the whole in a connective tissue capsule. The organ is fusiform, up to 2 mm long, and within it there are two types of muscle fiber — the "nuclear bag fibers" with numerous central nuclei and few peripheral myofibrils and "nuclear chain fibers" with a single row of nuclei and many small myofibrils. Sensory nerve fibers end as annulospiral endings around nuclear bag fibers and as flower-spray endings near the equators of nuclear chain fibers. Small motor fibers end at small, modified myoneural junctions on all intrafusal fibers. The annulospiral and flower-spray endings are mechanoreceptors, responding to stretch.

Specialized endings for taste and olfaction have been described previously in Chapters 11 and 12, respectively.

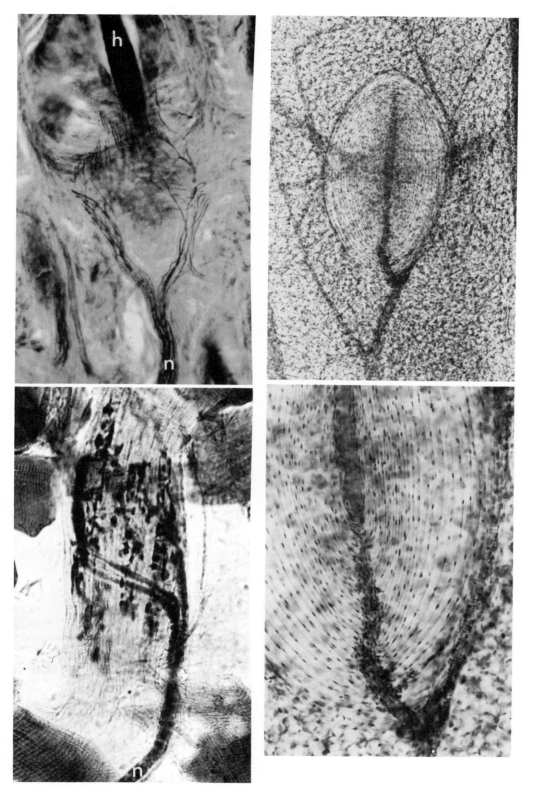

Figure 17–2. Photomicrographs of peritrichial nerve ending *(top left)* in relation to a hair follicle (hair labelled "h", nerve "n"), a neurotendinous ending *(bottom left),* and a lamellated corpuscle of Vater-Pacini *(top* and *bottom right).* Left figures, × 300; top right, × 40; bottom right, × 100.

THE EYE

Structurally, the eyeball often has been compared to a camera, but no analogy can be made about the nervous mechanisms involved. The essential component is the *retina,* the inner nervous layer that lines the posterior half of the eyeball. Developmentally and functionally, the retina is an isolated part of the central nervous system to which it remains connected by a tract of nerve fibers, the *optic nerve.* As in the CNS, the retina is nourished and protected by two coats or tunics, one of vascular and one of fibrous tissue. The outer fibrous coat, corresponding to dura mater, is white and opaque over the posterior five sixths of the eyeball (the *sclera*) and clear and transparent over the anterior one sixth (the *cornea*). Between the outer fibrous layer and the retina is a vascular, nutrient layer analogous to pia arachnoid. This *uveal* coat has three zones: a posterior *choroid,* the *ciliary body* just behind the corneoscleral junction, and, an-

teriorly, the *iris* that reflects inward to diverge from the cornea. In the iris is a central, spherical deficiency of variable diameter termed the *pupil.* The retina continues forward but as a non-nervous or non-photosensitive layer to line the inner surface of ciliary body and iris (the ciliary and iridial portions of the retina).

At the corneoscleral junction anteriorly and the exit of the optic nerve posteriorly, fibrous and vascular tunics are attached firmly to each other but elsewhere there is a potential space, the *perichoroidal (subchoroidal) space* across which pass nerves and blood vessels. Anteriorly where the iris reflects inward, the space between fibrous and vascular tunics is expanded as the *anterior chamber.* The lens lies immediately posterior to the iris supported by a *suspensory ligament* (the *zonule*) from the ciliary body. The *posterior chamber* is the slender space between iris and lens, and anterior and posterior chambers freely communicate through the pupil and

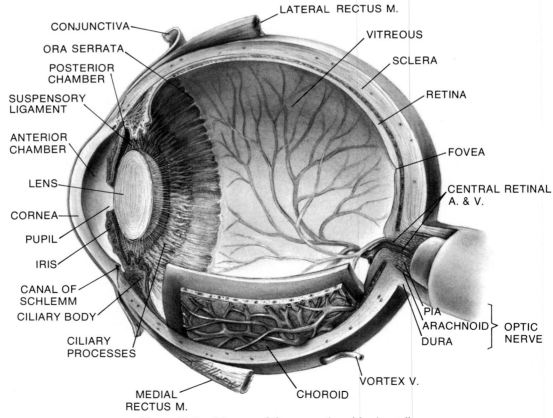

Figure 17–3.   Diagram of the eye sectioned horizontally.

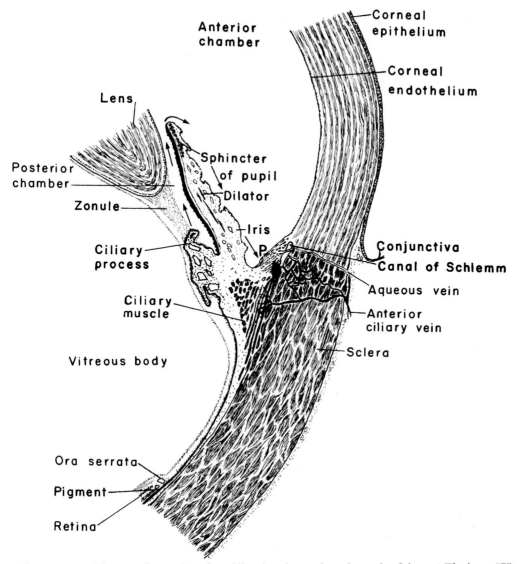

Figure 17–4. Diagram of a portion of meridional section to show the angle of the eye. The letter "P" indicates the pectinate ligament or trabecular meshwork. Compare with Figure 17–9. The arrows indicate the course of circulation of aqueous humor.

contain a clear fluid, the *aqueous humor,* secreted by the ciliary body. Posterior to the lens, the eyeball cavity is occupied by a transparent gel, the *vitreous humor.* Thus, to reach the sensory retina light rays pass through a series of transparent, refractive media consisting of cornea, aqueous humor, lens, and vitreous body.

The exit of the optic nerve is not at the posterior pole of the eyeball but is situated about 3 mm to the nasal side and 1 mm below it. The eyeball is a slightly asymmetrical sphere, somewhat flattened from above down. The central points of corneal and scleral curvatures are termed the *anterior* and *posterior poles,* and the line joining them is the *geometrical axis.* This differs from the *optic* or *visual axis,* which is a line between the center of the pupil and the fovea, the latter being the spot of most distinct vision. The posterior pole in fact lies between the fovea and the optic papilla. The *anatomical equator* is a circumferential line dividing the eyeball into anterior and posterior hemispheres. Any circle drawn through the poles and crossing the equator at a right angle is a *meridian,* of which two are important: the *vertical,* passing through the fovea and dividing the eye into nasal and temporal halves, and the *horizontal* or *transverse,* dividing the eye into upper and lower halves. The two meridians together divide the eye into four quadrants.

The cornea, the anterior one sixth of the eye surface, has a radius of about 8 mm, whereas the sclera has a radius of 12 mm. Thus, the cornea is curved more acutely. At the corneoscleral junction is a shallow circular sulcus, the *external scleral sulcus,* to which conjunctiva and bulbar fascia are attached. Around the exit of the optic nerve, the sclera is pierced in a ring fashion by ciliary nerves and short posterior ciliary arteries and, further anteriorly, one long posterior ciliary artery on each side pierces sclera with anterior ciliary arteries and veins passing through sclera just posterior to the corneoscleral junction. From each quadrant, just behind the equator, a vortex vein drains the choroid.

The eyeball in the adult has an anteroposterior diameter of about 24 mm, being slightly larger in the male.

Fibrous Coat

This outer layer of sclera and cornea provides a tough, fibroelastic support for the eye.

Sclera. The sclera is thickest at the posterior pole (1 mm), thinnest at the equator (0.3 to 0.4 mm), and anteriorly near the corneoscleral junction is 0.6 to 0.8 mm. It is composed of dense white connective tissue consisting of flat bundles of collagenous fibers running in various directions but mainly parallel to the surface, with flattened fibroblasts and fine networks of elastic fibers between the bundles. While quite uniform in structure, three layers are recognized. The outermost, the *episcleral tissue,* is loose fibroelastic tissue continuous externally with the dense connective tissue of *Tenon's capsule,* the two separated by loose tissue (Tenon's space). Tendons of extraocular muscles pass through Tenon's capsule to insert into the sclera. The eyeball can rotate because of this space, and because of orbital fat. The bulk of the sclera, the *sclera proper,* is formed by collagenous bundles and blends with the innermost layer, the *lamina fusca* (dark layer), where collagenous bundles are smaller, elastic fibers more numerous, and with branching chromatophores containing melanin between the fiber bundles. Posteriorly at the lamina cribrosa, the sclera is perforated by the fibers of the optic nerve. The sclera contains few blood vessels, no lymphatics, and a few ciliary nerve fibers.

Cornea. The cornea is clear and transparent with a smooth surface but is not uniformly curved. The central (opti-

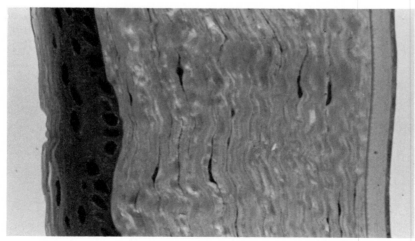 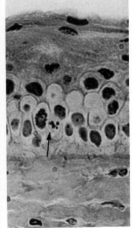

Figure 17–5. Photomicrographs of cornea. *Left:* The full thickness showing, from left to right, the epithelium resting upon Bowman's membrane, substantia propria (corneal stroma), Descemet's membrane, and endothelium. × 150. *Right:* The corneal epithelium with a mitotic figure (arrow) in the basal layer. × 375.

cal) zone has a smaller radius of curvature than the periphery, and the posterior surface is more strongly curved than the anterior; thus, it is thinner (0.7 to 0.8 mm) centrally than at its margin (1.1 mm). The refractive power of the cornea, a function of its refractive index and its radius of curvature, is greater than that of the lens. Anatomically, the cornea has two parts: the *cornea proper* and the *limbus,* a transition zone about 1 mm wide at the periphery. While the cornea proper is avascular, the limbus contains blood vessels and lymphatics.

Histologically, the cornea is composed of five layers. Externally is the *epithelium,* a stratified squamous nonkeratinizing epithelium, 50 to 70 μm thick, with 5 to 6 layers of cells. The basal layer is low columnar, then three or four layers of polyhedral ("wing") cells and one or two layers of surface squamous cells. The epithelium is highly sensitive, with numerous free nerve endings, and has excellent regenerative powers, mitoses occurring only in the basal layer. Beneath the epithelium is *Bowman's membrane,* 8 μm thick, structureless and acellular, formed by a condensation of intercellular substance with randomly distributed, fine collagenous fibrils. It ends abruptly at the limbus. The *substantia propria* forms the bulk of the cornea (90 per cent of its thickness), is transparent, and is composed of collagenous lamellae and cells. Lamellae are broad, tapelike bands of fibers, the fibrils in each lamella parallel, with lamel-

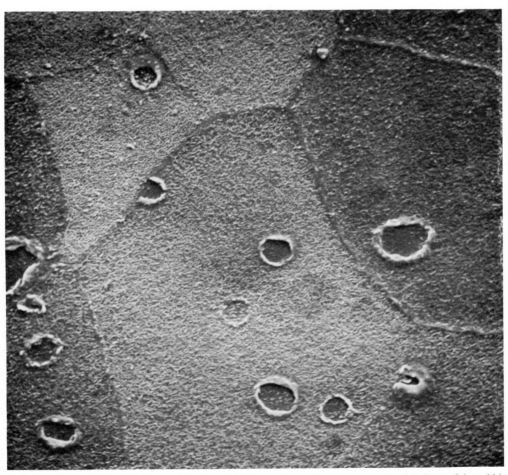

Figure 17–6. Scanning electron micrograph of the surface cells of the corneal epithelium of the rabbit. Cell boundaries are seen clearly, the cell surfaces show microvilli and microplicae (small folds), and the "craters" on the surface may represent secretory vacuoles. × 6500. (Courtesy of M. J. Hollenberg and B. J. Lewis.)

lae at different angles. Lamellae are held together by interchange of fibrils between adjacent lamellae. Fibrils are uniform in diameter (25 to 30 nm), show characteristic periodicity, and lie in mucoid intercellular substance. Stellate fibroblasts, flattened but with slender processes, lie between lamellae. *Descemet's membrane,* which appears homogeneous, lies internal to the substantia propria. It is 5 to 7 μm thick centrally but thickens to 8 to 10 μm peripherally, where it is continuous with material of the trabecular meshwork (pectinate ligament) of the iridial angle at the *ring of Schwalbe.* By electron microscopy, it contains small fibrils with a 100 nm periodicity arranged in a hexagonal pattern of great regularity. Chemically, the material is collagen. Descemet's membrane is the basement membrane for the *endothelium,* a single layer of cuboidal cells that lines the inner surface of the cornea. The cells show junctional complexes, irregular cell interfaces, and numerous pinocytotic vesicles. They transport fluid and solutes. The cornea is avascular, depending for nutrition on diffusion from peripheral blood vessels in the limbus and from aqueous humor centrally.

Limbus Corneae. This is the transitional or junctional zone, only 1 mm wide, between cornea and sclera. Here, corneal epithelium is thickened to 10 or more layers and becomes continuous with the conjunctiva, Bowman's membrane ends abruptly, Descemet's membrane tapers and splits up to become continuous with trabeculae of the pectinate ligament, and the corneal stroma becomes less regular and gradually changes from its characteristic lamellar arrangement to the less regular arrangement found in the sclera. The limbus is well vascularized.

Vascular Coat (the Uvea)

The vascular coat consists of choroid, ciliary body, and iris, all showing prom-

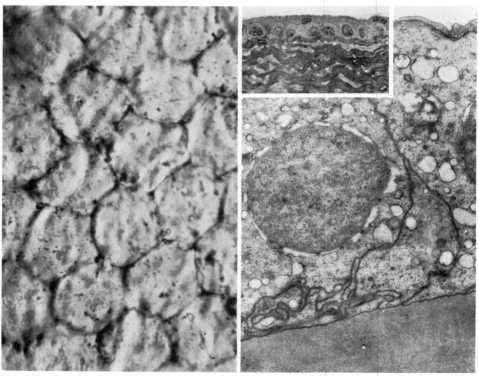

Figure 17–7. *Left:* Flat preparation of the corneal endothelium, showing the hexagonal cell pattern and penetration of the stain into the interdigitations between cells. × 950. (Courtesy of J. Speakman.) *Inset:* Plastic section of corneal endothelium. × 550. *Right:* Electron micrograph of the corneal endothelium with Descemet's membrane beneath. × 7500.

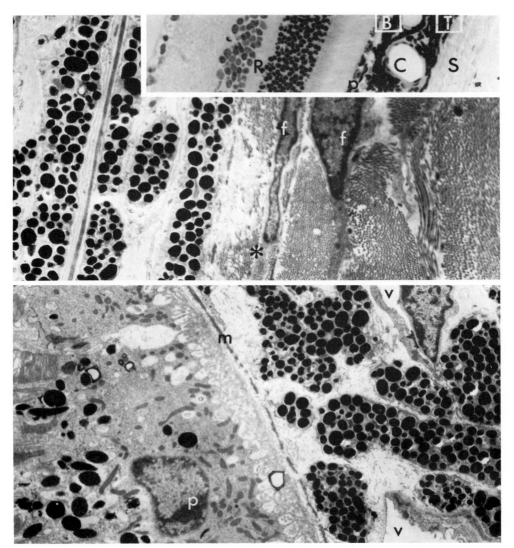

Figure 17–8. *Top right inset:* Photomicrograph showing all layers of the eyeball: S = sclera, C = choroid, R = retina, with "p" the pigment epithelium. The squares roughly indicate regions seen in the top (T) and bottom (B) electron micrographs. In sclera (top right), there are fibroblasts (f) and collagenous bundles, the region of the lamina fusca is marked with an asterisk, and in the choroid there are numerous melanocyte processes (left) containing melanin. *Bottom:* Deeper choroid is seen (right) with melanocytes and blood vessels (v), Bruch's membrane (m), and pigment epithelium (p.) Inset, × 250; top and bottom, × 6000.

inent blood vessels and pigment cells; hence the term "uvea," meaning grape-like.

    Choroid. This spongy, brown membrane contains extensive venous plexuses that usually collapse after death, thus making its thickness difficult to determine. It is about 0.1 to 0.3 mm thick with a potential *perichoroidal* (suprachoroidal) *space* separating it from sclera. Four layers usually are recognized. The *epichoroid* externally is only 20 to 30 μm thick and consists of loosely arranged collagenous and elastic fibrils partially bridging the perichoroidal space, with numerous stellate melanocytes between the fibrils. It blends internally with the *vessel layer,* the thickest part of the choroid, that consists of a mass of arteries and veins lying in loose connective tissue containing many melanocytes. The larger vessels lie more externally and only small vessels lie deep to the fovea. The venous plexuses are drained by four large whorls of veins, one in each quadrant, the efferent vein of each being a vortex vein. The third layer is the *choriocapillaris,* a layer of capillaries in which choroidal arteries terminate. This plexus supplies nutrition to the outer portion of the retina and is unique in that it is oriented in one plane and each capillary is of large diameter and lined by fenestrated (type II) endothelium. Between capillaries is a fine network of elastic and collagenous fibers with a few flattened fibroblasts and melanocytes. The choriocapillaris extends anteriorly only as far as the ora serrata. Internally, between choriocapillaris and the pigment epithelium of the retina is the *lamina elastica (Bruch's membrane),* a shiny homogeneous layer, 1 to 4 μm thick. It is formed by an external lamina of a dense elastic network and an inner, homogeneous basal lamina. The lamina extends anteriorly into ciliary body and posteriorly ends abruptly at the optic disk.

There are nerves in the choroid derived from ciliary (sympathetic) nerves and terminating on musculature of blood vessels. A few multipolar ganglion cells are associated with these nerve plexuses.

Ciliary Body.   The choroid extends anteriorly to the ora serrata where it is thickened as the ciliary body, encircling the eye. In meridional sections, it is triangular in shape, its base facing the anterior chamber, its outer surface separated from sclera by perichoroidal space, and its inner surface against the vitreous, covered by the ciliary (non-nervous) portion of the retina. This surface is irregular with shallow grooves (the ciliary striae) passing forward from the ora serrata, with deeper, radial grooves and ridges anteriorly (the ciliary processes). The outer angle is attached to the scleral spur (the inner, anterior extremity of the sclera that projects internally toward the anterior chamber), and the inner angle is free and juts internally just anterior to the equator of the lens. The ciliary body represents the anterior extension of the retina and the choroid, except the choriocapillaris.

The bulk of the ciliary body is the *ciliary muscle,* comprising three layers of

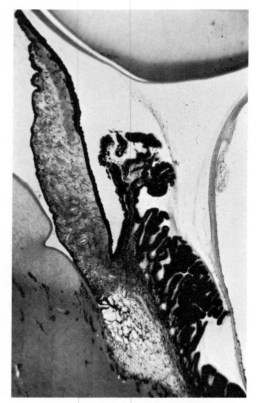

Figure 17–9.   Photomicrograph of a portion of a meridional section of the eye, showing corneoscleral junction, iris, ciliary processes, zonule, and part of the lens. Compare with Figure 17–4. × 25.

smooth muscle fibers with a common origin from the scleral spur and pectinate ligament. The fibers are meridional, radial, and equatorial in orientation and function in accommodation (discussed later), and probably aid also in drainage of aqueous humor. Between smooth muscle fibers is a rich elastic network containing melanocytes. The *vascular* (vessel) layer consists mainly of capillaries and veins lying in, and constituting the bulk of, the ciliary processes, with loose, elastic connective tissue around the vessels. These vessels probably are the site of formation of aqueous humor, the ciliary processes being covered by *ciliary epithelium.* The internal surface of the ciliary body facing the vitreous body (posteriorly) and the posterior chamber (more anteriorly) is covered by a double layer of cuboidal cells. The outer layer is the forward continuation of the pigment epithelium of the retina, supported by a basal lamina continuous with Bruch's membrane. The

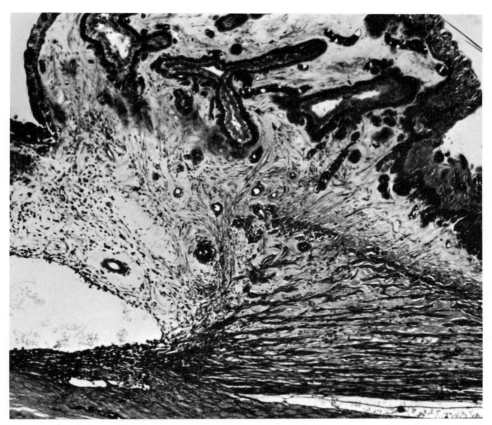

Figure 17–10. Photomicrograph of the angle of the eye, showing the root of the iris and ciliary processes above and the trabecular meshwork, canal of Schlemm, and ciliary muscle arising from scleral spur below. × 125.

inner layer, the ciliary epithelium, is nonpigmented with an irregular surface and represents the forward prolongation of the neural (sensory) retina. Both layers continue forward on the posterior surface of the iris, where the inner layer also becomes heavily pigmented. Internal to the epithelium is the internal limiting membrane, a thin membrane that follows the irregularities of the surface of the ciliary body. Anteriorly, it blends with the condensation of fibrillar material that forms the zonule of the lens.

Iris. This, the most anterior part of the uvea, literally means "rainbow," its central aperture, the pupil, meaning "little girl," so termed from the diminutive image reflected in the cornea against the black background of the

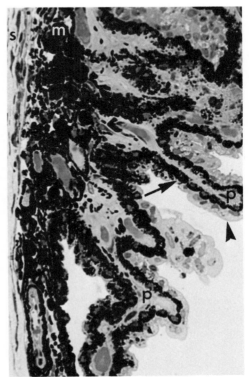

Figure 17–11. Photomicrograph of the ciliary body with sclera (s) to the left. Note numerous melanocytes (m) and ciliary processes (p) covered by ciliary epithelium, the basal layer pigmented (arrow), the internal layer nonpigmented (arrowhead). Plastic section. × 250.

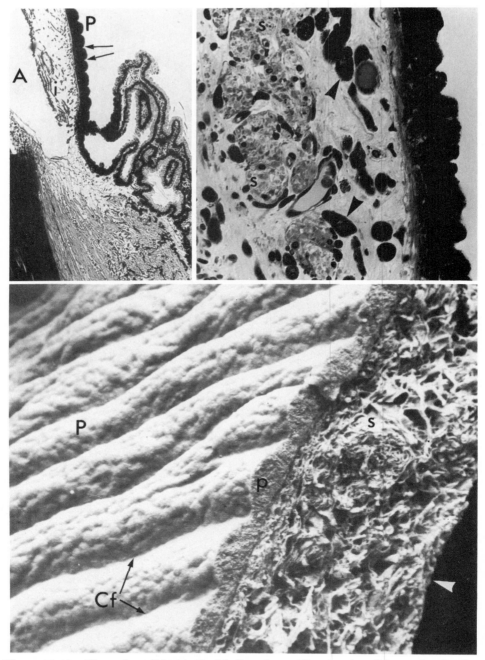

Figure 17–12.   Illustrations of the iris. *Top left:* Part of a meridional section of the eye showing the root of the iris (i) with posterior pigmented epithelium showing deep circular furrows (arrows). "*A*" and "*P*" are anterior and posterior chambers of the eye. (Compare with Figure 17–9.) × 40. *Top right:* The posterior portion of the iris with stroma containing circular smooth muscle of the sphincter pupillae (s), cut here in transverse section, and melanocytes (arrowheads): posterior pigmented epithelium at right edge. × 300. *Bottom:* Low-power SEM of a section through the iris showing deep circular furrows (Cf) of the posterior pigmented epithelium (P), the cells appearing granular in section (p). The iris stroma (s) is loose and irregular with the anterior surface of the iris at right (arrowhead). × 280. (SEM courtesy of Dr. D. H. Dickson.)

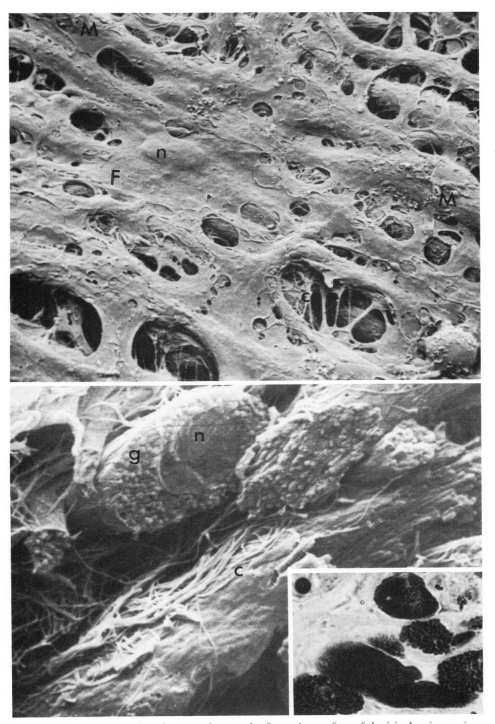

Figure 17–13.   *Top:* Scanning electron micrograph of anterior surface of the iris showing an incomplete surface layer of fibroblasts (F), much flattened, with a nucleus (n) seen, resting on successive layers of melanocytes (M), and collagen fibrils (c) in the stroma. × 900. *Bottom:* SEM of a freeze-fracture preparation of the iris stroma showing melanocytes with collagen fibrils (c). One melanocyte is fractured to show clearly the nucleus (n) and melanin granules (g) in its cytoplasm. × 6700. (Courtesy of Dr. D. H. Dickson and reproduced by kind permission of the editor, Canadian Journal of Ophthalmology). *Inset, lower right:* Melanocytes within the iris stroma. × 900.

pupil. It varies in color among individuals and with age. It is thin peripherally at its root where it attaches to the ciliary body, thicker centrally, and thin at its pupillary margin where it rests against the anterior surface of the lens. It has the form of a flat, truncated cone, inclining forward from its attachment to the ciliary body. Its anterior surface is irregular and divided into a peripheral ciliary zone and a central pupillary zone. The posterior surface is uniformly black and shows shallow furrows. Structurally, there are several layers, the anterior ones being part of the uvea (mesodermal) and the posterior ones being ectodermal (pars iridica). Most anteriorly is a single layer of flattened cells, considered by some continuous with corneal endothelium, but by others as a layer of fibroblasts. Beneath it is a delicate connective tissue stroma with fibroblasts and melanocytes, the quantity of pigment in these melanocytes determining the color of the iris. Little or no pigment gives a blue color and, with increasing pigment, shades of gray, green, brown, and black.

Beneath this stroma is a layer of blood vessels, running radially and in a spiral manner to accommodate easily to changes in length with changes in pupil diameter. The vessels have thick walls and lie in a delicate connective tissue stroma that contains chromatophores and primitive fibroblasts. Underlying this vessel layer are smooth muscle fibers arranged as sphincter and dilator pupillae. The sphincter muscle lies at the pupillary margin, supplied by parasympathetic fibers of the third nerve (Edinger-Westphal nucleus) that have synapsed in the ciliary ganglion. The dilator muscle is a thin, radially oriented, indeterminate layer just anterior to the posterior pigmented epithelium. It is not true muscle but consists of the basal processes of the basal (anterior) layer of this epithelium, i.e., these cells are myoepithelial. It is supplied by sympathetic fibers through the superior cervical ganglion. The epithelium of the posterior surface of the iris is heavily pigmented and consists of two layers of cuboidal cells. The basal (or anterior) layer adjacent to the stroma is formed by the apical parts of myoepithelial cells; the posterior layer shows junctional complexes and is separated from the posterior chamber by the limiting membrane of the iris, a thin basal lamina.

The Chambers of the Eye

Anterior Chamber. This is the space bounded anteriorly by the posterior surface of the cornea and posteriorly by the lens, iris, and anterior surface of the ciliary body. The lateral border of the anterior chamber is the iris angle or limbus occupied by the trabecular meshwork (pectinate ligament) through which aqueous humor is drained into the canal of Schlemm.

Posterior Chamber. This is bounded anteriorly by the iris, posteriorly by the anterior surface of the lens and zonule, and peripherally by the ciliary processes.

Both chambers contain *aqueous humor,* a thin watery fluid secreted partially by the ciliary epithelium and by diffusion from capillaries in ciliary processes. It contains diffusible materials of blood plasma but with a low protein content (0.02 per cent) compared to serum (7 per cent). It is secreted continuously into the posterior chamber, passes into the anterior chamber through the pupil, and is drained through the trabecular tissue into the canal of Schlemm. If the secretion rate is balanced by the drainage rate, intraocular pressure will remain constant at about 23 mm of mercury. However, if there is obstruction to drainage and secretion continues, intraocular pressure rises, a condition called *glaucoma,* which, if untreated, may result in damage to the retina and blindness. Drainage of aqueous thus is important and requires further description.

Canal of Schlemm. This annular vessel encircles the eye just anterior and external to the scleral spur, bounded externally by scleral tissue and internally by the deeper layer of trabecular tissue. It usually has a single lumen but may be double or even plexiform, with an endothelial wall only 1 μm thick. It has afferent connections for drainage of aqueous humor through trabecular spaces and efferent drainage via 20 to 30 endothelium-lined tubes leaving the canal around its circumference. They

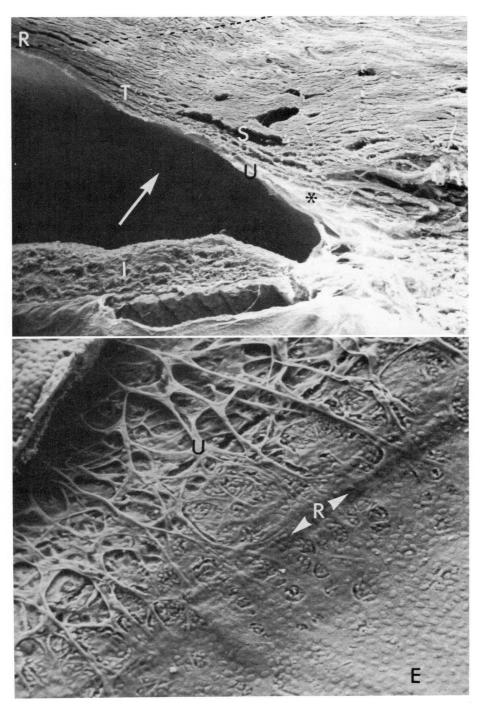

Figure 17–14. *Top:* Low-power scanning electron micrograph of a meridional section through the limbus (compare with Figure 17–12, top left). The corneolimbal junction is outlined by the dotted line commencing internally at the ring of Schwalbe (R). The trabecular meshwork, with the ropelike uveal meshwork (U) and the deeper scleral or trabecular meshwork proper (T), separates aqueous humor in the anterior chamber from the canal of Schlemm (S). The scleral spur (asterisk) and the iris (I) are seen also. × 100. (Courtesy of Dr. D. H. Dickson.) *Bottom:* SEM of the internal surface of the limbus as it would appear when viewed in the direction of the arrow in the top figure, with corneal endothelium (E) at lower right, showing nuclei, which become wider apart (i.e., the endothelial cells are larger) at the periphery of the cornea. × 180. (Courtesy of Drs. D. H. Dickson, N. Carroll, and G. W. Crock.)

pass into sclera and anastomose to form the deep scleral plexus. A few direct channels are present also and pass with efferent vessels from the deep scleral plexus to the episcleral venous plexus that lies external to the limbus. The more anterior channels of this plexus contain only aqueous and not blood ("aqueous veins").

Trabecular Meshwork (Pectinate Ligament). This spongelike tissue is interposed between the anterior chamber and the canal of Schlemm and is triangular in form in meridional sections. It is formed by trabeculae or beams with spaces between them in which aqueous humor drains, all the trabeculae arising anteriorly from the ring of Schwalbe, which marks the pos-

terior extremity of Descemet's membrane, and from subjacent corneal lamellae. Three zones are recognized.

The uveal meshwork is most internal and passes between Schwalbe's line and the root of the iris and its stroma. The trabeculae are thin and delicate. The scleral or main meshwork consists of thicker, flattened, perforated bands of tissue passing from Schwalbe's line and corneal lamellae to ciliary body and scleral spur. The endothelial (external) meshwork consists of perforated sheets of endothelium with little supporting connective tissue and forms the inner wall of the canal of Schlemm. The pores within it connect trabecular spaces internally with the lumen of the canal of Schlemm. All trabeculae are covered by

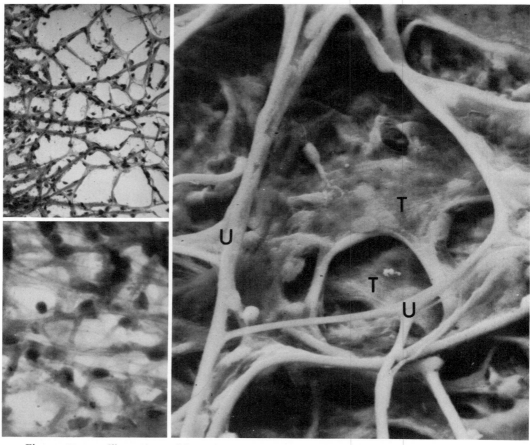

Figure 17–15. Illustrations of the trabecular meshwork. *Left:* Photomicrographs of flat preparations showing, *top,* the thin cords of the uveal meshwork with trabeculae covered by endothelium and trabecular spaces between, and *bottom,* the scleral meshwork with flat, lamella-like trabeculae. Top, × 225; bottom, × 350. (Courtesy of J. Speakman.) *Right:* SEM of the internal portion of the endothelium-covered trabecular meshwork with ropelike uveal trabeculae (U) and, more deeply, the flattened lamellae of the trabecular (scleral) (T) meshwork. × 1000. (Courtesy of Drs. D. H. Dickson, N. Carroll, and G. W. Crock.)

endothelium and the connective tissue core of the main scleral trabeculae is prominent and contains both ordinary collagen fibrils and "long-spacing" collagen with a periodicity of 105 to 125 nm. Present in the meshwork are fine nerve endings of the supraciliary plexus.

The Refractive Media

The refractive media include all transparent structures through which light rays must pass to reach the retina. The cornea and anterior and posterior chambers already have been described, and the remaining components are the lens and the vitreous body.

Lens. The crystalline lens is biconvex, the posterior surface being more highly curved than the anterior. Each surface has a pole. The line joining anterior and posterior poles is the axis, and the peripheral circumferential border is termed the equator. The lens is elastic in the young but becomes harder and sclerosed with age. It is surrounded by a strong, highly elastic capsule which is attached to the ciliary body by the zonule or suspensory ligament. The axis (thickness) is about 3.6 mm, increasing to 4.5 mm in accommodation; the equa-

torial diameter in the adult is about 9 mm.

The lens inherently tends to become spherical but is opposed by tension in the zonule.

Structurally there are three components. The *lens capsule* is a homogeneous, apparently structureless membrane, 10 to 20 μm thick, being thicker on the anterior surface, and composed of basal lamina material and reticular fibers. It is elastic, although it contains no elastic fibers, and the zonular fibers are attached to it. On the anterior surface only, beneath the capsule, is the *subcapsular epithelium,* a single layer of cuboidal cells. Towards the equator, these cells become columnar and transform into lens fibers. The *lens substance* is composed of lens fibers, each in the form of a six-sided prism, 8 to 10 mm long, 8 to 12 μm broad, and only 2 μm thick, with the long sides parallel to the lens surface. The external, younger fibers show a regular pattern, but the central, older fibers become more irregular. Younger fibers contain nuclei, but these are lost from central fibers. Fibers from opposite points of the equator meet at the poles in sutures or junctions to form a triradiate star figure in a Y form, the Y standing erect on the an-

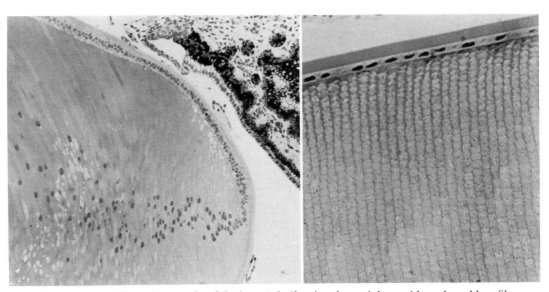

Figure 17–16. Photomicrographs of the lens. *Left:* Showing the periphery with nucleated lens fibers, homogeneous lens capsule, and subcapsular epithelium on the anterior (top) surface. Part of the ciliary body appears at top right. × 50. *Right:* The anterior surface of the lens with capsule, subcapsular epithelium, and closely packed, hexagonal lens fibers in transverse section. × 350.

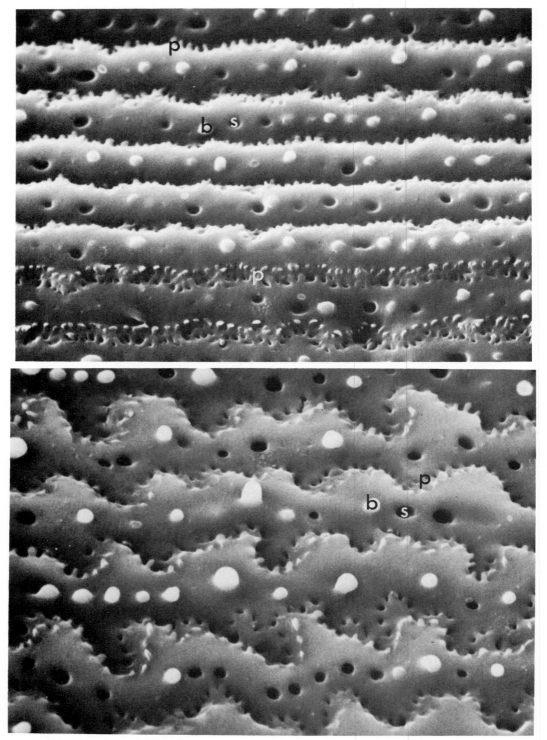

Figure 17–17.   Scanning electron micrographs of lens fibers. *Top:* The surface of cortical lens fibers (rat) close to the posterior pole of the lens, showing processes (p) of adjacent fibers which are closely interlocked. In addition, upper and lower surfaces of the fibers are held together by interlocking "ball (b) and socket (s)" processes. × 5200. *Bottom:* Outer surfaces of fibers close to the equator with similar interlocking but with the fibers in a zigzag arrangement. × 6000. (Courtesy of M. J. Hollenberg and B. J. Lewis.)

terior surface and inverted posteriorly. Between lens fibers is a small amount of cementing substance, and adjacent fibers show a complex interlocking of cytoplasmic processes.

The lens is held in place by the suspensory ligament or *zonule,* consisting of strands (zonular fibers) of fibrillar material passing from the ciliary body to the equator of the lens, thus covering the

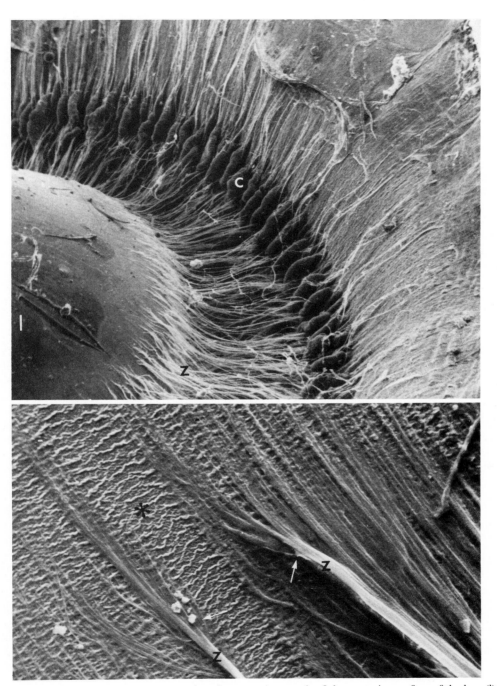

Figure 17–18. *Top:* Low-power scanning electron micrograph of the posterior surface of the lens (l), zonule (z), and ciliary body (c), with zonular fibers passing from the region of the ora serrata (top right) and ciliary body to the posterior surface of the lens. × 28. *Bottom:* A higher magnification showing that zonular fibers (z), as they approach the lens, splay out (arrow) before contacting the lens capsule, which is crenated (asterisk) by tension of the zonular fibers. × 660. (Courtesy of Dr. D. H. Dickson.)

lens. At their attachment to the lens, zonular fibers split into finer fibers that fuse with the lens capsule.

Vitreous Body. This is a clear, transparent gel that fills the space between the retina and the lens. Thus, it is spheroidal in shape with an anterior depression to accommodate the lens. It is adherent to the ciliary epithelium, particularly around the optic disc and the ora serrata. It is composed of hyaluronic acid and collagen fibrils in a fine network, the fibrils· being denser peripherally and around an anteroposterior, fluid-containing, tubular canal, the "hyaloid canal," which originally contained the embryonic hyaloid artery. A few cells are present, particularly at the periphery, and these are macrophages and cells ("hyalocytes") concerned in the synthesis and maintenance of collagen and hyaluronic acid. Peripherally, it is adherent to the internal limiting membrane.

The Retina

The retina is the innermost layer of the eyeball and comprises an anterior, nonsensitive portion (iridial and ciliary, already described) and a posterior, functional portion, the photoreceptor organ. It develops as an evagination of the forebrain, the optic vesicle, that retains its connection to the brain by the optic stalk, the future optic nerve. The optic vesicle becomes transformed into a two-layered optic cup, the outer layer forming the pigment epithelium, the inner becoming the neural retina or retina proper. A potential space remains between the two layers, traversed only by processes of the pigment cells. The outer, pigment layer is attached firmly to the choroid, but the inner layer is detached readily during histological preparation, and also in life following trauma ("clinical detachment" of the retina).

The optical or neural retina lines the choroid from the papilla of the optic nerve posteriorly to the ora serrata anteriorly and shows a shallow depression, the fovea centralis, situated about 2.5 mm to the temporal side of the optic papilla. Around the fovea is an area known as the yellow spot or *macula lutea*. The fovea is the area of most clear vision. There are no photoreceptors over the optic papilla, a region also called the *blind spot*.

Layers of the Retina. In cross section, from external to internal, the layers of the retina are as follows:

1. Pigment epithelium
2. Layer of rods and cones } 1st neuron
3. External limiting membrane
4. Outer nuclear layer
5. Outer plexiform layer
6. Inner nuclear layer } 2nd neuron
7. Inner plexiform layer
8. Ganglion cell layer
9. Optic nerve fiber layer } 3rd neuron
10. Internal limiting membrane

The retina is a complex structure, but the complexity becomes simplified with appreciation of the fact that it is only three neurons deep. Each rod or cone (the first neuron) has a sensory end organ lying outermost against the pigment epithelium, a nucleus, and an inner terminal fiber, and these parts of the cells account for the outer layers. The nuclei of the rods are placed more centrally than those of the cones. At the fovea, there are many layers of cone nuclei, but over the remainder of the retina, layer four is composed of a single outer row of cone nuclei with four rows of rod nuclei lying more centrally. The outer plexiform layer marks the junction between first and second (intermediate) neurons. The inner nuclear layer appears as a closely packed mass of nuclei of bipolar (second neuron) cells, association cells, and supporting elements. The inner plexiform layer is the site of junction between second and third neurons, the ganglion cell layer containing ganglion (third neuron) cells and neuroglia. The central processes of the ganglion cells form the optic nerve fibers, all of which pass to the optic papilla and thus to the optic nerve. These fibers are unmyelinated but obtain a myelin sheath as they pass through the cribriform plate at the optic papilla. Thus, it should be recognized that the retina is gray matter of the central nervous system and the optic nerve is white matter. The internal lim-

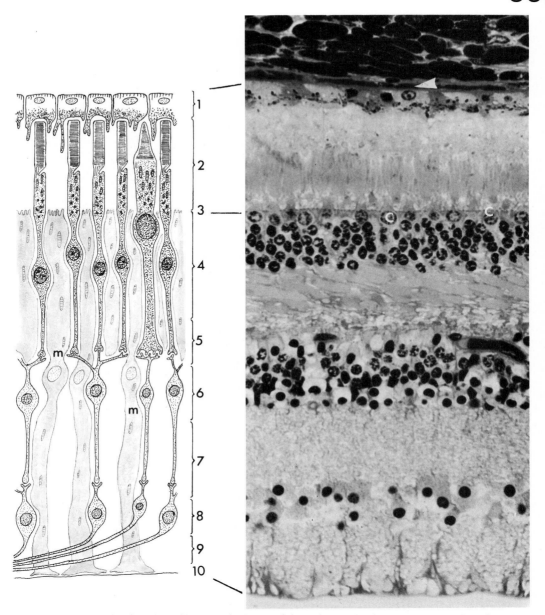

Figure 17–19. *Left:* Diagram to illustrate the layers of the retina. Only photoreceptors (rods and one cone), direct conducting neurons, and the fibers of Müller are illustrated. The numbers refer to the layers as listed in the text. *Right:* Photomicrograph of the same area. At top is the inner portion of the choroid with the choriocapillaris (dark, arrowhead). Cone nuclei are indicated (c). × 400.

iting membrane separates the retina from the vitreous body.

Pigment Epithelium. This is a single layer of polygonal cells, 10 to 14 μm high, and regular in shape; toward the ora serrata the cells become more flattened. Nuclei are spherical and lie toward the cell bases that show complex interdigitating cell processes typical of actively transporting epithelia. Lateral-

ly, there are junctional complexes and apically there are complex cylindrical outfoldings around photoreceptor outer segments with long microvilli between photoreceptors. Numerous mitochondria lie in basal cytoplasm and around nuclei with a well-developed agranular reticulum, some granular reticulum, a Golgi apparatus, and some lipofuscin granules. Prominent also are

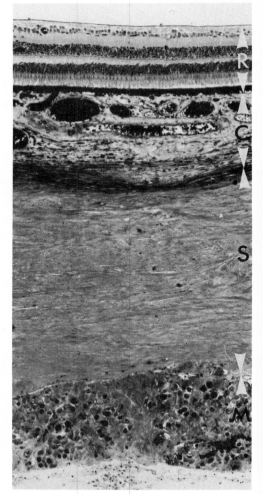

Figure 17–20. Photomicrograph of a section through the full thickness of the eye showing retina (R), choroid (C), sclera (S), and muscle (M) fibers of an extraocular muscle. × 50.

Figure 17–21. *Below.* Photomicrograph to show all layers of the retina. Compare with Figure 17–19. Part of the choroid appears below. ×350. *Inset:* Plastic section to show pigment epithelium (below), outer and inner segments of rods, and rod nuclei. ×1050.

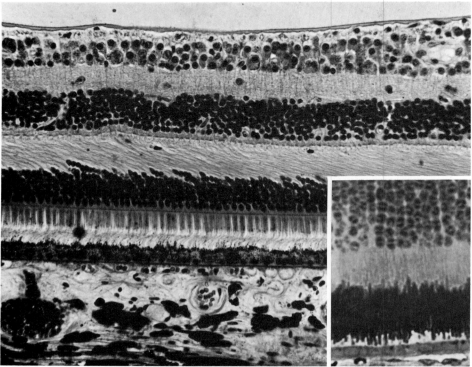

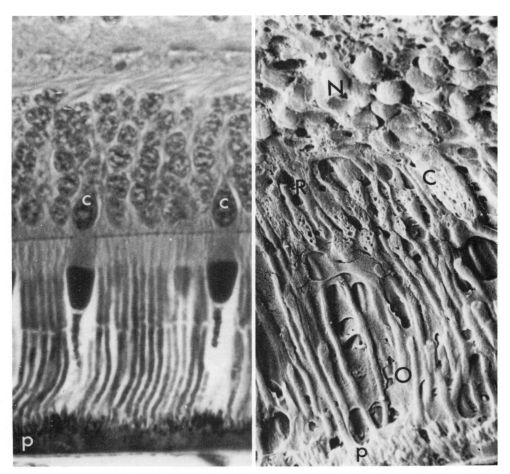

Figure 17–22. *Left:* Photomicrograph of part of the retina extending from Brüch's membrane (bottom) and pigment epithelium (p) to the outer plexiform layer (top). Note the two cone nuclei (c). × 1500. *Right:* Similar area shown by freeze-fracture scanning electron micrograph with nuclei of photoreceptors in the outer nuclear layer (N), inner segments of rods (R) and a cone (C), and outer segments (O). ×1500. (Scanning electron micrograph courtesy of Dr. D. H. Dickson.)

numerous melanin granules and premelanosomes and residual bodies or phagosomes containing lamellar debris resulting from phagocytosis of membrane lamellae from the external tips of photoreceptor outer segments.

Functionally, the pigment epithelium absorbs light and prevents reflection, is concerned in nutrition of the photoreceptors, is involved in the turnover of their membrane lamellae, and is essential for the formation of rhodopsin and its movement by storing and releasing vitamin A, a rhodopsin precursor.

Elements of the Neural Retina. Four cell groups are present: photoreceptors (rods and cones); direct conducting neurons (bipolar and ganglion cells); association and other neurons (horizontal, amacrine, and centrifugal bipolar cells); and supporting elements (Müller's fibers and neuroglia).

Photoreceptors. Both rods and cones are modified neurons and show inner and outer segments lying outside the external limiting membrane, an outer conducting fiber (physiologically a dendrite) passing to a cell body in the outer nuclear layer, and an inner conducting fiber (physiologically an axon) extending into the outer plexiform layer. It must be appreciated that light must pass through the thickness of the retina to reach photoreceptors.

The Rod. The rods are slender, specialized cells with cylindrical outer segments about 28 μm long containing the photopigment rhodopsin (visual purple)

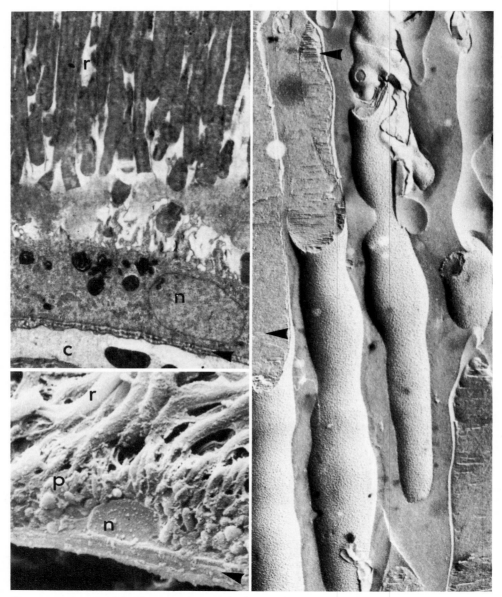

Figure 17–23.   *Top left:* Electron micrograph of rat retina showing outer segments of rods (r, above), pigment epithelium with a nucleus (n), Bruch's membrane (arrowhead) and choriocapillaris (c). × 3500. *Bottom left:* A similar area in a freeze-fracture scanning electron micrograph, with pigment granules (p) in the cytoplasm of the pigment epithelial cell. × 5000. (Courtesy of Dr. D. H. Dickson.) *Right:* Freeze-etch preparation of rod outer segments showing internal membrane lamellae (arrowheads). × 12,500.

and a slightly thicker inner segment of about 32 μm, both being 1.5 to 2 μm thick. The tip of the outer segment is "embedded" in pigment epithelium and shows transverse striations. The two segments are connected by a narrow "neck."

By electron microscopy, the outer segment is seen to be composed of trans-verse membrane lamellae or discs, 14 nm thick, with intervals of 10 nm. Rhodopsin is located on these lamellae. The neck region, which is eccentrically placed, contains a modified cilium that originates in a basal body located in the distal end of the inner segment, often with a striated rootlet. The inner segment shows an outer "ellipsoid" containing numerous mitochondria and an inner "myoid" with granular and agranular reticulum, microtubules, a Golgi apparatus, and particulate glycogen. The rod proper is connected to its perikaryon (in the outer nuclear layer) by a delicate outer rod fiber that traverses the external limiting membrane, from which an inner rod fiber extends into the outer plexiform layer to terminate in a small end knob, the rod spherule, which contacts dendrites of bipolar cells of the in-

ner nuclear layer and axons of horizontal cells. In rods, membrane lamellae constantly are synthesized and added to the outer segment with the oldest lamellae at their tips phagocytosed and destroyed by cells of the pigment epithelium, a cycle of total renewal occupying about 10 days.

The Cone. While similar to a rod, the cone shows a tapering outer segment swelling to a conical inner segment, the two being flask-shaped. Some lamellae of

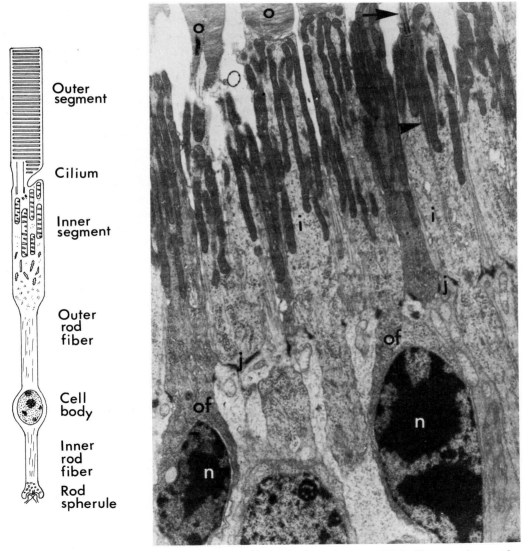

Figure 17–24. *Left:* Diagram of a rod as seen with the electron microscope. *Right:* Electron micrograph of the outer portion of rods showing outer segments (o); a connecting cilium in a neck region (arrow); inner segments (i), one showing a striated rootlet of a cilium (arrowhead); the external limiting membrane and its junctional complexes (j); outer rod fibers (of); and rod nuclei (n). × 4500.

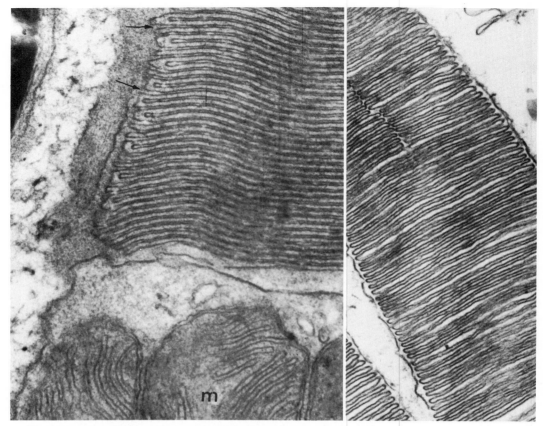

Figure 17–25.   Electron micrographs of the outer segments of a cone *(left)* and rods *(right)*. In the cone, some membrane lamellae appear to be infoldings of (i.e., continuous with) the covering plasmalemma (arrows). Part of the inner segment of the cone with mitochondria (m) is seen below. Left, × 56,000; right, × 52,000.

the outer segment, particularly the proximal ones, show membranes continuous with the covering plasma membrane so that their lumina are continuous with the extracellular space. Cone inner segments resemble those of rods, and inner and outer segments also are connected by a modified cilium. The cone nucleus is larger than that of the rod, shows less densely packed chromatin, and lies just internal to the external limiting membrane; thus, the outer cone fiber is short and the inner cone fiber is long. It is thicker too than that of the rod and widens at its termination in the outer plexiform layer to form a cone pedicle, from which small processes emerge. In the fovea, each cone pedicle is connected to a single bipolar cell. Cones vary in different regions of the retina: those at the fovea are long and slender with inner and outer segments of the same diame-

ter, viz., they are not truly cone-shaped. In peripheral retina, cones are shorter and thicker.

There are estimated to be 130 million rods and 6 to 7 million cones in the human retina.

Direct Conducting Neurons.   These comprise the bipolar and ganglion cells.

Bipolar Cells.   The cell bodies of these cells lie mostly in the central zone of the inner nuclear area. They can be divided into two main groups: the diffuse bipolars contacting several photoreceptors and the midget or monosynaptic bipolars connecting with a single cell. The dendrites of the diffuse bipolars contact rod spherules or groups of about six cone pedicles in the outer plexiform layer. The dendrites may be long ("mop" bipolars) or short ("brush" bipolars). As just stated, the dendritic expansions pen-

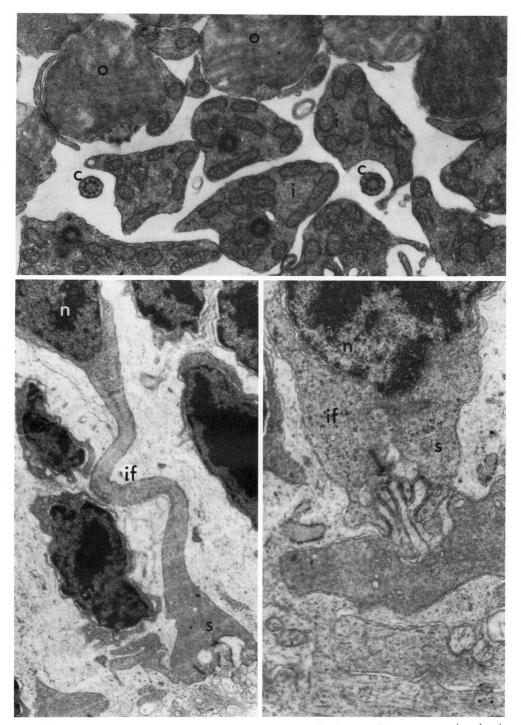

Figure 17–26. Electron micrographs to illustrate features of rods. *Top:* A transverse section showing outer segments (o) with membrane lamellae *en face,* inner segments (i), and neck regions with cilia (c). *Bottom left:* The central region of a rod showing nucleus (n), inner rod fiber (if), and rod spherule (s) in the outer plexiform layer. *Bottom right:* A rod nucleus (n) lying centrally in the outer nuclear layer has a short inner fiber (if) passing to a spherule (s). Note the dark, synaptic "ribbons" in spherules. Top, × 8,000; bottom left, × 4,500; bottom right, × 18,000.

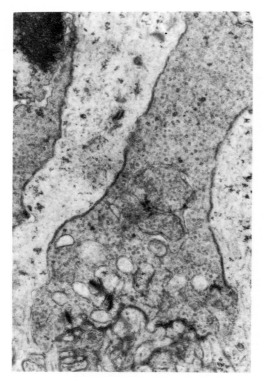

Figure 17–27. Electron micrograph of cone pedicle: note the dark, linear bodies (synaptic ribbons) in the pedicle. × 20,000.

etrate the rod spherules. Axons are straight and pass vertically into the inner plexiform layer where they contact dendrites of ganglion cells. The midget bipolars synapse with only a single cone pedicle. The axon passes into the inner plexiform layer and divides into several small telodendrons which synapse with the dendrites of a single midget ganglion cell, thus providing a one-to-one pathway from cone to optic nerve fiber.

Ganglion Cells. These are situated in the inner retina (layer 8, ganglion cell layer) with their dendrites in the inner plexiform layer and their axons constituting the optic nerve fibers. The axons never branch. They are large cells, closely resembling cerebral neurons with a mass of chromophil material (Nissl body) in the cell body. They are of two main types, the diffuse type with dendrites contacting several bipolar cells, and the small or monosynaptic type with dendrites synapsing with a single, midget, cone, bipolar cell.

Association and Centrifugal Neurons

Horizontal Cells. The bodies of these cells lie in the outer part of the inner nuclear layer with dendrites and axons in the inner part of the outer plexiform layer. The cell bodies are larger than most bipolar cells in the same layer. The dendrites terminate in cuplike "baskets" around numerous cone pedicles, and the single axon branches at its termination into an elaborate telodendron to synapse with both rod spherules and cone pedicles. The horizontal cells thus connect a group of cone cells in one area with a group of rods and cones in another area and perhaps raise or lower the functional threshold between rods and cones and the bipolar cells.

Amacrine Cells. These cells lie in the inner two or three rows of the inner nuclear layer. They are pear-shaped with a single process passing inward to terminate in the inner plexiform layer, where the process branches extensively and synapses with several ganglion cells.

Supporting Elements. In the retina, as in the brain, an elaborate framework of neuroglia serves functions of support, insulation, and nutrition. This framework consists of a main network of Müller's fibers with astroglia, perivascular glia, and microglia, the last being mesodermal in origin, the others ectodermal.

Cells of Müller. These cells, also called retinal gliocytes, are giant in size with their nuclei lying in the inner nuclear layer together with nuclei of bipolar cells. From the cell body, long, thin cytoplasmic processes extend to the inner and outer limiting membranes; i.e., they traverse nearly the full thickness of the retina. From these processes, subsidiary, sheetlike processes extend around photoreceptors, bipolar cells, and ganglion cells, and these gliocytes thus occupy much of the total volume of the retina, permitting little in the way of intercellular spaces. At the inner limiting membrane, broad, footlike processes abut against the membrane (and vitreous) while, externally, the processes meet rods and cones at junctional complexes to form the external limiting membrane. Here, the processes show a few microvilli.

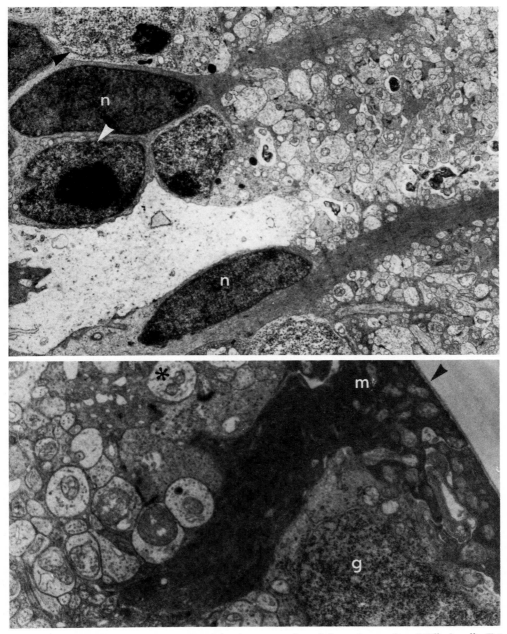

Figure 17–28. Electron micrographs of the deeper portion of the retina to show Müller's cells. *Top:* Müller's cell nuclei (n) lie in the inner nuclear layer with nuclei of bipolar cells (arrowheads), with processes passing to the right (centrally) in the inner plexiform layer. *Bottom:* A Müller's cell process (m) abuts against the internal limiting membrane (arrowhead) with the nucleus of a ganglion cell (g) and nerve fibers (asterisk) of the optic nerve fiber layer. Top, × 5,000; bottom, × 12,500.

Other Glial Elements. These form the finer neuroglial network and include "interstitial spongioblasts" in the inner nuclear layer and astrocytes, which are more numerous in the optic nerve and the region of the disk than in the retina itself. In the retina, the astrocytes are star-shaped cells in the ganglion cell layer and the inner and outer plexiform layers, and small cells usually only with two processes (the lemmocytes) situated in the nerve fiber layer. Microglia are found in all layers and are phagocytic.

The Limiting Membranes. As explained above, the external limiting membrane is formed by processes of Müller's cells and is perforate in the sense that photoreceptors traverse it. The internal limiting membrane is a basal lamina separating the central expansions of Müller's cells from the vitreous.

Central Area of Retina. The human retina can be divided into a central area 5 to 6 mm in diameter and a peripheral

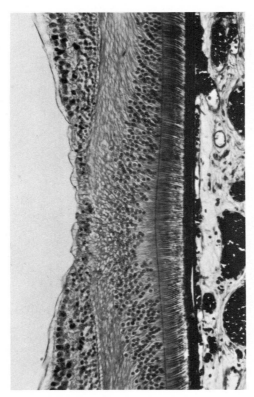

Figure 17–29. Section through the fovea centralis. Notice the disappearance of the inner layers of the retina and the closely packed, elongated cones in the floor of the depression. × 275.

area comprising the remainder of the retina. This distinction is both morphological and functional, the central area with a high concentration of photoreceptors being specialized for accurate diurnal vision, and the peripheral area being of coarser structure and more suitable for reception of weak stimuli in dim illumination.

Morphologically, in the central area there is an accumulation of ganglion cells in more than one row and a density of cones and bipolar cells. The *macula lutea* is a more vague area characterized by the presence of a yellow pigment in the inner layers of the retina. This is an area about 3 mm in diameter surrounding the *fovea,* which itself contains very little pigment and thus appears pale.

The fovea centralis is a shallow, rounded pit lying 4 mm to the temporal side of the optic disk and about 0.8 mm below the horizontal meridian. The depression is caused by the virtually complete absence of the inner layers of the retina in this region, the visual cells in the floor of the fovea all being cones, closely packed and longer than those in the peripheral retina. These cones synapse with bipolar cells obliquely placed around the margins of the fovea. There are no capillaries in the central area of the fovea.

Optic Papilla and Nerve. The retinal aspect of the optic nerve is termed the *optic disk.* This includes the slight prominence, the optic papilla, formed by the heaping up of nerve fibers as they leave the retina to enter the optic nerve, and a small central depression (the "physiological cup") through which the central artery and vein of the retina emerge. The central artery in the great majority of cases is the sole arterial supply to the retina, and its occlusion results in permanent blindness. In some people, the retina also is supplied partially by a cilioretinal artery to the macula. Occlusion of the central artery in these people causes only a loss of peripheral vision, the macula being spared. The optic disk usually is slightly oval, about 1.5 mm in diameter, situated to the nasal side of the posterior pole. At the margin of the disk all the retinal tissues except the optic nerve fibers cease abruptly. The opening in the sclera is filled by the lamina cribrosa, a dense fibrous plate

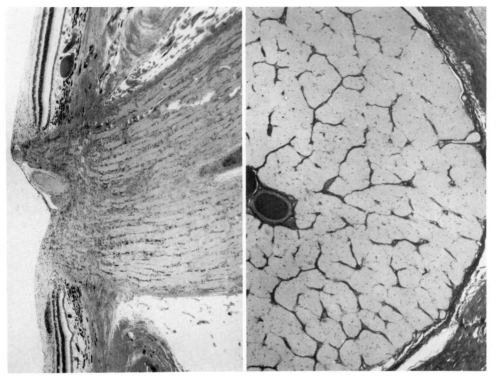

Figure 17–30. *Left:* Section through the optic disk and optic papilla with the central artery to the retina (dark, right center) within the optic nerve. × 25. *Right:* Part of the optic nerve in transverse section, central artery at center left. × 40.

perforated by bundles of optic nerve fibers, and continuous with the tissue of the sclera at its periphery.

The optic nerve itself is not a peripheral nerve but is a tract of the central nervous system between the retinal ganglion cells and the midbrain. It extends posteriorly to the optic chiasma and contains over 1000 bundles of myelinated nerve fibers supported by neuroglia (astrocytes) and not endoneurium. The meninges and subarachnoid space continue from the brain as sheaths of the optic nerve. In addition to afferent fibers from the retinal photoreceptors, the optic nerve also contains fibers running to the tectum of the brain for the pupillary reflex, fibers to the superior colliculus, some autonomic nerve fibers, and a few efferent fibers passing to the retina, of unknown function. The central artery and vein reach the retina by entering the optic nerve some distance posterior to the eyeball.

Accessory Organs of the Eye

The eyeball is situated in the bony orbit which, of course, is open anteriorly. This opening is closed by the upper and lower eyelids which, when they are opposed, meet at the transverse *palpebral fissure*. Conjunctiva covers the anterior surface of the cornea and is reflected from its perimeter to line the deep surface of the eyelids, the reflections being termed superior and inferior *fornices*. With the eyelids closed, the conjunctival sac is a closed space anterior to the eyeball filled with a small amount of fluid.

Eyelids. Essentially, each eyelid consists of a central supporting plate of connective tissue and skeletal muscle covered by skin externally and a mucous membrane internally. The skin anteriorly is thin with small hairs, sweat and sebaceous glands, and a dermis of delicate connective tissue rich in elastic

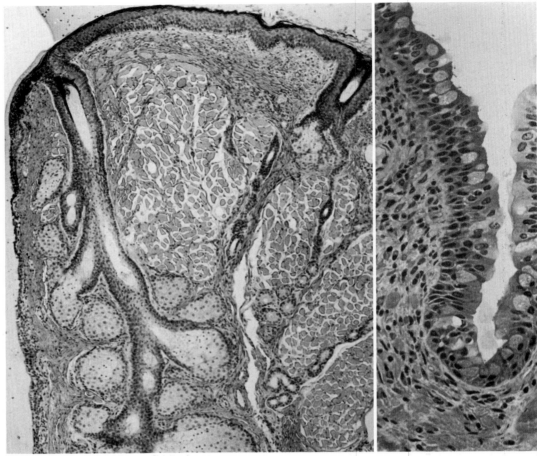

Figure 17–31. *Left:* Photomicrograph of part of an eyelid, showing conjunctiva (left), epidermis (above), and the large modified sebaceous glands (tarsal or meibomian glands). The striated muscle fibers (right) are part of the palpebral portion of orbicularis oculi muscle and between them are parts of three glands of Moll (apocrine type sweat glands). × 25. *Right:* The inferior conjunctival fornix with goblet, mucus-secreting cells (pale-staining) in the epithelium. × 200.

fibers. The dermis is more dense at the lid margin and here contains three or four rows of long, stiff hairs, the *eyelashes,* which penetrate deeply into the dermis. Between and posterior to the eyelashes are large, modified sweat glands characterized by straight and not coiled terminal ducts (the glands of Moll).

Beneath the skin is a layer of striated muscle fibers, this being the palpebral part of the orbicularis oculi muscle which is the bulk of the core of the eyelid, and the fibers of insertion of levator palpebrae superioris. Slender slips of smooth muscle, the palpebral muscles (of Müller), also are present.

Posterior to the muscle layer is a fibrous layer consisting of a thin sheet of fibrous tissue peripherally (the septum orbitale) and the tarsal plate. The tarsal plates are sheets of dense connective tissue curved to the shape of the eyeball, the upper being D-shaped with its lower horizontal border coextensive with the lid margin. The upper plate is 10 to 12 mm broad, but the lower plate is a narrow (5 mm) band lying in the central region of the lower lid. Present in both tarsal plates is a single row of very large sebaceous glands, the tarsal (meibomian) glands, the ducts of which open at the lid margin. From the main ducts, numerous lateral branches pass out to drain single or multiple secretory alveoli. The deep, posterior surface of each tarsal plate blends with conjunctiva which is continuous with epidermis at the inner edge of the lid margin.

Conjunctiva. The conjunctiva is the mucous membrane lining the inner surface of the eyelids from which it is reflected onto the anterior surface of the eyeball. It is continuous with corneal epithelium at the corneal margin and with skin at the lid margins.

The conjunctival epithelium varies with location but consists of a basal layer of cuboidal cells, a surface layer of cone or cylindrical shaped cells, and, particularly over the lower lid, one to three intermediate layers of polygonal cells. Scattered among the epithelial cells are some mucus-secreting goblet cells.

At the edge of the cornea, the conjunctival epithelium becomes stratified squamous identical to the corneal epithelium. Underlying the epithelium is a lamina propria, superficially composed of fine fibroelastic connective tissue with numerous lymphocytes (the "adenoid" layer) and deeply composed of dense fibroconnective tissue.

The Lacrimal Apparatus. The lacrimal apparatus comprises the lacrimal glands and their ducts draining into the conjunctival sac, and the lacrimal passages which drain excess tears from the conjunctival sac into the nasal cavity.

The main lacrimal gland lies in the superolateral corner of the orbit, just within the orbital margin, in relation to the tendon of levator palpebrae superioris and just beneath the conjunctiva of the superior fornix. It is the size of an almond, tubuloacinar, and serous, with prominent myoepithelial cells. The separate lobes of the gland drain via 10 to 15 excretory ducts into the lateral part of the superior conjunctival fornix. There also are numerous accessory lacrimal glands situated in the lamina propria of upper and lower eyelids.

After entering the conjunctival sac, the tears (the sterile secretion of the lacrimal glands) partially evaporate. They serve to keep the conjunctival epithelium moist, the blinking eyelids spreading the tears over the cornea like windshield wipers, and to wash out foreign matter, e.g., dust particles. Excessive evaporation is prevented by a film of mucus (from the tarsal conjunctival goblet cells) on the film of water and a film of oil (from the meibomian

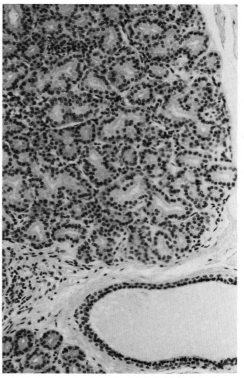

Figure 17–32. Photomicrograph of part of a lobe of the lacrimal gland, showing secretory serous acini and an interlobular duct (lower right). × 100.

glands). Excess tears pass medially to a slight expansion of the conjunctival sac (the lacus lacrimalis) and then into the lacrimal canaliculi, one in each eyelid, which open on the surface at a minute orifice termed the lacrimal puncta. These ducts pass to the lacrimal sac situated in the medial corner of the eye from which tears pass down the nasolacrimal duct to enter the inferior meatus of the nose.

Function of the Eye

The eye functions as the receptive organ of the visual system. Light rays entering the eye are focused by cornea and lens to form an inverted, real, reduced image of the object on the photosensitive layer of rods and cones of the retina. Focusing is accomplished by alteration of the convexity of the lens. In the position of rest with the ciliary muscle relaxed, the lens is flattened by elastic tension of the zonule. Contraction of the ciliary muscle, particularly of the outer, meridional fibers, pulls the choroid and ciliary body anteriorly. This relaxes the tension of the zonule and permits the lens, which is elastic, to become more convex, thus increasing the refractive power.

In the outer segments of rods and cones are two visual pigments: *rhodopsin* in the rods and *iodopsin* in the cones. These pigments consist of a specific protein bound to vitamin A aldehyde. Visible light falling on these pigments by a series of chemical changes results in depolarization of the receptor cell membrane and the formation of an action potential, which is then conducted by a series of neurons (including bipolar and ganglion cells) to the brain. The outer

segments of rods contain a greater quantity of photopigment than those of cones and are more photosensitive. Thus, they are used for dim light perception (night vision), while cones, being less photosensitive, are used for color perception and, with fewer interneuronal connections, for fine visual acuity. Hence the presence in the fovea centralis of cones only.

THE EAR

The ear is divided into three portions: the *external ear,* the *middle ear,* and the *inner ear,* the latter containing the organs both of hearing and of balance.

The external ear comprises the auri-

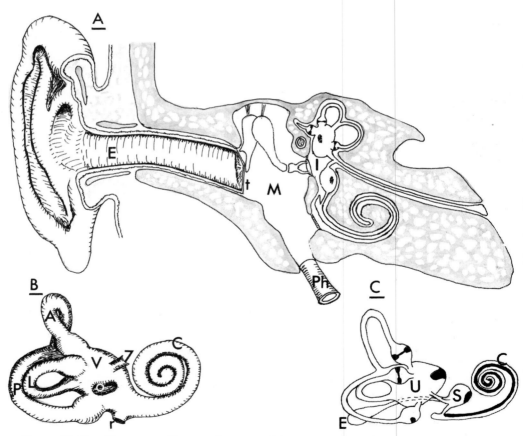

Figure 17–33. Diagrams to illustrate the parts of the ear. *A,* External ear consisting of pinna and external auditory meatus (E); middle ear (M), separated from the external ear by the tympanic membrane (t) and traversed by the three ossicles (malleus, incus, and stapes); and internal ear (I). The pharyngotympanic (eustachian) tube (Ph) extends inferomedially from the middle ear.*B,* Right osseous or bony labyrinth viewed from the lateral side. Anterior (A), posterior (P), and lateral (L) semicircular canals, vestibule (V), and cochlea (C) are shown. The oval (o) and round (r) windows and the canal for the facial nerve (7) also can be seen. *C,* Membranous labyrinth with semicircular canals, utricle (U), saccule (S), cochlear duct (C), and endolymphatic sac (E) and duct. Neuroepithelial (sensory) areas are indicated in black.

cle (the visible appendage), the external auditory meatus extending deep into the temporal bone, and the tympanic membrane or eardrum, which closes the deep extremity of the external auditory meatus. The middle ear is a cavity shaped like a biconcave lens, the lateral wall of which is the tympanic membrane and the medial wall of which is the external surface of the inner ear. Its cavity is traversed from tympanic membrane to inner ear by a chain of three small bones or ossicles (the malleus or hammer, the incus or anvil, and the stapes or stirrup). The inner ear consists of an irregular system of canals (the membranous labyrinth) walled in by bone (the bony labyrinth).

The External Ear

Auricle. The characteristic and complicated shape of the auricle is due to a plate of yellow elastic cartilage of 0.5 to 1 mm in thickness, covered by a perichondrium with a high content of elastic fibers. On all surfaces, it is covered by thin skin with a very thin subcutaneous layer (hypodermis) on the anterolateral surface. Hairs and sebaceous and sweat glands are present but in general are poorly developed. Contained in the subcutaneous layer and attached to perichondrium are a few small slips of striated muscle. These are vestigial in man, but in lower animals that are capable of ear movements they are more prominent.

External Auditory Meatus. The external auditory meatus extends from the auricle to the tympanic membrane. It is oval in section and held patent by the rigidity of its wall. The external third has a wall of elastic cartilage continuous with that forming the support of the auricle, and the inner two-thirds is of bone. The canal is lined by thin skin with no subcutaneous tissue, the deeper layers of the dermis blending with perichondrium or periosteum. Numerous hairs associated with sebaceous glands are present in the outer portion, and some small hairs and sebaceous glands are present in the roof only of the inner portion. Contained in the external meatus is *cerumen,* a brown, waxy material bitter to the taste and protective in

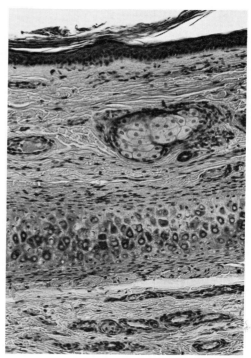

Figure 17–34. Photomicrograph of a section of the external auditory meatus. Note the thin epidermis, the sebaceous gland, and the elastic cartilage. × 100.

function. It is the combined secretion of the sebaceous and ceruminous glands, which are large, modified, coiled, tubular sweat glands, the ducts of which open either directly onto the skin surface or with sebaceous glands into the necks of hair follicles.

Tympanic Membrane. This is oval and placed obliquely to close the innermost extremity of the external meatus. It has a core of connective tissue in two layers, the fibers of the outer layer being radial, those of the inner layer being circular. Externally it is covered by very thin skin and internally by the mucosa of the middle meatus, here only 20 to 30 microns (μm) thick and with a cuboidal epithelium. Attached to the tympanic membrane is the malleus, one of the middle ear ossicles, the handle of which extends to the center of the membrane and causes it to bulge into the middle ear cavity. The upper portion of the tympanic membrane lacks collagenous fibers and is termed the flaccid part (Shrapnell's membrane).

The Middle Ear

The middle ear comprises a cleftlike cavity in the temporal bone, the *tympanic cavity,* and a canal or duct which connects it with the nasopharynx, the *auditory (eustachian) tube.*

The tympanic cavity is a flat, boxlike air space about 1.3 cm high and the same in length, but measuring only 2 to 3 mm transversely. The lateral wall is formed largely by the tympanic membrane, the medial wall by the inner ear. The bony roof separates it from the middle cranial fossa and temporal lobe of the brain, the floor from the retropharyngeal area and contents of the carotid sheath. Its posterior wall opens into another, smaller chamber, the tympanic antrum, into which open the numerous mastoid air cells. The anterior wall is partially deficient as the opening of the pharyngotympanic or auditory tube.

The epithelium lining the cavity and every structure it contains is squamous or low cuboidal over most of the area, but is columnar and ciliated anteriorly at the opening of the auditory tube. The lamina propria is thin and blends with periosteum.

The three ossicles, composed of compact bone without a marrow cavity, pass across the cavity of the middle ear, the malleus being attached to the tympanic membrane. Both the malleus and the incus are suspended by tiny ligaments from the roof. The base plate of the stapes is attached by a fibrous joint to an oval window or opening (the fenestra ovalis) in the medial wall. Between the three ossicles are two synovial joints. The thin periosteum of the ossicles blends with a thin lamina propria underlying the squamous epithelium lining the entire tympanic cavity. Associated with the chain of ossicles are two small muscles. The tensor tympani muscle lies in a canal above the auditory tube, its tendon passing at first posteriorly and then hooking around a small bony projection to cross the tympanic cavity from medial to lateral walls to insert into the handle of the malleus. The tendon of the stapedius muscle issues from a pyramidal bony projection in the posterior wall and passes anteriorly to insert into the neck of the stapes. These muscles are protective in that they "damp down" high frequency vibrations.

The oval window in the medial wall, occluded by the base plate of the stapes, separates the tympanic cavity from the perilymph in the scala vestibuli of the cochlea. Thus vibrations of the tympanic membrane are transmitted by the chain of ossicles to the perilymph of the inner ear. The perilymph spaces, however, are closed spaces and, because fluid is incompressible, a "safety valve" is necessary. This is the round window or fenestra rotunda, situated in the medial wall of the tympanic cavity below and behind the oval window and closed by an elastic membrane (the secondary tympanic membrane), separating the tympanic cavity from the perilymph of the scala tympani of the cochlea.

The auditory tube, connecting the tympanic cavity and the nasopharynx, is about 3.5 cm in length, the posterior third having a bony wall, the anterior two-thirds a cartilaginous wall. The lumen is flattened, and medial and lateral walls of the cartilaginous part usually are opposed to occlude the lumen. The epithelial lining varies from ciliated columnar near the tympanic cavity to pseudostratified, ciliated columnar with goblet cells near the pharynx. The lamina propria near the pharynx contains seromucous glands. By the act of swallowing, the walls of the tube are separated, thus opening the lumen and allowing air to enter the middle ear cavity to equalize pressure on both sides of the tympanic membrane.

The Inner Ear

The inner ear is a system of canals and cavities in the petrous part of the temporal bone, the osseous labyrinth, within which is a further series of canals and cavities, the membranous labyrinth. The membranous labyrinth is filled with fluid, the *endolymph,* the walls of the membranous labyrinth separating endolymph from *perilymph,* which fills the remainder of the osseous labyrinth.

Osseous Labyrinth. Centrally situated is the *vestibule* lying medial to the tympanic cavity, with the wall between the two containing the fenestra ovalis.

Posterior to the vestibule and opening into it are three *semicircular canals*. By their position, they are named anterior, posterior, and lateral, each being at right angles to the others. The two lateral canals of right and left ears are in approximately the same plane, and the anterior of one side is parallel to the posterior canal of the other side. Each canal has a dilatation or *ampulla* at one end. Those of the anterior and lateral canals lie close together above the fenestra ovalis; that of the posterior canal opens into the posterior part of the vestibule. Although there are three canals, there are only five and not six openings into the vestibule, the nonampullated posterior end of the posterior canal fusing with the nonampullated medial end of the anterior canal to open into the medial part of the vestibule by the *crus commune*. The nonampullated end of the lateral canal opens separately into the upper part of the vestibule. From the medial wall of the vestibule, a narrow canal extends inferoposteriorly to reach the posterior surface of the petrous temporal bone in the posterior cranial fossa.

Anteriorly, the cavity of the vestibule is continuous with the bony *cochlea*, a spirally coiled tube like a snail shell. Its total shape is conical with a base about 9 mm in diameter and a height from base to apex of 5 mm with two and three-quarter turns. The axial bony stem of the cochlea, the *modiolus,* is oriented across the long axis of the petrous temporal bone with the base toward the posterior cranial fossa and the apex pointing forward and laterally. A shelf of bone which projects from the modiolus forms a spiral ridge, the *spiral lamina,* like the thread of a screw around its stem.

It should be emphasized that the term "osseous labyrinth" may be confusing. It is *not* a separate bone, but simply a system of canals and cavities in the petrous part of the temporal bone, which, like the ossicles, is composed of compact bone.

Membranous Labyrinth. Within the osseous labyrinth is the membranous labyrinth, a system of interconnected parts lined by epithelium and containing endolymph. In a few regions, the wall of the membranous labyrinth is adherent to periosteum lining the osseous labyrinth, but in general it lies free and separated from the wall of the osseous labyrinth by perilymph. However, thin strands of connective tissue containing blood vessels pass across the perilymph space to suspend the membranous labyrinth within the osseous labyrinth.

The form of the membranous labyrinth is similar to that of the osseous labyrinth with the exception that the vestibule is occupied not by one but by two chambers and connecting channels. Posteriorly the *utricle* communicates via five orifices with the three membranous semicircular canals, which, like the osseous semicircular canals, have a crus commune between anterior and posterior canals. The ampullae of the membranous semicircular canals are large. Anteriorly the *saccule* is nearly spherical in shape and is joined to the utricle by a slim Y-shaped tube, the short stems being the utricular and saccular ducts. These ducts joint to form the *endolymphatic duct,* which passes posteroinferiorly to the posterior surface of the petrous temporal bone where it terminates as a blind sac, the *endolymphatic sac.* Anteriorly from its lower part, the saccule communicates with the *cochlear duct* by the short, narrow *ductus reuniens.*

There are sensory nerve endings in the ampullae of the semicircular canals (*cristae ampullares*) and in the utricle and saccule (*maculae utriculi* and *sacculi*) which subserve static and kinetic senses. The organ of hearing is the *organ of Corti* located along the length of the cochlear duct.

Utricle and Saccule. The connective tissue layer of the wall of the utricle and saccule is delicate and contains some fibroblasts and melanocytes. Fine trabeculae extend from its outer surface across the perilymphatic space to the inner surface of the periosteum lining the vestibule. They consist of a core of connective tissue covered by mesothelium. Interposed between the connective tissue layer of the wall of the utricle and saccule and the lining squamous epithelium is a fine basal lamina.

The macula utriculi lies in the lateral wall and is ovoid, 2 by 3 mm., and the macula sacculi is in the medial wall of the saccule and of similar size and shape. The two are oriented perpendicular to each other and have a similar structure. Three cell types are present in maculae. Supporting or sustentacular cells rest upon a basal lamina and are tall, columnar, and slender with apical microvilli and some cytoplasmic granules, possibly secretory in type. Two types of hair (sensory) cells are present. The *type I hair cell* is piriform in shape with a globular base containing a nucleus and a short neck. The *type II hair cell* is cylindrical, contains a central nucleus, numerous smooth-surfaced vesicles, and a prominent Golgi apparatus in a supranuclear position. In both types of hair cell, the apical surface shows 30 to 100 "hairs" or stereocilia (long, elongated microvilli) of varying length arranged in a regular, hexagonal pattern and a single *kinocilium*, always located at one border of the cell. This kinocilium resembles a cilium in structure with nine peripheral doublet microtubules, which form a basal body in apical cytoplasm. The central pair of microtubules present in cilia may be lacking in a kinocilium, and the motility of the kinocilium is doubtful. Covering the maculae is a surface, gelatinous layer about 22 microns (μm) thick. This is the *otolithic membrane,* and it contains numerous, small crystalline bodies, the *otoconia* or *otoliths,* composed of calcium carbonate and a protein. The microvilli of supporting cells and the stereocilia and kinocilia of hair cells are embedded in the otolithic membrane. Changes in position of the head result in changes in pressure or tension in the otolithic membrane and consequent stimulation of the hair cells. The stimulus is detected by nerve endings lying between the hair cells.

Semicircular Canals.   All are oval in cross section, the greatest convexity being closely apposed to periosteum, but each is smaller than the osseous semicircular canal and, on the opposite surface, there is a wide perilymph space traversed by trabeculae.

A crista is present in each ampulla. Each crista is oriented across the long axis of the duct and is formed by sustentacular cells and two types of hair cells similar to those described in maculae.

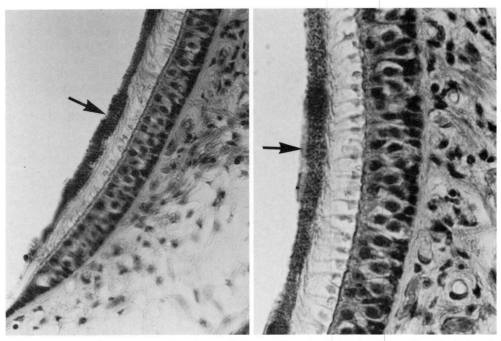

Figure 17–35. Photomicrographs of part of the macula utriculi showing hair cells with their apical sensory hairs extending into the otolithic membrane (arrow) that contains small crystalline bodies, the otoconia. Left, × 250; right, × 400.

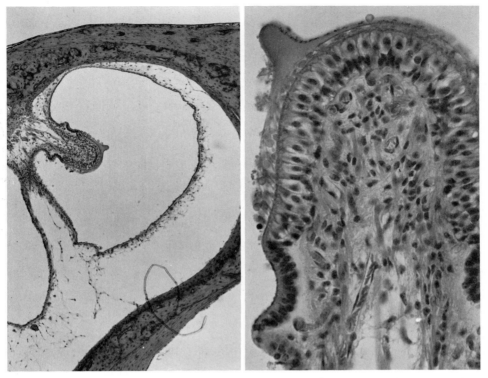

Figure 17–36. *Left:* Photomicrograph of the crista ampullaris of the lateral semicircular canal. × 40. *Right:* A higher magnification of the crista ampullaris. × 250.

Their microvilli, stereocilia, and kinocilia are embedded in a gelatinous mass termed a *cupula,* similar to the otolithic membrane but lacking otoconia.

Function. In cristae ampullaris, hair cells are stimulated by movement of endolymph following angular accelerations of the head. This movement of endolymph causes movement of stereocilia and kinocilia. In maculae, hair cells are similarly stimulated but by a change in position of the head in space, this resulting in an increase or decrease in pressure on the hair cells by the otolithic membrane.

Cochlea. The osseous cochlea, as explained previously, spirals for two and three-quarter turns around the modiolus, from which projects the spiral lamina. Extending from the spiral lamina to the outer wall of the cochlea is the *basilar membrane,* the cochlear periosteum being thickened at its outer attachment as the *spiral ligament.* A second membrane, the vestibular membrane (of Reissner) extends across the cochlea from the spiral lamina to the outer wall.

These two membranes thus divide the osseous canal into three cavities: an upper cavity, the *scala vestibuli,* a lower cavity, the *scala tympani,* and an intermediate cavity, the *cochlear duct.* The scala vestibuli and the scala tympani contain perilymph, and their walls, like those of other perilymph spaces, consist of connective tissue covered by a squamous layer of mesenchymal cells. The connective tissue blends externally with periosteum. The scala vestibuli is continuous with the perilymphatic space of the vestibule and thus reaches the inner surface of the fenestra ovalis. The scala tympani extends laterally to the fenestra rotunda and the secondary tympanic membrane which separates it from the tympanic cavity. At the apex of the cochlea, the scala vestibuli and scala tympani are in communication through a narrow canal termed the *helicotrema.*

The cochlear duct, via the ductus reuniens, connects with the saccule but terminates blindly near the helicotrema at the *cecum cupulare.*

At the junction of osseous spiral lami-

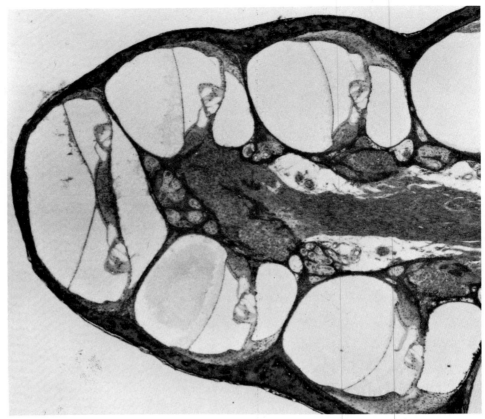

Figure 17–37. Photomicrograph of the cochlea of a guinea pig. × 25.

na and modiolus lies the *spiral ganglion,* incompletely surrounded by bone. From the entire length of the ganglion, bundles of nerve fibers perforate the bone of the spiral lamina to reach the organ of Corti. The periosteum above the spiral lamina is thickened and bulges into the cochlear duct as the *limbus spiralis.* Its lower part is continuous with the basilar membrane, which extends outward across the cochlear duct to attach to the spiral ligament. Contained in the basilar membrane are the *basilar fibers (auditory strings)* composed of compact bundles of minute collagenous fibrils embedded in some amorphous ground substance. Their length increases from the base to the apex of the cochlea (from about 0.2 to 0.36 mm), and they number about 24,000. The cochlear duct surface of the basilar fibers is covered by a thin, homogeneous basal laminar material, whereas its lower, tympanic surface is covered by delicate fibroconnective tissue in which there are a few blood capillaries.

The vestibular membrane is a thin sheet of connective tissue covered on its upper, vestibular surface by the mesenchymal, squamous lining of perilymph spaces. The lower, cochlear duct surface is covered by flat epithelium.

Cochlear Duct. The epithelium lining the cochlear duct varies with location. That over the vestibular membrane is squamous and may contain pigment. Over the limbus it is higher and irregular. Laterally, the epithelium is low columnar and is underlain by connective tissue containing many capillaries. This region is termed the *stria vascularis,* which is considered to be the site of secretion of endolymph. The epithelium over the basilar membrane is highly specialized as the organ of Corti.

Organ of Corti. As in other sensory areas in the inner ear, the organ of Corti comprises supporting and hair cells.

The *supporting cells* all are tall, columnar cells, but various groups are described. Within the organ of Corti is a

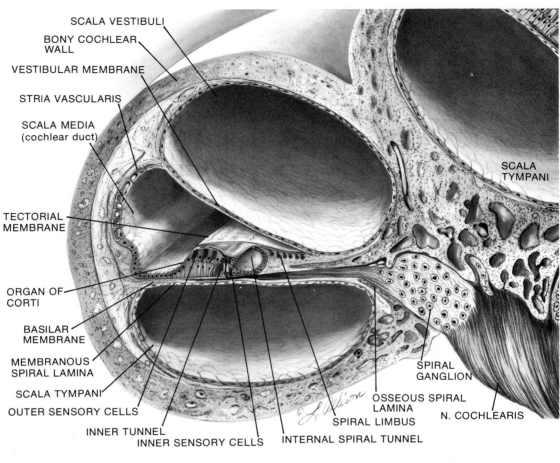

SCALA VESTIBULI

BONY COCHLEAR WALL

VESTIBULAR MEMBRANE

STRIA VASCULARIS

SCALA MEDIA (cochlear duct)

TECTORIAL MEMBRANE

ORGAN OF CORTI

BASILAR MEMBRANE

MEMBRANOUS SPIRAL LAMINA

SCALA TYMPANI

OUTER SENSORY CELLS

INNER TUNNEL

INNER SENSORY CELLS

INTERNAL SPIRAL TUNNEL

SPIRAL LIMBUS

OSSEOUS SPIRAL LAMINA

SPIRAL GANGLION

N. COCHLEARIS

SCALA TYMPANI

Figure 17–38. *Top:* Diagram of cochlea and the organ of Corti. *Bottom right:* Photomicrograph of the organ of Corti. ×40.

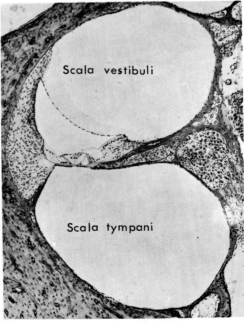

Scala vestibuli

Scala tympani

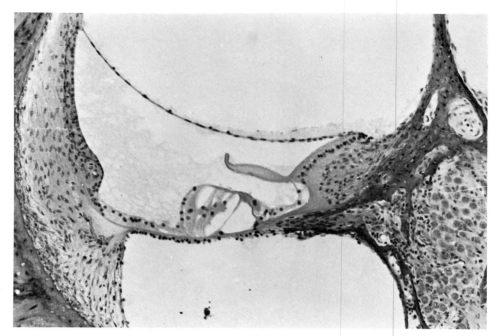

Figure 17–39. Photomicrograph of the organ of Corti. Compare with Figure 17–40. × 125.

tunnel extending the length of the cochlea, triangular in cross section and bounded basally by the basilar membrane and medially and laterally by the inner and outer pillar cells. The *inner pillar* cell is of a narrow cone shape with a broad base containing the nucleus lying against the basilar membrane and a narrow column expanding slightly at the apex. The apex overlies the outer pillar cell. The *outer pillar* cell is longer than the inner but of similar shape, with an expanded apex fitting into a depression on the undersurface of the head of an inner pillar cell. The inner pillar cells are more numerous than the outer,

roughly in the proportion of three to two.

The inner phalangeal cells and the outer phalangeal cells (of Deiters) lie on the basilar membrane adjacent to the pillar cells. The phalangeal cells are smaller; together with the pillar cells they surround the hair cells. However, there are spaces between the processes of phalangeal cells, although their bases fit tightly together along the basilar membrane. The innermost part of the basilar membrane near the limbus gives attachment to a slender row of border cells, whereas toward the spiral ligament there are elongated, polygonal cells ar-

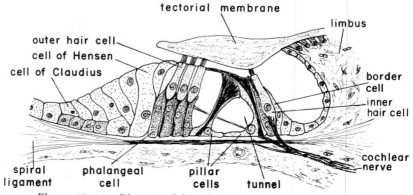

Figure 17–40. Diagram of the cellular types in the organ of Corti.

ranged in more than one row and decreasing in height. These are the cells of Hensen and of Claudius respectively.

The *hair cells* of the organ of Corti lie as a single row between the inner pillars on one side and the inner phalangeal and border cells on the other (the inner hair cells) and as three rows between the outer pillars and the outer phalangeal cells (the outer hair cells). The morphology of hair cells varies with location, but in general, the inner hair cells are similar to type I hair cells of maculae and ampullae. They are piriform in shape with nuclei lying in expanded bases with a slender, apical "neck" bearing 50 to 60 hairs or stereocilia but lacking kinocilia. The outer hair cells are more specialized, being longer and columnar with basal nuclei. They show about 100 stereocilia apically which are longer than the stereocilia of inner hair cells and, again, lack kinocilia.

The surface of the organ of Corti is covered by a ribbon of gelatinous material termed the *tectorial membrane*. This membrane, composed of homogeneous ground substance containing fibrillar material, in the living or fresh specimen rests upon the hairs (stereocilia) of the hair cells.

Spiral Ganglion. This is composed of bipolar neurons, the central processes (axons) being myelinated and running together to form the acoustic nerve. The peripheral myelinated processes (dendrites) run through canals in the bone surrounding the ganglion, lose their myelin sheaths, and terminate by entering the organ of Corti to lie between hair cells. The mode of stimulation remains uncertain. Sound waves are conducted from the perilymph of the scala vestibuli to the endolymph of the cochlear duct and in some manner affect the hair cells.

The eighth (acoustic) cranial nerve in addition to its cochlear division has a vestibular division for the sensory supply of the remainder of the labyrinth. Its ganglion is located in the internal auditory meatus of the temporal bone, and its axons run with those of the spiral ganglion. The peripheral dendrites pass to the three ampullae of the semicircular canals and to the maculae of the utricle and saccule. Additionally, some fibers join with those of the cochlear nerve. The function of these fibers is not understood.

Function. The external ear picks up sound waves which are converted to vibrations by the tympanic membrane. These vibrations then are transmitted by the chain of middle ear ossicles to the perilymph of the vestibule, setting up pressure waves in the perilymph with a movement of the fluid in both scala vestibuli and scala tympani. The secondary tympanic membrane of the round window moves freely as a safety valve in this movement of fluid, which also slightly displaces the cochlear duct and its basilar membrane. The displacement causes small shearing forces to develop between the stereocilia of hair cells and the tectorial membrane, thus stimulating the hair cells. It appears that the basilar membrane at the base of the cochlea is sensitive to high-frequency sounds, low-frequency sounds being appreciated in the remainder of the cochlear duct.

REFERENCES

Babel, J., Bischoff, A., and Spoendlin, H.: Ultrastructure of the Peripheral Nervous System and Sense Organs. London, J. & A. Churchill, Ltd., 1970.

Engstrom, H., and Ades, H. W. (editors): Inner ear studies. Acta Otolaryng., suppl. 301, 1973.

Feeney, L.: Lipofuchsin and melanin of human retinal pigment epithelium. Invest. Ophthalmol., *17*:583, 1978.

Fine, B. S., and Yanoff, M.: Ocular Histology. New York, Harper & Row, 1972.

Garant, P. R., Feldman, J., Chio, M. I., and Cullen, M. R.: Ultrastructure of Merkel cells in the hard palate of the squirrel monkey (Saimiri sciureus). Am. J. Anat., *157*:155, 1980.

Hogan, M. J., Alvarado, J. A., and Weddell, J. E.: Histology of the Human Eye. Philadelphia, W. B. Saunders Co., 1971.

Iurato, S.: Submicroscopic Structure of the Inner Ear. Oxford, Pergamon Press Ltd., 1967.

Last, R. J.: Wolff's Anatomy of the Eye and Orbit, 5th edition. Philadelphia, W. B. Saunders Co., 1968.

Leeson, T. S., and Leeson, C. R.: Choriocapillaris and lamina elastica (vitrea) of the rat eye. Br. J. Ophthalmol., *51*:599, 1967.

Leeson, T. S.: Rat retinal rods: freeze-fracture replication of outer segments. Can. J. Ophthalmol., *5*:91, 1970.

Leeson, T. S.: Lens of the rat eye: an electron microscope and freeze-etch study. Exp. Eye Res., *11*:78, 1971.

Leeson, T. S., and Leeson, C. R.: Myoepithelial cells in the exorbital lacrimal and parotid glands of the rat in frozen-etched replicas. Am. J. Anat., *132*:133, 1971.

Lindeman, H. H.: Studies on the Morphology of the Sensory Regions of the Vestibular Apparatus, Advances in Anatomy, Embryology and Cell Biology. Berlin, Springer-Verlag, 1969.

O'Rahilly, R.: The prenatal development of the human eye. Exp. Eye Res., *21*:93, 1975.

Quilliam, T. A., and Armstrong, J.: Mechanoreceptors. Endeavour, *22*:55, 1962.

Scheie, H. G., and Albert, D. M.: Adler's Textbook of Ophthalmology. Philadelphia, W. B. Saunders Co., 1969.

Sjöstrand, F. S., Kreman, M., and Crescitelli, F.: Freeze-fracture analysis of photoreceptor cell outer segment disks after minimal extraction of rhodopsin. J. Ultrastr. Res., *69*:53, 1979.

Smelzer, G. K. (editor): The Structure of the Eye (A Symposium). New York, Academic Press, 1961.

Spira, A. W., and Milman, G. E.: The structure and distribution of the cross-striated fibril and associated membranes in guinea pig photoreceptors. Am. J. Anat., *155*:319, 1979.

Steinberg, R. H., Wood, I., and Hogan, M. J.: Pigment epithelial ensheathment and phagocytosis of extrafoveal cones in human retina. Phil. Trans. R. Soc. B., *277*:459, 1977.

Vosteen, K. H.: Neue Aspekte zur Biologie und Pathologie des Innenohres. Arch. Ohr. Nas. Kehlkopfheilk., *178*:1, 1961.

Wislocki, G. B., and Ladman, A. J.: Selective and histochemical staining of the otolithic membranes, cupulae and tectorial membrane of the inner ear. J. Anat., *89*:3, 1955.

INDEX

Page numbers in *italics* indicate illustrations; (t) refers to tabular material.

583